Pediatric Emergency and Critical Care Ultrasound

Pediatric Emergency and Critical Care Ultrasound

Edited by

Stephanie J. Doniger, MD RDMS FAAP FACEP
Director of Emergency Ultrasound
Director of Pediatric Emergency Ultrasound Fellowship
Pediatric Emergency Medicine Physician
Division of Emergency Medicine
Children's Hospital and Research Center Oakland
Oakland, CA, USA
Clinical Instructor
Department of Emergency Medicine
University of California San Francisco School of Medicine
San Francisco, CA, USA

CAMBRIDGE
UNIVERSITY PRESS

CAMBRIDGE
UNIVERSITY PRESS

University Printing House, Cambridge CB2 8BS, United Kingdom

Cambridge University Press is part of the University of Cambridge.

It furthers the University's mission by disseminating knowledge in the pursuit of education, learning, and research at the highest international levels of excellence.

www.cambridge.org
Information on this title: www.cambridge.org/9781107062344

First published 2013
Reprinted 2016

Printed in the United Kingdom by Print on Demand, World Wide

A catalogue record for this publication is available from the British Library

Library of Congress Cataloguing in Publication data
Pediatric emergency and critical care ultrasound / [edited by] Stephanie J. Doniger.
p. ; cm.
Includes bibliographical references and index.
ISBN 978-1-107-06234-4
I. Doniger, Stephanie J., 1975–
[DNLM: 1. Ultrasonography – methods. 2. Child. 3. Critical Care – methods. 4. Emergency Medical Services – methods.
5. Infant. WN 208]
618.92′007543–dc23

2012047373

ISBN 978-1-107-06234-4 Hardback

I am so excited that such a talented and experienced group of authors contributed their wealth of knowledge to this text. I am fortunate to be a part of such a small, but growing field of Pediatric Emergency Ultrasound. I look forward to seeing the development of pediatric ultrasound, and how it can positively impact the care of our smallest and most vulnerable of patients.

First and foremost, I dedicate this text to my parents who have served as models and encouraged me along the way. To my father Marvin who has taught me the value of hard work and inspired me in his superhuman battle against all medical odds. To my mother Marsha who has dedicated her life to her family and over the years has become my very best friend.

Along the way, I have been fortunate to have some amazing mentors. To J. Christian Fox, who initially planted the idea of ultrasound eventually being useful in Pediatric Emergency Medicine, while in the Flying Samaritans clinic in El Testerazo, Mexico. To Resa Lewiss, who took a chance on me as the first Pediatric Emergency Medicine-trained physician to do an Emergency Ultrasound fellowship. To my mentor Ghazala Sharieff whose invaluable advice, guidance, and mentorship have helped shape my career, and who has become a close friend. To my colleagues at Children's Hospital Oakland – I am so privileged to have joined your family, and am constantly inspired by all of you. It has been such a joy to see that even the most experienced of physicians is excited by ultrasound. I look forward to continuing to teach you, and to learn from you. To all of my colleagues that I am constantly learning from, this text would not have been possible without you.

A special thank you to Wendi Karam and Kelly Kroll, who provided their beautiful children to be photographed in this text; to Ricky Knack, the talented nurse, photographer, and friend who photographed them. To Laura Berg, MD, also did a tremendous last-minute job rescuing the illustrations. To my international colleagues who constantly inspire me and remind me why I went into medicine in the first place. I will always have a particular place in my heart for the people in El Testerazo, Mexico and Roatan, Honduras.

And last but certainly not least, to my patients and their families who give me the unique opportunity to enter their lives and help them in their most vulnerable times of need. Thank you for letting me into your lives to treat your most precious gifts – your children.

Contents

Section 4 Special populations

Foreword

The chief religious and political authority of the 1600s was the Roman Catholic Church. It is under their traditional worldview that Galileo's heliocentric planetary model constituted the heart of the debate among his scholarly colleagues. While this rift between Church and State is the one popularized, the real conflict was between conservative and progressive attitudes of the scientists themselves. Though no invention of his own, the telescope that Galileo used was admired throughout Europe. Initially, many other respected scholars of his time such as Johannes Kepler did not own, or even know how to use, this "spyglass." This lack of familiarity transformed into an excuse for others not to fully *believe* what Galileo had seen with his own eyes. The key word here is "initially." Once others learned how to grind the lenses to develop their own telescopes, they (grudgingly) swallowed their pride and confirmed his observations that the moon did indeed have a rocky surface and Jupiter had four moons.

In 1816, the stethoscope was invented and to this day serves as the current method of performing a physical examination of a patient in a doctor's office, hospital bed, or in the emergency room. In fact not much about the physical examination has really changed substantially since the time of Hippocrates. When a patient complains of pain, presently, physicians examine the patient based on their knowledge of human anatomy. In the doctor's mind are images of organs beneath the skin that may be related to an ailment; the physician seeks to probe or listen to those organs by manual palpation or listening with a stethoscope. But only the most obvious of abnormalities are detected in this manner.

What if physicians instantly had access to more precise visual information about those organs? With the advent of compact, battery-powered, handheld ultrasound machines, doctors can now peer through the skin at internal organs to see abnormalities even without having to expose patients to radiation. These devices are truly revolutionary tools that are profoundly enhancing the doctor/patient relationship throughout diagnostic medicine. Handheld ultrasound units, unlike their cart-based older siblings, can be deployed in every clinical arena, easily carried about by the physician. The time it takes to perform the examination is similar to what would be required for a routine standard hand/stethoscope examination, while the return on this small investment is significantly greater. More specifically, handheld ultrasound devices can uncover many diseases and pediatric conditions at an earlier time before the patient is in crisis. In any healthcare setting, portable ultrasound devices *transform* the typically passive role of the physician, family, and patient alike into one that engages all in proactive and, at times, even preventative healthcare. This is satisfying for both the practitioner and patient, and can lead to effective and more cost-efficient health outcomes. This has far-reaching implications, not only in large urban medical communities but also in rural medicine and in telemedicine, where ultrasound imaging may be the only definitive link to a patient's illness or injury.

This incoming wave of innovation changes the way patients and physicians work together to address medical issues that may not be revealed by the manual physical examination. To demonstrate how point-of-care ultrasound has revitalized the pediatric physical examination, Stephanie Doniger and colleagues have done an outstanding job in bringing these concepts to life by supplying us with high-quality images. These images can be referred to in our busy clinical areas, or when studied separately may trigger a consideration in the differential diagnosis of a clinical conundrum not possible without the knowledge of the capabilities inherent in this powerful device.

Other ways to image our patients involve exposing them to radiation. A single computed tomography (CT) scan of the abdomen and pelvis is roughly equivalent to receiving 500 chest-X-rays-worth of ionizing radiation. Of course, one must always consider risk/benefit when evaluating the ill child; however, if the answer can come via sound instead of beta rays then we should be ashamed to NOT reach for ultrasound in these children. After all, it was Hippocrates who first told us to "do no harm." In no other place is our oath more relevant than in our youngest patients who have no voice in the matter.

In the end, humans are creatures of habit, and thus, as doctors, we find ourselves complacent and happy with our daily routine. We show up to work and engage in a familiar pace and role with our nurses and patients, well within a comfort zone that was established way back in residency training. Yet it is our responsibility to achieve more. Galileo permanently changed humankind's perception of the planets in our universe because he knew a feasible, revolutionary invention when he saw one, and the story today about ultrasound is not so different. Ultrasound has the capacity to alter thinking in powerful ways that will shape the future for years to come. The physicians of tomorrow will wonder how we ever got by without this knowledge.

J. Christian Fox, MD RDMS
Rebecca Kasl, BS

Contributors

Alyssa Abo, MD
Director, Pediatric Emergency Ultrasound
Division of Pediatric Emergency Medicine
Cohen Children's Medical Center
Department of Emergency Medicine
North Shore University Hospital
Assistant Professor of Emergency Medicine
Hofstra North Shore-LIJ School of Medicine
Manhasset, NY, USA

Faiza Al Talaq, MD
Division of Ultrasound in Emergency Medicine
Massachusetts General Hospital
Boston, MA, USA

Alexander C. Arroyo, MD FAAP
Director, Pediatric Emergency Medicine
Director, Pediatric Emergency Medicine Ultrasound Research
Division of Emergency Medicine
Maimonides Medical Center
Brooklyn, NY, USA

Laura J. Berg, MD
Department of Emergency Medicine
North Memorial Medical Center
Robbinsdale, MN, USA

Tony Berger, MD MS
Department of Emergency Medicine
Staff Physician
Department of Emergency Medicine
Kaiser South Sacramento Medical Center
Sacramento, CA, USA

Lei Chen, MD MHS
Associate Fellowship Director
Section of Emergency Medicine
Associate Professor of Pediatrics
Yale University School of Medicine
New Haven, CT, USA

Roberto Copetti, MD
Emergency Department
Latisana General Hospital
Latisana, Italy

Stephanie J. Doniger, MD RDMS FAAP FACEP
Director of Emergency Ultrasound
Director, Pediatric Emergency Ultrasound Fellowship
Division of Emergency Medicine
Children's Hospital and Research Center Oakland
Oakland, CA, USA
Department of Emergency Medicine
University of California San Francisco School of Medicine
San Francisco, CA, USA

Mahmoud Elbarbary, MD PhD MSc
Consultant and Assistant Professor of Critical Care Medicine
National Guard Health Affairs
King Saud Ben Abdulaziz University for Health Sciences
Riyadh, Saudi Arabia

Alaa A. Eldemerdash, MD FAAP
Consultant Neonatologist
Head of Neonatal Intensive Care Unit
Latifa Hospital
Dubai, UAE

Jason W. Fischer, MD MSc
Director, Emergency Ultrasound Program
Division of Emergency Medicine
The Hospital for Sick Children, Toronto
Assistant Professor of Paediatrics
University of Toronto
Toronto, Ontario, Canada

John Christian Fox, MD, RDMS
Professor of Clinical Emergency Medicine
Director of Emergency Ultrasound
Department of Emergency Medicine
University of California Irvine Medical Center
Orange, CA, USA

Katja Goldflam, MD
Assistant Residency Director
Director, Emergency Ultrasound Education
Yale School of Medicine
New Haven, CT, USA

Beatrice Hoffmann, MD PhD RDMS
Emergency Ultrasound and Fellowship Director
Department of Emergency Medicine
Beth Israel Deaconess Medical Center
Harvard Medical School
Boston, MA, USA

Jamie A. Jenkins, MD RDMS FAAEM
Regional Emergency Ultrasound Director, FHS/Team Health
Division of Emergency Medicine
St. Joseph Medical Center
Tacoma, WA, USA

David Kessler, MD MSc RDMS FAAP
Director of Clinical Operations
Director of Pediatric Emergency Ultrasound
Division of Pediatric Emergency Medicine
New York Presbyterian Morgan Stanley Children's Hospital of New York
Assistant Professor of Pediatrics
Columbia University Medical Center
New York, NY, USA

Heidi Ladner, MD
Associate Chief
University of California Davis Medical Center
Kaiser Permanente, Vacaville,
Vacaville, CA, USA

Samuel H. F. Lam, MD RDMS FACEP
Assistant Ultrasound Director
Department of Emergency Medicine
Advocate Christ Medical Center/Advocate Children's Hospital
Oak Lawn, IL, USA
Clinical Assistant Professor of Emergency Medicine
University of Illinois at Chicago
Chicago, IL, USA

Jason A. Levy, MD RDMS FAAP FACEP
Director of Emergency Ultrasound
Fellowship Director, Pediatric Emergency Ultrasound
Division of Emergency Medicine
Boston Children's Hospital
Assistant Professor in Pediatrics
Harvard Medical School
Boston, MA, USA

Resa E. Lewiss, MD RDMS
Director of Emergency Ultrasound
Department of Emergency Medicine
St. Luke's-Roosevelt Hospital Center
New York, NY, USA

Andrew S. Liteplo, MD RDMS FACEP
Emergency Ultrasound Fellowship Director
Department of Emergency Medicine
Massachusetts General Hospital
Assistant Professor
Harvard Medical School
Boston, MA, USA

Jennifer R. Marin, MD MSc
Director of Pediatric Emergency Ultrasound
Division of Emergency Medicine
Children's Hospital of Pittsburgh
Assistant Professor of Pediatrics and Emergency Medicine
University of Pittsburgh School of Medicine
Pittsburgh, PA, USA

Arun Nagdev, MD
Director, Emergency Ultrasound
Alameda County Medical Center
Highland General Hospital
Oakland, CA, USA
Assistant Clinical Professor
University of California San Francisco
School of Medicine
San Francisco, CA, USA

Vicki E. Noble, MD
Director, Division of Emergency Ultrasound
Massachusetts General Hospital
Associate Professor
Harvard Medical School
Boston, MA, USA

Daniela Ramirez-Schrempp, MD
Director of Pediatric Emergency Ultrasound
Division of Pediatric Emergency Medicine
Boston Medical Center
Assistant Professor
Boston University
Boston, MA, USA

Joshua Rempell, MD
Division of Emergency Medicine
Brigham and Women's Hospital
Boston, MA, USA

Randall T. Rhyne, MD, RDMS
Director of Emergency Ultrasound
Carolinas Medical Center – University
Charlotte, NC, USA

Antonio Riera, MD FAAP
Director, Pediatric Emergency Medicine Ultrasound Curriculum
Section of Emergency Medicine
Assistant Professor of Pediatrics
Yale University School of Medicine
New Haven, CT, USA

Dana R. Sajed, MD FAAEM
Division of Emergency Medicine
University of Washington School of Medicine
Seattle, WA, USA

Fernando Silva, MD MSc
Department of Emergency Medicine
Kaiser Permanente Northern California
Napa/Solano, CA, USA

Adam B. Sivitz, MD
Medical Director, Pediatric Emergency Medicine
Newark Beth Israel Medical Center
Children's Hospital of New Jersey
Clinical Assistant Professor of Emergency Medicine
New Jersey Medical School
University of Medicine and Dentistry of New Jersey
Newark, NJ, USA

Dave Spear, MD
Clinical Assistant Professor
Department of Surgery
University of Texas Southwestern Medical Center
Dallas, TX, USA

Rebecca L. Vieira, MD RDMS FAAP
Associate Director of Emergency Ultrasound
Division of Emergency Medicine
Boston Children's Hospital
Instructor in Pediatrics
Harvard Medical School
Boston, MA, USA

S1 Introduction

Stephanie J. Doniger

Pediatric Emergency Medicine is a relatively new field of medicine developed in the 1980s. Since its inception, several advancements have been made in order to improve the emergency care of children. In 2007, an Institute of Medicine report described the deficit of pediatric-centered emergency care, calling for the need for more resources to be dedicated towards the emergency care of children. The mere existence of this field of medicine embodies the idea that children are not just "small adults" but have distinct pathology, and need care and equipment tailored to their size and physiology.

Ultrasound technology was originally introduced in the 1950s, and portable scanners made their way into the adult emergency department in the 1980s. The first "ultrasonic stethoscope" was introduced to make rapid decisions and perform estimation of the sizes of left-sided heart structures. Initially, point-of-care ultrasonography has become an extension of the physical examination, and provided the ability for more expeditious diagnoses at the bedside (Figure S1.1). More recently, it has become much more – a powerful diagnostic tool. The advent of portable machines allowed for the performance of ultrasonography by the clinician at the bedside. Since that time, machines have rapidly evolved and offer possibilities for the expansion of these applications. In 1994, the first emergency ultrasound curriculum was introduced, and it is now a requirement that Emergency Medicine residency programs offer training and credentialing for ultrasound in their residencies. Most recently, the Accreditation Council for Graduate Medical Education (ACGME) has developed a new system of accreditation, which involves the development and implementation of specific milestones for each medical specialty. The ACGME has designated ultrasound as one of the 24 Emergency Medicine milestones (Figure S1.2).

In addition, point-of-care ultrasound (POCUS) has also become prevalent in multiple other subspecialties (Table S1.1). Point-of-care ultrasound has become part of the standard of practice in adult critical care; a recent national survey showed that it is starting to be used in pediatric critical care as well. While vascular access is the most common use for point-of-care ultrasound in the intensive care unit (ICU), it is also commonly used to identify pleural effusions and pericardial effusions. Unfortunately, formal training in critical care is rare, with only 20% of responding surveyed hospitals reporting formal ultrasound training. Point-of-care ultrasound has even been

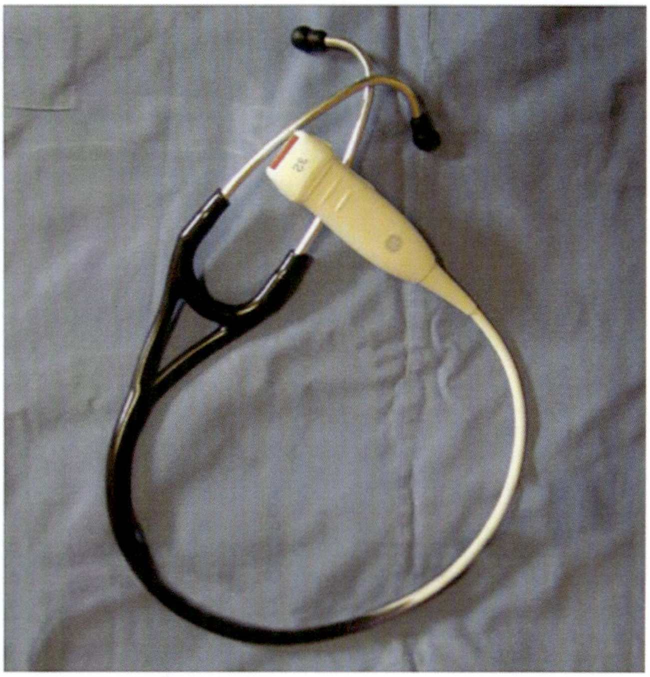

Figure S1.1 **"Ultrasonoscope."** Point-of-care ultrasonography can best be conceptualized as an extension of the physical examination, but also serves as an important diagnostic tool. *Image courtesy of Mahmoud Elbarbary, MD MSc PhD.*

introduced into the care of the smallest of children, in the neonatal intensive care unit (NICU; see Chapter 23).

The use of point-of-care ultrasound is only beginning to emerge in the field of Pediatric Emergency Medicine, but has not yet been formally incorporated into the subspecialty fellowship curricula, though recently consensus educational guidelines were published. While numerous applications for pediatric patients are being realized, there is a strong desire for pediatric-specific training. Thus far, the majority of obstacles have been identified as lack of equipment, resources, training, and individuals to oversee quality assurance and credentialing. Further, there are few well-established indications for children. It has been argued that several of the indications for point-of-care ultrasound are different for children. However, the adult applications of FAST (focused assessment with sonography for trauma), first trimester pregnancy, limited echocardiography, and as a procedural adjunct have been extended for use in pediatric and adolescent patients. It is an

Pediatric Emergency and Critical Care Ultrasound, ed. Stephanie J. Doniger. Published by Cambridge University Press.

Table S1.1 Selected applications of point-of-care ultrasonography, according to medical specialty.

Specialty	Ultrasound applications
Anesthesia	Guidance for vascular access, regional anesthesia, intraoperative monitoring of fluid status and cardiac function
Cardiology	Echocardiography, intracardiac assessment
Critical care medicine	Procedural guidance, pulmonary assessment, focused echocardiography
Dermatology	Assessment of skin lesions and tumors
Emergency medicine	FAST[a], focused emergency assessment, procedural guidance
Endocrinology and endocrine surgery	Assessment of thyroid and parathyroid, procedural guidance
General surgery	Ultrasonography of the breast, procedural guidance, intraoperative assessment
Gynecology	Assessment of cervix, uterus, and adnexa; procedural guidance
Obstetrics, maternal–fetal medicine	Assessment of pregnancy, detection of fetal abnormalities, procedural guidance
Neonatology	Cranial and pulmonary assessments
Nephrology	Vascular access for dialysis
Neurology	Transcranial Doppler, peripheral-nerve evaluation
Ophthalmology	Corneal and retinal assessment
Orthopedic surgery	Musculoskeletal applications
Otolaryngology	Assessment of thyroid, parathyroid, and neck masses; procedural guidance
Pediatrics	Assessment of bladder, procedural guidance
Pulmonary medicine	Transthoracic pulmonary assessment, endobronchial assessment, procedural guidance
Radiology, interventional radiology	Ultrasonography taken to the patient with interpretation at the bedside, procedural guidance
Rheumatology	Monitoring of synovitis, procedural guidance
Trauma surgery	FAST[a], procedural guidance
Urology	Renal, bladder, and prostate assessment; procedural guidance
Vascular surgery	Carotid, arterial, and venous assessment; procedural assessment

[a] FAST denotes focused assessment of sonography with trauma.
Source (copyright): Moore, C. L., Copel, J. A. (2011) Point-of-care ultrasonography. N Engl J Med *364: 749–57.*

Uses ultrasound for the bedside diagnostic evaluation of emergency medical conditions and diagnoses, resuscitation of the acutely ill or injured patient. and procedural guidance

Level 1	Level 2	Level 3	Level 4	Level 5
Describes the indications and limitations of limited, goal-directed emergency ultrasound	Explains how to optimize ultrasound images and identify the proper probe for each of the focused ultrasound applications Performs an E-FAST Correctly interprets acquired images Uses ultrasound for procedural guidance for central venous access	Performs focused ultrasound examinations such as intrauterine pregnancy, AAA, cardiac, biliary, urinary tract, soft tissue/musculoskeletal, and thoracic procedures, and procedures for ocular complaints	Performs a minimum of 150 focused ultrasound examinations	Expands ultrasonography skills to include: advanced echo, TEE, bowel, adnexal and testicular pathology, and transcranial Doppler

Comments:

Figure S1.2 Emergency medicine milestones. The ACGME named ultrasound as one of the 24 milestones in Emergency Medicine. Therefore, Emergency Medicine residents must attain competency through their training, through various evaluation methods. E-FAST, extended focused assessment with sonography for trauma; AAA, abdominal aortic aneurysm; TEE, transesophageal echocardiogram. *Used with permission by the American Board of Emergency Medicine and the Accreditation Council for Graduate Medical Education.*

especially attractive modality for children, since it involves no ionizing radiation and has the potential to decrease the use of radiographs and computed tomography (CT) scans.

This textbook is meant to serve as a comprehensive review of the techniques to perform point-of-care or point-of-care ultrasonography. Each chapter involves a literature review and details of the techniques of how to perform the ultrasound examinations, and highlights important pathology. Finally, case presentations will help serve to incorporate the point-of-care ultrasound assessment into the care of patients.

Selected references

American College of Emergency Physicians. (2009) Emergency ultrasound guidelines. *Ann Emerg Med* **53**: 550–70.

Beeson, M., Christopher, T., Heidt, J., *et al.* (2012) *Emergency Medicine Milestones.* Chicago, IL: Accreditation Council for Graduate Medical Education.

Chamberlain, M. C., Reid, S. R., Madhok, M. (2011) Utilization of emergency ultrasound in pediatric emergency department. *Pediatr Emerg Care* **27**: 628–32.

Chen, L., Baker, M. (2007) Novel applications of ultrasound in pediatric emergency medicine. *Pediatr Emerg Care* **23**: 115–25.

Hegenbarth, M. (2004) Bedside ultrasound in the pediatric emergency department: basic skill or passing fancy? *Clin Pediatr Emerg Med* **5**: 201–16.

Institute of Medicine's Committee on the Future of Emergency Care in the United States Health System. (2007) *Emergency Care for Children: Growing Pains.* Washington, DC: The National Academies Press.

Logtvoet, C., Rusterborgh, H., Kappen, L., Bom, N. (1978) Real time ultrasonic imaging with a hand-held scanner. Part I – technical description. *Ultrasound Med Biol* **4**: 91–2.

Ludwig, S., Fleisher, G. (1985) Pediatric emergency care: a new journal. *Pediatr Emerg Care* **1**: 1–2.

Mateer, J., Plummer, D., Heller, M., *et al.* (1994) Model curriculum for physician training in emergency ultrasonography. *Ann Emerg Med* **23**: 95–102.

Roelandt, J., Bom, K., Hugenholtz, P. (1980) The ultrasound cardioscope: a hand-held scanner for real-time cardiac imaging. *J Clin Ultrasound* **8**: 221–5.

Chapter 1

Physics and "knobology"

Alyssa Abo

Ultrasound, as an imaging modality, has been in existence for decades (Figure 1.1a,b). Over the last half century, technology has significantly improved, providing enhanced image quality with compact machines at more affordable pricing (Figure 1.1c). These advances have broadened its spectrum of use in the medical field, and expanded its applicability. Ultrasound is an integral part of not only radiology but also other specialties including obstetrics and gynecology, anesthesiology, and cardiology to name a few. In the acute care setting, such as the emergency and critical care departments, the field of bedside or point-of-care ultrasound is rapidly expanding.

Point-of-care ultrasound provides the clinician with real-time, non-invasive data, making it an asset in the emergency and critical care departments. Its lack of ionizing radiation makes it particularly valuable for use in pediatric patients. For the abovementioned reasons, ultrasound is gaining momentum in the pediatric acute care setting as an adjunct to patient evaluation, as well as an adjunct for invasive procedures.

It is important for providers performing ultrasound to understand the basic concepts behind the complicated technology. Simply stated, ultrasound is based on sound waves and their physical principles. While audible sound is in the range of 20–20,000 Hertz (Hz), medical ultrasound uses sound waves in the range of 2–20 mega or million Hertz, MHz. Appreciating the fundamentals of ultrasound as well as the system functions, or "knobology," will guide the clinician in better image acquisition.

Basic ultrasound principles, physics

The general principle of medical ultrasound is the "**pulse echo principle,**" which is best described using the analogy of sonar. SONAR, which is the acronym for sound navigation and ranging, is a technique based on sound propagation where devices generate and receive sound. For example, in submarine navigation, sonar capability allows a submarine to emit an acoustic pulse and then receive the returning sound after it strikes an object. Since the acoustic pulse has a known speed in a known medium (water), the elapsed "flight" time, the time from when the sound is transmitted to when it is received, can be used to calculate how far away the object of interest is located.

In medical ultrasound, the transducer emits pulsed longitudinal sound waves into the patient's body and "listens" for returning echoes. The transducer contains ceramic crystals that, via the "**piezoelectric effect**" (Figure 1.2), convert electrical energy into mechanical energy (i.e. sound waves). Electricity is generated that vibrates the crystals to release sound waves at a speed of 1540 m/s, which is the average speed of sound in humans at body temperature. The transducer then listens for returning echoes, accounting for the time elapsed as well as intensity of the returning echoes. The returning sound vibrates the crystals and is converted back to electrical energy, to finally produce an image.

Sound is a form of mechanical energy that is characterized as a cycle of an upward and downward deflection. Frequency (Hertz, Hz) is the number of cycles that are repeated in one second. The amplitude (decibels, dB) is the height of the deflection and correlates with the "loudness" or intensity of the echo. The wavelength (mm) is the distance traveled in a single cycle (Figure 1.3).

Attenuation

As ultrasonic waves travel through the body, the path and intensity of the sound change. Attenuation, which is the loss of energy, weakens the sound waves. Some energy is absorbed by the surrounding tissues and released as heat. Sound waves are also attenuated through reflection, refraction, and scattering. The degree to which the path changes is related to the acoustic impedance of the neighboring tissues through which it is traveling. **Reflection** is the redirection of the sound wave back to its source. **Refraction** is the redirection of part of the sound wave, as it crosses a boundary of two mediums with different propagation speeds. **Scattering** occurs when the sound waves encounter an irregular interface or one that is smaller than the sound beam. As sound waves encounter tissues of different densities, the path may be bent or refracted. The sound waves that are reflected back to the transducer are ultimately translated into an image.

Acoustic impedance

Acoustic impedance is the resistance of the tissue to molecular movement. Acoustic impedance is directly related to the density

Pediatric Emergency and Critical Care Ultrasound, ed. Stephanie J. Doniger. Published by Cambridge University Press.

(a)

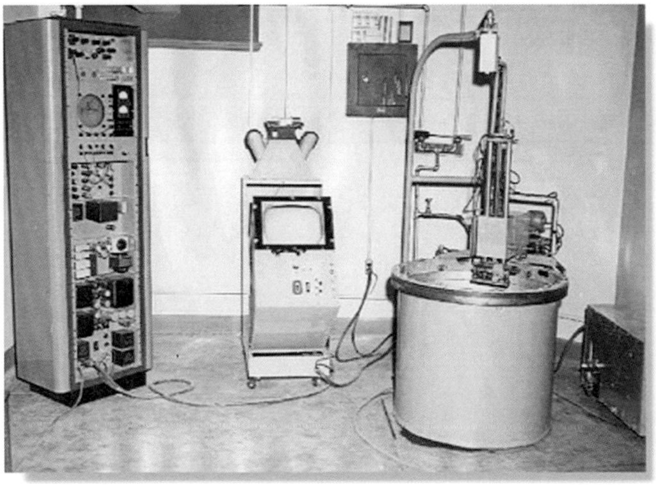

(b)

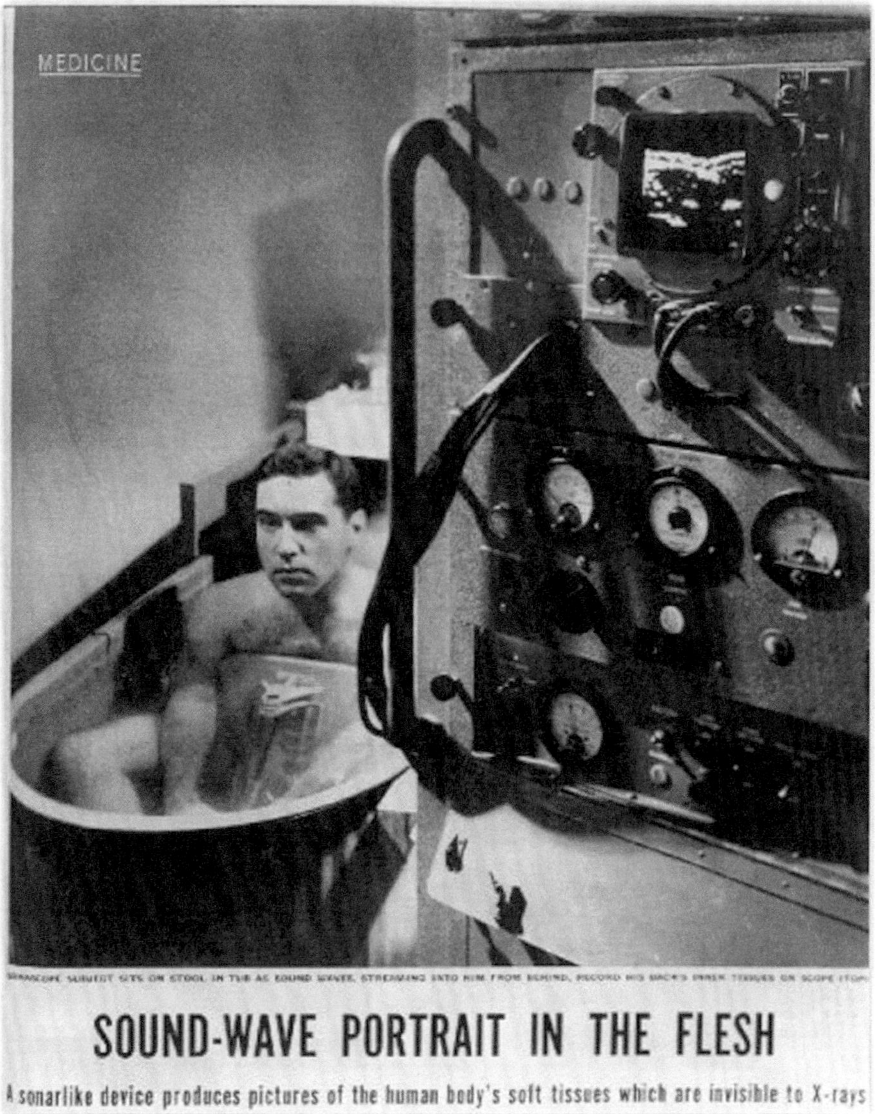

Figure 1.1 The evolution of ultrasound. When ultrasound was introduced, it was (a) a large apparatus that required (b) the immersion of a patient into a waterbath. (c) and (d) Current point-of-care ultrasound machines are portable and may be used at the patient's bedside.

(c)

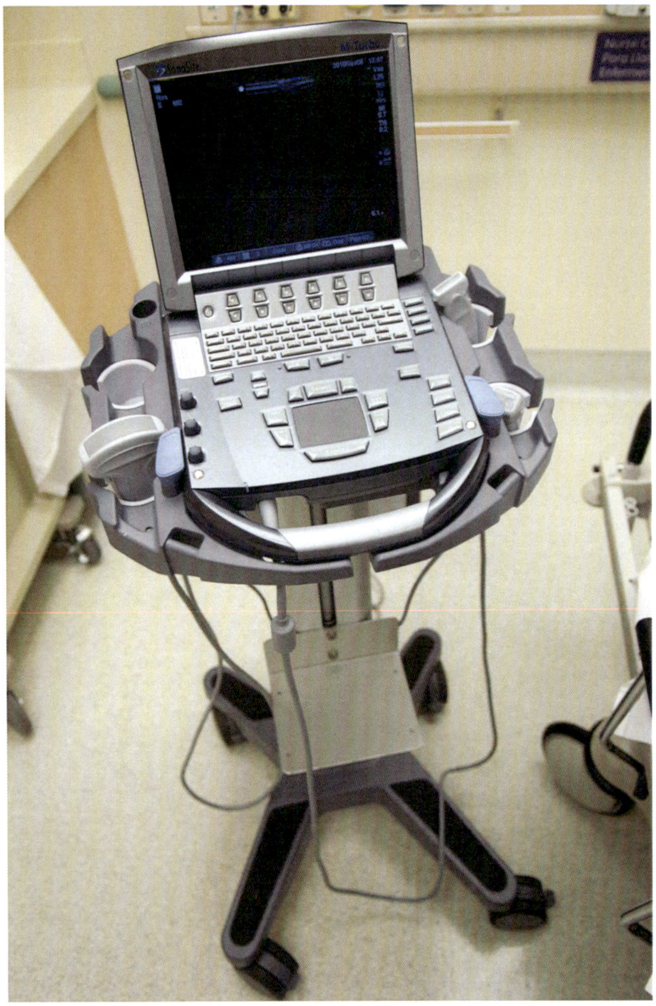

Figure 1.1 (cont.)

(d)

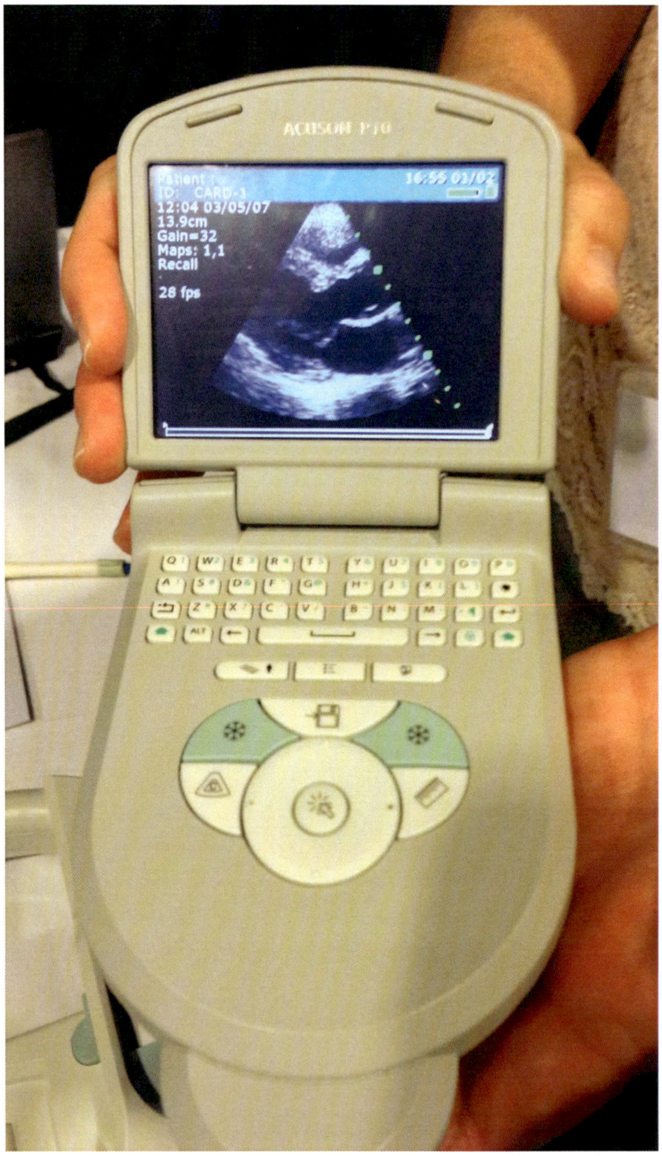

Figure 1.1 (cont.)

as well as the propagation of sound through that specific tissue. The greater the difference in acoustic impedance from one tissue to another, the louder the echo produced. Greater changes in acoustic impedance require more energy; thus, sound waves will have less energy to interrogate deeper structures. When the difference in acoustic impedance is the largest (i.e. soft tissue next to bone or air) this is referred to as **acoustic mismatch**. In this scenario, sound waves are scattered, and little information is reflected back to the transducer. In contrast, tissues with similar acoustic impedance allow sound to penetrate and interrogate deeper structures and are referred to as **acoustic windows**. The bladder is an example of an acoustic window.

Equipment

Transducers

Ultrasound transducers, or probes, are manufactured in assorted shapes and sizes (Figure 1.4). They are broadband devices that work over many frequencies. For example, the "abdominal probe" has a range from 2 to 5 MHz. The user can switch that transducer's frequency to 2MHz, 3MHz, 4 MHz, or 5MHz. The lower frequencies offer penetration, while the higher frequencies offer resolution.

The choice of a particular transducer should reflect the clinical indication and the patient population. Each transducer has a marker, or indicator, on it, correlating to a marker on the screen. This allows for proper orientation by the sonographer when performing and interpreting ultrasound (Figure 1.5). Spatial orientation is directly related to the transducer position and the two-dimensional plane being interrogated (see S2, Introduction).

A thorough investigation requires movement of the transducer. **Fanning or sweeping** of the transducer is accomplished by moving the transducer along an imaginary arc. **Rocking** the probe will tilt it, while **rotating** the probe is achieved by twisting the transducer clockwise or counterclockwise. Applying

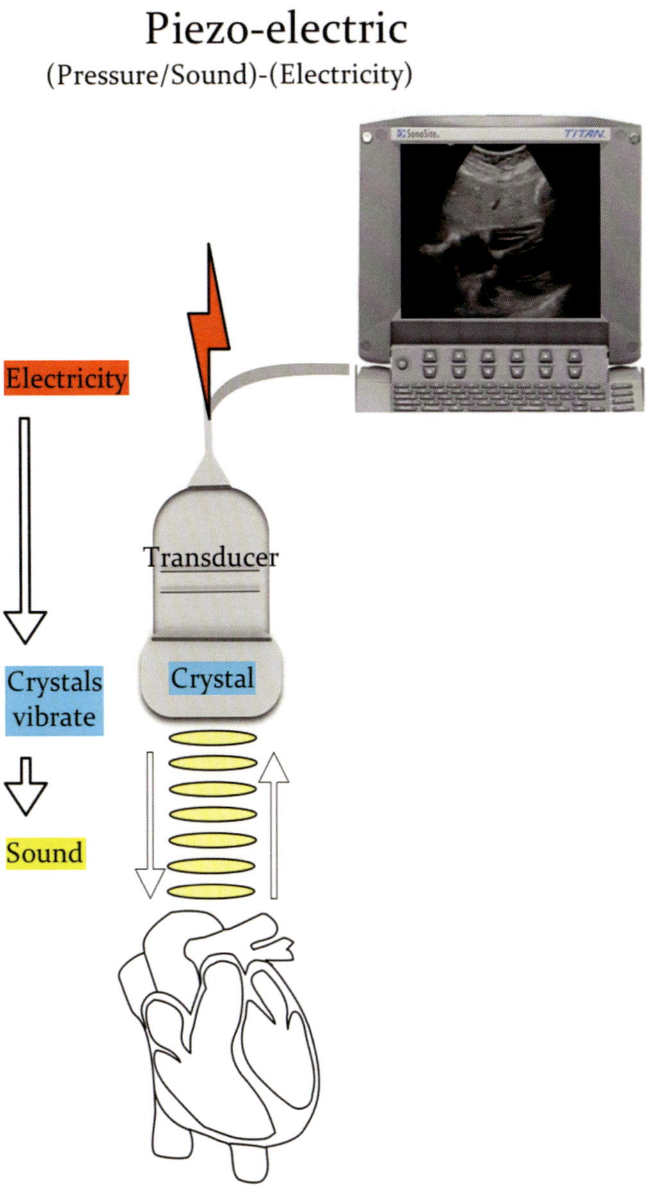

Figure 1.2 The piezoelectric effect. Electricity causes the crystals within the transducer to vibrate, creating sound. The sound reaches the organ of interest and returns to the transducer. The transducer spends 99% of the time "listening" to the returning sound waves. These are then converted into an image that can be seen on the ultrasound monitor. *Illustration by Laura Berg, MD.*

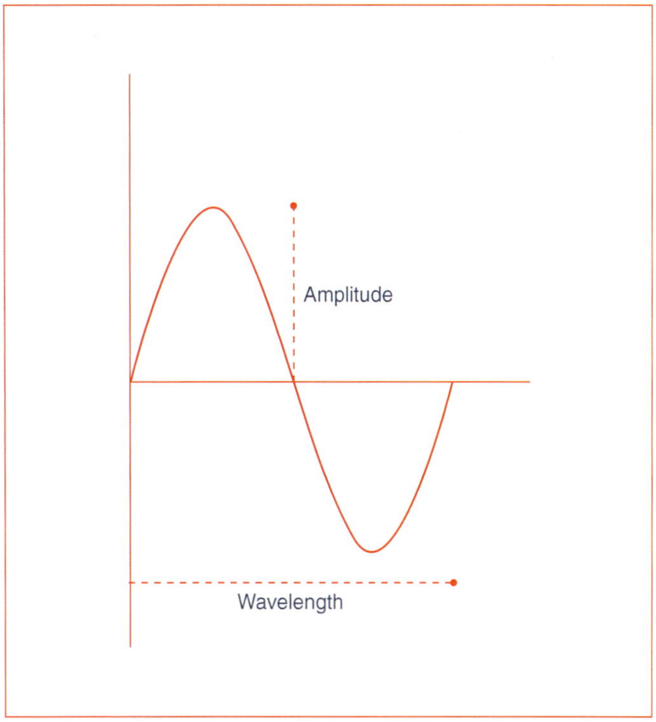

Figure 1.3 The cycle of sound. Frequency (Hz) is the number of cycles repeated in one second, amplitude (dB) is the height of the deflection, and the wavelength (mm) is the distance traveled in a single cycle.

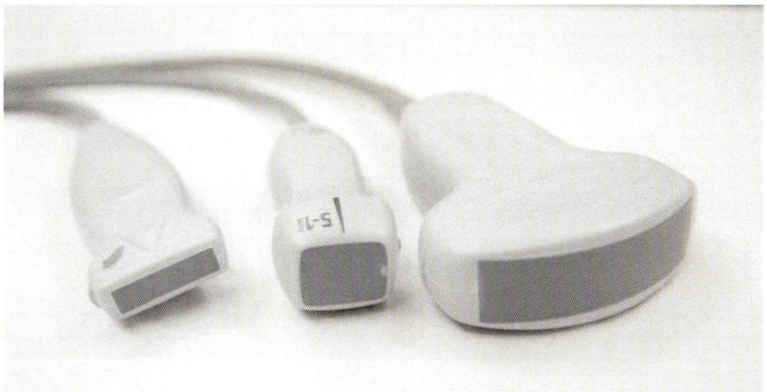

Figure 1.4 Various types of transducers.

pressure on the transducer and pushing downward may displace bowel gas that interferes with image acquisition.

There are different types of ultrasound transducers: linear, curvilinear (or convex), phased array/sector, and endocavitary. They are characterized by shape, arrangement of the piezoelectric crystals, frequency range, footprint, and shape of the image produced. The footprint is the area of the transducer that comes in contact with the patient.

Linear transducers have a flat footprint that is rectangular in shape, and they therefore produce a rectangular image. The piezoelectric crystals are arranged in a linear fashion. There are various types of linear transducers that have different sized footprints; there is a particular linear transducer known as the "hockey stick" (Figure 1.6a). The frequency range varies among transducers and is approximately 5–10 MHz. Linear transducers often have higher frequencies, providing better resolution for shallow structures. However, with higher frequencies penetration and depth are sacrificed. These transducers are appropriate for visualizing superficial structures and as an adjunct for performing procedures such as vascular access, musculoskeletal applications, and abscess evaluation (see Section 3, Procedural ultrasound).

Convex (curvilinear)-array transducers have a curved end (Figure 1.6b). They produce a sector-shaped image, with a curved area at the top. The piezoelectric crystals are arranged alongside one another along the curved face. These transducers have lower frequencies (2–5 MHz), allowing for better penetration of deeper structures. They are commonly used for the examination of the abdomen and pelvis. Smaller

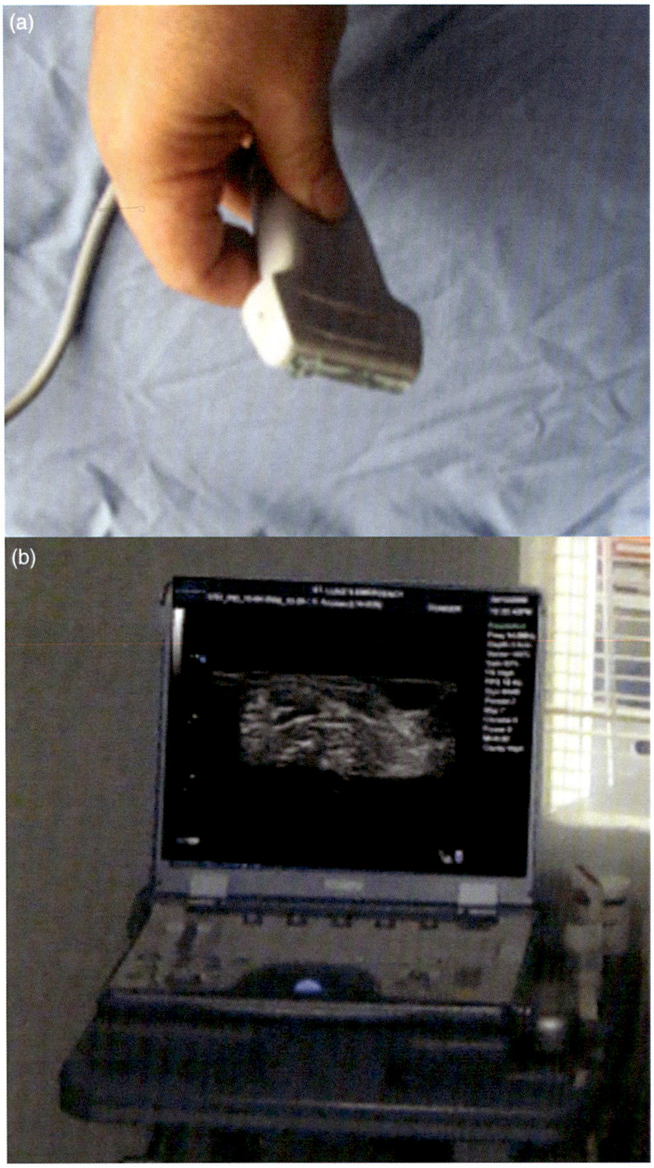

Figure 1.5 Indicator and screen orientation. (a) Each transducer has an indicator mark, which corresponds to the indicator mark on the ultrasound image. (b) In the standard views, the indicator corresponds with the left-hand side of the image.

versions of the curvilinear transducers are referred to as microconvex, and have a smaller footprint that is especially useful in the pediatric population. **Endocavitary transducers** are a type of microconvex transducer with a long handle (Figure 1.6c). These transducers are appropriate for endovaginal evaluation of the female pelvis. Other indications include evaluation of the oral cavity; i.e. assessing peritonsillar abscesses.

Phased-array (sector) transducers have a flat end that is square or rectangular in shape, producing an image that is pie-shaped (Figure 1.6b). The piezoelectric crystals are grouped into a very small cluster and are steered electronically. These transducers emit lower-frequency (2–8 MHz) acoustic pulses and are useful for cardiac, thoracic, and abdominal imaging. Similar to the microconvex transducers, they have smaller footprints that are beneficial for pediatric scanning.

Monitors

Monitor considerations include flat-panel and cathode-ray tube monitors. Flat-panel monitors provide better image quality and are lighter, but also more expensive. Monitor size varies from 5 to 15 inches. Regardless of the type of monitor, it is important to remember to adjust the room lighting, in order to view images properly and identify subtle findings.

Maintenance of equipment

Ultrasound machines and equipment must be properly maintained. For the most part, transducers are extremely delicate. Care must be taken to not drop or damage them. Cracks in the crystals may appear as a vertical or horizontal line, depending on the type of transducer (Figure 1.7). Care must also be taken in cleaning the probes. A non-alcohol-based germicidal wipe may be used, or water and a non-abrasive soap. Note that when alcohol is used on the transducer footprint it may cause cracking. A cracked footprint should not be used on a patient, as it could expose both the patient and clinician to an electrical current. If footprint cracking occurs, the transducer should not be used and should be replaced. Special consideration should be taken in the sterilization of endocavitary probes. Due to the potential disruption of the barriers used, the transducers should be soaked in high-level disinfectants such as a glutaraldehyde product or Cidex OPA® solutions.

It is not uncommon in the chaotic emergency department and critical care settings to overlook the maintenance of machines. Special care must be taken to avoid running over electrical and transducer cords. When a cord is frayed, it should be replaced and not used further.

Accessories

There are several accessories needed for successful ultrasound use. As previously discussed, the acoustic impedance of air makes ultrasound virtually impossible. Gel placed between the transducer and skin forms a barrier, thereby reducing air interference, and allowing the transmission of sound. Gels are made commercially, and standard gels are for external use only (Figure 1.8a). They should not be used if the integrity of the skin is compromised. Standard gels should also not be used in oral or endovaginal ultrasound as they can irritate the mucous membranes. A sterile sheath without overlying gel is sufficient and essential in performing endovaginal ultrasonography.

When performing ultrasound-guided procedures, it is often necessary to maintain a sterile field. Commercially available sterile probe covers are available (see S3, Introduction). In order to properly prepare the transducer, a layer of standard gel is placed on it, followed by a sterile sheath, with sterile gel on top (see S3, Introduction). Sterile gel is manufactured and can be placed on top of the sterile sheath. Alternatively, a

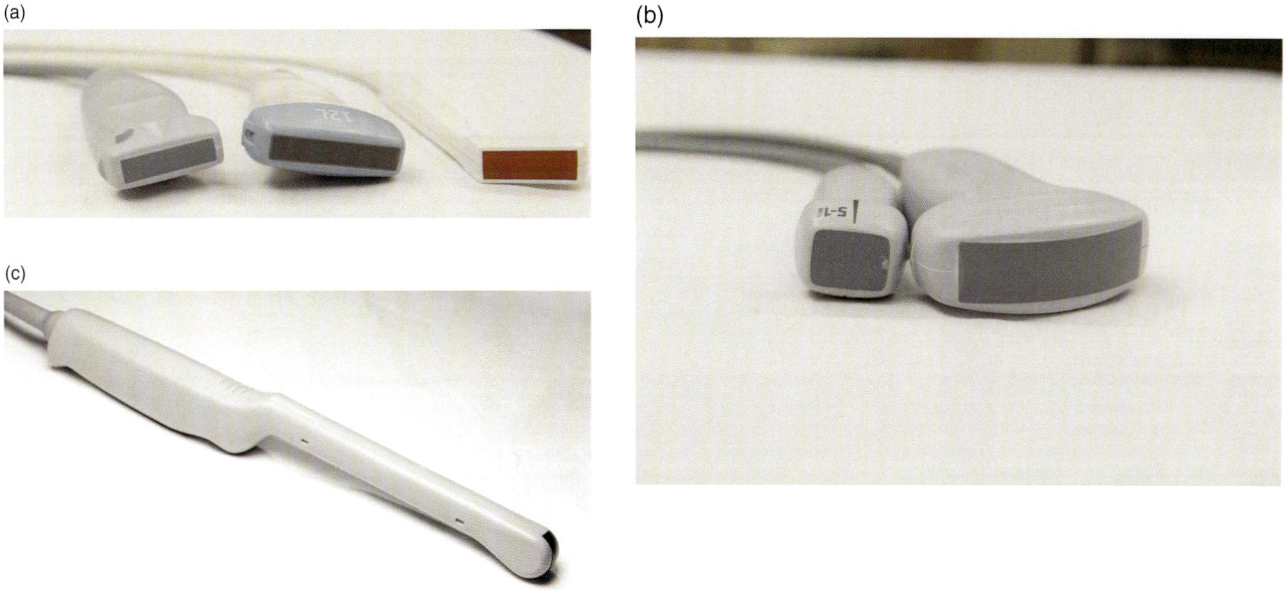

Figure 1.6 Transducers. (a) Linear high-frequency transducers. Note the different-sized footprints. The transducer on the right is a "hockey stick" linear transducer. (b) Low-frequency transducers used for cardiac and abdominal examinations. The transducer on the left is a phased array and the transducer on the right is the curvilinear. (c) Endocavitary transducer which is used for transvaginal ultrasonography and for the evaluation of peritonsillar abscesses.

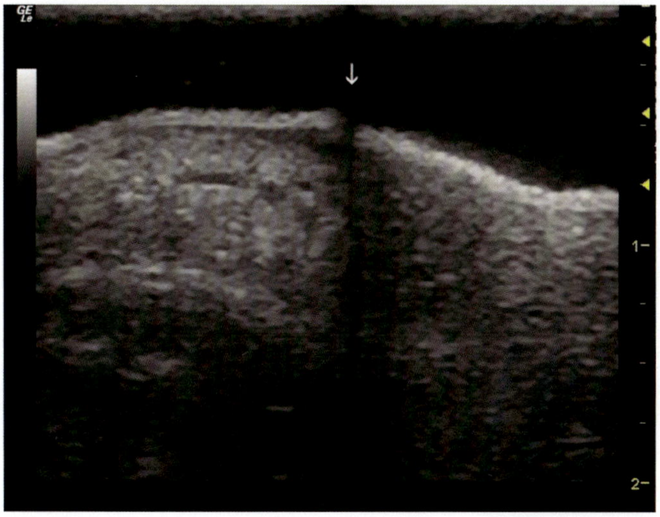

Figure 1.7 A damaged transducer. For the most part, transducers are extremely delicate. Dropping a transducer may result in a cracked crystal. In this linear transducer, there is a crack in a crystal, creating a vertical black line in the center of the image. When crystals are cracked, the transducer needs to be replaced.

sterile lubricant may be utilized (Figure 1.8b). This type of set up is used for sterile procedures, including central line placement. In addition, many manufacturers offer a needle guide that attaches to the transducer to assist with ultrasound-guided procedures. These may be beneficial but are not a necessity.

Image storage

There are several options for image storage of both video clips and still images. Through a USB port, images can either be transferred to a flash drive, external hard drive or another computer. Some machines have a burner for CDs or DVDs, to which images can be stored. There are also the options of network storage, where images and videos can be transferred via an Ethernet port or WiFi and stored on a remote computer. Digital imaging and communication in medicine (DICOM) is the format that allows for transmission and storage of the images. This format is a standard among many departments and allows the user to manage the images within the available software applications. Disadvantages include the relative cost associated with DICOM packages and associated software. Lastly, images can be printed and stored as hard copies. Machines may come with either a black and white or color printer (Figure 1.9).

Modes of scanning

In order to produce an image, the transducer accounts for the time–distance relationship as well as intensity of the returning sound. The data can be displayed differently depending on the mode of scanning.

A-mode

A-mode, or "amplitude" mode, is one of the original modes of medical ultrasound. In A-mode, sound travels along a path where the ultrasound beam encounters different tissues of different acoustic impedances. The information received by the transducer is plotted on an x–y graph where the y-axis is amplitude or intensity and the x-axis is time. The image produced is a tracing. This mode has been utilized in medicine for evaluation of the eye as well as the fetal head.

(a) (b)

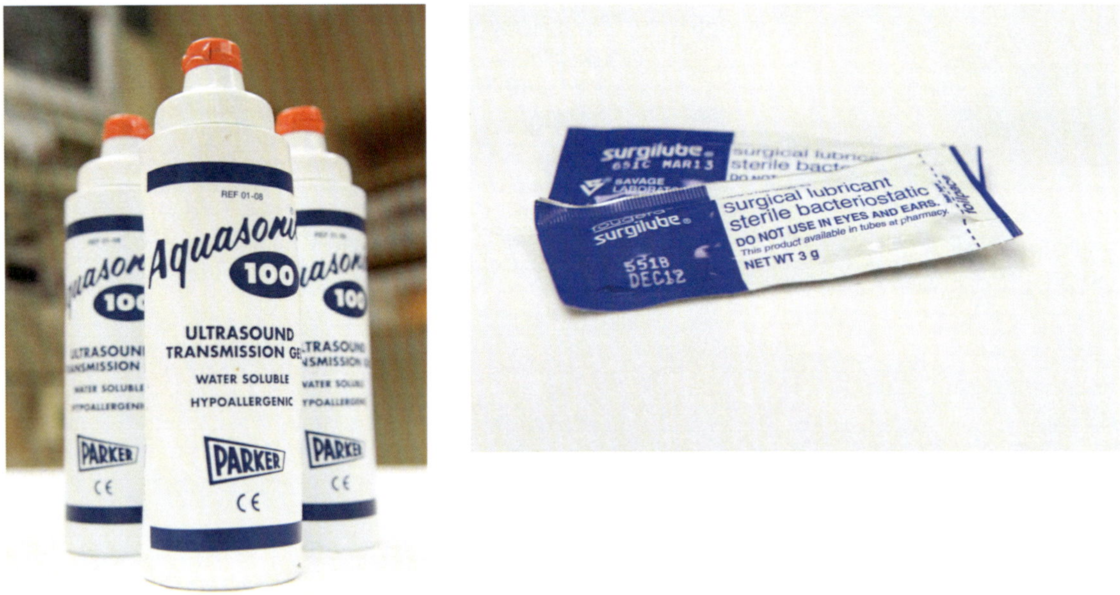

Figure 1.8 **Gel.** In order to transmit ultrasound waves, gel must be placed on the transducer footprint. (a) Commercially available gels are available, but are not sterile. (b) In order to maintain a sterile field while performing procedures, sterile lubricant may be utilized as an alternative.

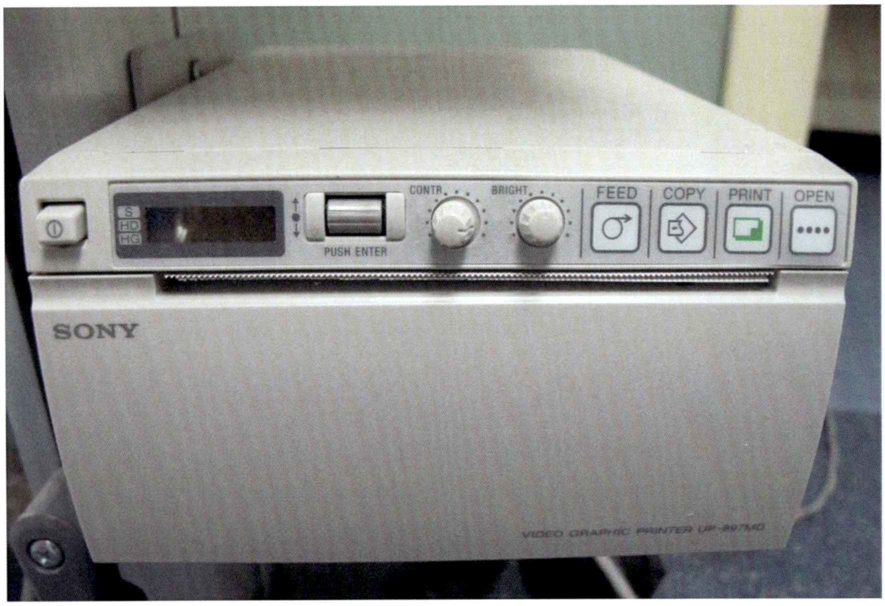

Figure 1.9 **Ultrasound printer.** Images may be stored digitally. However, a printed copy is often required for billing purposes.

B-mode

B-mode, or "brightness" mode, is the primary imaging modality in medical ultrasound. B-mode is similar to A-mode in that the time–distance relationship is fundamental in interpreting the returning sound waves. It differs, however, in how it translates the intensity of that sound. The returning echo is translated into a dot where the amplitude or intensity of the sound determines the brightness of the dot. The greater the intensity, the brighter the dot appears. Structures that produce stronger echoes are termed **hyperechoic** and appear "brighter" or "whiter," as opposed to structures that do not produce echoes and are termed **anechoic**, appearing black. **Hypoechoic** is a relative term describing structures that give off weaker echoes than the surrounding tissues, and **isoechoic** refers to tissues of similar echogenicity (Figure 1.10). The standard two-dimensional image produced is therefore based on a series of dots and a gray scale of 256 shades of gray (Figure 1.11).

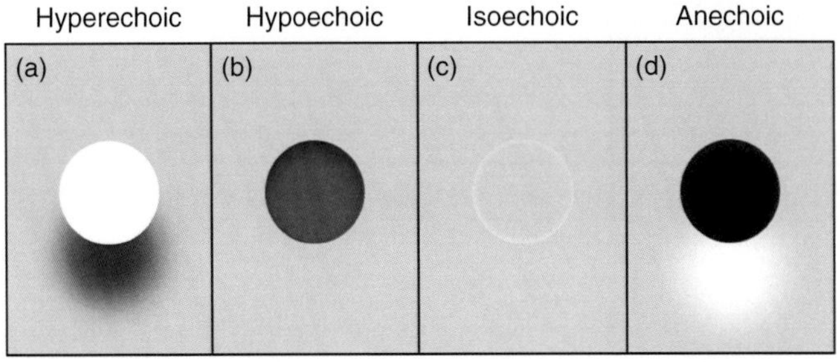

Figure 1.10 Echogenicities. (a) Hyperechoic tissue has greater echogenicity, or is brighter than surrounding tissue. (b) Hypoechoic tissue is less echogenic, or darker than surrounding tissue. (c) Isoechoic tissue has the same echogenicity in relation to surrounding tissue. (d) Anechoic tissue produces no echoes and appears black. *Illustration by Laura Berg, MD.*

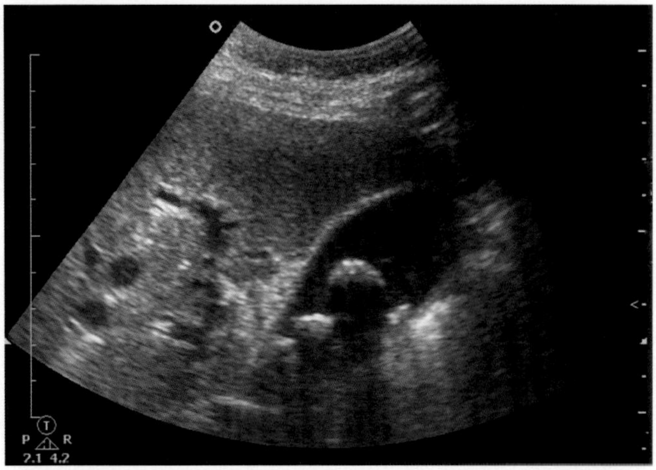

Figure 1.11 B-mode image that is created from 256 shades of gray. This is an image of a gallbladder with a large hyperechoic stone within the gallbladder lumen.

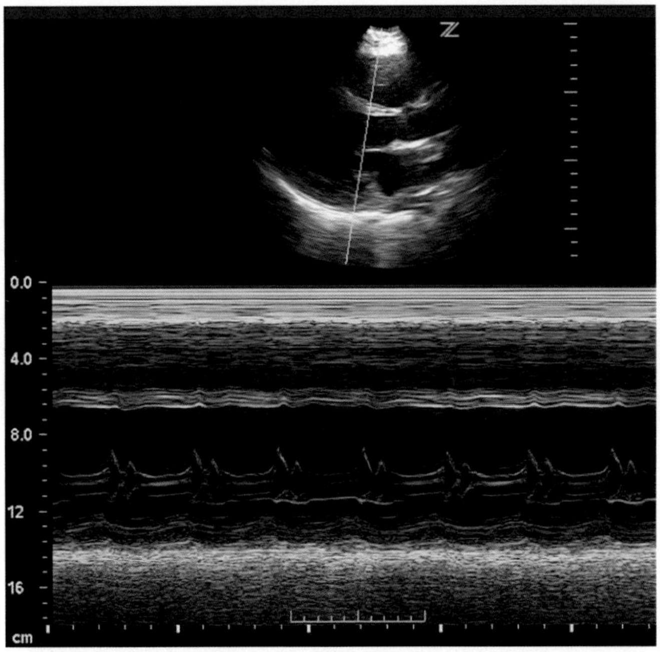

Figure 1.12 M-mode, or "motion" mode detects tissue movement over time. This is an example of an evaluation of cardiac activity with M-mode, showing cardiac contractions.

M-mode

M-mode, or "motion" mode, provides additional information to the sonographer during B-mode imaging. In M-mode, the transducer records motion changes along one path of the B-mode image and displays the result in a graphical format on an x–y plot. The y-axis represents the distance from the transducer, while the x-axis represents time. M-mode is beneficial as an adjunct to B-mode imaging, particularly in the evaluation of the heart, lungs, and fetus. For example, in cardiac imaging the B-mode image will provide an overall picture of the heart, while M-mode can assess the motion of the mitral valve along a given axis (Figure 1.12).

Doppler

Doppler ultrasound measures the change in the frequency of the acoustic wave: the frequency shift. By assessing the frequency shift, Doppler ultrasound analyzes both the velocity and the direction of objects in motion, such as red blood cells. The information is displayed in an audible, spectral, or color Doppler format. **Audible Doppler** does not provide a visual component; it simply creates an audible sound from the shift. **Spectral** or **pulse wave Doppler**, graphically displays the change in graphical format with time on the x-axis and velocity on the y-axis. Characteristic arterial and venous waveforms may aid in the differentiation of vessels.

Color Doppler provides information on both the intensity and direction of movement by displaying color over a grayscale image (Figure 1.13). Duplex ultrasound consists of a grayscale image with color or spectral Doppler, and a triplex ultrasound displays all three (Figure 1.14a,b). **Power Doppler** is similar to color Doppler, except that the information displayed regarding motion is non-directional information. Power Doppler is more sensitive in detecting frequency shifts of low-flow states (Figure 1.15).

Pulsed wave, or spectral Doppler displays the velocity of moving structures on the vertical axis (y-axis), with respect to time as the horizontal axis (x-axis). The resulting graph quantifies flow, such as through vascular structures and the heart (Figure 1.16).

"Knobology," system controls

Frequency

Ultrasound transducers each have a specific range of **frequencies** preset by the manufacturer. The degree to which the sonographer can manipulate the transducer's frequency is also predetermined. Sonographers may alter the frequency to optimize the relative balance between resolution and penetration for the object of interest.

Resolution

Resolution of an ultrasound image is similar to the resolution of a photograph and is interpreted as overall image quality.

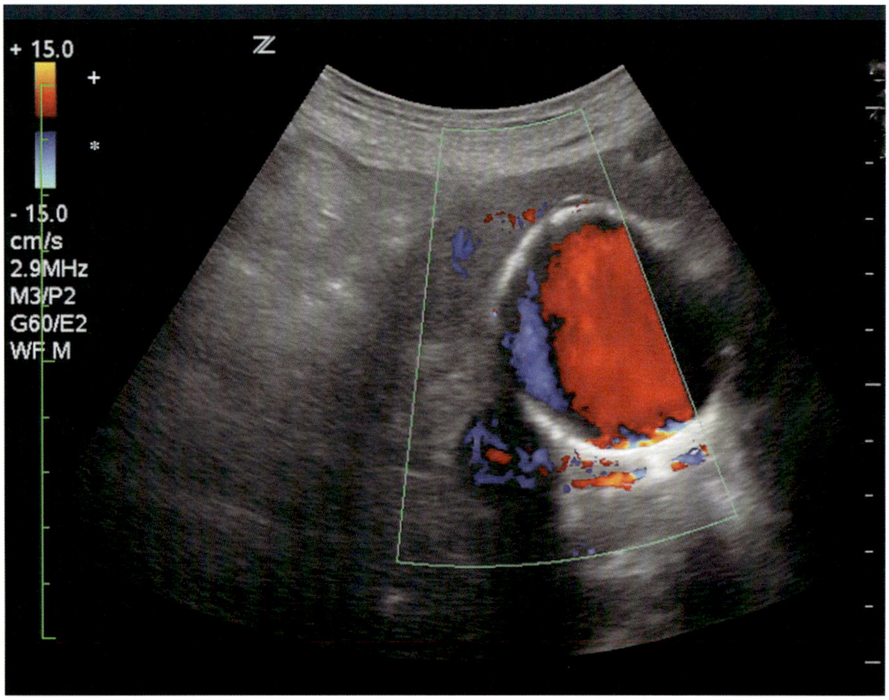

Figure 1.13 Color Doppler provides information on intensity and direction of movement. In this image of the aorta, red indicates flow towards the transducer, while the blue indicates flow away from the transducer. The bar on the left upper side of the image depicts the direction of flow. Above the midline is towards the transducer (+), while below the midline is away from the transducer (*).

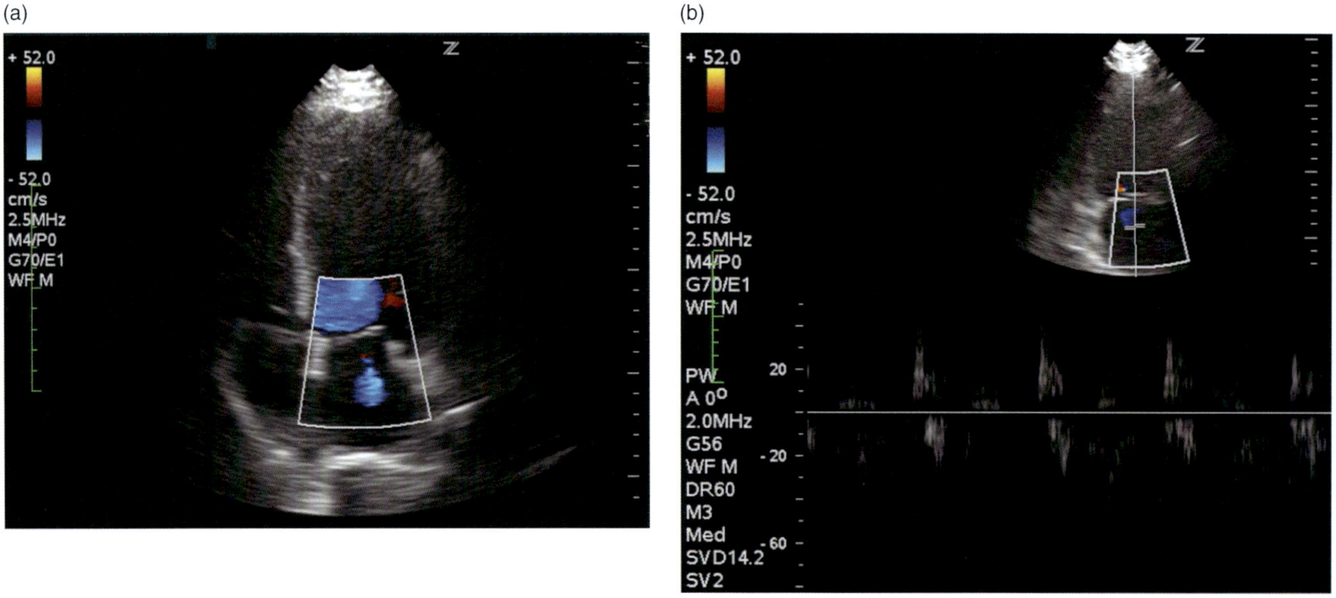

Figure 1.14 Duplex and triplex Doppler imaging. (a) Duplex imaging of the heart, which consists of a grayscale image with color or spectral Doppler. (b) Triplex Doppler imaging consists of a grayscale image with color Doppler and spectral Doppler all on the same image.

Technically, resolution is defined as the ability to discriminate two separate objects. In ultrasound, there is spatial and temporal resolution. **Spatial resolution** is further characterized by axial and lateral resolution, where **axial resolution** refers to discriminating objects in the scanning plane of the ultrasound beam and **lateral resolution** refers to discriminating objects perpendicular to the ultrasound beam. **Temporal resolution** is related to the rate at which images are acquired, i.e. the frame rate (frames per second). At a higher frame rate, the image will appear smoother.

The relationship between frequency, axial resolution, and depth is fundamental. Ultrasound transducers with higher frequencies provide better resolution; however, as frequency increases so does attenuation. Therefore, the ultrasonic wave loses its ability to penetrate deeply and is thus limited to interrogating at shallow depths. The contrary is also true: transducers that emit lower frequencies will have greater penetration (i.e. depth), but at the cost of resolution. Consider the analogy of a telephone cord. If the telephone cord is bunched up, it is not very long but it is easy to count the number of coils. If you

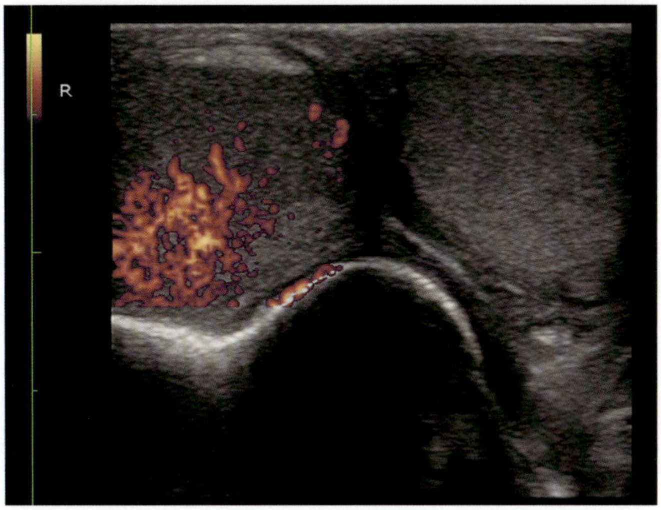

Figure 1.15 **Color power Doppler (CPD)** displays information regarding non-directional motion. In this image of the testicles, CPD is more sensitive in detecting low flow. Note the absence of flow in the left testicle, which is concerning for a testicular torsion.

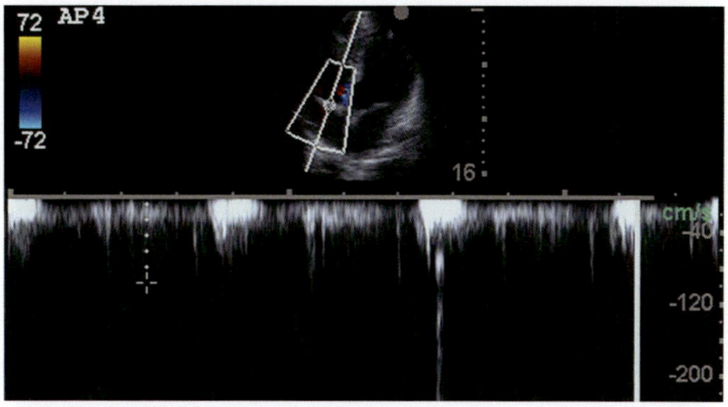

Figure 1.16 **Pulsed wave or spectral Doppler** displays the velocity of moving structures with respect to time. This is an apical four-chamber view of the heart, using pulsed wave Doppler to measure the tricuspid jets.

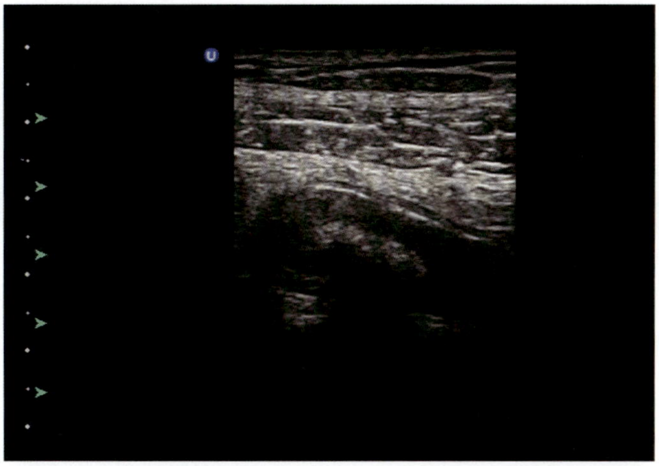

Figure 1.17 **Focal zones** provide the best lateral resolution. They are represented by a triangle or line on the right hand or left-hand side of the image. Machines often have the capability of "focusing" the ultrasound beam and changing the focal zone. This is a longitudinal view of an enlarged appendix with an appendicolith. The blue arrows on the left of the image indicate multiple focal zones.

stretch out the same cord, it will cover a greater distance, but it is more difficult to count the number of coils. The trade off between resolution and depth is related to the frequency of the transducer.

Focus

Ultrasound waves transmitted by the transducer create a cylindrical beam. The beam is similar in shape to an hourglass with the narrowest portion being the focal or transition zone between the near and far fields. The focal zone provides the best lateral resolution; therefore, objects of interest should be interrogated at the focal zone. The focal zone is often represented by a triangle or line on the right or left-hand side of the image (Figure 1.17). Machines may provide the capability of adjusting the focal zone by "**focusing**" the ultrasound beam. Ultrasound machines may also have the ability to create multiple focal zones; however, the more focal zones, the lower the frame rate. In other words, improving the lateral resolution will be at the expense of the temporal resolution.

Gain

Gain is related to the brightness of the image, similar to the brightness function on a computer monitor. As sound travels, it is attenuated and the beam weakens. The ultrasound machine has internal functions to counteract attenuation by making deeper images appear brighter. By adjusting the gain, the sonographer can artificially amplify the echoes that return to the transducer and are processed by the machine. The gain function is similar to an amplifier: increasing the gain will make the entire image brighter, whereas decreasing it will make the image darker (Figure 1.18).

Time gain compensation

Time gain compensation (TGC) is the ability to adjust the gain at specific depths (Figure 1.19). Manufacturers determine the modality (i.e. knob or button) that controls the overall gain and TGC. Options include one dial for overall gain, as well as a two-dial system for near and far field gain. Adjusting the near field gain will adjust the top half of the screen, while the far field gain is responsible for the bottom half of the image. Other machines will have a linear row of buttons, where each button corresponds to a given depth from the top of the image downward. The buttons move from side to side, which increases and decreases the gain respectively at the specific depth, similar to a stereo equalizer. Alternatively, some machines have an "optimize" function that will attempt to optimize the overall image, automatically adjusting several functions, including the gain.

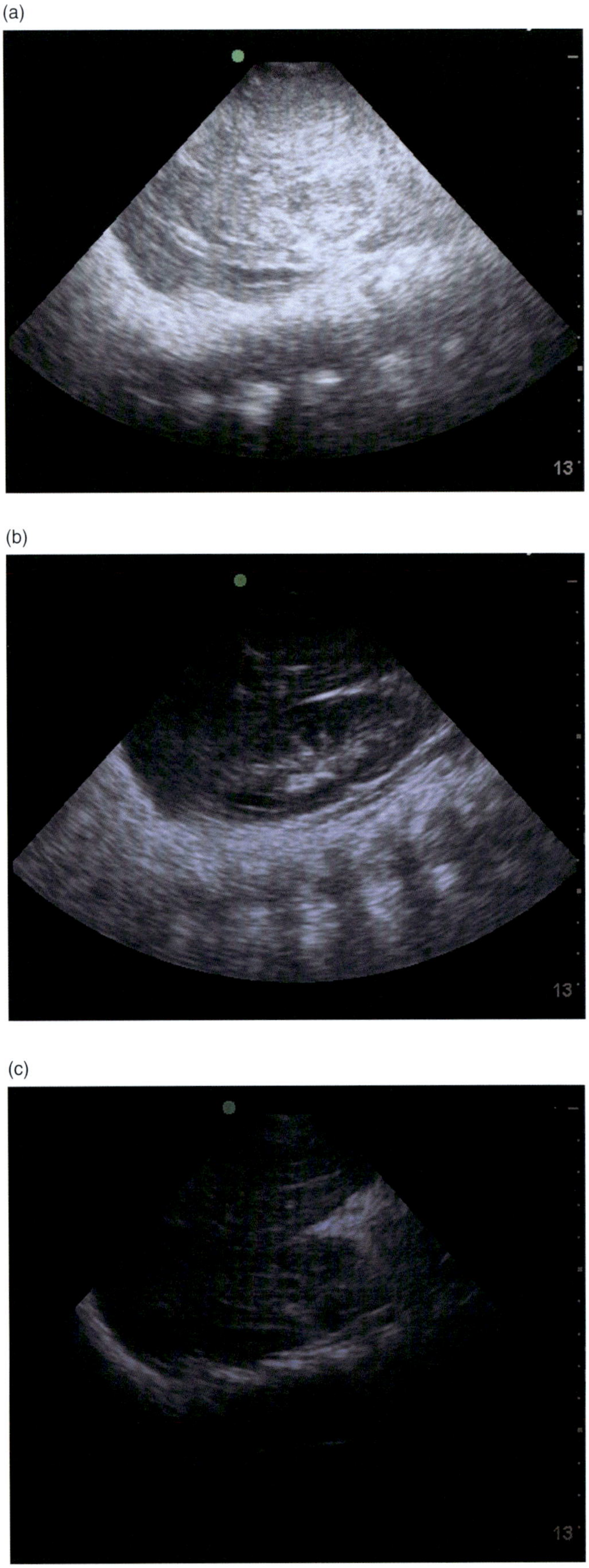

Figure 1.18 **Gain** is the overall brightness of an image. (a) The image has too much gain, or is too bright. (b) The image is properly gained. (c) The image has too little gain, or is too dark.

Depth

Adjusting the **depth** modifies the area of interrogation between shallow and deep structures. Increasing the depth lengthens the time of flight of the ultrasound wave, in turn decreasing the imaging frame rate. If shallow structures are imaged with increased depth settings, the image displayed will be a smaller absolute size on the monitor. It is important to maximize the depth settings, since excessive depth will result in an inefficient use of the monitor's display (Figure 1.20).

Zoom

The **zoom** function enlarges a select portion of the image (Figure 1.21). Differing from adjusting depth, this function actually "zooms" in on a portion of the image, making the image larger, but with a decreased resolution. The number of pixels is constant; thus enlarging the image may make it appear blurry or grainy.

Freeze

The **freeze** button holds the image on the screen. After freezing the image, the sonographer can scroll through the frames leading up to the still image. The number of still images frozen at a given time is referred to as the **cine loop** and is predetermined by the manufacturer. Freezing an image allows for measuring structures on the image. It also allows for saving a specific image.

Harmonics (THI)

Ultrasound waves are transmitted and received by the transducer at a certain frequency. When receiving the returning sound wave, the transducer also receives other signals scattered from different points on the image, at different frequencies. The transducer receives the primary frequency, and harmonic frequencies, which are multiples of the original frequency (i.e. 2×, 4×, etc.). The **tissue harmonic imaging (THI)** filters these echoes returning at the primary frequency and uses the harmonic frequency to create the image (Figure 1.22). Harmonic frequencies create less scatter and side-lobe artifact, creating a cleaner image.

Measurements and calculations

Nearly all portable ultrasound machines have the capability of performing measurements. Calipers are used which automatically calculate measurements when positioned properly (Figure 1.23). Additionally, preset calculations including volume, gestational age, fetal heart rate, and cardiac output can all be measured, depending on the transducer utilized and the preinstalled calculation package.

Artifacts

Acoustic shadowing

Acoustic shadowing is one of the most common artifacts in ultrasound. It occurs when sound encounters highly reflective

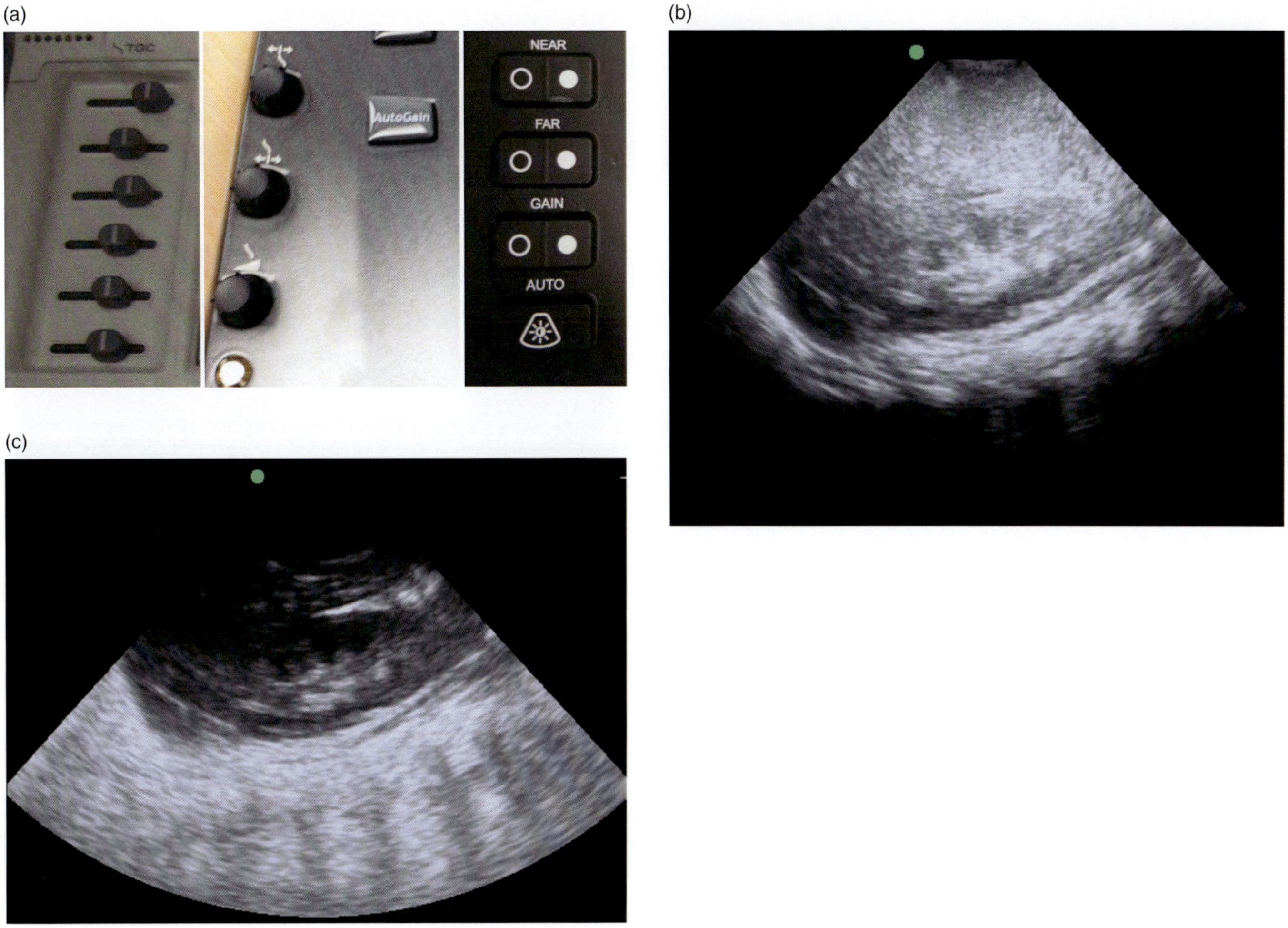

Figure 1.19 Time gain compensation (TGC) is the ability to change the gain at different depths. (a) Various machines have a slide, knob, or buttons to adjust the overall gain and TGC. (b) In this image of Morison's pouch, the near field gain is too high, or too bright. (c) The far field gain is too high, or too bright. These can be corrected by adjusting the TGC at the near and far fields.

surfaces that absorb much of the sound energy, leaving essentially no energy to penetrate deeper structures. Structures that have high attenuation (highly reflective), i.e. bone and calcifications, reflect about 30% of the sound and absorb the rest, thereby producing "**clean**" or black shadows. "**Dirty**" shadowing is often a result of acoustic impedance mismatch (i.e. air and soft tissue) producing shadows filled with shades of gray (Figure 1.24).

Edge artifact is another example of acoustic shadowing. Also known as "**lateral cystic shadowing**," this artifact arises due to a change in the ultrasound beam when it encounters a curved surface such as a cyst. Part of the beam is refracted and scattered, thereby producing a thin shadow on the lateral sides of the structure (Figure 1.25).

Posterior acoustic enhancement

Posterior acoustic enhancement occurs when sound traverses areas of low attenuation (i.e. fluid-filled structures), allowing more energy to penetrate deeper structures. Since the ultrasound beam attenuates as it propagates, the machine compensates for this phenomenon by amplifying the returning echoes of deeper structures. Sound waves traveling through the bladder will be subject to less attenuation, allowing more acoustic energy to penetrate and return to the transducer. Therefore, the amplification of echoes deep to the bladder will be overcompensated and appear artificially enhanced, or brighter (Figure 1.26). This can be corrected by decreasing the far gain, or TGC.

Reverberation artifacts

Reverberation artifacts are a result of sound reverberating or "bouncing" between two reflective surfaces. This is displayed as repeating bright arcs that are equidistant from one another. In lung ultrasound, A-lines are repetitive horizontal lines resulting from sound that is reverberating between the lung pleura and the transducer. The first bright line is the pleural line, and the subsequent lines are due to the reverberation artifact (Figure 1.27).

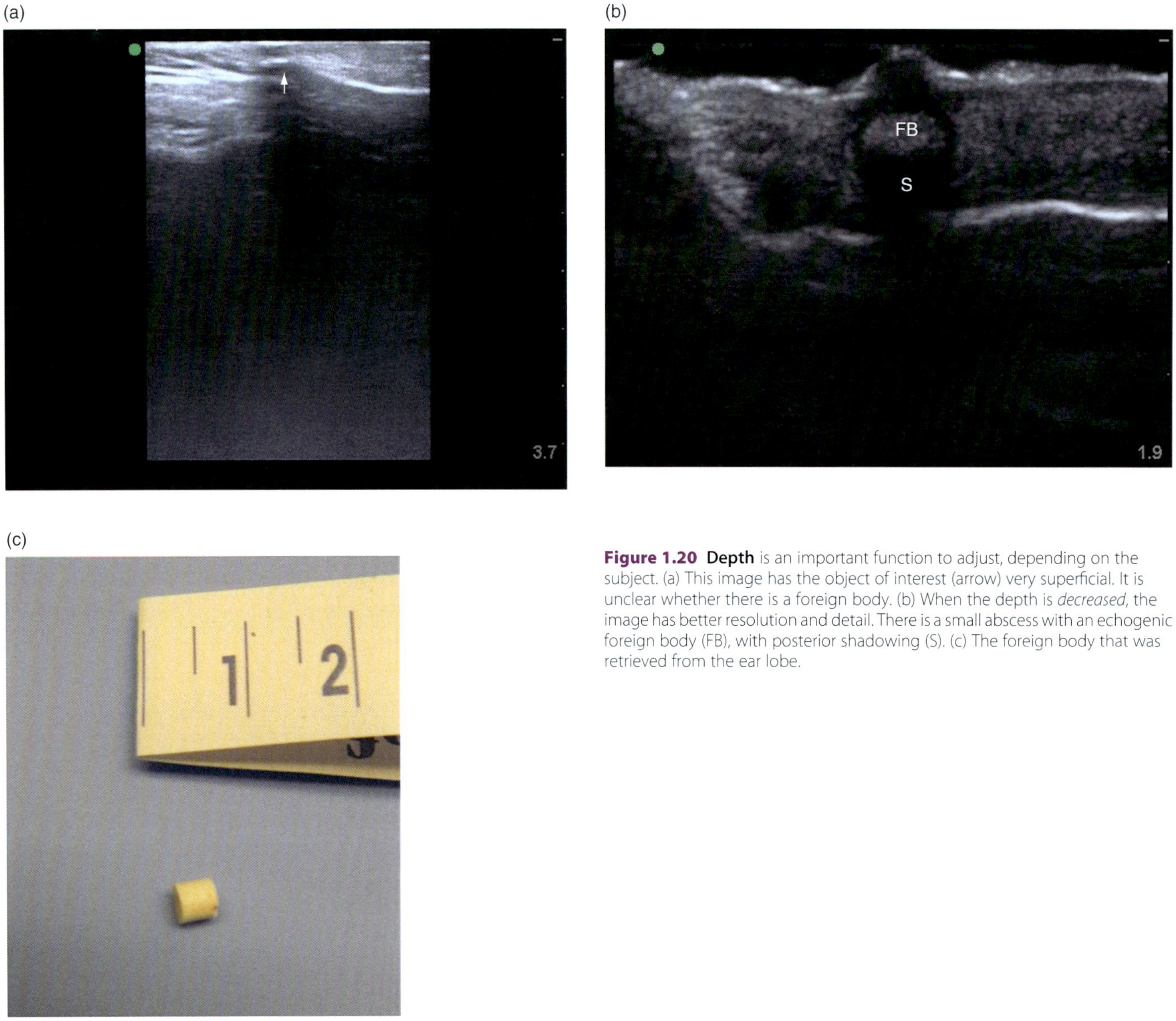

Figure 1.20 **Depth** is an important function to adjust, depending on the subject. (a) This image has the object of interest (arrow) very superficial. It is unclear whether there is a foreign body. (b) When the depth is *decreased*, the image has better resolution and detail. There is a small abscess with an echogenic foreign body (FB), with posterior shadowing (S). (c) The foreign body that was retrieved from the ear lobe.

Ring-down, also referred to as a "**comet tail**," is a type of reverberation artifact. It appears deep to highly reflective surfaces, linear to the ultrasound beam, with narrow spacing between reverberating echoes. Ring-down may result at interfaces between tissue and air (e.g. bowel with intraluminal air), as well as foreign material such as metal (e.g. needle tip, BB gun pellet). With regard to lung ultrasound, B-lines are a type of comet-tail artifact. Multiple B-lines within an image are referred to as "**lung rockets**" and suggest an interstitial process (Figure 1.27).

Mirror-image artifacts

Mirror-image artifacts occur when ultrasound encounters a strong reflective surface that produces a mirror image. In abdominal imaging, the diaphragm is a strong reflector because of air in the lungs. When imaging the liver, sound is reflected and refracted by the diaphragm. The refracted sound may encounter nearby reflective surfaces before returning to the transducer. Thus, the transducer will interpret the initial, "real," image as well as the reflected, "false," image. The false image is the result of multiple echo paths, delaying travel back to the transducer, and therefore appears in the far field of the image (Figure 1.28).

Side-lobe artifacts

Side-lobe artifacts are a result of low-energy, extraneous ultrasound beams, adjacent to the main ultrasound beam, and interfere with lateral resolution (Figure 1.29). They can be counteracted, by focusing the main ultrasound beam. Otherwise, the echoes produced by the side lobes return false information to the transducer, hence side-lobe artifacts.

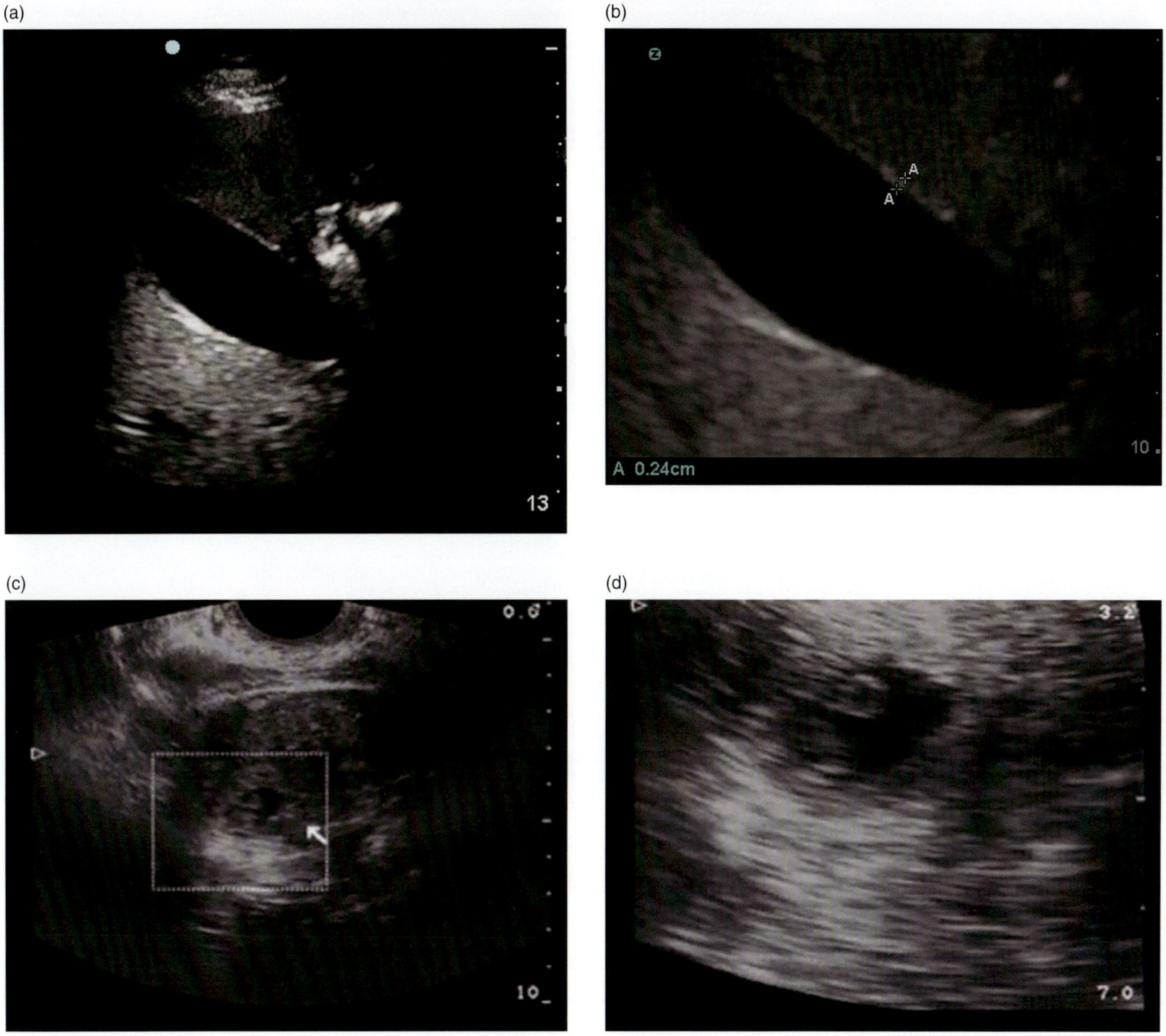

Figure 1.21 Zoom is used to focus on the subject of an image. This is commonly utilized to focus on a fetus in order to better visualize and perform measurements. (a) In this image, the gallbladder wall is difficult to appreciate and measure. (b) After the image is "zoomed" in, the gallbladder wall is more easily measured. In zoom, there is a "z" on the image. (c) "Zoom" is commonly used to identify a fetus and to evaluate for cardiac activity. (d) Though the resolution is lost, one can focus on the fetus to evaluate further.

Summary

1. Basic comprehension of ultrasound fundamentals and system controls will facilitate image acquisition and improved image quality.
2. Ultrasound is an imaging modality based on sound waves that provides real-time, non-invasive data. The mode of ultrasound determines how the information is displayed. The major modes utilized today are B-mode, M-mode, and Doppler.
3. The relationship between resolution and penetration, as it relates to frequency, should be considered when selecting an ultrasound transducer.
4. Ultrasound transducers account for the time elapsed as well as the intensity of returning echoes in order to produce an image. A wide variety of transducers exist, including linear, curvilinear (or convex), phased array/sector, and endocavitary.
5. Artifacts do not exist in real life, but aid in image interpretation. These artifacts include edge, reverberation, ring-down, side-lobe, and mirror-image artifacts. Other artifacts include acoustic shadowing and posterior acoustic enhancement.

(a) (b)

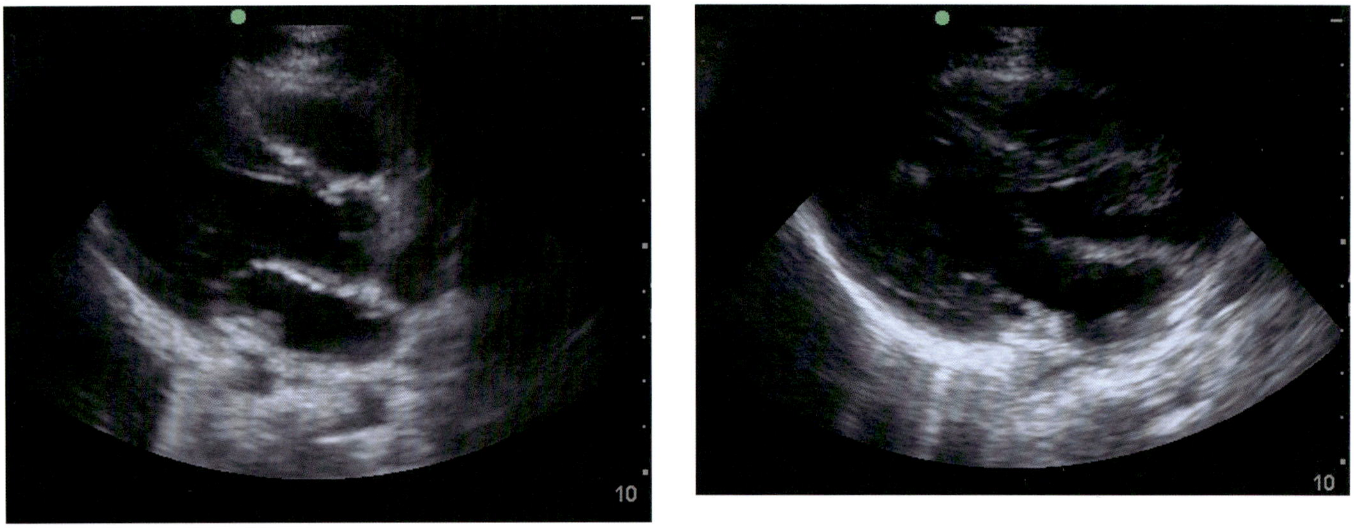

Figure 1.22 Tissue harmonic imaging (THI). Tissue harmonic imaging filters echoes returning at the primary frequency and uses the harmonic frequency to create the image with less scatter. This is an example of the parasternal long-axis view of the heart (a) without THI and (b) with THI.

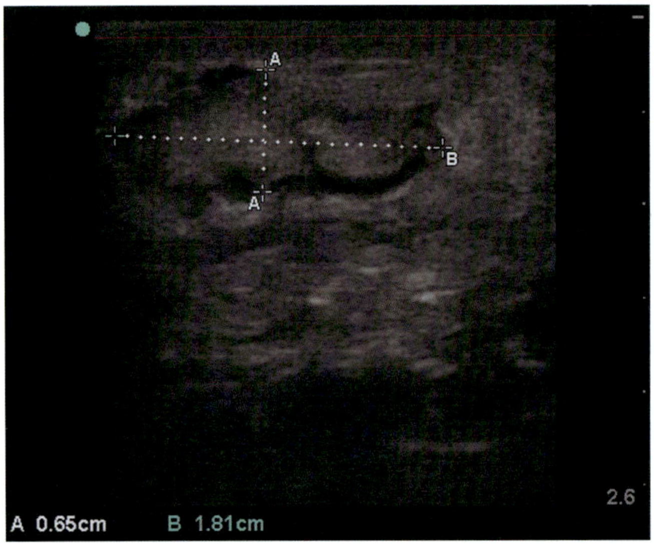

Figure 1.23 Measurements are performed with calipers. In this image, the dimensions of an abscess are measured.

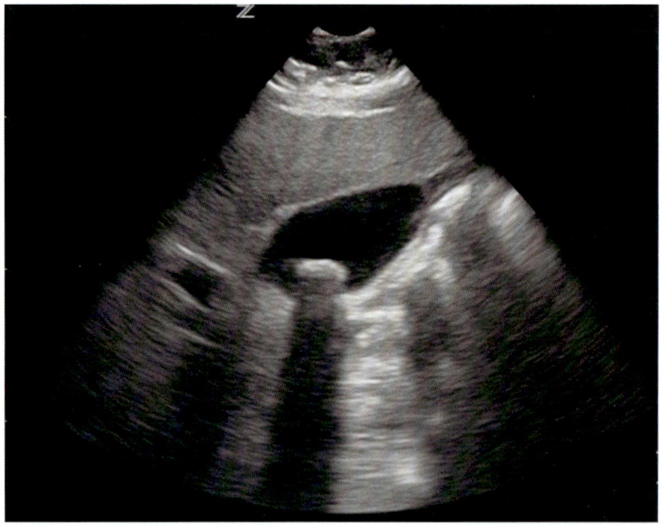

Figure 1.24 Acoustic shadowing occurs when sound waves encounter a reflective surface, and leaves no energy to penetrate to deeper structures. This is an example of a large, dense gallstone with a posterior acoustic shadow.

(a) (b) (c)

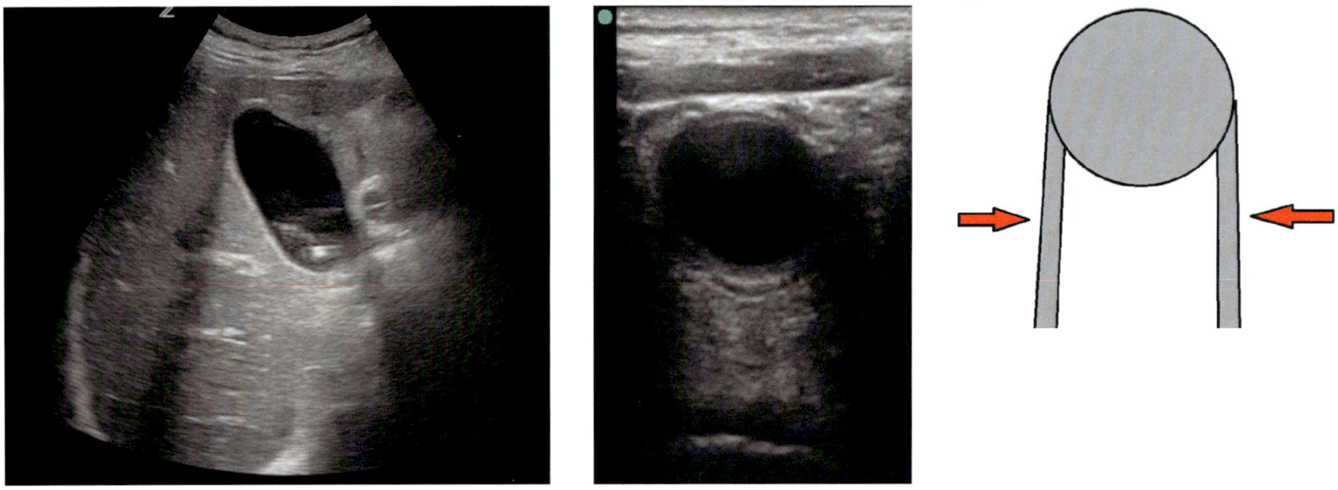

Figure 1.25 Edge artifact, or lateral cystic shadowing occurs when a sound wave encounters a curved, fluid-filled structure. This artifact may help in locating the gallbladder and other cystic structures. (a) This is an example of the gallbladder with thin shadows on the lateral sides. (b) Transverse view of an inflamed appendix with lateral cystic shadowing. (c) Illustration depicting lateral cystic shadowing. *Illustration by Alexander Arroyo, MD, FAAP.*

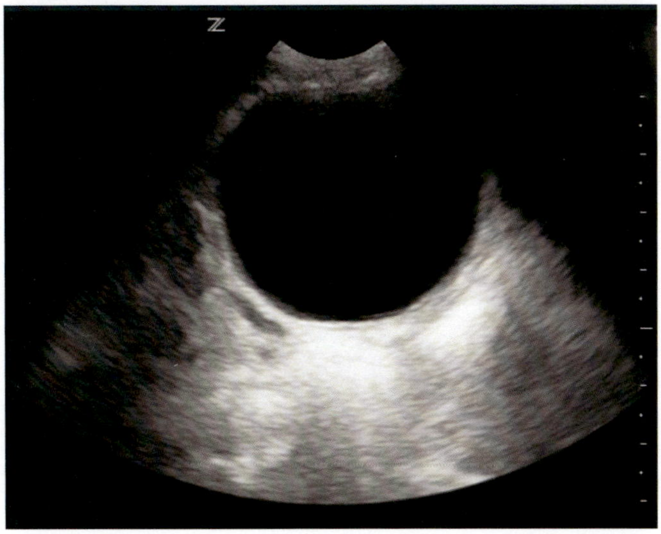

Figure 1.26 Posterior acoustic enhancement. As sound waves traverse fluid-filled structures such as the bladder, the sound waves attenuate proportionally less, allowing more energy to return to the transducer. The echoes deep to the bladder will be overcompensated and artificially brighter. Changing the TGC may correct this.

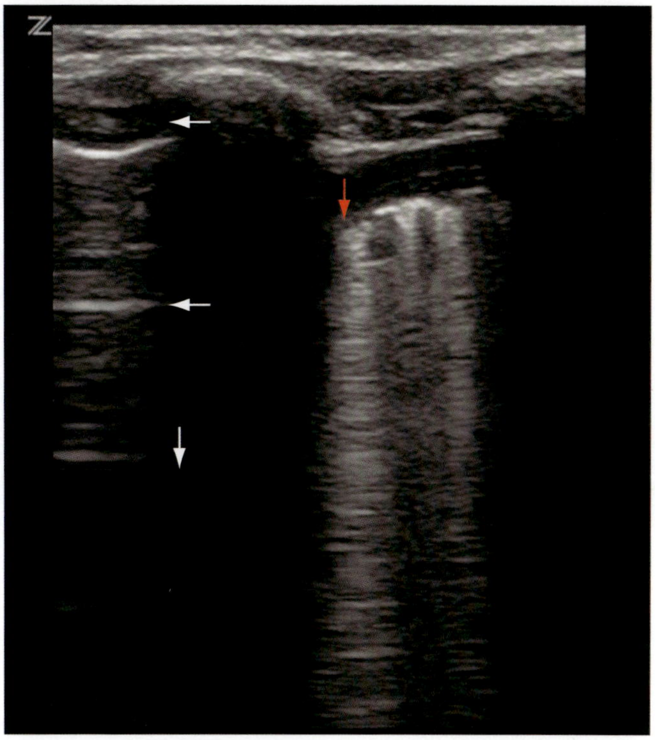

Figure 1.27 Reverberation artifacts. A-lines are a type of reverberation artifact resulting from sound that is reverberating between the lung pleura (*). A-lines (white arrows) appear as horizontal lines deep to the pleural line (top white arrow). Comet-tail artifacts (red arrow) are vertical lines that arise from the pleural line.

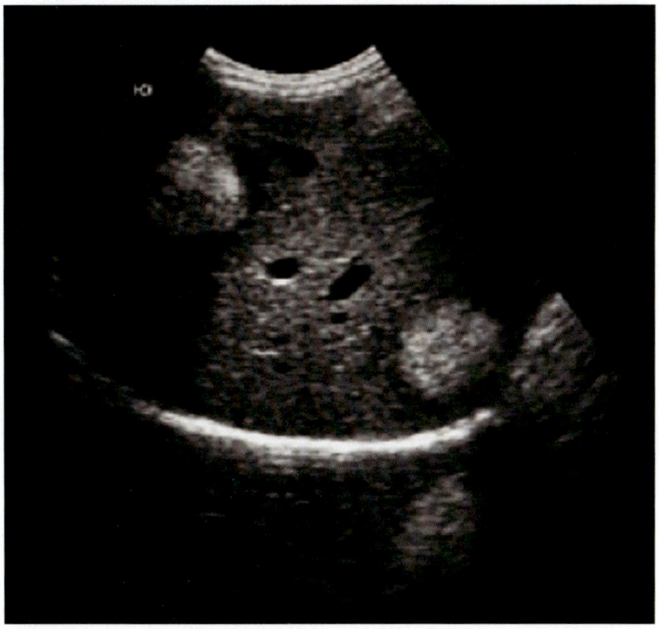

Figure 1.28 Mirror-image artifacts occur when ultrasound encounters a strong reflective surface, such as the diaphragm. In this ultrasound image, hyperechoic tumors are reflected across the diaphragm. It appears that there are tumors superior to the diaphragm, but this is just artifact. *Image courtesy of St. Luke's Roosevelt Hospital, Emergency Ultrasound Division.*

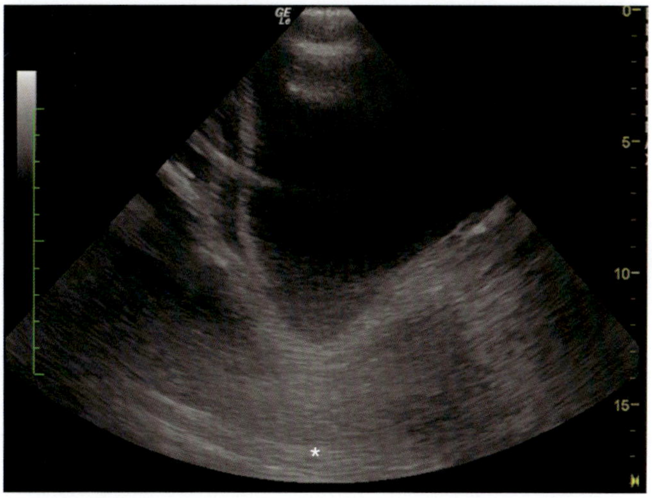

Figure 1.29 Side-lobe artifacts are a result of low-energy, extraneous ultrasound beams adjacent to the main ultrasound beam, which interfere with lateral resolution. This is commonly encountered with imaging of the bladder and may be corrected by focusing the main ultrasound beam.

Selected references

American Institute of Ultrasound in Medicine. (June 4, 2003) AIUM Official Statement: Guidelines for cleaning and preparing endocavitary ultrasound transducers between patients. Laurel, MD: American Institute of Ultrasound in Medicine. Available at http://www.aium.org/resources/statements.aspx (accessed November 16, 2012).

Blaivas, M., Brannam, L., Theodoro, D. (2004) Ultrasound image quality comparison between an inexpensive handheld emergency department (ED) ultrasound machine and a large mobile

ED ultrasound system. *Acad Emerg Med* **11**(7): 778–81.

Fowlkes, J.B. (2008) American Institute of Ultrasound in Medicine consensus report on potential bioeffects of diagnostic ultrasound: executive summary. *J Ultrasound Med* **27**: 503–15.

Fox, J.C., ed. (2008) *Clinical Emergency Radiology*. 1st edn. Cambridge: Cambridge University Press.

Lawrence, J.P. (2007) Physics and instrumentation of ultrasound. *Crit Care Med* **35**: S314–22.

Lichtenstein, D.A., Meziere, G., Lascols, N., *et al.* (2005) Ultrasound diagnosis of occult pneumothorax. *Crit Care Med* **33**: 1231–8.

Ma, O.J., Mateer, J.R., Blaivas, M. (2008) *Emergency Ultrasound*. 2nd edn. New York, NY: McGraw-Hill.

Mcgahan, J.P., Goldberg, B.B. (1998) *Diagnostic Ultrasound: A Logical Approach*. Philadelphia, PA: Lippincott-Raven.

Moore, C.L., Copel, J.A. (2011) Point-of-care ultrasonography. *N Engl J Med* **364**: 749–57.

Rumack, C.M., Wilson, S.R., Charboneau, W., *et al.* (2005) *Diagnostic Ultrasound*. 4th edn. St. Louis, MO: Mosby Elsevier.

Chapter 2

Getting started

Jason A. Levy

Point-of-care ultrasound has been a tool for physicians for nearly three decades, and has expanded considerably since its early stages. The beginnings are rooted in the adult emergency department, but point-of-care ultrasound now has gained widespread acceptance across multiple subspecialties, with an ever-broadening range of evidence-based applications. Beginning to incorporate ultrasound as a routine skill can be exciting and have immediate impacts on clinical decision-making and patient safety. However, when first encountering an ultrasound machine, it can become daunting. We recommend a stepwise approach, and taking "baby steps" (Figure 2.1) in order to acquire the skill and develop an ultrasound program.

The initial implementation of an ultrasound program is often fraught with administrative, political, and technical obstacles. Overcoming these hindrances can be facilitated by following a well-thought-out, comprehensive plan. While there is no single formula for success, addressing the issues outlined in this chapter early in the process will lead to greater benefit and allow for smoother transition incorporating ultrasound into everyday practice. Although the recommendations set forth here are based on the experience in an emergency department, the points outlined may be applied across multiple different specialties.

Step 1: identifying a point person

Before starting any ultrasound program, an **ultrasound program director** must be identified. Ideally, this person should be within the department or division starting the program and should already be well trained in point-of-care ultrasound, or be prepared to undertake additional ultrasound training. Their ultrasound skills must be sufficient such that they will be able to teach machine basics, ultrasound physics, and instrumentation, acquire images, and recognize clinical indications for ultrasound use. Once the faculty begins to incorporate ultrasound into clinical practice, the director will review all training images and provide feedback with respect to image acquisition and interpretation. The director will also assume roles involving quality assurance and interdepartmental communication. Without an ultrasound director, staff and trainees will become frustrated without the necessary guidance and assistance in troubleshooting.

The ultrasound director should have acquired additional ultrasound skill and knowledge during the course of his/her training. This can be accomplished by various means: having a focus on ultrasound during residency or fellowship, extra training as a faculty member, or completing a dedicated point-of-care ultrasound fellowship. Completing a fellowship is not an absolute requirement, but often provides a useful comprehensive background in establishing and running an ultrasound division. Regardless of his/her training, the director needs to have an adequate understanding of ultrasound principles such that that knowledge can be imparted to the rest of the faculty, fellows, and residents. If not, sufficient time will need to be devoted to training the ultrasound director. This can be accomplished in a variety of ways, but should include a point-of-care ultrasound course, in addition to a considerable amount of time performing hands-on training with an experienced sonographer.

There is some debate with regard to the requisite credentials of the ultrasound director. Currently, there exist no strict qualifications for ultrasound directors, and it is up to division leadership to decide on the necessary experience. Many directors have chosen to pursue the Registered Diagnostic Medical Sonographer (RDMS) certification, which is generally what ultrasound technologists have obtained. While this certification may be of some value both educationally and to hospital leadership, it is by no means necessary as it encompasses a much broader range of ultrasound imaging knowledge than should be necessary for point-of-care ultrasound applications. In the future, more specific point-of-care ultrasound certification may be available.

Step 2: program planning

Choose the indications

The first step in program planning is to consider what type of ultrasound scans will be performed. Several factors should be considered when making this decision. First, determine which indications will have the greatest impact on patient care. Choosing a core set of applications that may identify life-threatening conditions or improve the safety of a commonly performed procedure will be an easier sell to not only the departmental faculty, but also hospital leadership. Those conditions in which significant morbidity or mortality may result from a delay in diagnosis (e.g. hemopericardium from a stab wound to the chest) should be strongly considered. Second, consider the patient population. For centers that see a high volume of trauma, incorporating the FAST (focused assessment

Pediatric Emergency and Critical Care Ultrasound, ed. Stephanie J. Doniger. Published by Cambridge University Press.

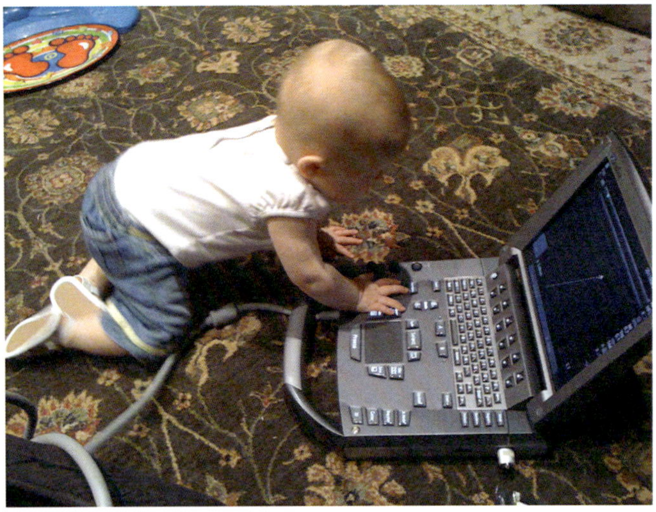

Figure 2.1 **Baby steps**. When starting to perform point-of-care ultrasonography, it is best to use a stepwise approach.

with sonography for trauma) examination would seem prudent. For centers that see a high rate of pregnancy-related complications, pelvic ultrasound would be appropriate. Third, consider what services are already available. While few hospitals have ultrasound technologists 24 hours per day, many do have overnight radiology residents and fellows. It can be a more difficult task convincing departmental and hospital leadership of the need for an ultrasound program based on non-urgent conditions when sonography is available at all hours.

Determining the type of examinations to be performed will set the foundation for the training and credentialing process, as well as direct the purchasing of the ultrasound system. The ultrasound director should attempt to identify all potential ultrasound indications in the initial development of the program. For each type of ultrasound examination chosen, trainees will need to be exposed to didactic sessions, participate in hands-on practice sessions, and be required to obtain a minimum number of images reviewed by the ultrasound director or other appropriately trained staff member.

Set the training requirements

Once an ultrasound director has been identified and an ultrasound system has been purchased, a well-thought-out training plan must be in place before education may begin. Each ultrasound practitioner in the department must learn when to use ultrasound appropriately, how to obtain and interpret these images for each indication, and be able to apply their findings to individual clinical scenarios.

Certain subspecialties have published minimal standards and requirement for ultrasound training within their respective fields. Other subspecialties in which ultrasound may be a new tool have left training requirements more nebulous. Guidelines from the American College of Radiology and the American Institute of Ultrasound in Medicine (AIUM) are geared towards comprehensive, diagnostic examinations and may be too extensive for point-of-care ultrasound. Therefore, the American College of Emergency Physicians (ACEP) published consensus training guidelines, based upon expert opinion and previous published data, which have now become the current standard in emergency medicine. A collaborative group consisting of the American Academy of Pediatrics (AAP), Society for Academic Emergency Medicine (SAEM), and AIUM is in the process of creating pediatric-specific guidelines. Generally speaking, programs should establish a minimum number of didactic hours, a minimum number of overall ultrasound examinations, and a minimum number of specific studies to look for a particular finding. Whenever possible, specialty-specific guidelines pertaining to essential requirements should be followed.

Credentialing and privileging

Credentialing or privileging (terms often used interchangeably) defines a physician's scope of practice. It is the process by which hospitals allow physicians to join the medical staff, and the pathway by which the hospital approves an individual department's delineation of privileges for physicians within that department. For example, any physician who performs procedural sedation must have sedation privileges and be credentialed by the hospital for such. The pathway to achieve this credentialing may be varied, specialty-specific, and based on either prior experience obtained in training or internal departmental training. Similarly, point-of-care ultrasound credentialing will be hospital specific and based on specialty-specific guidelines. In support of point-of-care ultrasound, the American Medical Association (AMA) passed resolution HR 802.99.2001 (Privileging for ultrasound imaging), which states that "privileging of the physician to perform ultrasound imaging procedures in a hospital setting should be a function of the hospital medical staff and should be specifically delineated on the Department's Delineation of Privileges form … and that each hospital medical staff should review and approve criteria for granting ultrasound privileges based upon background … and training standards developed by each physician's respective specialty." In this manner, point-of-care ultrasound falls under the purview of each specialty, and no one specialty has jurisdiction over all of ultrasound imaging. Accordingly, departmental leadership should request general point-of-care ultrasound privileging for its faculty, with specific requirements and maintenance to be monitored internally.

Credentialing goes hand-in-hand with training, and should be based upon meeting the minimum requirements set forth in the training plan. The departmental leadership and the ultrasound director should agree upon the credentialing plan. Expert recommendations exist, but in general credentialing requirements should entail the following:

1. A one- to two-day ultrasound course that teaches point-of-care ultrasound fundamentals and physics, and the various relevant ultrasound applications (Figure 2.2). For each application, there should be some didactic time devoted to the fundamentals of image acquisition and interpretation of positive and negative results. Additionally, there should be some hands-on time where the participant may apply what they have just learned (Figure 2.3). Clinicians should not be considered proficient and credentialed after a one- to two-

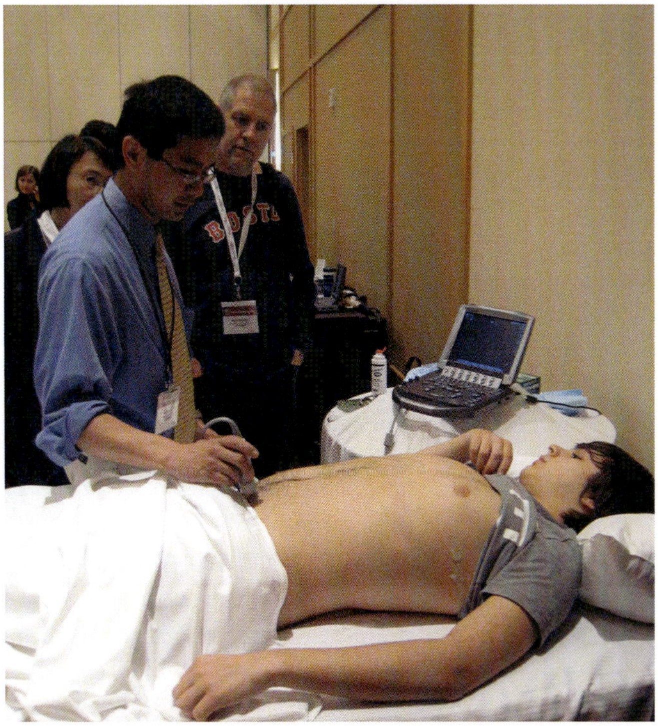

Figure 2.2 Ultrasound courses. Courses that include didactic and hands-on instruction are a helpful basis for acquiring knowledge and initial skills. Lei Chen, MD MPH performs hands-on instruction as part of a brief course at a Pediatric Academic Society meeting.

day course. This instruction merely serves as a foundation for further learning in ultrasonography.

2. Experiential training in which the physician performs ultrasounds and interprets the images in real clinical scenarios. Each of these images should be reviewed for quality and interpretation as outlined below in the quality assurance section of this chapter. A minimum number of ultrasound images should be obtained. For example, according to ACEP, the majority of the basic indications require a clinician to perform 25 scans for each individual application, with a proportion of those scans having pathology.
3. If not covered in the ultrasound course, a didactic session for each application, reviewing image acquisition and the interpretation of both positive and negative findings. A minimum number of didactic hours should be outlined.

Until the predetermined credentialing requirements are met, the physician should be considered in training mode and, consequently, no patient management decisions should occur based on ultrasound images obtained. Definitive studies, such as formal radiographic studies, should be obtained in order to confirm findings obtained on point-of-care ultrasonography. Patients and families should be made aware that these scans are educational and for learning purposes only and are not meant to guide clinical decision-making.

Create a quality assurance plan

A robust quality assurance (QA) plan is a fundamental component of any ultrasound program. As faculty members develop

(a)

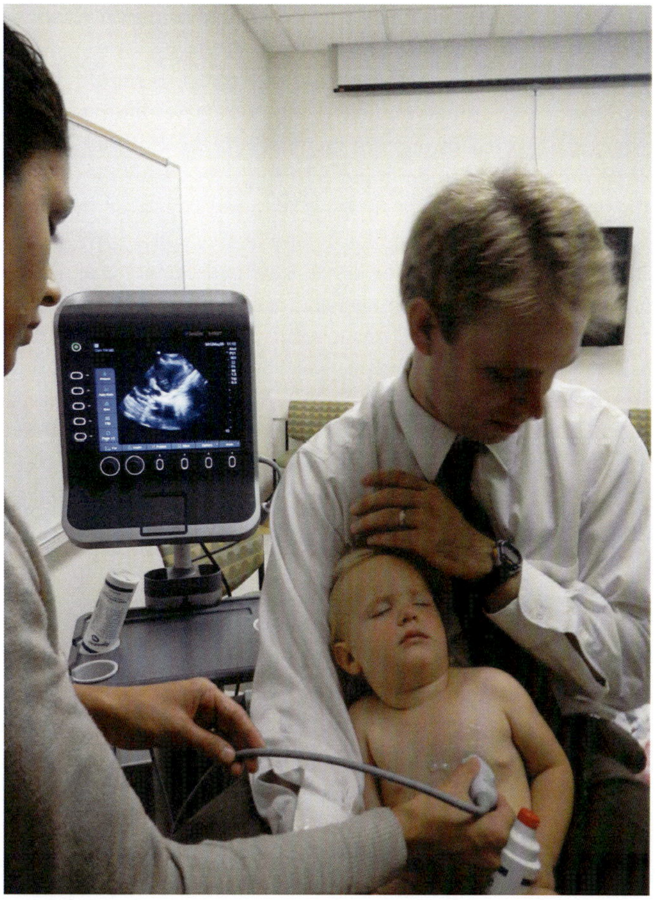

(b)

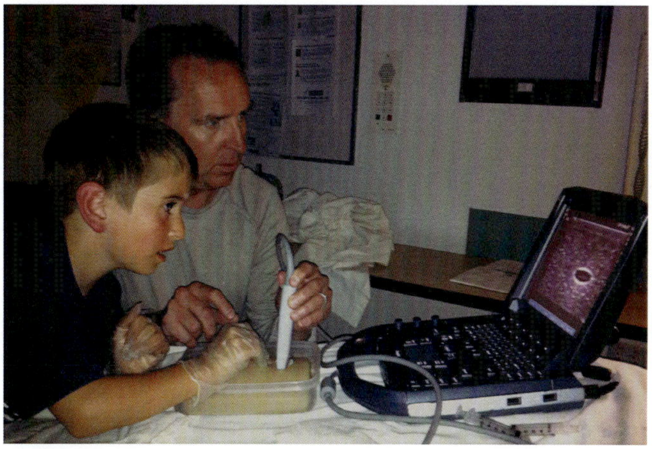

Figure 2.3 Hands-on. A key component to ultrasound instruction is gaining the opportunity to practice scanning. (a) A medical student practices ultrasound on a child at UC Irvine's Ultrafest Medical Student workshop. It is important to practice on pediatric models. (b) Practicing procedural guidance is also an important component of hands-on instruction.

the necessary skills for image acquisition, prompt evaluation of the scans that they perform will facilitate both technical and interpretative skills. Timely review by the ultrasound director can also lessen the frustration experienced by the staff. All too often, proactive faculty members will practice and perform the requisite scans, but will become discouraged by the lack of timely feedback. This is likely one of the most common reasons leading to failure of program implementation.

Generally speaking, the ultrasound director should have either sufficient time or sufficient help to review all ultrasound images performed by faculty members in the training stage. While the staff are undergoing training, every scan should be interpreted at the time the image is acquired and saved in some fashion (either as a printed hard copy or electronic copy). The ultrasound director and/or other qualified faculty members should then review each image and provide feedback in terms of both technical aspects (image quality, proper settings/transducers) and image interpretation. Specific suggestions for improvement should be included. Maintaining this "scan-feedback loop" throughout the training process will do wonders for encouraging the staff and promoting ultrasound use. Because of the number of examinations that will potentially be reviewed and the need to keep track of faculty scans, a QA database should be built. The system should have the capability to tally total numbers for individual practitioners, as well as keep track of positive, negative, and misread images.

Once the staff have reached the minimum required number of scans to be hospital-credentialed in ultrasound, each and every image no longer needs to be reviewed. However, it is at the discretion of the ultrasound director. Several well-established ultrasound programs choose to continue to review all ultrasound scans in order to ensure quality and education. Regardless, the ultrasound director, in concert with division leadership, should continue to review a minimum percentage of scans for each application and faculty member. In addition, all studies in which a major discrepancy exists between a point-of-care ultrasound examination and another study (e.g. radiologist-performed ultrasound, CT, MRI, echocardiography) should be reviewed.

Ongoing ultrasound education and experience is a requirement for any credentialed staff. While no well-established guidelines exist, it is imperative that faculty members maintain their skills by attending educational conferences and performing ultrasound examinations routinely. The ultrasound director should decide how much continuing medical education (CME) time is required and set a minimum number of scans per year in order to maintain credentialing.

Create a plan for documentation

Documentation of image interpretation for credentialed physicians should be straightforward. Any interpretation should be written in the chart, and medical decision-making based on such should be noted. Point-of-care ultrasound documentation should echo the purpose of the examination, which is limited and seeks to answer a simple (usually "yes" or "no") question. Pertinent findings should be communicated to other teams caring for the patient. In order to receive reimbursement for scans performed by credentialed physicians, a hard copy or printed image should be retained in the medical record. For paperless, electronic charting systems, images are typically stored within departmental systems, but may also be archived within the hospital imaging database. Factors to consider include hospital policies around patient privacy, access to patient records by other services, and maintenance of the server on which images are kept. All scans that are performed should additionally be saved in a database that is easily accessible.

Evaluate administrative and maintenance issues

Starting any departmental program brings with it a host of administrative matters, and ultrasound is no different. Addressing these issues early on in the process, and devising a plan to deal with them, is of paramount importance. Questions that will need to be addressed include:

1. How will the ultrasound machine be maintained, stocked, and cleaned?
2. Who will download images from the system?
3. How will a quality assurance database be built and updated?
4. Who will maintain the image storing system database?

In general, tasks assigned should match skill sets. For example, physicians performing scans should not have to input their findings and interpretations into the database. Hiring administrative help dedicated to the ultrasound program may be considered.

Consider hospital policies and politics

It is strongly recommended to involve hospital leadership early in the process, when starting an ultrasound program. Whenever possible, it is advised to collaborate with colleagues at other institutions and investigate other successful programs. While this may lead to additional inquiry into the program structure and organization, such scrutiny will lead to a better understanding and communication between departments down the line.

In the initial stages of point-of-care ultrasound, there were many opponents to its use. The strongest resistance most often comes from those in radiology departments, who feel that point-of-care ultrasound practitioners may not have the proper training or fear that point-of-care ultrasound may encroach on their territory. This hesitancy frequently stems from a lack of understanding of the indications for point-of-care ultrasound as well as the limited nature of the point-of-care examinations. A frank and honest conversation early in the process can allay their fears and lead to improved communication between departments as the program matures. Indeed, many of those who were opposed to point-of-care ultrasound in the beginning now recognize a role for point-of-care, focused examinations. As medicine places an increasing focus on patient safety, efficiency and the concepts of ALARA (as low as reasonably achievable radiation), point-of-care ultrasound will continue to gain greater acceptance.

Step 3: purchasing equipment

Purchasing an ultrasound system is an important step in setting up an ultrasound program and should be done prior to initiating ultrasound education for the division. Staff and trainees must be able to put into use the abilities they have acquired.

Without ongoing practice, their recently learned skills will diminish quickly. Only those who perform ultrasound scans routinely will gain sufficient facility to incorporate it into their everyday practice.

There are now many companies that recognize the need for portable point-of-care ultrasound machines, and make specific products catering to specific needs. When choosing a machine, the most important aspect guiding the purchase should be the anticipated type of ultrasound scans to be performed. For example, if a machine were being purchased for vascular access only, then one with a high quality cardiac application would not be justified. Given the wide range of ultrasound systems that are tailored to the practice of emergency and critical care medicine, other features should be considered. All machines should be portable and maneuverable enough to fit into the cramped spaces of a patient room. A cart-based system is ideal for ease of movement, changing of probes, storage space, and housing considerations. Additionally, ease of use should weigh heavily in the decision-making process. Ultrasound directors and those with advanced skill often forget how daunting an ultrasound machine can be to the novice user. An advanced system with multiple buttons and knobs will likely intimidate the novice ultrasonographer, and may ultimately be a roadblock to gaining further experience.

In addition to the system itself, transducers (or probes) will need to be purchased. Generally speaking, transducers are classified based on frequency. Low-frequency transducers have greater penetration but poorer image quality, and high-frequency transducers have superior image resolution but weaker penetration into deep tissue (see Chapter 1). Similar to the purchasing of the system, transducers should be purchased based on the anticipated type of examinations to be performed. If a significant percentage of patients present with pregnancy-related complaints, an endocavitary probe may be warranted. However, if the system is being purchased primarily for procedures, a linear, high-frequency transducer should be purchased. Transducers can always be added at a later date if the range of applications goes beyond what is initially expected. The footprint of the transducer, which is the portion of the transducer that comes into contact with the skin, should also be considered. Large-footprint transducers can display a wider field of view, but can sometimes be difficult to fit into the small intercostal spaces of infants and children. Generally speaking, at least two transducers should be considered essential when purchasing an ultrasound system: a low-frequency transducer to be used for abdominal and cardiac examinations, and a high-frequency, linear transducer, to be used for procedural applications.

Step 4: train the faculty

Now that the program plan has been established, training of the group may commence. Training should be performed in a focused, stepwise fashion. All ultrasound indications should not be implemented at once, since this can be overwhelming to both faculty members and the ultrasound director. Starting with one or two applications, and learning these comprehensively, will lead to a greater acceptance and more expeditious implementation of ultrasound into everyday practice. Additionally, the skills learned for one indication are transferrable and make learning each subsequent indication less onerous and time-consuming. We recommend that, at the very least, all staff participate in a one- to two-day point-of-care ultrasound course covering ultrasound fundamentals and physics, as well as both didactic and hands-on sessions for the various core applications to be implemented. Hands-on sessions should be performed on live models. The course should be limited in numbers to allow for all participants to obtain significant scanning time, with no more than four to five participants per instructor. Models with positive findings are ideal, but not necessary as faculty members are learning the machine buttons and basic skills of image acquisition in this introductory course. There are numerous courses given nationwide, and several companies that will provide in-hospital courses catering to a program's particular need. Alternatively, if the ultrasound director has sufficient experience and training, he or she may create the course, with the help of additional instructors for the hands-on portion.

After attending the basic course, faculty members will have attained the basic skills to push forward with their training. By no means will anyone become an expert, and subsequent practicing of what he or she has learned will be of paramount importance. It is this critical junction where staff are often "lost to follow-up" because either they were not pushed to continue their learning, or became frustrated by their lack of skill, or the ultrasound director was unavailable for continued preceptorship. It is often helpful for the ultrasound director to schedule dedicated hands-on scanning time with faculty members. Becoming proficient in ultrasound is a slow process. However, staff should be encouraged as much as possible at this point and made aware that, over a short time, the curve begins to steepen considerably and the skill becomes second nature. Continued didactic sessions as part of educational conferences and short hands-on sessions will still be required. Initially, the more available the ultrasound director or other qualified staff are, the more likely individuals will maintain their momentum.

From this author's experience, it may be advantageous to integrate ultrasound education of residents and fellows into a program simultaneous with teaching of staff. Recent published educational guidelines suggest ways to integrate training into Pediatric Emergency Medicine fellowship training programs. As the trainees begin to learn and develop their ultrasound skill as a program requirement, faculty members will have both greater exposure and increased incentive to incorporate ultrasound into their skill set. As faculty members and trainees begin to incorporate ultrasound into everyday practice, they will begin to wonder how they ever functioned without it, and ultrasound will gradually become routine and commonplace.

Summary

1. Starting a point-of-care ultrasound program may be a daunting task, but the rewards and improvements to patient care far outweigh any obstacles encountered along the way.

2. Departmental leaders should remember that the course of action should be both structured and stepwise, and make every attempt not to rush through the development process before the ultrasound director or staff are ready.
3. Thinking about program implementation in terms of years instead of months will set the proper tone and timeline, lead to greater satisfaction, and ultimately create the environment most conducive to success.
4. It is important to consider the clinical setting and patient population when developing an ultrasound program. It is often useful to introduce the training and implementation of ultrasound applications in a stepwise fashion.
5. It is crucial to establish didactic and hands-on training. Continued education may be provided through regular lectures, and hands-on scanning with the ultrasound director.

Selected references

American College of Emergency Physicians. (2009) Emergency ultrasound guidelines. *Ann Emerg Med* **53**(4): 550–70.

American College of Radiology. (March 23, 2012) Physician qualifications. In Ultrasound Accreditation Program Requirements, pp. 3–4. Reston, VA: American College of Radiology. Available at http://www.acr.org/Quality-Safety/Accreditation/Ultrasound (accessed November 16, 2012).

American Institute of Ultrasound in Medicine. (November 5, 2011) AIUM Official Statement: Training guidelines for physicians who evaluate and interpret diagnostic ultrasound examinations. Laurel, MD: American Institute of Ultrasound in Medicine. Available at http://www.aium.org/resources/statements.aspx (accessed November 16, 2012).

American Medical Association. (2001) Policy H-230.960: Privileging for ultrasound imaging. Chicago, IL: American Medical Association. Available at: http://www.ama-assn.org (accessed November 16, 2012).

Dietrich, A.T., Coley, B.D. (2008) Bedside pediatric emergency evaluation through ultrasonography. *Pediatr Radiol* **38** (Suppl 4): S769–84.

Marin, J.R., Zuckerbraun, N.S., Kahn, J.M. (2012) Use of emergency ultrasound in United States pediatric emergency medicine fellowship programs in 2011. *J Ultrasound Med* **31**(9): 1357–63.

Moore, C.L. (2011) Credentialing and reimbursement in point-of-care ultrasound. *Clin Pediatr Emerg Med* **12**(1): 73–7.

Ramirez-Schrempp, D., Dorfman, D., Tien, I., *et al.* (2008) Bedside ultrasound in pediatric emergency medicine fellowship programs in the United States: little formal training. *Pediatr Emerg Care* **24**: 664–7.

Stein, J., Nobay, F. (2009) Emergency department ultrasound credentialing: a sample policy and procedure. *J Emerg Med* **37**(2): 153–9.

Vieira, R. L., Hsu, D., Nagler, J., *et al.* (2013) Pediatric emergency medicine fellow training in ultrasound: consensus educational guidelines. *Acad Emerg Med* **20**(3): 30–6.

Chapter 3

Ultrasound in austere environments

Dana R. Sajed and Vicki E. Noble

Objectives

The delivery of medical care in the austere environment is often defined as the practice of medicine in conditions of limited resources. This can be the result of economic austerity, remote geographic location, or from natural disasters and mass-casualty incidents. While access to medical resources may be limited under such conditions, recent technologic advances have improved the delivery of care in extreme settings. In particular, the expanding field of point-of-care ultrasound has created new opportunities for having diagnostic imaging capability, where nothing was previously available.

Point-of-care applications of ultrasound are varied, and continuously evolving. In situations, where diagnostic imaging capabilities are limited, ultrasonography may have its greatest impact. Thus far, the majority of studies have focused on the utilization of point-of-care ultrasonography for trauma and obstetrics. Additional applications include procedural guidance, biliary ultrasound, cardiac ultrasound, the inferior vena cava (IVC) assessment for dehydration, appendicitis, and fracture reduction. All of these applications, if disseminated to areas with limited resources, could greatly impact the care of the ill or injured child. The increased familiarity of providers with this technology and its relative portability make hand-carried ultrasound ideal as a tool for both diagnostic measures and interventional guidance in the medically austere setting. In this chapter, we review what research exists, looking at the use of ultrasound in a few selected austere environments, namely in the developing world, in the prehospital settings, wilderness, and disasters. We will review those applications that are most likely to have the greatest impact in these settings.

Ultrasound in the developing world

In the majority of the developing world, there is a lack of diagnostic equipment available to the medical practitioner. Clinicians are required to make medical decisions with limited objective data, thereby increasing the risk of inadequate or inappropriate therapy. Diagnostic imaging, in particular, is relatively scarce. Only about 10% of the world's population has access to CT, and the World Health Organization (WHO) estimates that about 60% of people lack the ability to obtain any form of X-ray. These constraints are usually a result of fiscal and maintenance issues. The cost of MRI and CT machines is prohibitive, and X-ray technology, while less expensive, still requires maintenance and continuing financial investment in the form of film, image development, and machine maintenance. Added to this, there is a paucity of trained radiologists in much of the developing world. In light of these factors, ultrasound technology, particularly point-of-care ultrasound, has emerged as a viable solution to the imaging needs in resource-poor settings.

Commercially available compact, or hand-carried, ultrasound units have been used in clinical practice for at least 20 years. These smaller devices have made ultrasound broadly accessible outside of traditional locations. While becoming more readily available, portable ultrasound units have placed the technology in the hands of the primary practitioner, making the clinician responsible for image acquisition, interpretation, and subsequent clinical decision-making. This paradigm differs from the usual practice pattern in the United States, where a clinician orders a diagnostic imaging test, which is performed by a technician, interpreted by a radiologist, and finally the results are communicated back to the ordering clinician. In addition, with the decrease in size of these machines and increased competition in the marketplace, the purchase price has consequently decreased as well, from more than $150,000 for full-size ultrasound units to around $20,000 to 30,000 for compact units, making the technology more affordable to a diverse group of practitioners. There are also various grant programs such as Soundcaring™, which provides donations and matching grants to organizations in resource-poor areas. In addition to low cost, portable ultrasound machines are typically simple to operate, robust, and have rechargeable-battery power options. These features are ideal for low-resource settings with unreliable power grids. A novel solution for machinery in this type of setting may be solar energy. While battery powered machines are the standard, solar-voltaic panels have been used to run ultrasound machines during prolonged journeys without access to a power source. This approach has been tested during expeditions to Mount Kilimanjaro, where an external solar panel harvested photoelectric energy through a battery, used to power a machine, which successfully ran on the generated electricity (Figure 3.1).

Finally, in developing ultrasound programs in resource-poor regions, it is important to consider the maintenance and sustainability of a program. Machine and transducer maintenance,

Pediatric Emergency and Critical Care Ultrasound, ed. Stephanie J. Doniger. Published by Cambridge University Press.

(a) (b)

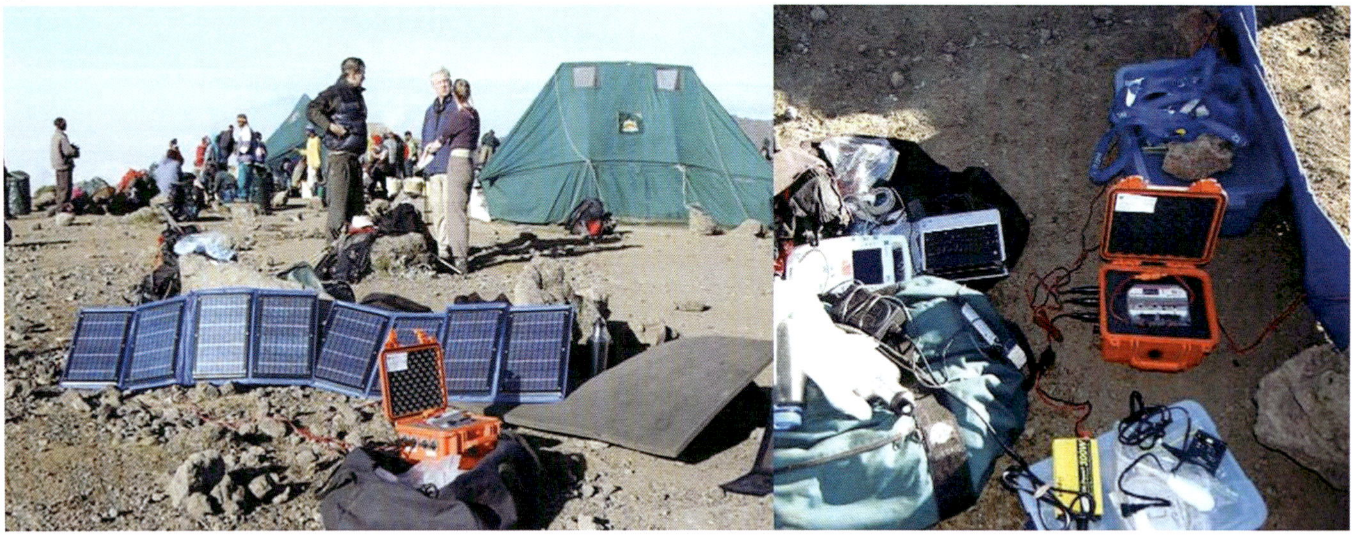

Figure 3.1 Solar energy used to charge and power medical equipment in the remote environment. (a) Photovoltaic panels are used to charge a battery. (b) The charged battery is then used to power various equipment, including a portable ultrasound machine and netbook computer. *Image courtesy of N. Stuart Harris, MD.*

contact gel, and cleansing solution do add a small but continued financial commitment to ultrasound use. Likely of greatest concern and need in the developing world is the adequate training of providers in the use and interpretation of sonography. Any sustainable program requires a continued experienced presence in the field to maintain the use and quality assurance of clinical ultrasound; this is often the greatest challenge as well-trained personnel are few and far between. Ultrasound training should include the long-term planning of projects with a concern for sustainability. Ideally these programs should involve trainees becoming trainers themselves, and creating a self-maintained ultrasound program.

Applications in the developing world

The various uses of ultrasound add to its utility in a setting where X-ray availability may be limited or non-existent and more advanced imaging may require transfer to far-off tertiary care centers. With a variety of transducers, one portable ultrasound machine may be used for multiple common indications such as echocardiography, obstetrics, and trauma. Other diagnostic abilities include long-bone fracture detection, pulmonary sonography, musculoskeletal, and soft tissue imaging. Sonography is also commonly used for procedural guidance. These applications include venous access, lumbar puncture, thoracentesis, paracentesis, pericardiocentesis, arthrocentesis, and nerve blocks for painful procedures. This "multi-use" phenomenon makes portable ultrasound particularly well adapted for the austere setting. While most of these studies can be performed with a single curvilinear transducer, optimal performance and diagnostics would be accomplished with a variety of transducers, including linear, phased-array, and endocavitary probes, which unfortunately add to the cost of a machine.

Despite having so many potential applications, there has been little focused, long-term research looking at the clinical

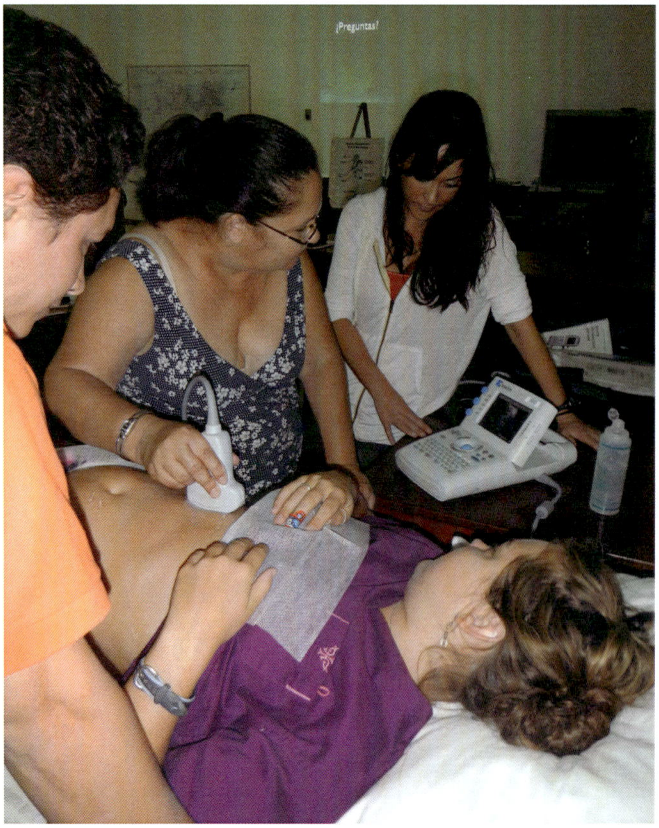

Figure 3.2 Training courses abroad should be tailored to the needs of the local clinicians. A point person should be identified, and continuing education and oversight should be established. This course was performed in Roatan, Honduras. Dr. Suzanne Hiramatsu instructs local physician Dra. Cibeles Mejia in the evaluation of the E-FAST examination, aorta, gallbladder, and pregnancy.

and cost outcomes when adding diagnostic ultrasound to various practice settings in the developing world. Obstetric ultrasound has received particular attention, since it has the potential to improve maternal and fetal outcomes in the

(a) (b)

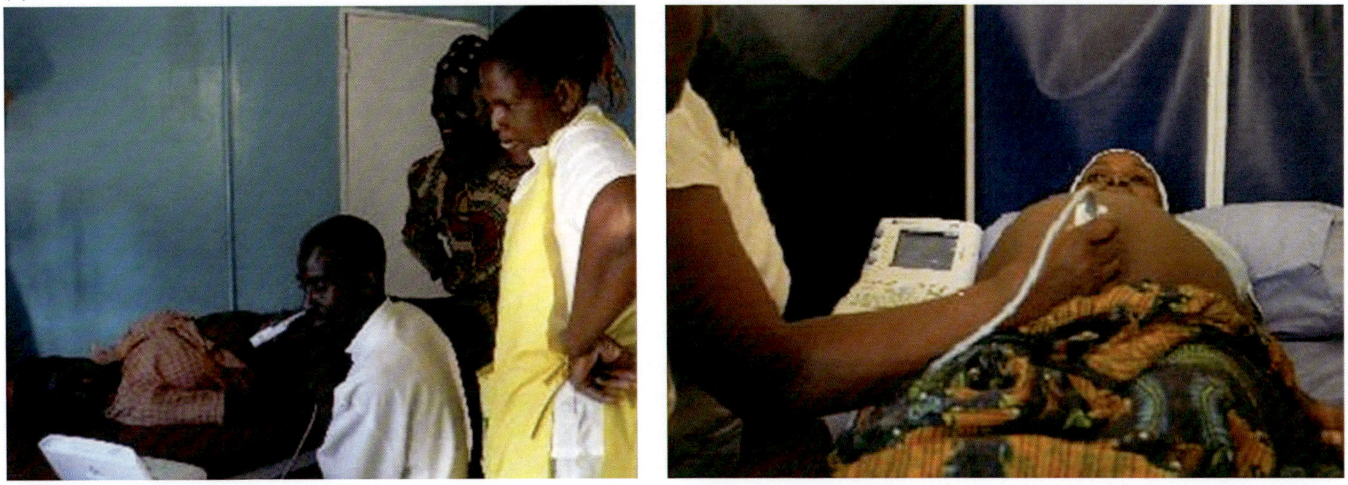

Figure 3.3 Prenatal sonography taught to midwives in rural care centers in Zambia. (a) A portable machine is used to estimate gestational age. (b) Ultrasound plays a vital role in prenatal care in the developed world. In resource-limited settings, the availability of an ultrasound machine and skilled operator aid in the detection of high-risk pregnancies and the decision to refer high-risk patients for further care.

developing world. In contrast to childbearing in industrialized nations, pregnancy and childbirth remain perilous in the developing world. Almost all maternal deaths in a 2005 estimate by the WHO occurred in the developing world. Maternal mortality is the leading cause of death for women of childbearing age, and accounts for more than 15% of deaths in this age group. Estimating the lifetime risk of maternal death highlights the disparity between developed and underdeveloped nations: 1 out of 7 women in some parts of Sub-Saharan Africa who become pregnant will eventually die of a maternal-related cause; in most of Europe, this rate is about 1 per 48,000. The risk to the fetus is even more pronounced and equally disproportionate. Current estimates of annual perinatal deaths stand at approximately six million, with the developing world accounting for about 98% of this number. With minimal training, point-of-care sonography can prevent potential obstetric emergencies in resource-restricted settings. Although there is a lack of large studies that indicate a change in mortality as a result of obstetric ultrasound use, there is evidence that indicates a significant change in patient management as a result of point-of-care obstetric sonography performed by health providers (physicians and midwives). Common findings with ultrasound in rural and remote settings include non-vertex lie of the fetus, multiple gestation, lack of fetal heart rate, and abnormal placenta positioning. Additionally, ultrasound can be used to assess for intrauterine fetal demise, ectopic pregnancy, and gross fetal anomalies. Although many developing countries have restrictive abortion laws, therapeutic abortion for major fetal malformation is permitted in many places. Routine ultrasound can therefore influence perinatal and infant mortality, through the early discovery and abortion of fetuses with major malformations. For less severe fetal abnormalities, the early diagnosis and awareness can help formulate a clear management plan, which may include the place of delivery (e.g. at a tertiary hospital with adequate neonatal care facilities), mode of delivery (e.g. planned cesarean section), and, sometimes, timing of delivery (Figure 3.3).

Trauma is one of the leading causes of death and disability worldwide. A lack of trained specialists in trauma and resuscitation is coupled with the lack of availability of advanced diagnostic imaging, limiting trauma care in developing countries. In addition, equipment shortage, facility disrepair, and improper maintenance of resources compound existing challenges. The FAST examination is frequently used to assess the presence of intraperitoneal or pericardial bleeding in trauma. It has been introduced to developing nations and is identified by the WHO as desirable in their *Guidelines for Essential Trauma Care*. While CT scanning remains the gold standard in terms of radiologic assessment in trauma, it has been proposed that FAST may be an acceptable alternative in resource-poor facilities where CT scans are unavailable. The early ultrasound detection of free fluid in the trauma patient could be used as an indication to expedite transfer to a center that has advanced imaging capabilities, thereby reducing overall morbidity and mortality. Additionally, at the peripheral hospitals with no CT scanning and limited radiology, the results of the FAST could be communicated to the surgeon or specialist at the referral hospital, providing useful information to surgeons in referral centers (Figure 3.4).

Another useful application of handheld ultrasound in the developing world is point-of-care echocardiography for the detection of structural cardiac anomalies. In particular, rheumatic heart disease (RHD) is estimated to affect 15.6–19.6 million people worldwide and causes 233,000–492,000 deaths each year, 95% of which occur in developing countries. While Africa has about 10% of the world's population, as many as half of the 2.4 million children affected by RHD globally live on the continent. Rheumatic heart disease accounts for a major proportion of all cardiovascular disease in children and young adults throughout Africa, Asia, and South America. While acute rheumatic fever is on the decline in the developing world, there are still a large number of chronic rheumatic heart disease cases, often detected as an incidental finding on clinical examination or undetected until the disease is complicated by chronic congestive heart failure and recurrent thromboembolic phenomena. Echocardiography is a highly accurate method for diagnosing and characterizing valvular lesions. With appropriate training, care providers in remote settings have been able to detect valvular lesions not heard on clinical examination. In fact, the use of portable ultrasound machines has resulted in the detection of more RHD in developing nations over the last few years; over 80% of lesions noted on point-of-care ultrasound were inaudible to experienced auscultators. In addition to being a tool to diagnose cardiac lesions, ultrasound may be also used in the management of heart disease. Combining echocardiography and pulmonary ultrasound to detect pulmonary edema can be used to target optimal diuresis and fluid management in patients with heart failure and valvular insufficiency. In places where central venous pressure monitoring and chest X-ray are unavailable, sonographic assessment may be critical in patient management (Figure 3.5).

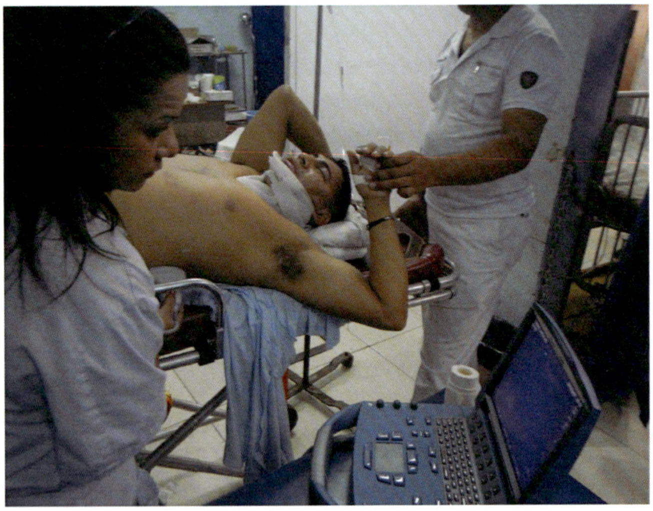

Figure 3.4 Ultrasound in locations where advanced imaging is unavailable. This trauma surgeon, Dr. Indira Sanchez in Roatan, Honduras, uses point-of-care ultrasound to determine whether this patient needs to be operated on. She is the only surgeon on the entire island with a population of 70,000+ and no CT scanner.

Beyond these applications, ultrasound may serve as the first and only diagnostic examination a patient may receive. As such, ultrasound may need to be used to assess orthopedic injuries, thyroid disease, pulmonary complaints, and general abdominal illnesses. Interestingly, many infectious diseases have characteristic sonographic findings as well. Tuberculosis (TB) is known to cause pericardial and pleural effusions; abdominal TB has been noted to show lymphadenopathy with hypoechoeic/necrotic echotexture and hypoechoic splenic lesions. *Ascaris lumbricoides* intestinal infestations have characteristic sonographic appearance of two parallel echogenic lines with a central anechoic area (Figure 3.6). Dengue fever, with and without hemorrhagic symptoms, often shows perisplenic and perihepatic fluid collections as a result of plasma leakage. Some authors have noted that the degree of severity of Dengue fever in children may be proportional to the degree of wall thickening and the amount of free fluid present in the abdomen. In patients with cerebral malaria, increased optic nerve sheath diameter is almost uniformly noted, and splenomegaly can be measured sonographically as well.

Ultimately, the most important question is whether patient outcomes are altered by the use of point-of-care ultrasound. A number of studies have estimated that the performance of a point-of-care ultrasound added to a diagnosis in about two-thirds of cases, and altered the course of patient management in a comparable number of cases. Some reports note that up to approximately 80% of ultrasound studies performed in some developing world settings are abnormal and pathological. Additionally, although abnormal findings may not result in actual management change, they are of prognostic value, and

(a)

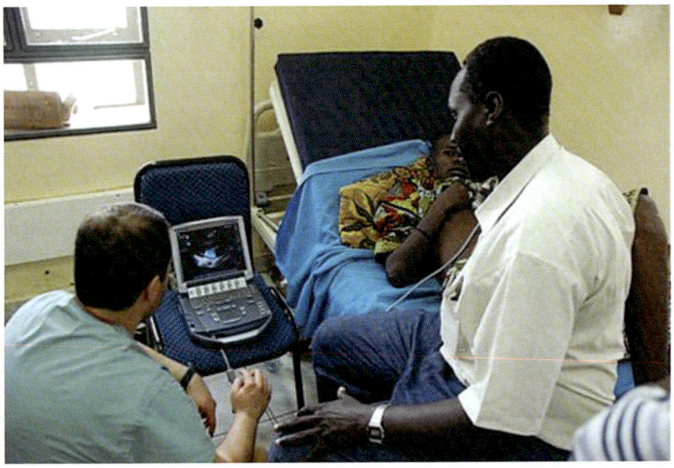

(b)

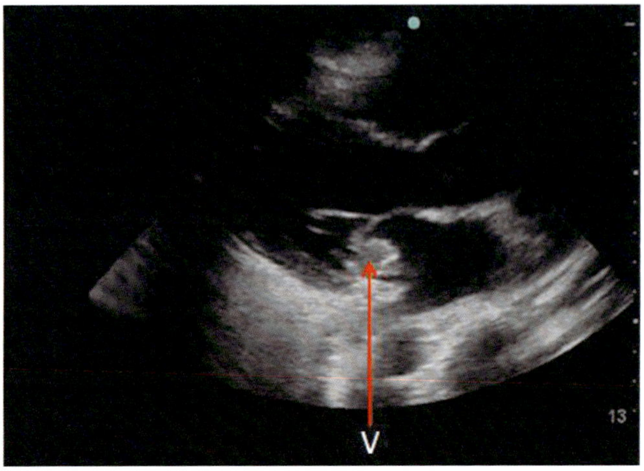

Figure 3.5 Ultrasound for the detection of rheumatic heart disease. (a) A young adult male receives an echocardiogram after presenting with fever and hemiparesis in Juba, South Sudan. (b) The patient was found to have a large vegetation (V) with regurgitant flow across his mitral valve, consistent with the diagnosis of endocarditis and rheumatic heart disease.

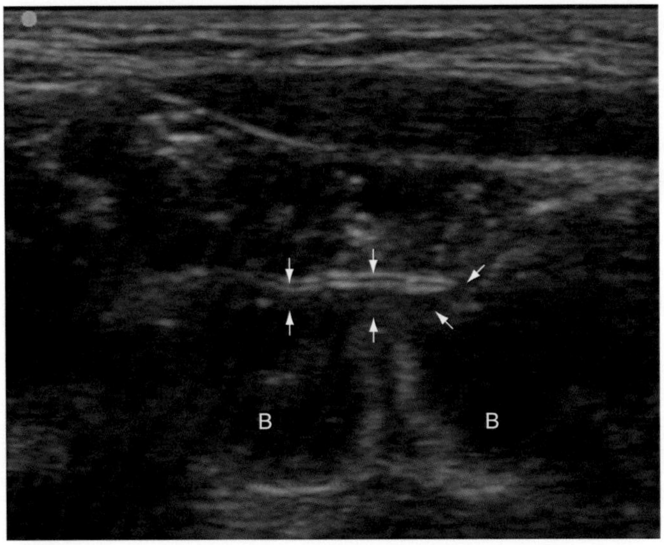

Figure 3.6 ***Ascaris lumbicoides***. Ultrasound image obtained with the linear high-frequency transducer. The bowel (B) can be visualized, as well as hyperechoic parallel lines (arrows) consistent with an Ascaris worm. *Image courtesy of David Kessler, MD MSc RDMS.*

may confirm an already suspected clinical diagnosis. It is assumed that early detection of certain disease processes could lead to decreased morbidity and mortality. However, further rigorous research and program development is needed to take advantage of this potential and to identify those applications with the biggest impact.

Prehospital ultrasound

While point-of-care sonography has been employed in emergency departments for nearly 20 years, the use of ultrasound by prehospital personnel has recently gained interest. The compact nature, durability, and portability of newer machines have allowed for their expanded use in helicopter and ambulance prehospital care. Portable ultrasound has already been deployed by emergency medical services (EMS) in Europe, Australia, and the United States. With appropriate training, EMS personnel have used portable ultrasound in the field to diagnose a variety of emergent conditions, both medical and surgical. A slight difference in practice patterns between European countries and North American countries illustrates the variety of users and uses for ultrasound by prehospital services. In the United States, EMS crews are typically non-physician personnel, and the focus of patient care is on rapid transport to emergency departments. In other nations, there are often physicians who serve as field responders and spend more time in on-scene evaluation and management.

The German Air Rescue Organization (*Deutsche Rettungsflugwacht*), as well as several ground-based ambulance services in Germany, have used ultrasound in the field since 2002 to perform FAST examinations and cardiac sonography for non-traumatic illness. Their crews are comprised of both physicians and paramedics. French prehospital clinicians have adopted ultrasound in certain areas as well. During helicopter medical evacuation, the feasibility of using portable ultrasound has been reported. Beyond the FAST examination, physicians in aeromedical units have used sonography to assess for the diagnosis of hemothorax, pneumothorax, hemoperitoneum, hemopericardium, and collapse of the IVC (a marker for hypovolemia). Experiences in both countries have further illustrated the feasibility of ultrasound on a helicopter, without significant interference from vibration, yielding accurate and reproducible results. In Italy, prehospital ultrasound has been used since 2005. Specifically in Milan, helicopter and ground EMS units are equipped with portable ultrasound devices, and use sonography in both medical and traumatic illness. Prehospital personnel are trained to look for reversible causes of pulseless electrical activity (PEA) and cardiac arrest, and perform FAST examinations in trauma. They also receive training in basic pulmonary sonography including the detection of pneumothoraces, pleural effusions, pulmonary edema, and a variety of other cardiopulmonary disorders. Results of ultrasound performed by prehospital personnel are often used in patient triage and transfer decision-making. Stateside, the focus of EMS systems is on rapid transport to medical facilities, since EMS crews typically do not have physicians as part of the team. Portable ultrasound has slowly been adopted in the training of paramedics and has been shown to be sufficient for FAST examinations and basic echocardiography. After receiving limited training (three to seven hours), prehospital personnel have become proficient in abdominal sonography. They have even found that EMS providers retain these skills months after initial training.

Furthermore, improvements in telecommunication and cellular technology now allow for the remote transmission of images from the field to a centralized medical center. This model has been investigated as a substitute for traditional triage algorithms, image acquisition, and interpretation. The ultrasound images obtained in ambulances can be reviewed remotely by clinicians in a variety of locations. For example, a paramedic can retrieve a patient at an incident scene, perform a FAST examination, and transmit the images to a central site, where image interpretation and triage decisions can be made. As a result, patients can be directed and transported to the appropriate medical centers. This method is already in place for echocardiography and FAST. In Taiwan, the EMS system utilizes tele-ultrasound to transfer echocardiography images via 3G from dispatch to control centers and receiving hospital emergency departments. Further research has evaluated image clarity and diagnostic accuracy of transmitted FAST images performed in a field environment. FAST examinations were performed on patients with handheld units; a video transmitter attached to the ultrasound unit transmitted wireless ultrasound video to a receiving antenna. The ultrasound images were then redirected via satellite to a medical center, which reliably reproduced images in real time without a deterioration in quality or interpretability.

In the military setting, echocardiographic images have been sent from a remote field hospital via wireless and satellite transmission in patients with known structural heart disease. Cardiac ultrasound was performed with a handheld instrument. Images were then transmitted via a commercial satellite to a medical center, where they were interpreted in real time by a board-certified cardiologist. On-site and satellite-transmitted images had a 95% concordance rate, with a high degree of agreement in technical quality and assessments of left-ventricular ejection fraction, the presence of a pericardial effusion, and left-ventricular size. The investigators demonstrated that they could reliably transmit and interpret normal and abnormal echocardiographic images without any deterioration in quality. This technology has already been applied to mass-casualty incidents, and helps to redirect the triage of trauma cases. FAST images obtained by first responders are sent via satellite to a receiving hospital. As a result of the image interpretation, patients are diverted to appropriate trauma centers, where operative teams are armed with the ultrasound examinations' results.

Wilderness, remote settings

Ultrasound has also been used in wilderness and geographically remote settings. In remote locations, sonography is often the only available diagnostic imaging test available, and, much like in the developing world, necessity requires its use for a variety of applications. Again, the development of small portable systems that are rugged has allowed the machines to be taken with teams on long expeditions or used by medical personnel in wilderness expeditions.

Expeditions at elevation face unique medical conditions. Acute mountain sickness can cause significant morbidity and, in extreme cases, leads to high-altitude cerebral edema (HACE). A hallmark of this disease process is increased cranial pressure, which can reliably be predicted with ultrasound, by measuring the optic nerve sheath diameter (ONSD) (see Chapter 8). Following the treatment for cerebral edema, serial ONSD measurements have shown decreased diameters, correlating with improved symptoms (Figure 3.7). In addition, at elevation, portable ultrasonography has been successfully used to diagnose high-altitude pulmonary edema (HAPE). The presence of pulmonary "comet tail" artifacts, or "B-lines," is characteristic of edematous lung, whereas a horizontal pattern, "A-lines," indicates a dry lung (see Chapter 6). A predominantly B-line pattern on lung ultrasound during mountain expeditions has been shown to be highly predictive of HAPE. Additionally, symptom resolution correlated with decreased B-line artifacts when serial assessments were made during and following therapy. Finally, handheld ultrasound has been utilized to evaluate adult and pediatric long-bone injuries (see Chapter 19). For those fractures that require immediate reduction in the field, sonography may be repeated to assess for adequate reduction and appropriate position after splinting.

There is the potential to utilize the transmission of ultrasound via satellite to larger centers. For example, medical control for Mount Everest expeditions has included telemedicine and portable ultrasound. The mountain medical team uses ultrasound to obtain images, which are then transmitted to a computer on site via a local area network (Figure 3.7). The computer then transmits medical data and ultrasound imaging from Everest to a tele-operation center at another location (the Canadian Science Administration) via satellite. Clinicians can subsequently review the images and provide real-time medical control to non-physician personnel. Unfortunately, this sort of system is limited by cellular network availability and may not be suitable in all regions.

Disasters

Another arena where ultrasound has tremendous impact is during medical deployments to natural disasters. Disaster scenes and mass-casualty events often involve less than ideal environmental locations. With the development of compact,

(a) (b)

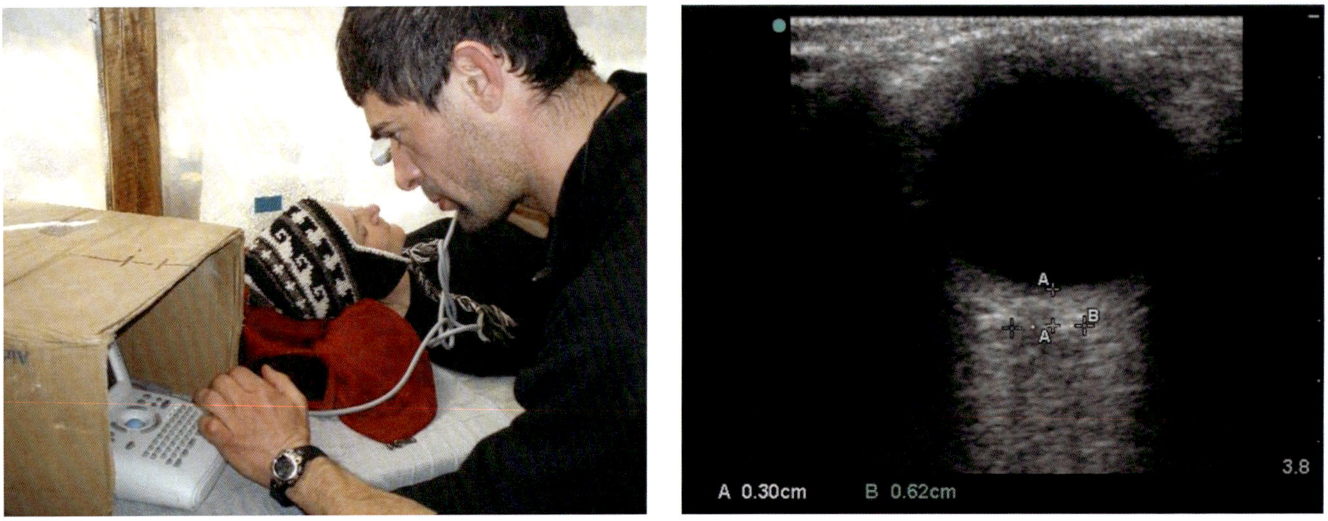

Figure 3.7 Ultrasound used to detect elevated intracranial pressure by measuring the optic nerve sheath diameter (ONSD) at Mount Everest base camp. (a) A high-frequency transducer is placed on the eye. (b) Calipers are used to measure the width of the optic nerve sheath 3 mm from the globe. A measurement of greater than 5 mm is considered abnormal, and elevated intracranial pressure should be suspected. *Image courtesy of Peter J. Fagenholz, MD.*

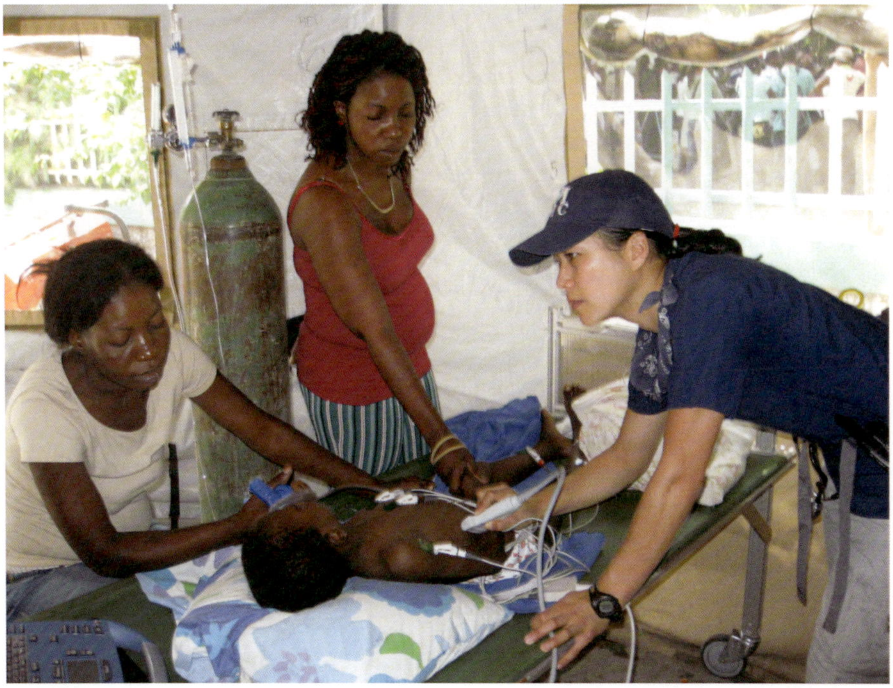

Figure 3.8 Ultrasound is invaluable in disaster situations. Following the earthquake in Haiti, physicians utilized point-of-care ultrasound to identify acute life-threatening illness as well as chronic conditions. *Image courtesy of Jessica Ngo, MD.*

durable, and robust portable machines, they have been able to withstand the harsh environments which they were traditionally not able to withstand.

Among the first incidents where ultrasound was used during disaster management was following a magnitude 6.9 earthquake which devastated northwestern Armenia in December 1988. This incident resulted in more than 25,000 deaths and roughly 150,000 injuries. To deal with the high volume of patients following the earthquake, two triage rooms were set up in the Republic Hospital, each with an ultrasound machine. In a 72-hour period, 400 patients received 530 ultrasound examinations, of which about 25% demonstrated some form of pathology. Sixteen patients had operative intervention, usually laparotomy, based solely on clinical examination and ultrasound findings. Four false-negative cases (<1%) were reported among the 530 studies performed. These false negatives illustrate the limitations of point-of-care sonography in trauma. Ultrasound is known to have a low sensitivity for detecting hollow viscous or retroperitoneal injuries. Obesity and subcutaneous emphysema also decrease examination accuracy. Despite these limitations, however, the use of ultrasound proved to be highly sensitive and specific in this resource-limited circumstance. More recently, hand-carried ultrasound was used following devastating mudslides in Guatemala in October 2005, where 99 patients received 137 ultrasound examinations: 58 pelvic, 34 right upper quadrant, 23 renal, 6 other abdominal, 5 orthopedic, 4 cardiac, 3 pleura and lung, 3 soft tissue, and 1 FAST. In Australia, disaster medical assistance teams (DMATs) use ultrasound for field triage decisions. Following a cyclone in Western Australia during March 2007, the need to transport patients from their remote location for tertiary-level care necessitated rapid diagnostic capabilities. With the region's only CT scanner felled by the cyclone, hand-carried ultrasound was used in a number of patients to determine the acuity of their illness. The primary studies performed were the FAST examination and thoracic ultrasound. Other authors have described the use of ultrasound in disaster response following the Tsunami in Banda Aceh in 2004, the Wenchuan earthquake in 2008, and the Haitian earthquake in 2010 (Figure 3.8).

In addition to natural disasters, ultrasound has played an increasing role in the evaluation of patients following terrorist attacks. Emergency responders and hospital personnel used ultrasound to perform FAST examinations following the Madrid train bombing in 2004, the London Underground bombing in 2005, and during the second Lebanon war in 2006. During these events, ultrasound was used for the initial assessment of degree of injury and surgical decision-making. In these settings, a negative FAST examination in a stable patient allowed the trauma team to determine which patients could receive delayed CT scans and transfer to distant medical facilities. Most importantly, ultrasonography was able to identify those patients who were of higher priority, who needed more immediate surgical care. In this setting, ultrasound was invaluable in streamlining patient care.

Summary/key points

1. The use of ultrasound is ideal in an austere environment due to its rapidity, portability, and durability. A variety of applications can be performed including the FAST and limited echocardiography. Obstetric ultrasonography is especially useful in the developing world, where maternal and fetal mortality is high.
2. In resource-limited settings, sonography often replaces other imaging modalities that are frequently unavailable. Ultrasound can be used for both screening medical

examinations and the immediate response to medical or traumatic illness.

3. For first responders to disaster and mass-casualty events, ultrasound offers a rapid, portable triage and diagnostic tool; in the remote environment, ultrasound is a multifunctional tool that may be used to assess illness from head to toe.
4. With the development of telecommunication, ultrasound examinations can be performed by prehospital providers and those in remote settings. Images may be sent via satellite or wireless transmission to centers where images can be interpreted. Results from these studies can expedite care and direct patients towards appropriate medical centers.
5. As the ultrasound machines become more compact and less expensive and providers become more comfortable with their use, it is likely that this technology will continue to find new applications.

Selected references

Dyer, D., Cusden, J., Turner, C., *et al.* (2008) The clinical and technical evaluation of a remote telementored telesonography system during the acute resuscitation and transfer of the injured patient. *J Trauma* **65**(6): 1209–16.

Fagenholz, P.J., Gutman, J.A., Murray, A.F., *et al.* (2007) Chest ultrasonography for the diagnosis and monitoring of high-altitude pulmonary edema. *Chest* **131**(4): 1013–18.

Fagenholz, P.J., Gutman, J.A., Murray, A.F., *et al.* (2009) Optic nerve sheath diameter correlates with the presence and severity of acute mountain sickness: evidence for increased intracranial pressure. *J Applied Physiol* **106**(4): 1207–11.

Kimberly, H., Murray, A., Mennicke, M., *et al.* (2009) Teaching focused obstetric ultrasound to midwives in rural Zambia. *Ann Emerg Med* **54**(3 Suppl): S87.

Levine, A.C., Shah, S.P., Umulisa, I., *et al.* (2010) Ultrasound assessment of severe dehydration in children with diarrhea and vomiting. *Acad Emerg Med* **17**: 1035–41.

Mock, C., Lormand, J.D., Goosen, J., Joshipura, M., Peden, M. (2004) *Guidelines for Essential Trauma Care*. Geneva: World Health Organization.

Nelson, B.P., Chason, K. (2008) Use of ultrasound by emergency medical services: a review. *Intl J Emerg Med* **1**(4): 253–9.

Shah, S.P., Epino, H., Bukhman, G., *et al.* (2009) Impact of the introduction of ultrasound services in a limited resource setting: rural Rwanda 2008. *BMC Int Health Hum Rights* **9**: 4.

Shah, S., Price, D., Bukhman, G., *et al.*, eds. (2011) *Manual of Ultrasound for Resource-Limited Settings*. 1st edn. Boston, MA: Partners in Health.

Sippel, S., Muruganandan, K., Levine, A., *et al.* (2011) Review article: use of ultrasound in the developing world. *Intl J Emerg Med* **4**(72): 1–11.

S2

Introduction

Stephanie J. Doniger

Since its inception, the American College of Emergency Physicians (ACEP) has developed guidelines for the utilization of point-of-care ultrasonography in the emergency department. ACEP recommends the six basic diagnostic applications that are the most immediately life-saving and include the FAST, cardiac, abdominal aortic aneurysm (AAA), gallbladder, pelvic, and renal examinations. These diagnostic applications can be extended for use in pediatric and adolescent populations. More recently, pediatric-specific diagnostic applications have been developed and studied and include the "pediatric abdomen," which consists of intussusception, appendicitis, and pyloric stenosis. New applications for children continue to be developed and rapidly evolve.

This overview for diagnostic ultrasound describes the general imaging practices and general planes of imaging. These fundamentals are important to understand prior to learning individual scanning applications. With additional experience, research, and a steep learning curve, we have been able to expand the applications of point-of-care ultrasound and decrease the risks of ionizing radiation. This is especially important in pediatric patients, for whom, over a lifetime, cumulative radiation exposure can lead to cancers.

Technique

Transducer selection and orientation

The majority of diagnostic applications utilize a low-frequency curvilinear or phased-array transducer (2–5 MHz). The exception, however, is the "pediatric abdomen" (Chapter 10), which utilizes the high-frequency linear transducer (5–10 MHz). Whenever possible, a smaller-footprint transducer should be utilized.

When performing diagnostic ultrasonography, it is important to understand and maintain proper transducer orientation. Standard terminology will be utilized throughout the text, with regards to transducer orientation and the different scanning planes. The coronal, sagittal, and transverse orientations are in relation to the long-axis of a patient's body:

Coronal orientation: The transducer is oriented lateral to the patient's body. The indicator is towards the patient's head (Figure S2.1a).

Sagittal orientation: The transducer is oriented along the long-axis of the patient's body, with the indicator oriented towards the patient's head (Figure S2.2a). This is somewhat similar to the coronal view, since the indicator is oriented towards the patient's head.

Transverse or axial orientation: The transducer is oriented perpendicular to the long-axis of the patient's body (Figure S2.3a). This is rotated 90° from the sagittal view. The indicator is oriented towards the patient's right-hand side.

Patient position and preparation

When performing ultrasonography on pediatric patients, positioning and comfort are paramount to obtaining an adequate scan. In babies, it is often helpful to have the child lying in the parent's lap (Figure S2.4a). Older children benefit from distraction techniques such as videos (Figure S2.4b).

Ultrasound imaging

Coronal orientation: Cephalad structures appear on the left-hand side of the ultrasound image where the screen indicator is (Figure S2.1b).

Sagittal orientation: Cephalad structures will appear on the left-hand side of the image, where the screen indicator is (Figure S2.2b).

Transverse or axial orientation: Structures on the right side of the body will be on the left-hand side of the ultrasound image, where the screen indicator is (Figure S2.3b).

Summary

Point-of-care ultrasound may be utilized as a bedside diagnostic tool. It has become incorporated into several subspecialties and continues to evolve. It is important to become familiar with the anatomic planes of imaging. With pediatric patients in particular, it is important to properly position a patient in order to obtain adequate imaging.

Pediatric Emergency and Critical Care Ultrasound, ed. Stephanie J. Doniger. Published by Cambridge University Press.

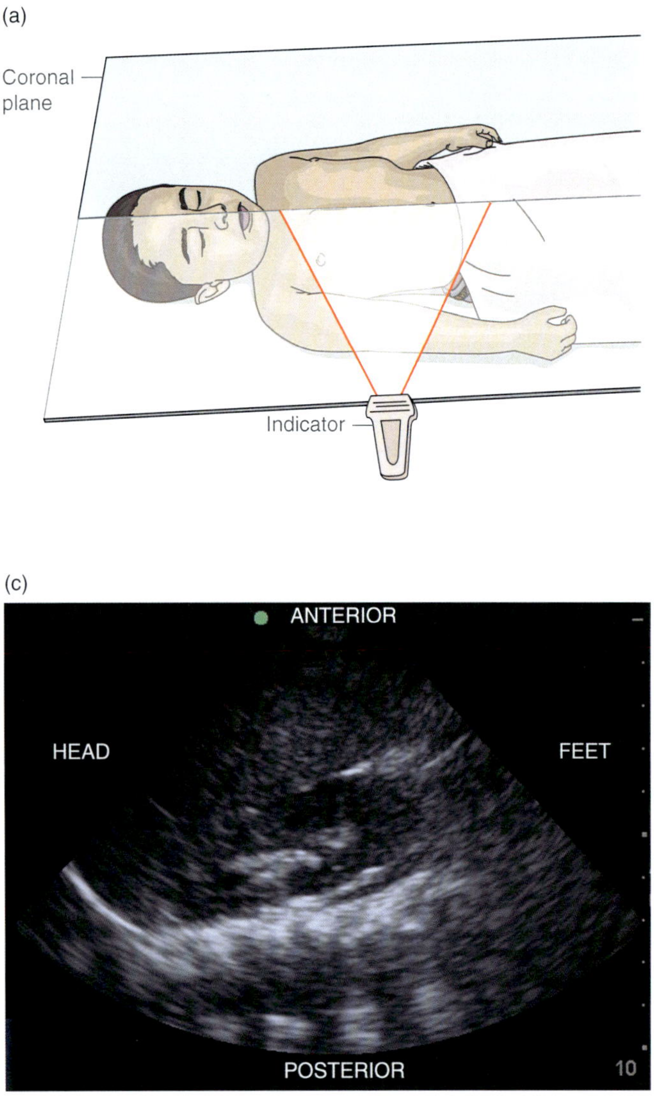

Figure S2.1 Coronal orientation. (a) The transducer is placed laterally and divides the patient's body into anterior and posterior. The indicator is oriented towards the patient's head. (b) Photo showing transducer placement for the coronal orientation. This orientation is used for the right upper quadrant view of the E-FAST. (c) The corresponding ultrasound image has the patient's head on the left-hand side of the image and the feet on the right-hand side.

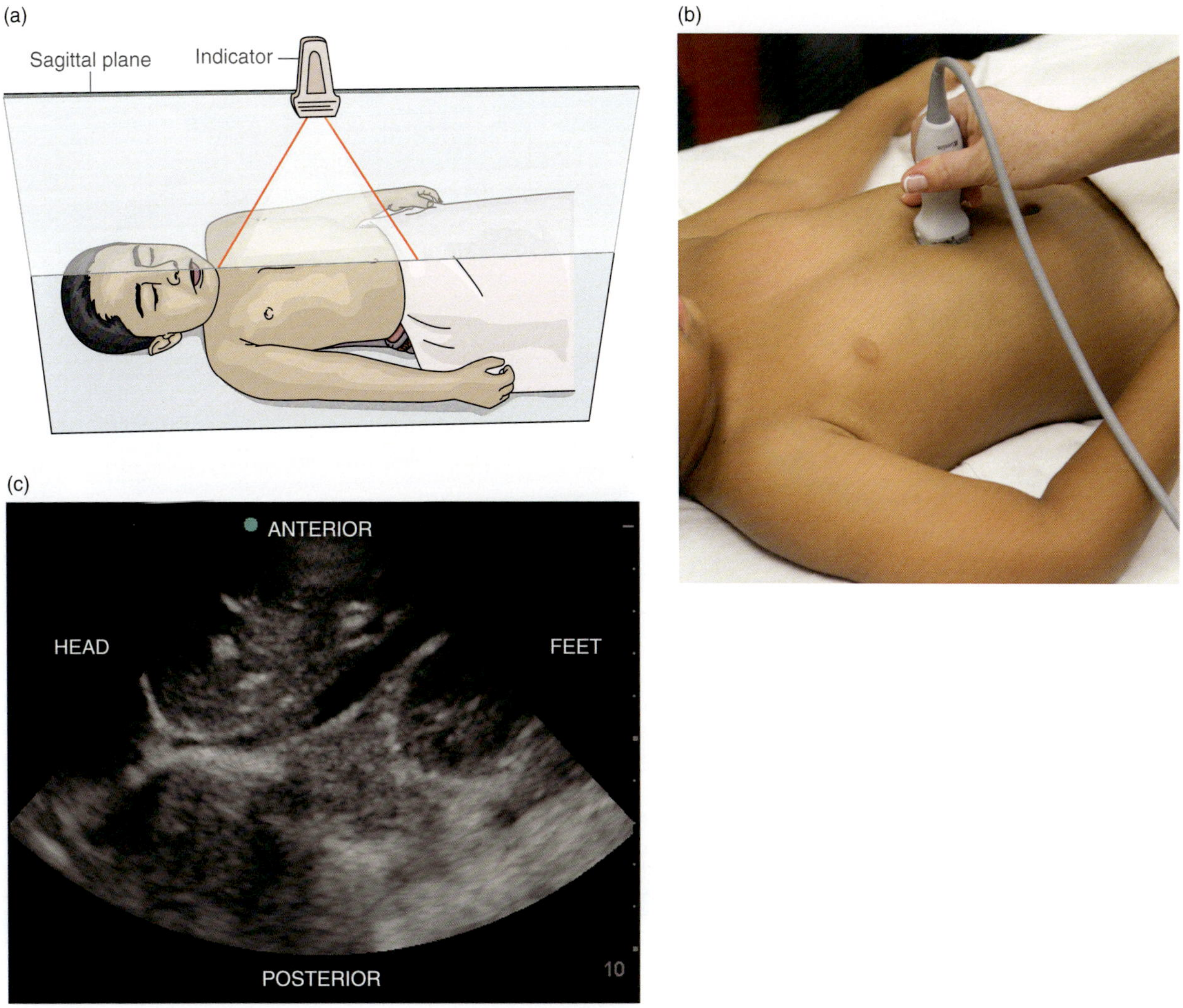

Figure S2.2 Sagittal orientation. (a) The transducer is oriented along the long axis of the patient's body, and divides the body into right and left sides. The indicator is oriented towards the patient's head. (b) Photo showing transducer placement for the sagittal orientation. This orientation is used for the longitudinal view of the IVC. (c) The corresponding ultrasound image has the patient's head on the left-hand side of the image, and the feet on the right-hand side.

(a)

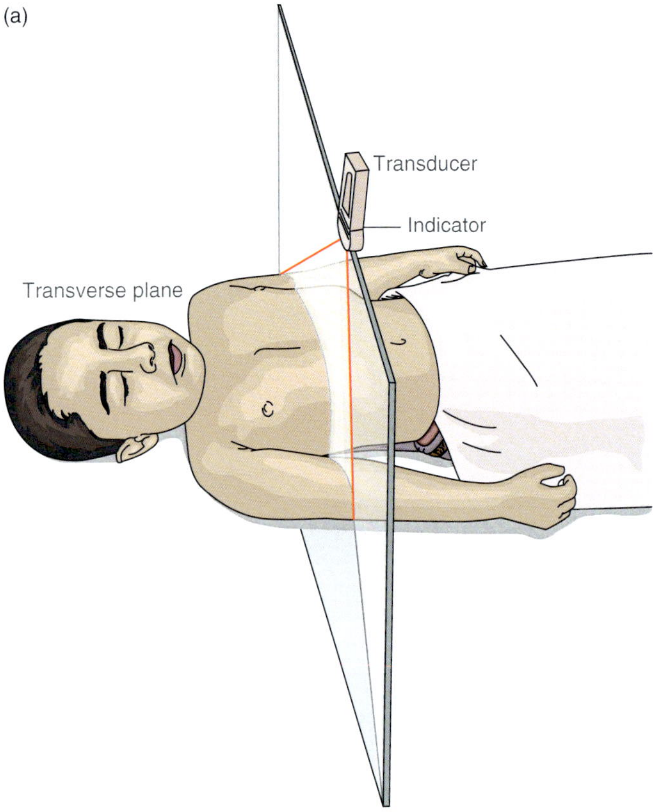

(b)

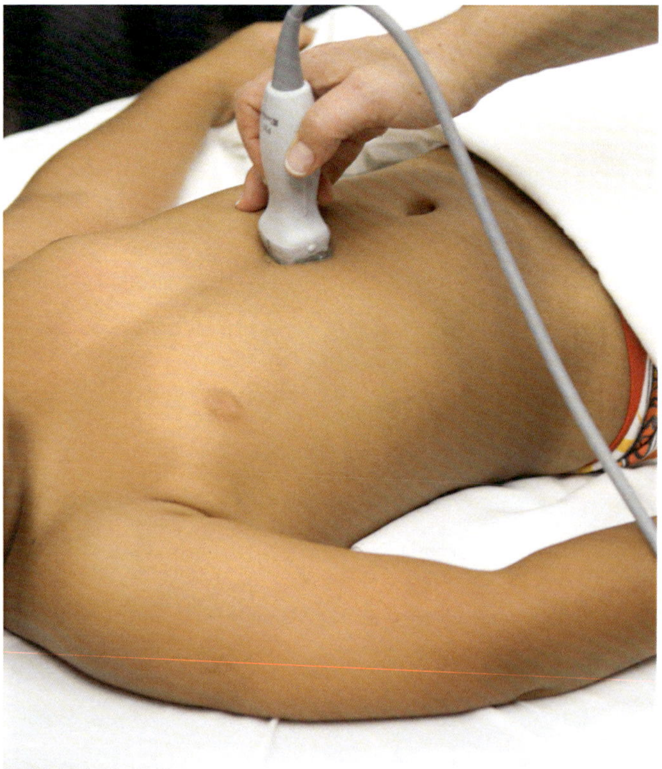

(c)

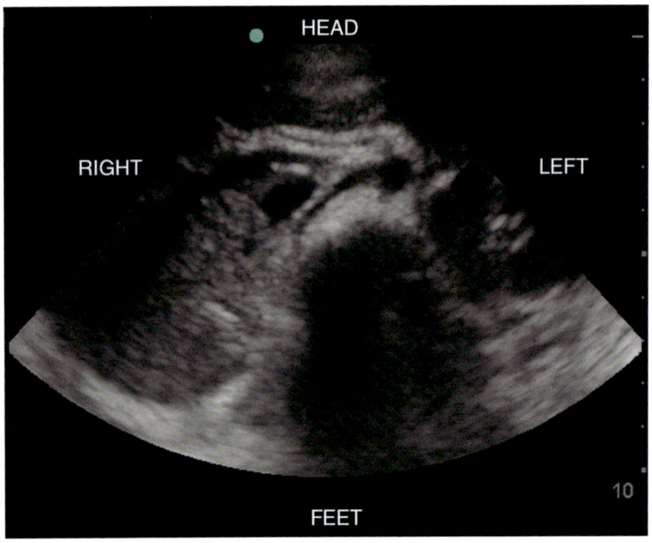

Figure S2.3 Transverse or axial orientation. (a) The transducer is oriented perpendicular to the long axis of the body. The indicator is oriented towards the patient's right side. (b) Photo showing transducer placement for the transverse, or axial orientation. This orientation is used for the transverse view of the IVC. (c) The corresponding ultrasound image is divided into the right-hand side and left-hand side.

(a)

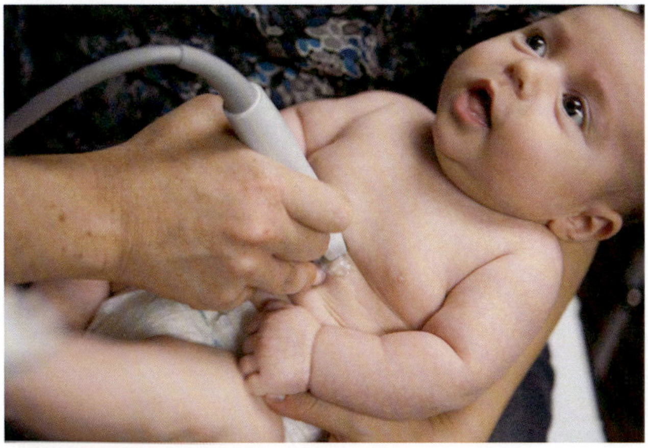

(b)

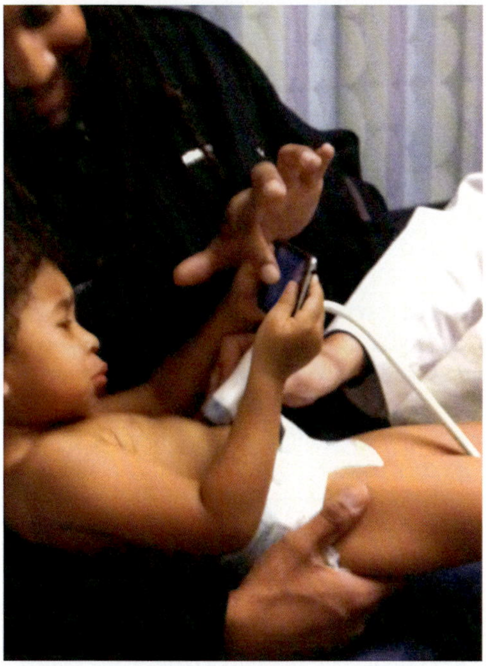

Figure S2.4 Patient preparation. (a) In infants and small children, it is often helpful to have the patient lying supine in a parent's lap. (b) Older children benefit from distraction techniques, such as videos.

Selected references

American College of Emergency Physicians. (2006) ACEP Policy Statement: Ultrasound imaging criteria compendium. Irving, TX: American College of Emergency Physicians. Available from http://www.acep.org/_Ultrasound-Section-Microsite/Policy-Statements/ (accessed November 16, 2012).

American College of Emergency Physicians. (2008) Policy Statement: Emergency ultrasound guidelines. Irving, TX: American College of Emergency Physicians. Available from http://www.acep.org/_Ultrasound-Section-Microsite/Policy-Statements/ (accessed November 16, 2012).

Chen, L., Santucci, K. (2006) Probing the availability of emergency ultrasound in pediatrics [abstract]. *Pediatr Emerg Care* **22**: 688.

Cohen, J. S., Teach, S. J., Chapman, J. L. (2012) Bedside ultrasound education in pediatric emergency fellowship programs in the United States. *Pediatr Emerg Care* **28**(9): 845–50.

Evans, N., Gournay, V., Cabanas, F., *et al.* (2011) Point-of-care ultrasound in the neonatal intensive care unit: international perspectives. *Semin Fetal Neonatal Med* **16**: 61–8.

Lambert, R.L., Boker, J.R., Maffei, F.A., *et al.* (2011) National survey of bedside ultrasound use in pediatric critical care. *Pediatr Crit Care Med* **12**(6): 655–9.

Levy, J.A., Noble, V.E. (2008) Bedside ultrasound in pediatric emergency medicine. *Pediatrics* **121**: e1404–12.

Marin, J.R., Zuckerbraun, N.S., Kahn, J.M. (2012) Use of emergency ultrasound in United States pediatric emergency medicine fellowship programs in 2011. *J Ultrasound Med* **31**(9): 1357–63.

Moore, C.L., Copel, J.A. (2011) Point-of-care ultrasonography. *N Engl J Med* **364**: 749–57.

Ramirez-Schrempp, D., Dorfman, D., Tien, I., *et al.* (2008) Bedside ultrasound in pediatric emergency medicine fellowship programs in the United States: little formal training. *Pediatr Emerg Care* **24**: 664–7.

Chapter 4

The extended focused assessment with sonography for trauma (E-FAST)

Samuel H.F. Lam

Objectives/indications

Trauma is the leading cause of pediatric mortality in the developed world. Among the causes of pediatric unintentional injuries, traffic collisions and falls are the most common mechanisms of injury, often leading to blunt abdominal trauma. Ultimately, the majority of pediatric patients with blunt abdominal trauma are managed non-operatively, even when they suffer from liver and splenic lacerations. When intra-abdominal injuries are suspected, children often undergo CT scans, which involve significant radiation exposure.

The focused assessment with sonography for trauma (FAST) was first introduced as a screening tool in adults, in order to identify free fluid in the abdominal cavity and around the heart. The goal of the FAST is to detect free intra-abdominal fluid in dependent areas, which most likely represents blood in the acute trauma patient. In recent years, the extended focused assessment with sonography for trauma (E-FAST) began to incorporate lung ultrasound into the traditional four views, in order to identify a hemothorax or pneumothorax. Several published studies have concluded that emergency physician-performed point-of-care lung ultrasonography is actually more sensitive than a supine chest X-ray in identifying pneumothorax in the adult trauma patients. Overall, the E-FAST has been widely adopted and incorporated into adult trauma algorithms, due to its ease of use and skill acquisition, its non-invasive nature, and its ability to make rapid diagnoses at the bedside of an unstable patient. It is also easily reproduced and repeated and involves no ionizing radiation. While the E-FAST is useful, it is important to recognize its limitations. Though it might occasionally reveal solid organ injuries, the operator should not assume that a negative E-FAST can rule out such injuries. Similarly, E-FAST cannot reliably detect retroperitoneal and hollow viscous injuries. In a hemodynamically stable patient with a normal E-FAST examination, the patient may potentially be observed without undergoing further radiologic studies. In the hemodynamically unstable patient, definitive care may be facilitated, especially when operative intervention is required.

For the pediatric trauma patient in particular, the E-FAST can be an effective screening tool for prioritization of life-saving procedures (e.g. pericardiocentesis, thoracostomy, thoracotomy, laparotomy) in those with unstable vital signs, and prioritization of imaging studies in those with stable vital signs. The individual clinician is advised to consider each clinical scenario, available resources, and local practices when incorporating the E-FAST into their trauma practice. Further prospective studies need to be performed in pediatric patients in order to thoroughly evaluate the effectiveness of the E-FAST in the pediatric trauma evaluation.

This chapter reviews the literature and indications for performing the E-FAST examination. While the literature is robust for the utility of the E-FAST examination in adults, it is unclear as to the role the E-FAST will play in pediatric trauma. Specific techniques are reviewed, with specific locations for transducer placement in order to master the E-FAST examination. Throughout the text, FAST and E-FAST may be used interchangeably, noting that the E-FAST includes the additional lung evaluation.

Background

The FAST examination has been used in emergency trauma resuscitation for the past 20 years in North America, and for even longer in Europe and Japan. Studies have demonstrated that the FAST examination has a sensitivity of 69–90% and a specificity of 83–100%, in detecting free abdominal fluid in adult trauma patients. In adult trauma patients, the FAST examination has been shown to decrease time to operative care, decrease the number of CT scans performed, decrease hospital lengths of stay, generate lower hospital charges, and decrease patient complications. As a result, the FAST has been incorporated into many adult trauma algorithms. According to the American College of Surgeons' Advanced Trauma Life Support certification course, with appropriate equipment and in experienced hands, FAST has a sensitivity, specificity, and accuracy comparable to CT and diagnostic peritoneal lavage (DPL) in detecting intra-abdominal fluid. As a result, the FAST has largely replaced DPLs, and a positive FAST often leads to exploratory laparotomy in adult patients.

Recently, a number of studies have investigated the utility of the FAST in blunt abdominal trauma in pediatric patients. The reported sensitivity varies widely from 30 to 100%, and specificity from to 79 to 100%. This large discrepancy may in part be due to the FAST being compared to disparate definitions of gold standards and outcomes. Some studies utilized CT or laparotomy as the gold standard, while others used patient observations without further studies or interventions. In addition, in calculating the sensitivities and specificities, some studies only included the presence or absence of free intra-abdominal fluid, while others included the presence or absence

Pediatric Emergency and Critical Care Ultrasound, ed. Stephanie J. Doniger. Published by Cambridge University Press.

of solid organ injuries. Direct comparison among the various studies is further complicated by different study designs and inclusion criteria. For instance, some studies only recruited hemodynamically stable children, while others included both hemodynamically stable and unstable children. A recent meta-analysis of 25 relevant articles by Holmes concluded that abdominal ultrasonography was 80% sensitive and 96% specific, with a positive likelihood ratio of 22.9, and a negative likelihood ratio of 0.2 for identifying hemoperitoneum in pediatric blunt-trauma patients. In conclusion, FAST is most helpful when the result is positive (i.e. intra-abdominal fluid is visualized), but only moderately helpful when it is negative (i.e. intra-abdominal fluid is not seen). Most importantly, a negative FAST cannot be solely relied upon to rule out hemoperitoneum, in all but the lowest of risk patients.

Controversy exists regarding the utility of FAST in pediatric trauma patients, since their mechanisms of injury and the management are different from adult trauma patients. In grossly unstable, injured children, the presence of abdominal fluid on the FAST examination is likely an indication for emergency laparotomy. Studies suggest that the sensitivity of FAST increases drastically in hypotensive blunt-trauma patients. Nevertheless, there is controversy regarding the role of FAST in hemodynamically stable pediatric trauma patients. Since a negative FAST cannot completely rule out any abdominal solid organ injury, and a positive FAST often does not indicate the actual location and extent of the injury, many experts argue its utility is limited in making management and disposition decisions in the stable pediatric trauma patient. On the other hand, limited studies have suggested that with a negative FAST, combined with careful clinical examination and close observation, most children recover uneventfully. By selectively ordering CT scans for those with positive FAST or moderate to high clinical suspicion for intra-abdominal injury, radiation may be spared in up to 75% of pediatric blunt-trauma patients.

Anatomy

In the supine patient, free intraperitoneal fluid tends to accumulate in three dependent regions: the hepatorenal recess (Morison's pouch), the splenorenal recess, and the rectouterine space (pouch of Douglas in females, the rectovesicular pouch in males) (Figure 4.1). The pelvic cavity is connected to the hepatorenal recess by the right paracolic gutter. Fluid can also flow along the left paracolic gutter but is limited cranially, by the phrenicocolic ligament. Free fluid can also flow between the splenorenal and hepatorenal recesses via the epiploic foramen (Figure 4.2).

Theoretically, free intraperitoneal fluid would collect first in the lowest point of the supine abdominal cavity (i.e. the pelvic cavity) (Figure 4.1b). In reality, however, this potential space is quite small, and any clinically significant intraperitoneal fluid will overflow into the right upper quadrant via the right paracolic gutter. With fluid originating from the left upper quadrant (LUQ), free fluid often accumulates first in the subphrenic space before overflowing into the splenorenal recess, and subsequently the Morison's pouch (Figure 4.2).

Technique

Point-of-care questions

1. Is free fluid/blood in the abdomen present?
2. Is fluid/blood in the pericardium present?
3. Is fluid/blood in the thorax present?
4. Is a pneumothorax present?

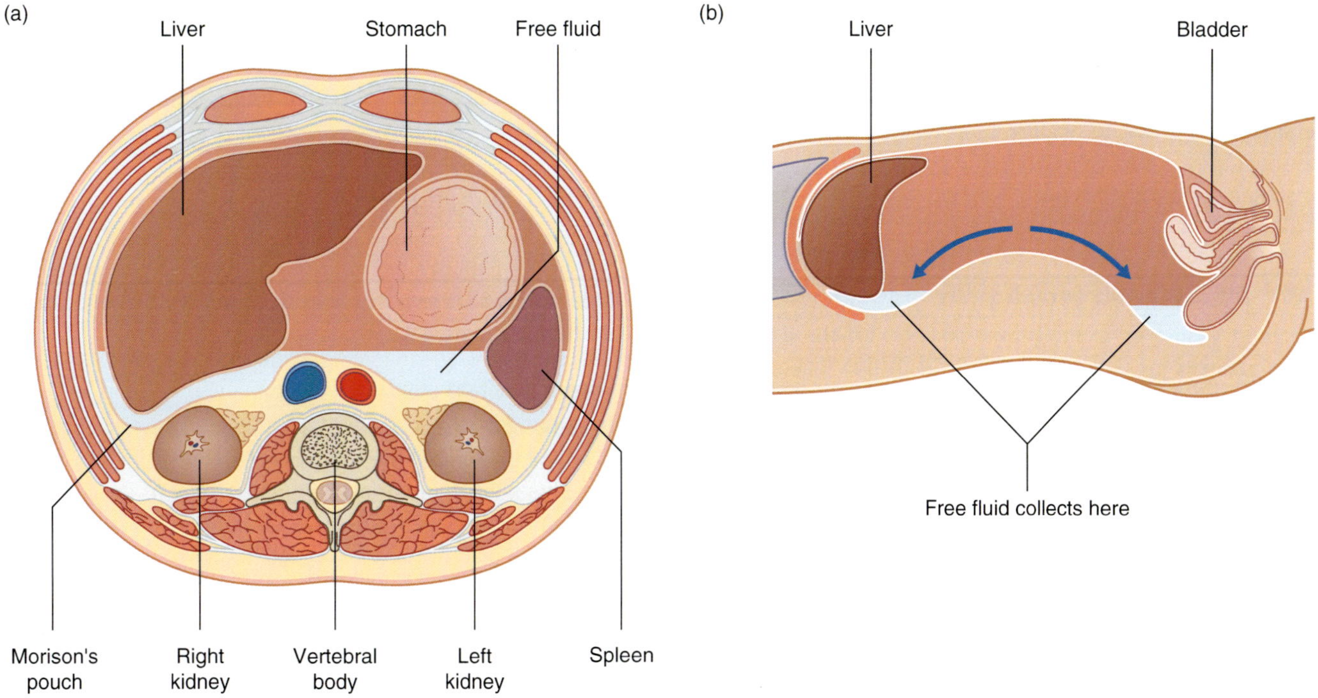

Figure 4.1 Potential spaces in the peritoneal cavity. (a) Transverse and (b) midline longitudinal views. *Artwork created by Emily Evans © Cambridge University Press.*

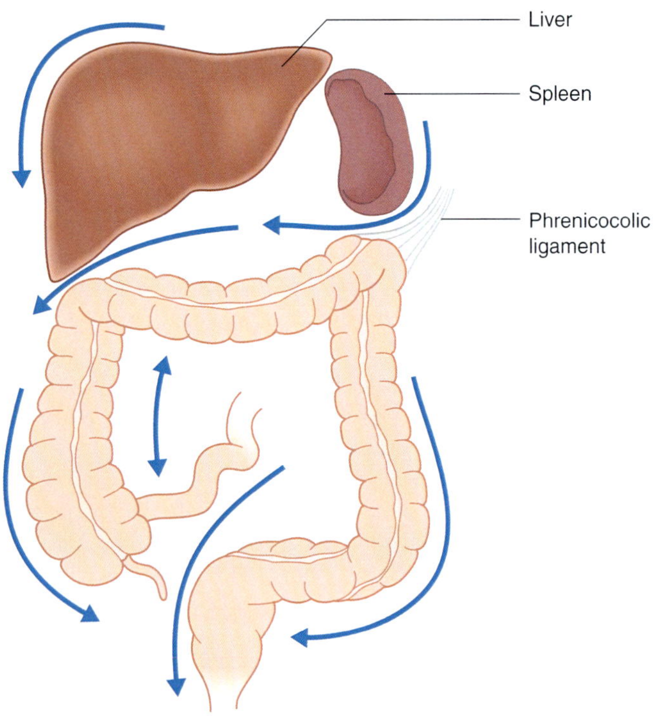

Figure 4.2 Gutters in the abdominal cavity. *Artwork created by Emily Evans © Cambridge University Press.*

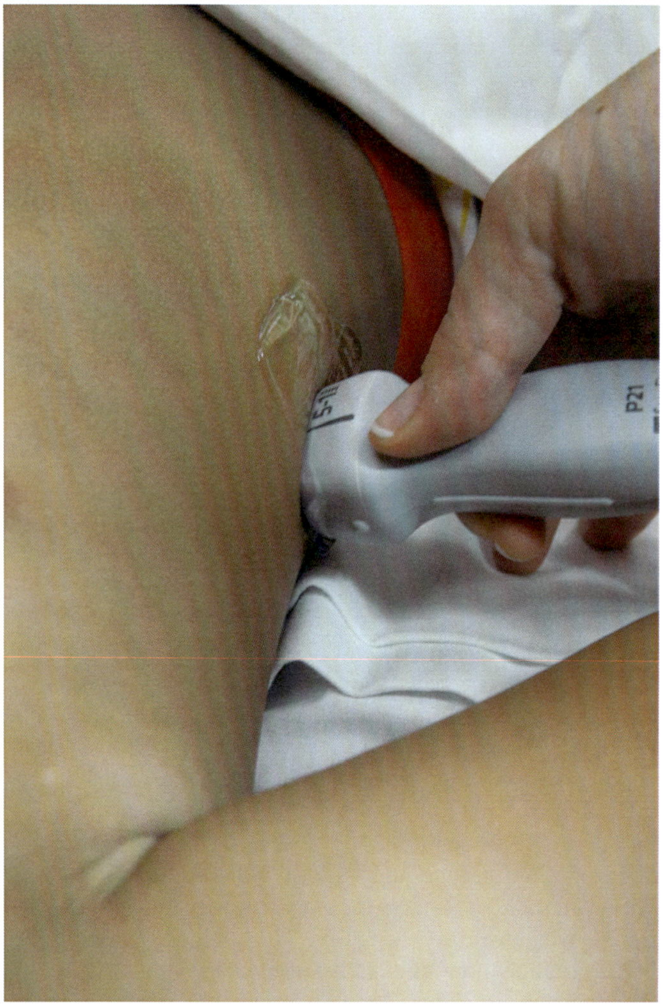

Figure 4.3 Transducer orientation. In order to obtain proper right upper quadrant and left upper quadrant views of the FAST examination, the indicator should be obliquely oriented, and angled posteriorly approximately 10° in order to scan along the long-axis of the kidneys.

Transducer selection and orientation

For the most part, the abdominal portion of the E-FAST examination is performed with a low-frequency (2–5 MHz), curvilinear ultrasound transducer. This ensures good penetration and adequate visualization of the anatomical structures in question. For smaller children, the phased-array transducer (2–8 MHz) may also be used since it has a smaller footprint and a higher frequency. Finally, since the lungs are more superficial compared to the abdominal solid organs, a higher frequency linear transducer (5–10 MHz) is preferable for this part of the E-FAST examination. Alternatively, the low-frequency abdominal transducer may be utilized to acquire lung images. In performing ultrasonography at the right and left upper quadrants, the indicator should be angled posteriorly, approximately 10°, in order to scan along the longitudinal axis of the kidneys (Figure 4.3).

Patient position and preparation

The patient should be in the supine position for the E-FAST. For the majority of patients, the most sensitive location for detecting intra-abdominal fluid is at the most dependent portion of the peritoneal cavity – Morison's pouch, or the right upper quadrant. It is important to note that, in smaller children, their most dependent portion may actually be the pelvis rather than Morison's pouch.

In order to improve the sensitivity for detecting fluid in the abdominal cavity, the patient may be in 5–10° Trendelenburg position. Likewise, positioning the patient in a reverse Trendelenburg position may increase the sensitivity of the subxiphoid and suprapubic views. The right upper quadrant scan should be completed prior to log-rolling a trauma patient, in order to maximize its sensitivity for detecting intra-abdominal fluid.

Ultrasound imaging: views

Ideally the E-FAST should be completed in less than five minutes at the patient's bedside. The E-FAST is performed in the four standard views, in addition to the bilateral lung examinations (Figure 4.4).

Right upper quadrant (Morison's) view

The purpose of the right upper quadrant view is to visualize the region where the right kidney is adjacent to the liver (Morison's pouch). This is likely the most important view of the E-FAST examination, since free fluid from abdominal organ injuries usually collects here first. Approximately 85% of positive FAST examinations have fluid in the right upper quadrant. As little as 250 mL of intra-abdominal fluid can be visualized. Start by placing the transducer in the longitudinal/coronal orientation, with the indicator towards the patient's head (Figure 4.5a). Begin imaging at the costal margin, at approximately the

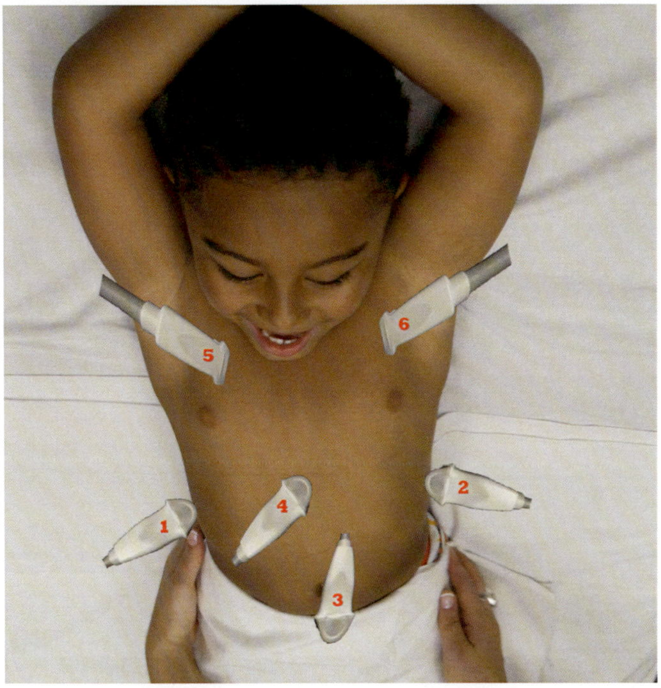

Figure 4.4 Probe positioning for the E-FAST examination. The recommended order is to first obtain Morison's view at the right upper quadrant, since it is the most sensitive. Then, the left upper quadrant view. The kidney on the left is located more superior and posterior than the right. Next, obtain the suprapubic windows. Then, the subxiphoid view, since depth will need to be increased. Finally, the lung examinations are performed with the linear high-frequency transducers.

midaxillary line. Once the hepatorenal junction is visualized, sweep through the entire kidney – anterior to posterior, superior to inferior – to complete the scan. By moving the transducer slightly cephalad, the diaphragm can be visualized as well on this view.

Normally Morison's pouch appears as a bright white line between the liver and the right kidney (Figure 4.5b–d). Free fluid, most commonly from intra-abdominal blood in the case of trauma, would appear anechoic. The diaphragm, if visualized, appears as another hyperechoic, or bright white, structure cephalad to the liver. When encountering difficulties visualizing Morison's pouch, it is often helpful to move the transducer longitudinally along the rib cage or anteriorly/posteriorly to try to bring the right kidney then the liver into view.

Left upper quadrant (splenorenal) view

The purpose of the left upper quadrant (LUQ) view is to visualize the region where the left kidney is adjacent to the spleen (splenorenal junction) and to detect fluid collection there. Start by placing the transducer in a longitudinal/coronal orientation, with the indicator oriented towards the patient's head (Figure 4.6a) on the patient's left side. Begin imaging at the costal margin, *posterior* to the midaxillary line. It is important to note that the left kidney is located more superior and posterior than the right kidney. Once the splenorenal junction is visualized (Figure 4.6b–d), sweep through entire kidney – anterior to posterior, superior to inferior – in order to complete the scan. Move the transducer slightly cephalad to visualize the diaphragm. Note that free fluid can accumulate medial or cephalad to the spleen in addition to the splenorenal interface. Therefore the left upper quadrant should not be considered complete until the diaphragm is visualized on this view. The left upper quadrant view tends to be technically more difficult since the spleen is smaller, more cephalad, and more mobile compared to the liver. Given the location of the left kidney, one often encounters more rib shadows that obscure the view of the splenorenal interface. In order to improve visualization of this region, the transducer can be placed more posterior (to the point that it almost touches the bed) while maintaining the wrist in a neutral (as opposed to a flexed) position.

Similar to the right upper quadrant view, the splenorenal junction normally appears as a hyperechoic line, and free fluid would appear anechoic on ultrasound. However, the phrenicocolic ligament prevents free fluid from actually accumulating between the spleen and kidney. Therefore, fluid often collects inferior or superior to the kidney, or beneath the diaphragm.

Suprapubic view

The purpose of the suprapubic view is to visualize the rectovesicular pouch in males and rectouterine pouch (pouch of Douglas) in females. It is interesting to note that, due to the anatomic differences between children and adults, this is often the most dependent portion of the abdominal cavity in children. Start by placing the transducer in a transverse orientation immediately superior to the pubic symphysis, with the indicator towards the patient's right. Angle the transducer slightly towards the feet in order to adequately visualize the entire bladder (Figure 4.7a). Once the bladder is visualized (Figure 4.7c,d), rotate the transducer 90° clockwise towards the patient's head in order to obtain the sagittal view (Figure 4.8).

Anechoic free fluid may be visualized posterior to, or adjacent to, the bladder. In order to improve the visualization of free fluid, it is often necessary to decrease the far field gain (time gain compensation), which minimizes posterior acoustic enhancement artifact (see Chapter 1). False positives in this view can be due to physiologic fluid in menstruating women, the prostate in men, or fluid within the bowel loops. Ideally, the suprapubic view should be performed prior to the insertion of a Foley catheter, whenever feasible. Otherwise, it may be difficult to identify the bladder itself and distinguish it from surrounding free intraperitoneal fluid. Alternatively, the Foley catheter may be clamped after its insertion, or saline can be instilled in order to help visualize the bladder and the structures posterior to it (Figure 4.9).

Cardiac (subxiphoid) view

The purpose of the subxiphoid view is to evaluate cardiac activity and to detect pericardial effusions. Begin by placing the transducer at the subxiphoid region, with the indicator oriented towards the patient's right side (Figure 4.10a). The transducer should be placed relatively flat on the abdomen, and slightly angled up towards the patient's left shoulder. It is

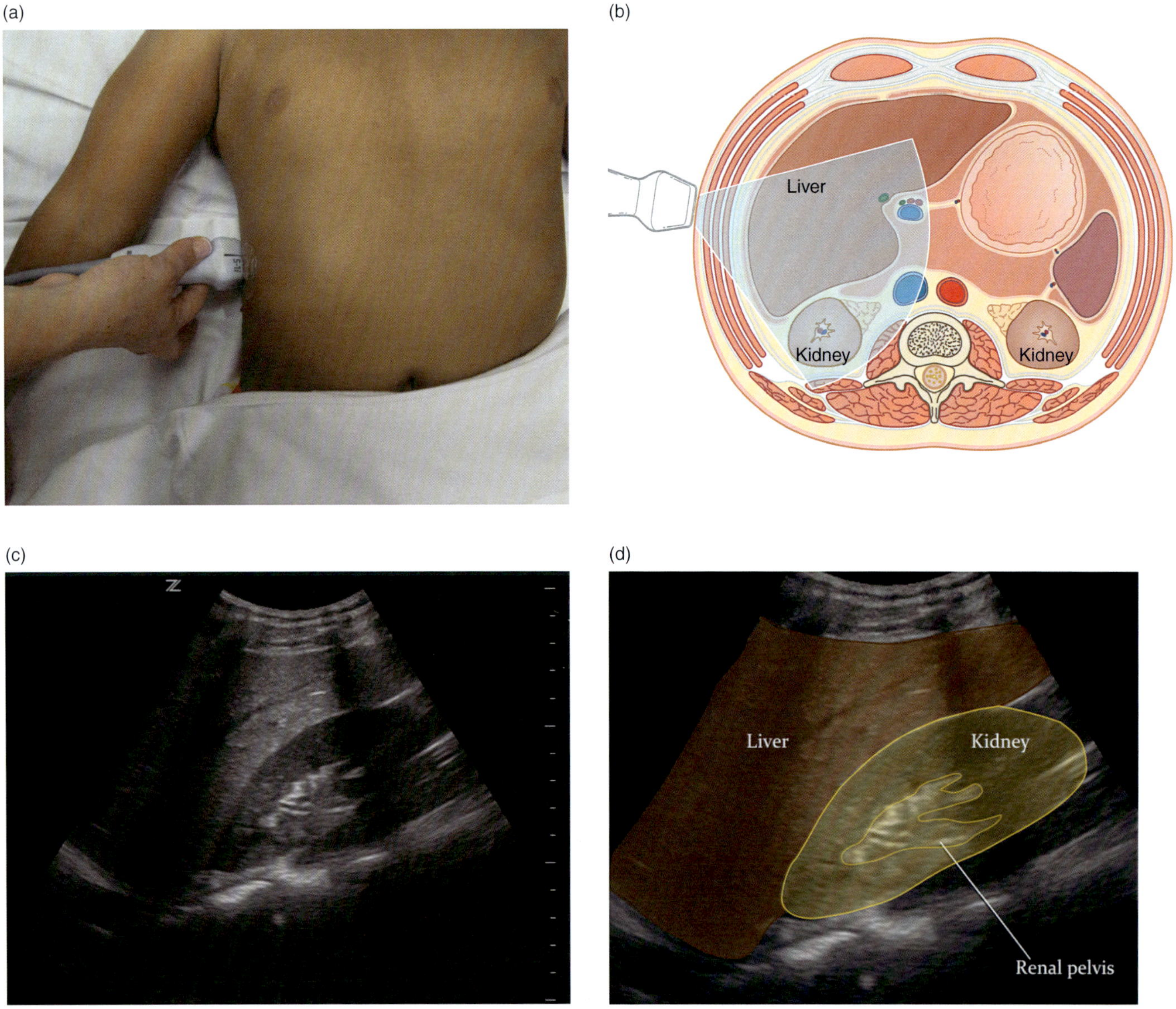

Figure 4.5 Right upper quadrant (Morison's) view. (a) Transducer placement at the right upper quadrant (RUQ). (b) Illustration of transducer placement and relevant anatomy *Artwork created by Emily Evans © Cambridge University Press.* (c) Normal ultrasound image of Morison's pouch. (d) Illustration of important structures visualized in the ultrasound image including the kidney, diaphragm, and liver. *Illustration by Laura Berg, MD.*

suggested to hold the transducer from above, in order to attain the appropriate plane of imaging (Figure 4.10b). Steady pressure might be required to displace interfering bowel gas. With this positioning, the left lobe of the liver acts as an acoustic window to enhance imaging of the heart. Further, image depth often needs to be adjusted (increased) in order to completely visualize the posterior pericardium. If the subxiphoid view is difficult to obtain, a parasternal long view should be attempted as an alternative cardiac view (see Chapter 5).

In the subxiphoid view, the right ventricle (RV) is the most anterior chamber, and the left atrium (LA) is the most posterior chamber (Figure 4.10d,e). A pericardial effusion would be expected to first collect posteriorly in a supine patient. A moderate pericardial effusion would extend towards the apex of the heart, and a larger effusion would circumscribe the entire heart. A pericardial fat pad, which is also hypoechoic or anechoic on ultrasound, can often be confused with a pericardial effusion. However, a pericardial fat pad is almost always located anterior to the right ventricle, rather than at the posterior pericardium. If the alternative parasternal long-axis view is obtained, free fluid appears as an anechoic pocket between the heart and descending aorta. Cardiac tamponade is a clinical diagnosis made based on the patient's hemodynamics and clinical picture. However, the clinical Beck's triad is often absent. Therefore, sonographic signs of cardiac tamponade are helpful. These signs include a circumferential pericardial effusion, paradoxic diastolic collapse of the right ventricle, and, in severe cases, a "swinging heart." Unstable patients with cardiac tamponade warrant emergent pericardiocentesis. Ultrasound guidance may be utilized in order to improve the safety and efficacy of pericardiocentesis (see Chapter 21).

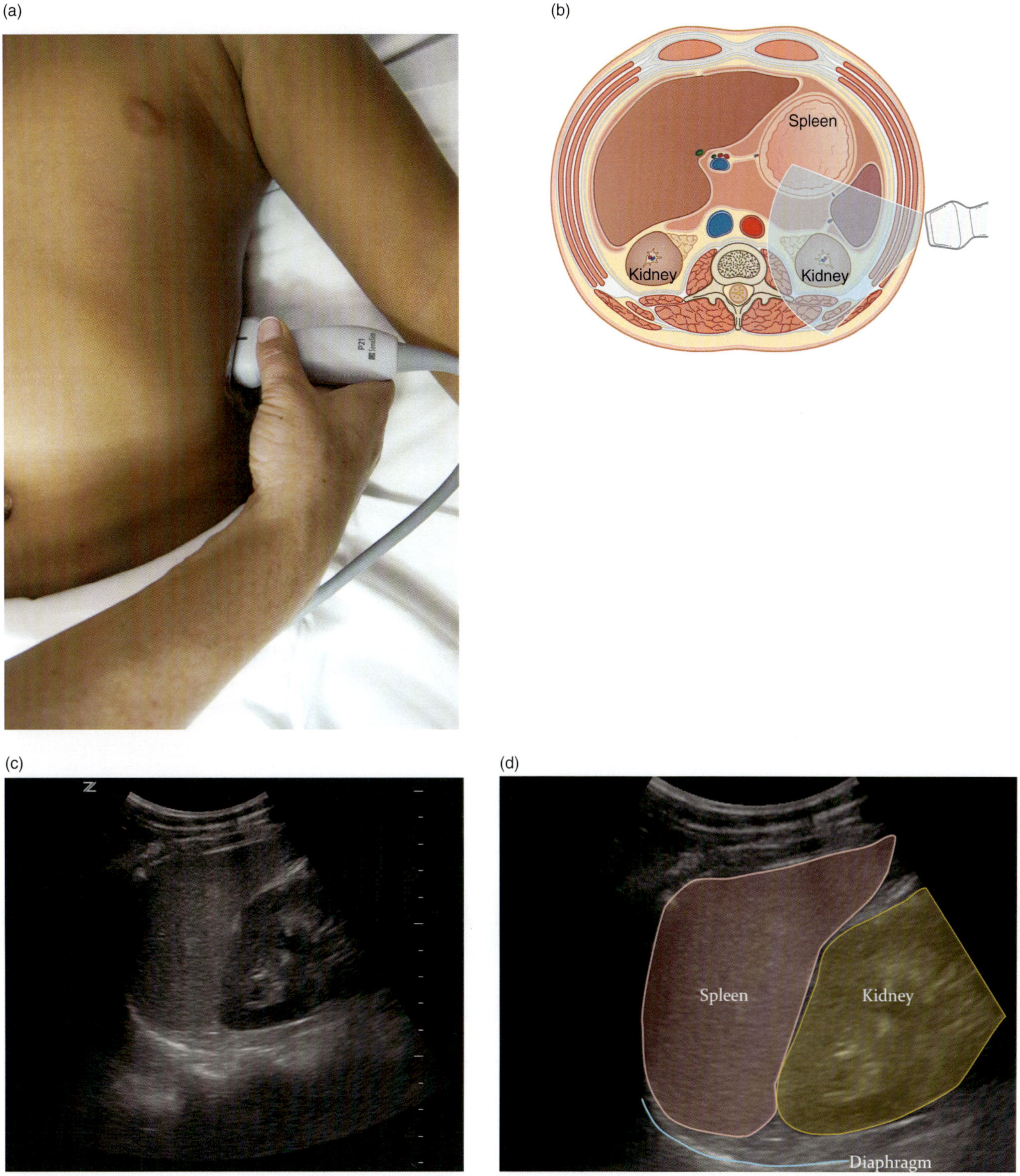

Figure 4.6 Left upper quadrant (splenorenal) view. (a) Transducer placement at the left upper quadrant (LUQ). (b) Illustration of transducer placement and relevant anatomy. *Artwork created by Emily Evans © Cambridge University Press.* (c) Normal ultrasound image of the splenorenal space or left upper quadrant. (d) Illustration of important structures visualized in the ultrasound image including the kidney, diaphragm, and spleen. *Illustration by Laura Berg, MD.*

Lung views

The additional lung windows in the E-FAST enable the examiner to make timely diagnoses of potentially life-threatening conditions, such as a hemothorax or pneumothorax. In order to detect a hemothorax or pleural effusion, place the transducer in the longitudinal orientation (coronal plane) identical to the positions for the right upper quadrant and left upper quadrant views (Figures 4.5a, 4.6a). Then move the

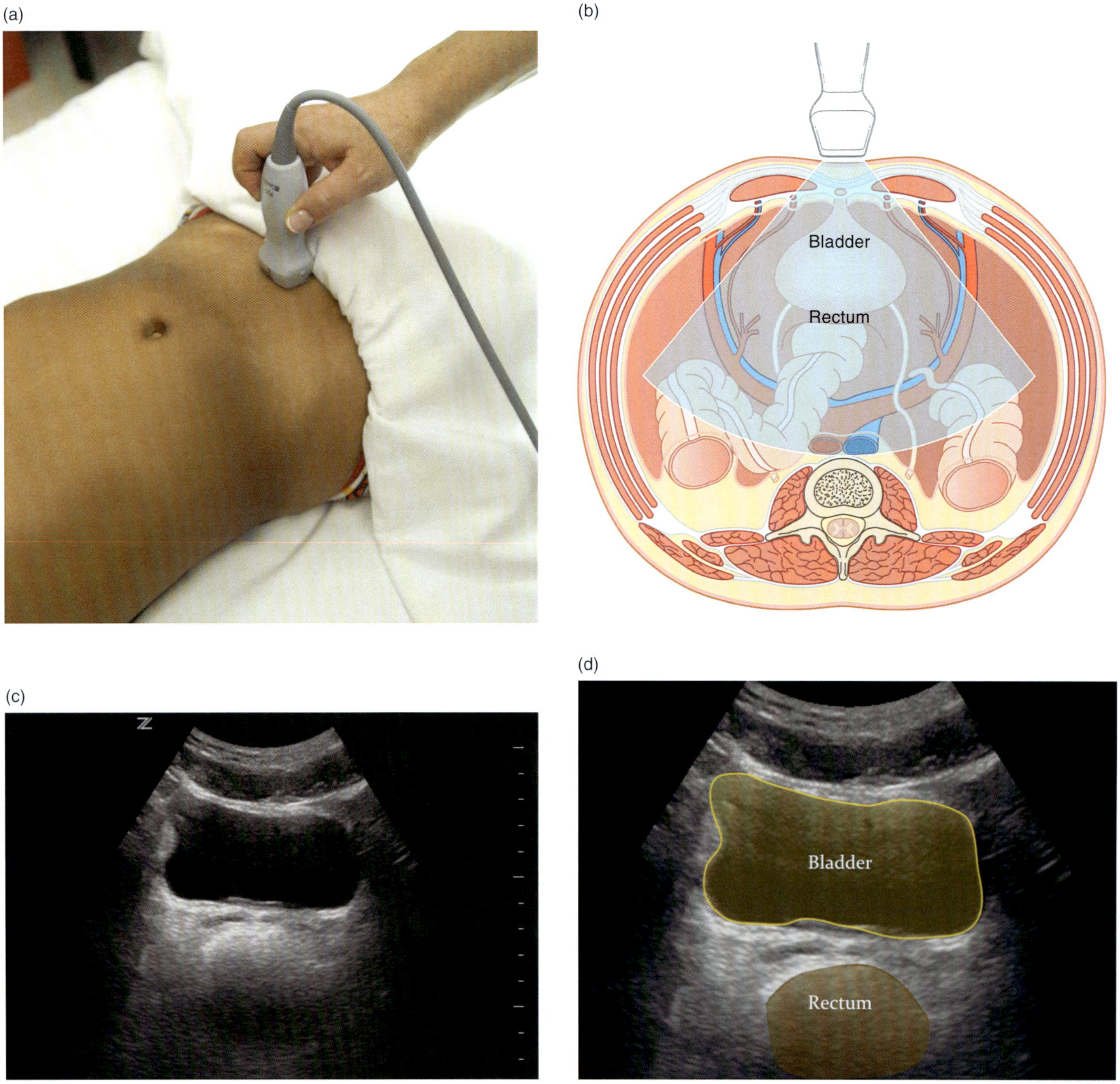

Figure 4.7 Suprapubic view, transverse orientation. (a) Transducer placement at the suprapubic region with the indicator oriented towards the patient's right side. (b) Illustration of transducer placement and relevant anatomy. *Artwork created by Emily Evans © Cambridge University Press.* (c) Normal ultrasound image of the transverse suprapubic view. (d) Illustration of important structures visualized in the ultrasound image, including the bladder and rectum. *Illustration by Laura Berg, MD.*

transducer cephalad until the hyperechoic diaphragm is visualized. If a mirror image artifact of the liver or spleen is seen, there is likely no fluid present in the pleural cavity (Figure 4.11a). Alternatively, if the mirror image artifact is absent, and an anechoic area cephalad to the diaphragm is visualized, a fluid collection is present (Figure 4.11b). The etiology of a pleural effusion superior to the diaphragm largely depends on the clinical scenario. In trauma situations, this pleural effusion is presumed to be a hemothorax until proven otherwise.

In order to detect a pneumothorax, a linear, high-frequency transducer is preferred (Figure 4.12a,b), though a low-frequency, curvilinear or phased array transducer may also be used (Figure 4.13). In the supine patient, a pneumothorax is often visualized anteriorly as air tends to rise to the top of the rib cage. Begin imaging in the midclavicular line, at the third

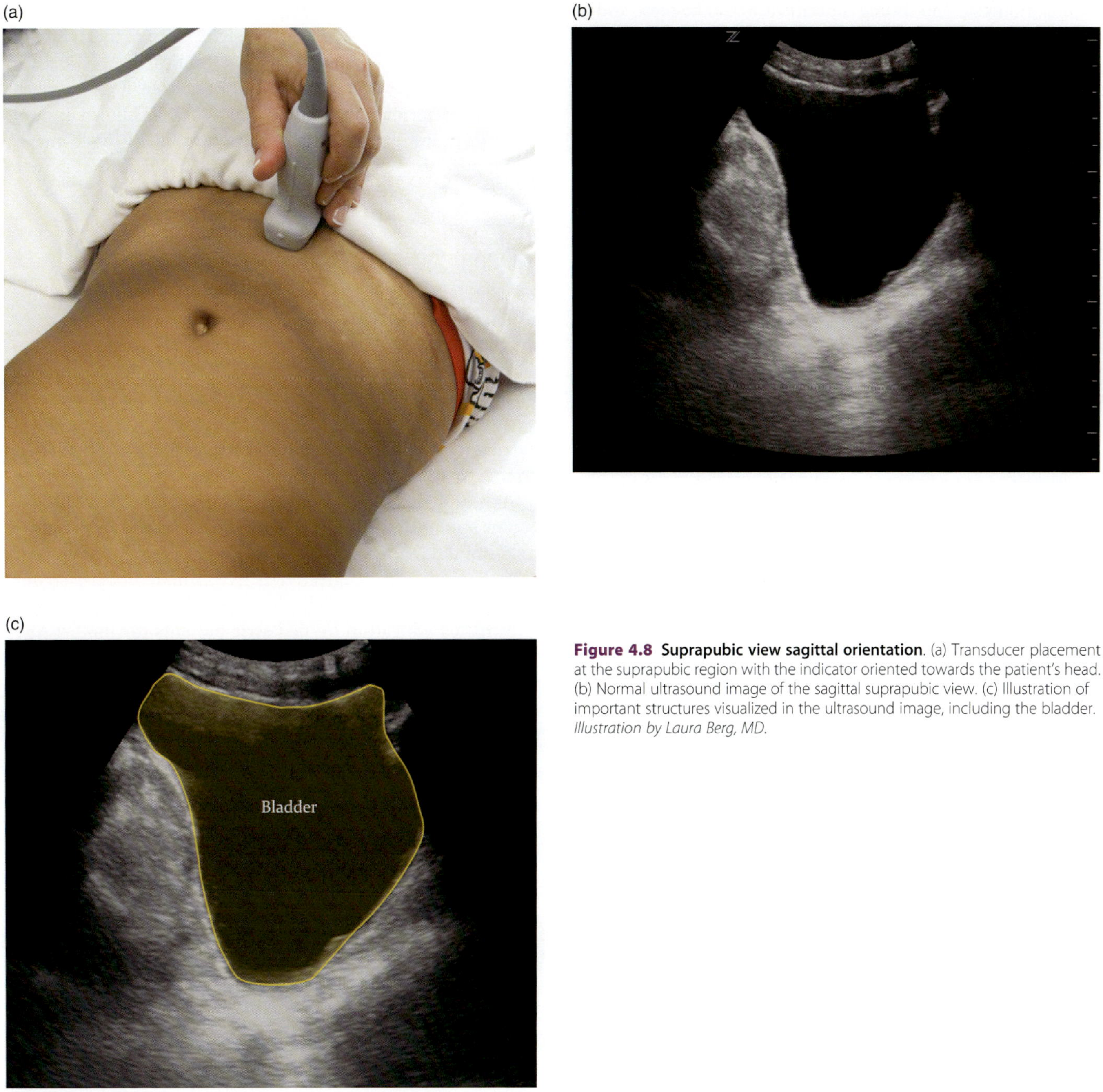

Figure 4.8 Suprapubic view sagittal orientation. (a) Transducer placement at the suprapubic region with the indicator oriented towards the patient's head. (b) Normal ultrasound image of the sagittal suprapubic view. (c) Illustration of important structures visualized in the ultrasound image, including the bladder. *Illustration by Laura Berg, MD.*

to fifth intercostal space (Figure 4.12a,b). Place the transducer perpendicular to the ribs and scan the area between two adjacent rib shadows. The pleural line will be in between the rib shadows, otherwise known as the "bat sign" (Figure 4.12c,d). Additional views can be obtained at the fourth intercostal space at the anterior axillary line, and the sixth intercostal space at the posterior axillary line if necessary. The transducer should be kept steady for three to four respiratory cycles, in order to avoid a false-positive examination. Both B-mode and M-mode imaging can be utilized in order to detect patterns consistent with normal lung and conversely a pneumothorax:

1. **Lung sliding** – the movement of the parietal against the visceral pleura at their interface during normal respiration, can be visualized in real-time B-mode imaging. "Comet tails" are normal artifacts that arise from the pleural line (Figure 4.14a) (see Chapter 6). This lung sliding may be highlighted by utilizing the Power Doppler function (the "**power slide**," see Figure 4.15). In the case of a

pneumothorax, no sliding movement would be seen, and there would be an absence of "comet tail" artifacts (Figure 4.14b).

2. Lung movement can be further visualized in the M-mode. The cursor is oriented perpendicular to the pleural line. The movement of the normal lung and pleura over time during respiration would produce a granular artifact, giving the characteristic "**seashore sign**" (Figure 4.16a). The absence of these movement artifacts in the case of a pneumothorax would produce a "**stratosphere sign**" or "**bar-code sign**" (Figure 4.16b). Further, the actual location where the pneumothorax begins can often be detected. This interface between normal lung and pneumothorax is known as the "**lung point.**" This can be visualized on the M-mode image, where both the "seashore sign" and "stratosphere sign" are seen on the same M-mode image (Figure 6.11).

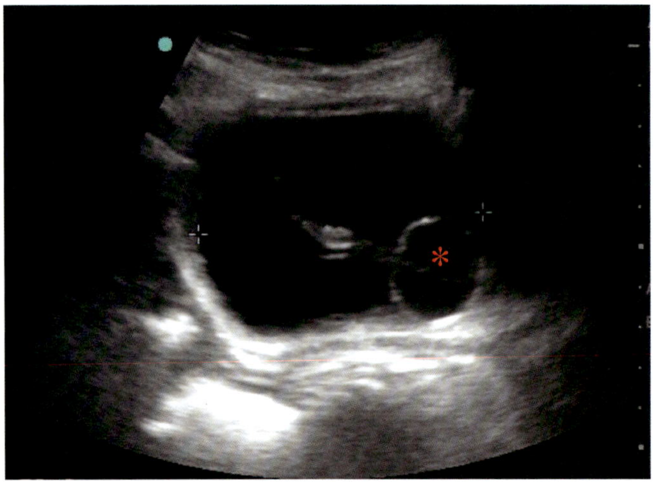

Figure 4.9 Transverse view of the bladder with a Foley catheter. In order to visualize the bladder once a Foley (*) is in place, the catheter may be clamped and/or saline instilled into the bladder.

Training and education

It is generally agreed that E-FAST instruction should include a didactic portion, hands-on practical, and experiential components. Recently, instruction in the E-FAST examination has been introduced into both medical student education and the training of prehospital providers. Studies have also examined various models of hands-on practical teaching. Most instructors utilize healthy models. However, it is often challenging to gain experience with pathology. Patients with peritoneal dialysis and simulator models have been utilized. Recent studies have suggested that multimedia and mannequin simulator models, such as the UltraSim® sonographic training model, are as effective as live human models. To our knowledge there have been no studies that have specifically investigated education on pediatric patients for the E-FAST examination.

(a)

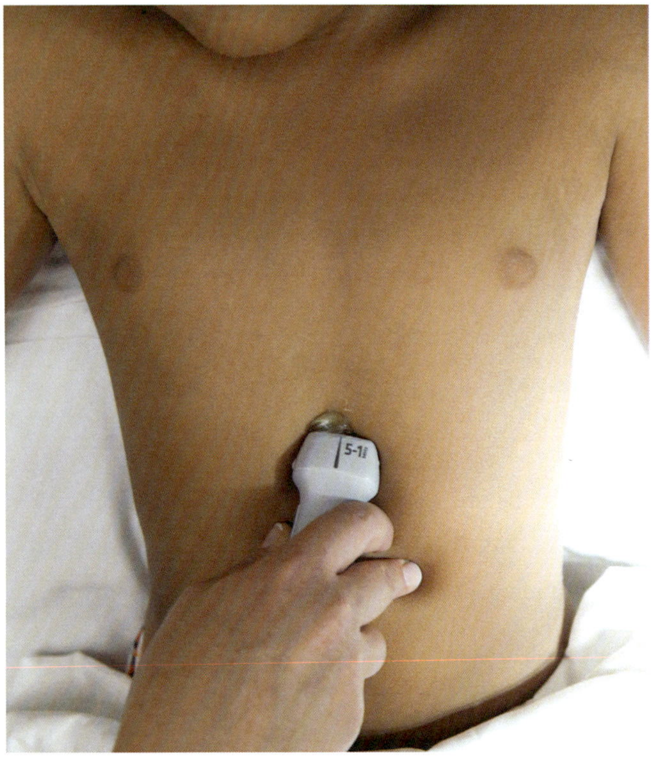

(b)

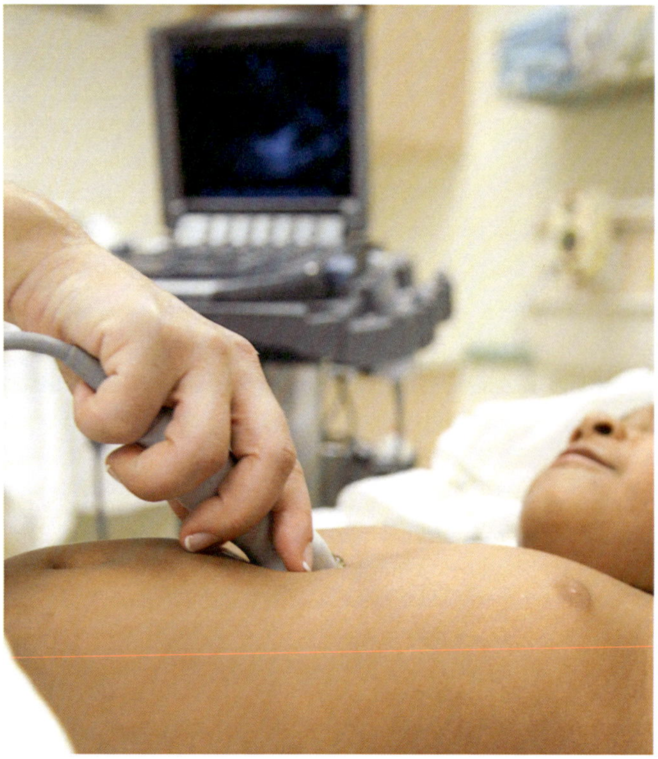

Figure 4.10 Cardiac (subxiphoid) view. (a) Transducer placement below the xiphoid process, with the indicator oriented towards the patient's right side. (b) The transducer is placed relatively flat in relation to the patient's body. (c) Illustration of the cardiac anatomy in the subxiphoid view. *Artwork created by Emily Evans © Cambridge University Press.* (d) Normal ultrasound image of the heart in the subxiphoid view. *Image courtesy of Christopher Kerwin, MD.* (e) Illustration depicting the structures visualized in the subxiphoid view: right ventricle (RV), left ventricle (LV), left atrium (LA), right atrium (RA), and liver. *Illustration by Laura Berg, MD.*

(c)

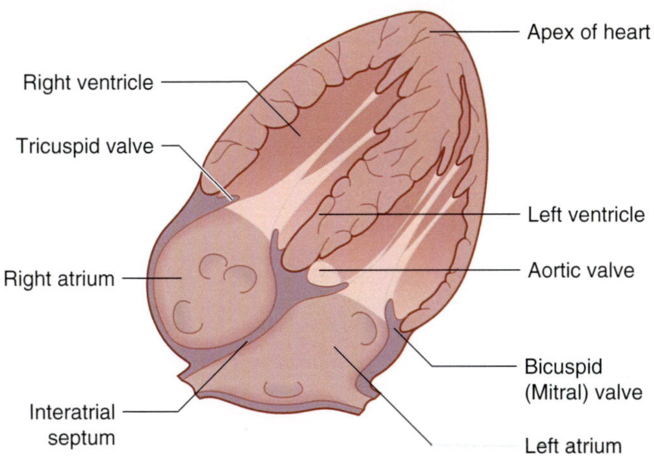

(d)

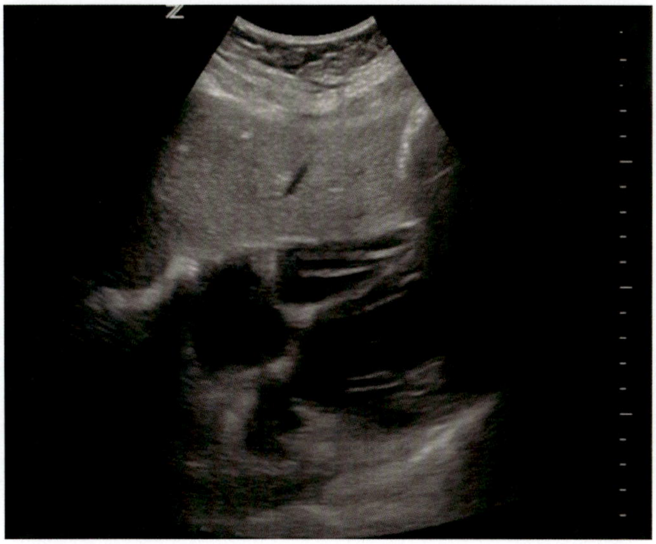

(e)

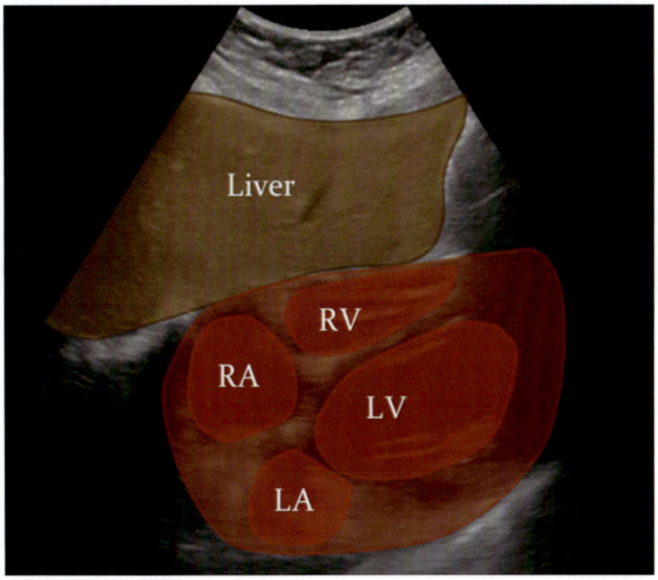

Figure 4.10 (cont.)

Scanning tips

Pitfalls

- The E-FAST should not solely be relied upon for medical decision-making in trauma situations. It is only moderately sensitive in detecting solid abdominal organ injuries, and does not identify the actual location of injury.
- At times E-FAST images may be suboptimal due to body habitus, the presence of subcutaneous emphysema, or other technical reasons. It is important to remember a suboptimal study is NOT equivalent to a negative E-FAST.
- In delayed presentation of trauma, clotted blood may appear hyperechoic, and can easily be missed.
- While free fluid collection on the E-FAST examination is most likely due to blood, under the right circumstances, ascites, continuous ambulatory peritoneal dialysis fluid, urine from a ruptured bladder, and physiologic fluid in a female can all appear identical to blood.
- Blood sometimes collects only at the inferior or superior poles of the kidneys, especially in the left upper quadrant. Make sure to visualize both kidneys in their entirety.
- Perinephric fat can sometimes mimic free fluid collection. If in doubt, always compare the two sides.
- A pericardial fat pad may be mistaken for a pericardial effusion. However, the pericardial fat pad is generally located anterior rather than posterior to the heart.

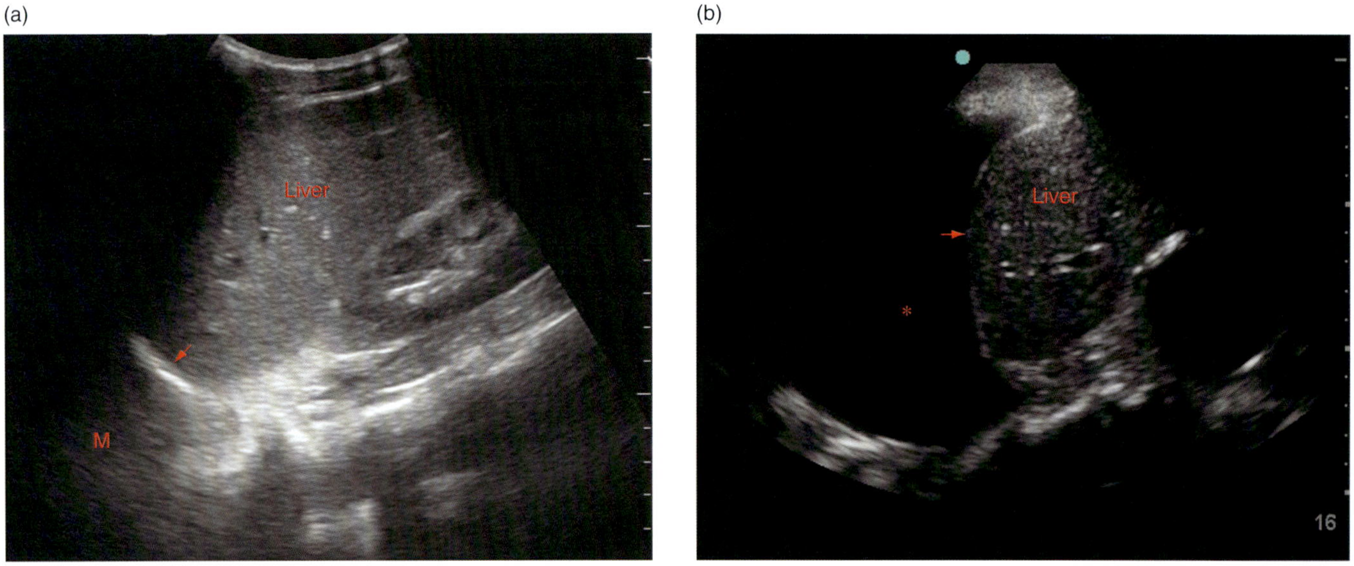

Figure 4.11 Pleural effusion and loss of mirror-image artifact (a) Normal right pleural cavity view with the mirror image artifact (M) of the liver seen. The diaphragm (arrow) appears as a hyperechoic, bright white line. (b) The absence of the mirror-image artifact above the diaphragm (*) indicates a pleural effusion.

Tips to improve scanning

✓ Having the patient placed in 5–10° Trendelenburg position will increase the sensitivity of detecting free fluid at Morison's pouch.

✓ Rotating the transducer approximately 10° in a posterior oblique orientation will allow for ideal imaging along the long-axis of the kidney. The left kidney is located more superior and posterior in relation to the right kidney.

✓ Asking a cooperative patient to inhale deeply can help bring the liver/spleen/heart down into view.

✓ Repeating E-FAST at intervals, or when the patient's hemodynamics changes, can increase its sensitivity.

✓ Remember to increase image depth to completely visualize the posterior pericardium of the heart, when evaluating for a pericardial effusion.

✓ In order to evaluate adequately for a hemothorax, it is important to visualize above the diaphragms on the left and right upper quadrant views.

✓ In order to assess for a pneumothorax, visualize lung sliding on B-mode. The M-mode pattern of the "seashore sign" signifies a normal lung; while "stratosphere sign" represents a pneumothorax.

Cases

1. An eight-year-old male is hit by a car while riding a bicycle, and is thrown over the hood of the vehicle. On arrival at the emergency department, the child has a Glasgow Coma Scale (GCS) score of 15. Vital signs are: heart rate (HR) 160 bpm, blood pressure (BP) 98/63 mmHg, respiratory rate (RR) 45/mm. He appears pale and anxious, with a distended and diffusely tender abdomen. Advanced Trauma Life Support (ATLS) protocol is followed, and primary and secondary surveys reveal no other significant findings. An initial E-FAST is performed, which reveals no free fluid. The patient becomes less responsive while being evaluated in the emergency department. His abdomen becomes progressively more distended. Repeat vital signs are: HR 175 bpm, BP 78/33 mmHg, RR 60/min. Despite adequate intravenous crystalloid fluid resuscitation, and blood transfusion, the patient remains hypotensive and his mental status deteriorates. A repeat E-FAST is performed, which reveals new intra-abdominal free fluid (Figure 4.17). The decision is made to intubate the child and take him to the operating room. On laparotomy, a grade 5 splenic laceration and several small liver lacerations are found. Splenectomy is performed. The child makes an otherwise uneventful recovery.

   This is a classic example of the utility of the E-FAST, and the importance of repeating the E-FAST. Though not as common in the pediatric population as adults, the E-FAST can quickly detect intraperitoneal bleeding and facilitate operative management in the unstable trauma patient, due to its high specificity and positive likelihood ratio. It is non-invasive, and can be quickly and easily performed at the patient's bedside while other resuscitation efforts are ongoing.

2. A 16-year-old male, unrestrained driver is brought in to the emergency department after a head-on collision with a telephone pole at high speed. On examination, the patient

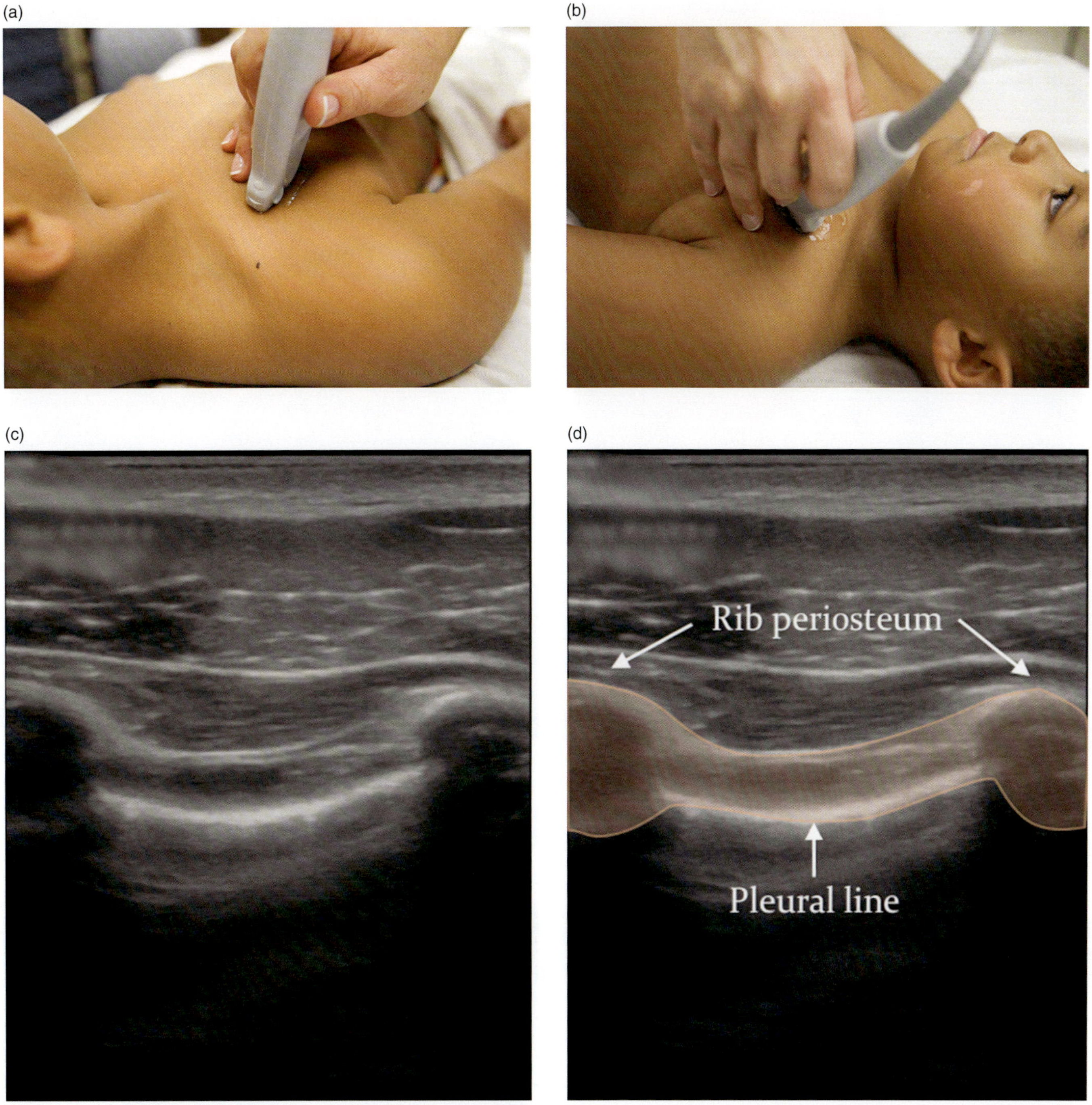

Figure 4.12 Lung views. (a) Transducer placement at the right chest, with the indicator towards the patient's head. (b) Transducer placement at the left chest, with the indicator towards the patient's head. The left placement should be slightly superior and lateral, to avoid cardiac movement being confused for lung sliding. (c) Normal ultrasound image of the pleural line in between two rib shadows, otherwise known as the "bat sign." (d) Illustration of important structures visualized in the ultrasound image including the pleural line, ribs, and rib shadows. *Illustration by Laura Berg, MD.*

has agonal respirations, and a GCS score of 7. Vital signs are: HR 130 bpm, BP 95/45 mmHg, RR 6/min. The patient is quickly intubated after intravenous access is established. Post-intubation breath sounds are equal and clear bilaterally. Secondary survey reveals multiple facial injuries, and chest and abdominal wall contusions. Repeat vital signs are: HR 150 bpm, BP 70/35 mmHg. The E-FAST show relevant findings (Figure 4.18). As a result, emergency needle decompression of the chest and pericardiocentesis are performed, with improved vital signs. The patient is taken to the operating room for emergent thoracotomy and pericardial window. He survives the surgery, but

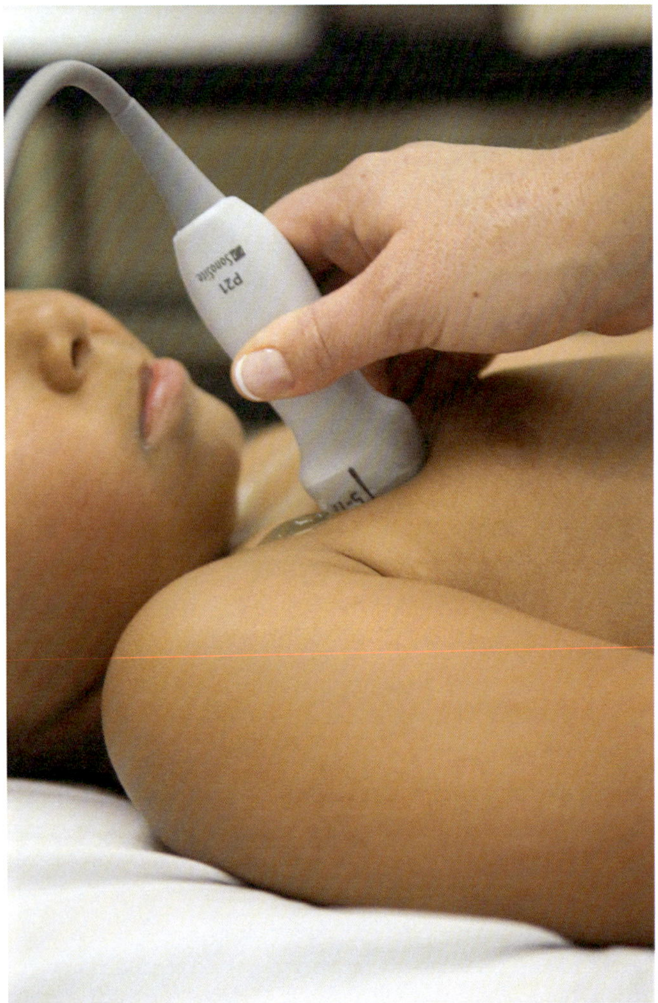

Figure 4.13 Low-frequency transducers may also be utilized in the lung portion of the E-FAST examination.

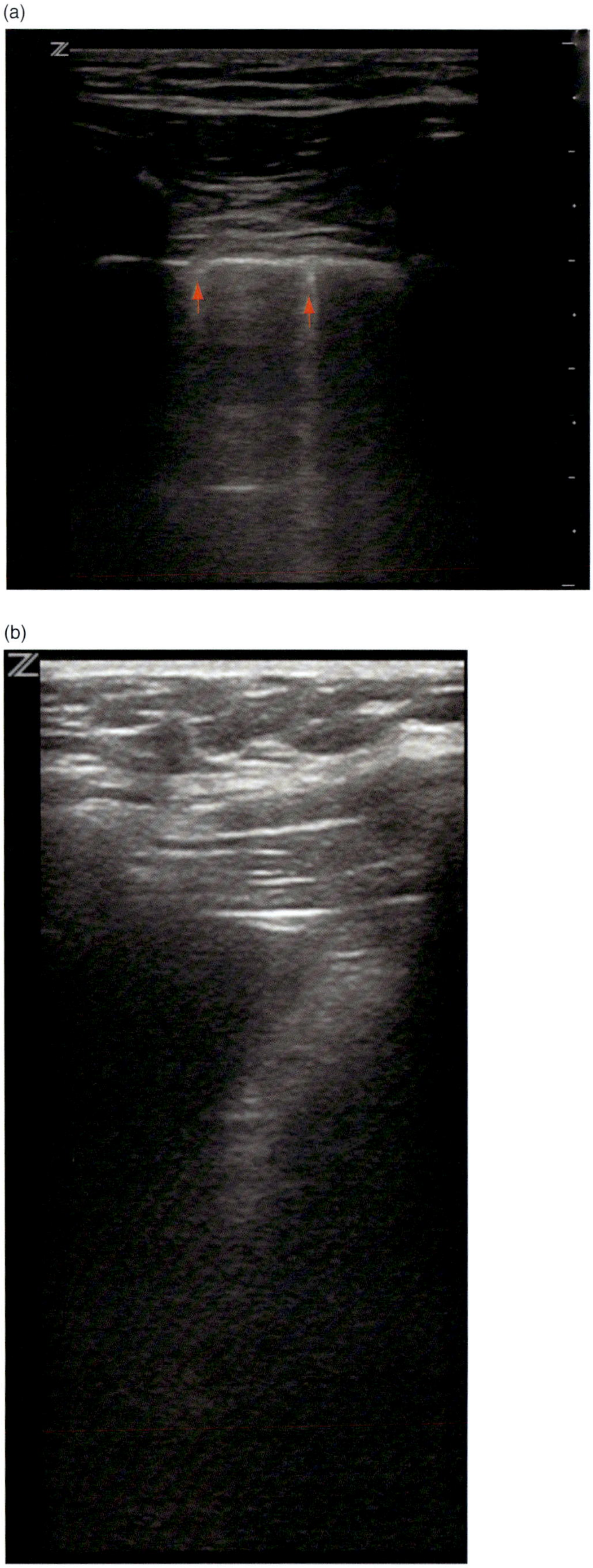

Figure 4.14 Comet-tail artifact. (a) This is an artifact (arrow) that arises from the pleural line of a normal lung, with normal lung sliding. (b) Comet-tail artifacts are absent when there is no lung sliding, as is seen with a pneumothorax.

eventually succumbs to complications from severe brain injury.

This is an example of how E-FAST can help detect and manage life-threatening injuries in the thoracic cavity. In this case, the patient likely sustained a hemopericardium and cardiac tamponade from impact of the chest on the steering wheel. The classic Beck's triad of hypotension, muffled heart sound, and jugular venous distension may be absent in up to 60% of patients with cardiac tamponade. Though its benefit has only been proven by research in adult penetrating-trauma patients, the cardiac views of the E-FAST play an important role in the management of pediatric as well as adult blunt thoracic trauma patients.

3. A six-year-old child falls about 15 feet out of a tree house. She is brought into the emergency department in full spinal immobilization. On arrival, she has a GCS score of 9, HR 140 bpm, BP 100/70 mmHg, RR 8/min. Her lung and cardiovascular examinations are unremarkable. Intravenous access is obtained, and rapid-sequence intubation is performed in order to protect the patient's

airway. On secondary survey, she has a large parietal scalp hematoma, multiple facial abrasions, a left abdominal wall abrasion, and obvious right forearm and right thigh deformities. The rest of her examination is unremarkable. Repeat vital signs are: HR 120 bpm, BP 88/58 mmHg, RR 20/mm. The E-FAST examination reveals no abnormal findings in the chest cavity, but some free fluid at Morison's pouch (Figure 4.19). The patient is then brought to the radiology suite, where a large subdural hematoma and a grade 2 liver laceration are found on CT scans. She is also found to have right mid-femur and distal right radius and ulnar fractures. The patient is taken to the operating room, where her various injuries are managed by neurosurgeons and orthopedic surgeons. The liver laceration is managed non-operatively.

This is an example where E-FAST can help prioritize studies and intervention in a multi-organ-system trauma patient, with an unobtainable examination and the potential for clinical deterioration. Though it has limitations, a hemodynamically stable patient with a negative bedside E-FAST can help rule out life-threatening diagnoses such as hemothorax, pneumothorax, and significant intra-abdominal hemorrhage. While a positive E-FAST might not warrant immediate surgical intervention, a stable patient should have additional studies obtained such as a CT scan. However, in an unstable patient, a positive E-FAST might indicate emergent surgical intervention.

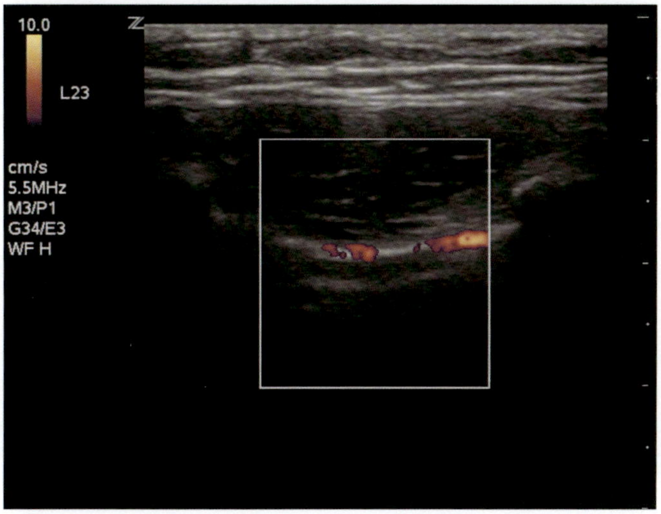

Figure 4.15 Power Doppler. Normal lung sliding as seen with color power Doppler.

Summary

1. The FAST examination includes the right upper quadrant, left upper quadrant, suprapubic, and subxiphoid views to detect free intraperitoneal free fluid. The E-FAST includes the traditional four views in addition to lung windows in order to detect a pneumothorax or hemothorax.
2. The E-FAST examination is limited in detecting hollow abdominal organ/retroperitoneal injuries, and generally cannot pinpoint the source of free intra-abdominal fluid.
3. The E-FAST has a high positive likelihood ratio but only moderate negative likelihood ratio. Therefore, a positive E-FAST can rule in intra-abdominal organ injuries, but a negative E-FAST cannot completely rule them out.

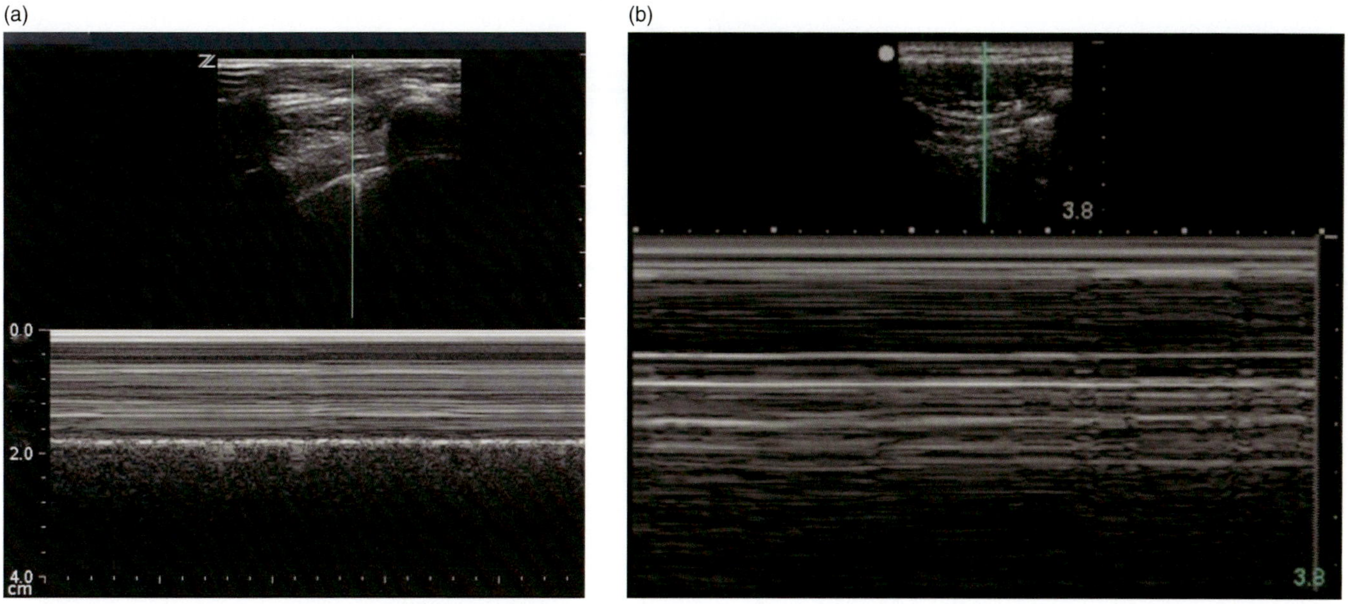

Figure 4.16 M-mode. (a) The normal lung shows lung sliding, a characteristic pattern in M-mode known as the "seashore sign." (b) A pneumothorax will have an absence of lung sliding. The characteristic M-mode pattern is known as the "stratosphere sign."

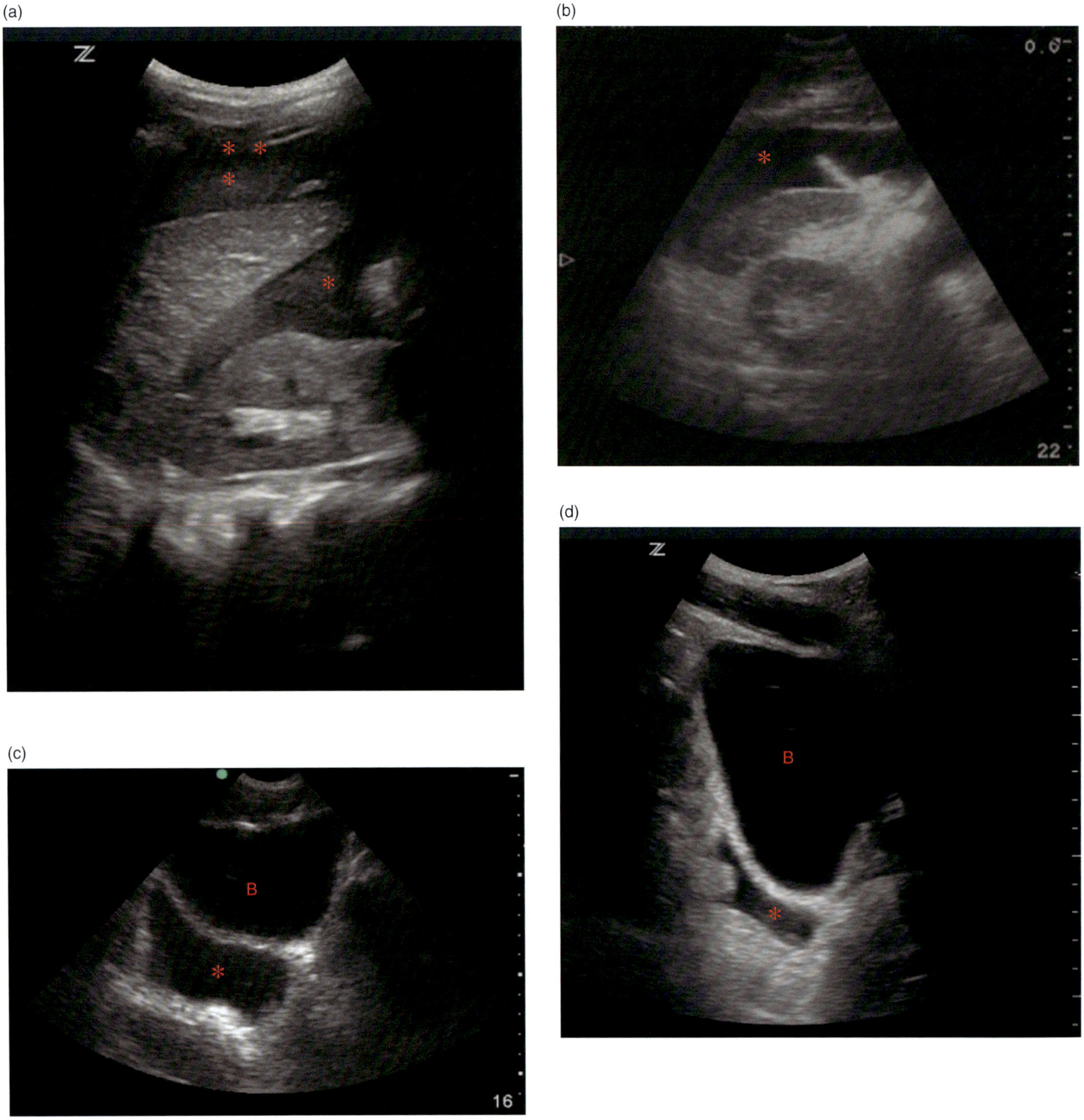

Figure 4.17 **Case 1**. (a) Right upper quadrant view, with fluid (*) visualized in Morison's pouch. *Image courtesy of Christopher Kerwin, MD.* (b) Left upper quadrant view, with fluid (*) visualized around the spleen. *Image courtesy of Michael Lambert, MD.* (c) Fluid (*) visualized in the rectovesicular space on the transverse suprapubic view. (d) Fluid (*) visualized surrounding the bladder (B) on the sagittal suprapubic view.

4. The right upper quadrant view, or Morison's pouch, gives the highest yield for detecting intra-abdominal free fluid. Placing a patient in Trendelenburg positioning can further increase the sensitivity of detecting fluid at the right upper quadrant.
5. Clinical judgment should take precedence over any E-FAST results. The E-FAST is best utilized in conjunction with the clinical scenario, and should be repeated when a patient's clinical status changes.

(a)

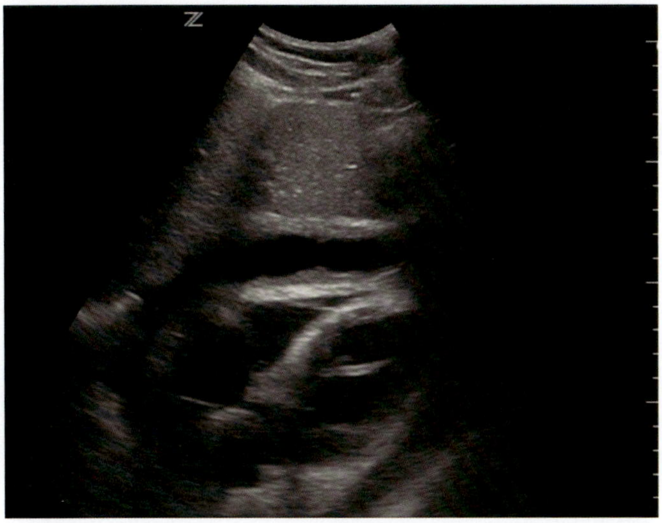

(b)

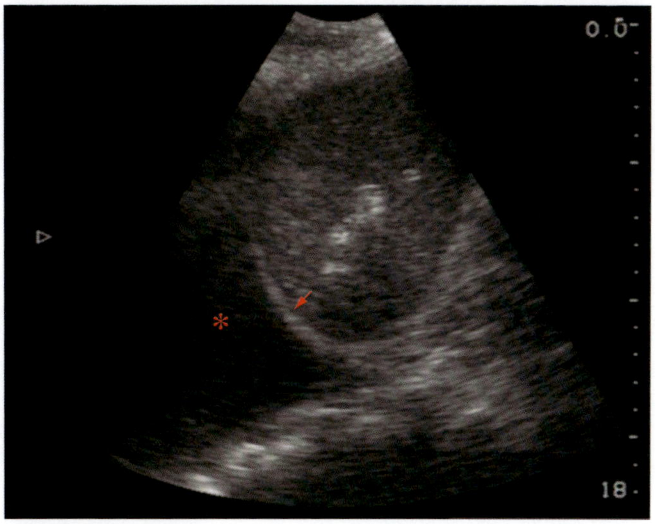

(c)

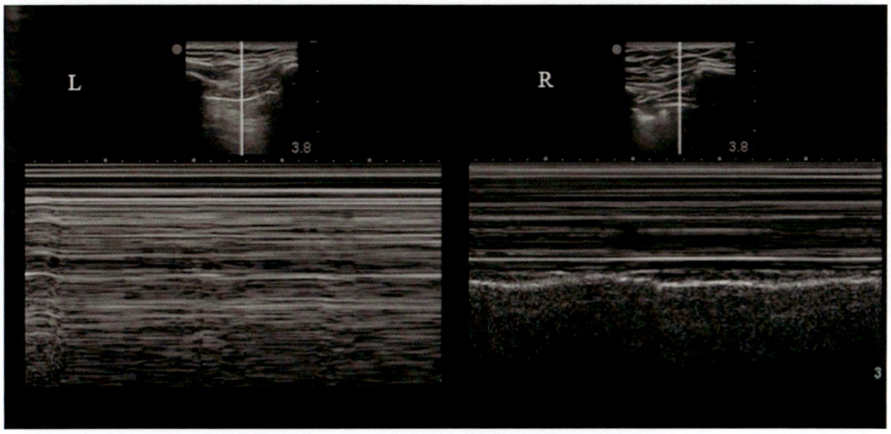

Figure 4.18 **Case 2: Pericardial effusion.** (a) Circumferential pericardial effusion (*) visualized on the subxiphoid cardiac view. (b) Hemothorax (*) visualized superior to the diaphragm (arrow). Note the loss of the mirror-image artifact superior to the diaphragm. *Image courtesy of Michael Lambert, MD.* (c) Lung windows were also obtained in M-mode, which showed a normal "seashore" sign on the right, and a "stratosphere" sign on the left, indicative of a pneumothorax.

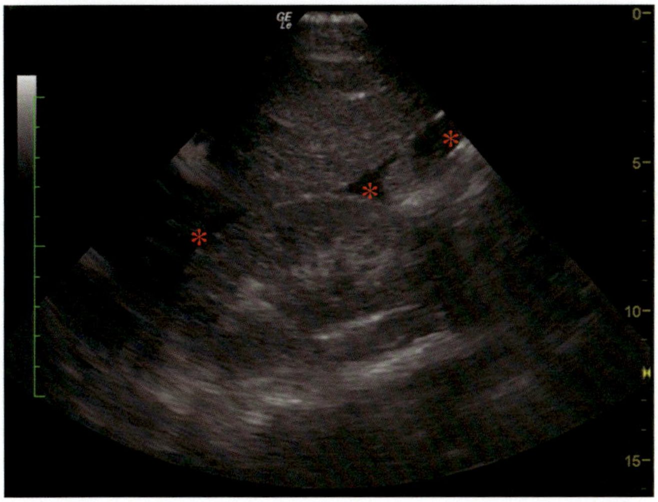

Figure 4.19 **Case 3: positive right upper quadrant view.** Free fluid is visualized in Morison's pouch. The remainder of the E-FAST was negative. While the patient ended up having a grade 2 liver laceration, lacerations of the liver and spleen are often difficult to identify on the E-FAST.

Selected references

Coley, B.D., Mutabagani, K.H., Martin, L.C., *et al.* (2000) Focused abdominal sonography for trauma (FAST) in children with blunt abdominal trauma. *J Trauma* **48**(5): 902–6.

Corbett, S.W., Andrews, H.G., Baker, E.M., *et al.* (2000) ED evaluation of the pediatric trauma patient by ultrasonography. *Am J Emerg Med* **18**: 244–9.

Damewood, S., Jeanmonod, D., Cadigan, B. (2011) Comparison of a multimedia simulator to a human model for teaching FAST exam image interpretation and image acquisition. *Acad Emerg Med* **18**: 413–19.

Fox, J.C., Boysen, M., Gharahbaghian, L., *et al.* (2011) Test characteristics of focused assessment of sonography for trauma for clinically significant abdominal free fluid in pediatric blunt abdominal trauma. *Acad Emerg Med* **18**(5): 477–82.

Holmes, J.F., Gladman, A., Chang, C.H. (2007) Performance of abdominal ultrasonography in pediatric blunt trauma patients: a meta-analysis. *J Ped Surg* **42**: 1588–94.

Melniker, L.A., Leibner, E., McKenney, M. G., *et al.* (2006) Randomized controlled clinical trial of point-of-care, limited untrasonography for trauma in the emergency department: the first sonography outcomes assessment program trial. *Am Emerg Med* **48**(3): 227–35.

Scalea, T.M., Rodriguez, A., Chiu, W.C., *et al.* (1999) Focused assessment with sonography for trauma (FAST): results from an international consensus conference. *J Trauma* **46**(3): 466–72.

Soudack, M., Epelman, M., Maor, R., *et al.* (2004) Experience with focused abdominal sonography for trauma (FAST) in 313 pediatric patients. *J Clin Ultrasound* **32**(2): 53–61.

Suthers, S.E., Albrecht, R., Foley, D., *et al.* (2004) Surgeon-directed ultrasound for trauma is a predictor of intra-abdominal injury in children. *Am Surg* **70**: 164–8.

Wilkerson, R.G., Stone, M.B. (2010) Sensitivity of bedside ultrasound and supine anteroposterior chest radiograph for the identification of pneumothorax after blunt trauma. *Acad Emerg Med* **17**(1): 11–17.

Chapter 5

Focused cardiac ultrasound

Stephanie J. Doniger

Objectives/indications

Approximately 16,000 American children suffer out-of-hospital cardiac arrest per year (8–20/100,000). When compared with adults, children are more likely to survive arrest, with greater than 10% of children surviving to hospital discharge. Among those treated for in-hospital cardiac arrest, two-thirds can be successfully resuscitated with return of spontaneous circulation, and greater than 25% survive to hospital discharge. Overall, cardiac arrests presenting with asystole or pulseless electrical activity (PEA) have worse survival outcomes when compared with patients presenting with ventricular fibrillation or pulseless ventricular tachycardia. When compared with adults, children have better outcomes even following asystole and PEA. However, it is difficult to predict survival outcomes from pulseless cardiac arrest. Pediatric resuscitations may be carried out for extended periods of time, often requiring considerable resources.

Point-of-care ultrasonography has rapidly developed over the past several years, and has now become part of the standard of care in adult patients for several applications. While point-of-care ultrasonography has only recently been applied to critically ill pediatric patients, several of the well-established adult indications may be applied to pediatric patients. One of the most important and life-saving applications is focused cardiac ultrasound, or echocardiography. Clinicians may rapidly and effectively assess for the presence of a pericardial effusion, tamponade, and asystole. In patients presenting in PEA, the emergency physician can expeditiously differentiate cardiac standstill from correctable causes of PEA. These assessments may be performed often simultaneously with the physical examination, and during resuscitation. In addition, in those patients presenting with undifferentiated hypotension, the emergency physician can easily assess global cardiac wall function by visual interpretation, and estimate central venous pressure (CVP) by measurements of the IVC.

In the approach of the cardiac assessment in the emergency department, it is important to note that focused cardiac ultrasound is not meant to replace formal, comprehensive echocardiography. Rather, it is best seen as an extension of the physical examination, and is meant to answer specific binary yes/no questions such as "Is there a pericardial effusion? Is cardiac activity present?" The goal of the point-of-care focused cardiac ultrasound is to answer these basic questions, rather than to identify complex congenital heart disease lesions. This chapter reviews the indications for point-of-care focused cardiac ultrasound as well as the techniques to perform this examination.

Background

Echocardiography is the gold standard for the diagnosis of cardiac and pericardial abnormalities, and is a non-invasive modality for detecting life-threatening cardiac conditions. The incorporation of point-of-care focused cardiac ultrasound in adult populations has been shown to have a significant impact on medical decision-making and be a useful adjunct to the clinical examination, when radiologic and laboratory studies are often unreliable and nonspecific. A recent comprehensive literature review (1978–2004) reported a remarkable increase in the diagnostic accuracy by cardiologists and non-cardiologists, when a cardiac ultrasound study was added to the physical examination. Overall, it has been shown that non-cardiologists can be quickly and effectively trained to perform and interpret focused echocardiograms. Even trainees with limited ultrasound experience have been shown to be able to successfully assess left ventricular function and pericardial effusions.

One of the earliest and most well-recognized applications for point-of-care, limited cardiac ultrasound is for the identification of pericardial effusions in traumatic and non-traumatic conditions. It is especially crucial to promptly identify pericardial effusions and tamponade, since this may lead to life-saving interventions. Mandavia *et al.* studied echocardiography (echo) performed by emergency physicians in patients at high risk for pericardial effusions, revealing an overall accuracy of 98%, sensitivity of 96%, and specificity of 98%. In trauma patients, Ma *et al.* reported a 100% sensitivity, 99% specificity, and 99% overall accuracy for the identification of pericardial effusions in patients with chest trauma. In a 10-year retrospective review, Plummer *et al.* showed that point-of-care echo improved the outcome of patients with penetrating chest trauma with shorter time to diagnosis (15.5 vs. 42.4 min) and better overall survival (100% vs. 57%). In a case series, Schiavone *et al.* highlighted the importance of the ability to identify pericardial effusion and early signs of tamponade in facilitating surgical management of patients with cardiac rupture secondary to blunt non-penetrating chest trauma. These results contributed to the

Pediatric Emergency and Critical Care Ultrasound, ed. Stephanie J. Doniger. Published by Cambridge University Press.

American College of Surgeons revising the Advanced Trauma Life Support (ATLS) course to incorporate the rapid point-of-care ultrasound assessment to identify pericardial effusions.

In addition, focused cardiac ultrasound has tremendous utility in resuscitation. In a study of adult patients with out-of-hospital cardiac arrest, no patients who required greater than two doses of epinephrine or who had greater than 20 minutes of resuscitation without return of spontaneous circulation (ROSC) survived. Blaivas *et al.* and Salen *et al.* showed that no patients with sonographic cardiac standstill had ROSC, regardless of initial presenting rhythm. Conversely, the presence of sonographic-identified cardiac activity at any point during the resuscitation was associated with 37% survival to hospital admission. During this particular study, 96% of physicians reported that cardiac ultrasonography provided useful information about the resuscitation, and that it could be performed with ease without interfering with resuscitation efforts. It has been further suggested that a low capnography reading in conjunction with sonographic cardiac standstill may be associated with poor resuscitation outcomes.

Focused cardiac ultrasound is also useful in patients presenting with undifferentiated hypotension. Point-of-care ultrasound may aid in monitoring the effectiveness of ionotropic support or vasopressor infusion, and aid in the optimization of therapy. Randazzo *et al.* reported that, with limited focused training, emergency physicians could assess the left ventricular (LV) ejection fraction accurately. The undifferentiated hypotensive patient (UHP) ultrasound protocol utilized the three locations for identifying abdominal free fluid, qualitative cardiac assessment, and the abdominal aorta assessment as part of the evaluation of an adult patient in PEA or with undifferentiated hypotension. In pediatric patients, Pershad *et al.* presented the "BLEEP" (bedside limited echocardiography by emergency physicians), which combined a protocol of LV function estimation and IVC measurement to apply to the assessment of a pediatric patient presenting with undifferentiated hypotension or shock. When over-read by pediatric cardiologists, emergency physicians were able to obtain acceptable quality images and accurately assess LV function and IVC volume.

To date, there is limited research dedicated towards the application of point-of-care, focused cardiac ultrasound in pediatric patients. However, Longjohn *et al.* recently evaluated the overall accuracy of point-of-care cardiac ultrasound performed by pediatric emergency medicine (PEM) physicians. The focused cardiac ultrasound included an assessment of LV systolic function, the presence or absence of a pericardial effusion, and IVC collapsibility to estimate cardiac preload. The overall sensitivity and specificity of point-of-care echocardiography compared with formal echo were 95% and 83% respectively. The PEM ultrasound agreed with the pediatric cardiologist's with a kappa of 0.87. Further research remains to be performed in pediatric patients with regards to resuscitation outcomes, and congenital heart disease.

Anatomy

It is important to be familiar with the cardiac anatomy prior to performing point-of-care, focused cardiac ultrasound. In addition to the four chambers of the heart and their corresponding valves (Figure 5.1), it is important to recognize the descending thoracic aorta and the IVC. The right ventricle is the most anterior structure, and can easily be identified on ultrasonography.

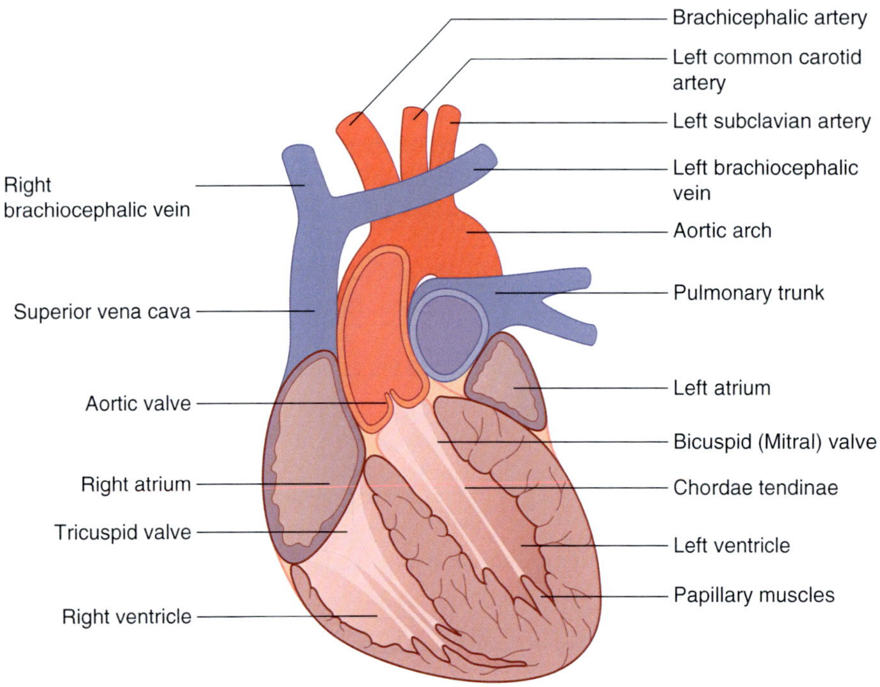

Figure 5.1 **Anatomy of the heart.** *Artwork created by Emily Evans © Cambridge University Press.*

Technique

Point-of-care questions

1. Is cardiac activity present? Asystole?
2. Is a pericardial effusion present? Are there signs of tamponade?
3. What is the global cardiac function (hyperdynamic, normal, depressed)?
4. Is there normal preload (IVC)? (See Chapter 7.)

Transducer selection and orientation

Low-frequency transducers should be utilized for the cardiac assessment. A 2–5 MHz phased-array or microconvex transducer with a small footprint is most often used in order to allow for imaging between ribs. For smaller children and neonates, a higher frequency (4–8 MHz) microconvex transducer is often required (Figure 5.2). While there is much controversy surrounding transducer orientation, emergency ultrasonographers often suggest utilizing the abdominal setting on the machine to avoid confusion. It is important to note that the "cardiac" settings on machines flip the image on the screen. Therefore, in order to create a screen image that is consistent with formal echocardiography and cardiologists, the indicator needs to be rotated 180° in relation to those transducer positions traditionally used by cardiologists. To complicate matters further, pediatric cardiologists flip the image vertically in order to most closely mirror the patient's anatomy, which is especially useful in complex congenital heart disease (Figure 5.3d). This is not routinely recommended in the emergent and critical care settings.

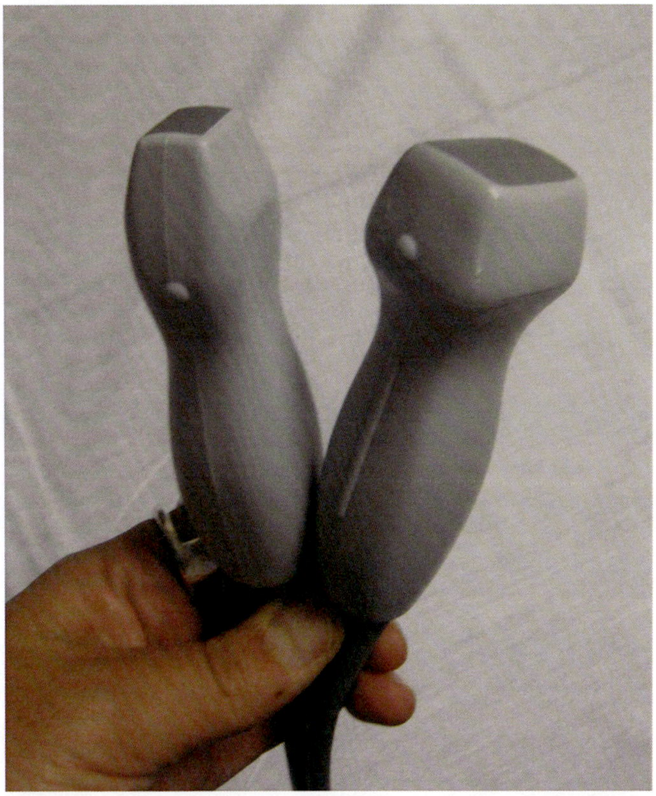

Figure 5.2 Microconvex and phased-array transducers (2–8 MHz), ideal for point-of-care cardiac ultrasonography. Note the small footprints, which can easily scan in between rib spaces. The transducer on the left is a higher-frequency (2–8 MHz) microconvex transducer, while the one on the right is the phased-array transducer.

Patient position and preparation

When approaching a pediatric patient in particular, positioning and patient comfort are paramount. Smaller children often require more preparation and patience. Measures to improve patient comfort and compliance with examinations include: warmed gel, lying in the parent's lap, and pacifiers or feeding during the examination. Since children have much smaller and superficial structures than adult patients, it is important to adjust the depth of the images accordingly.

Ultrasound imaging: views

Standard views for point-of-care, focused cardiac ultrasound include subxiphoid, parasternal long-axis, parasternal short-axis, and apical four-chamber views. Angling and tilting of the transducer may be necessary in order to obtain proper images (Figure 5.4). It is important to note that all abnormal findings should be confirmed with multiple cardiac views. Additional assessments involve IVC measurements for preload and hydration status (see Chapter 7).

Subxiphoid view

The subxiphoid view is the preferred view in the EFAST examination, and is the most useful during resuscitation, since it does not typically interfere with resuscitation and procedures. The indicator should be oriented to the patient's right side and is placed subcostally, just below the xiphoid process, directing the indicator towards the patient's left shoulder (Figure 5.5a). The transducer itself is quite flat (Figure 5.5b), and should be held at a 15° angle to the patient's body, in contrast to most other positionings which are perpendicular to the patient's body.

The subxiphoid view utilizes the liver as an acoustic window and readily visualizes all four chambers of the heart (Figure 5.5c–e). It is the most accurate in identifying pericardial effusions, especially at the posterior pericardium where effusions begin to develop. It may be difficult to obtain in obese patients or patients with abdominal distension.

Parasternal long-axis view

The parasternal long-axis view is the preferred view for the assessment of left ventricular contractility, and the identification of pericardial effusions when adequate subxiphoid images cannot be obtained. The transducer is placed perpendicular to the chest wall, immediately to the left of the sternum, between the third and fourth intercostal space, above the level of the nipple line. The indicator should be directed towards the patient's left hip, or 4 o'clock (Figure 5.6a). A distinguishing feature is that the aortic outflow tract is stacked on top of the left atrium (Figure 5.6a–d).

The parasternal long-axis view is best utilized to measure contractility. The left ventricular shortening fraction (SF),

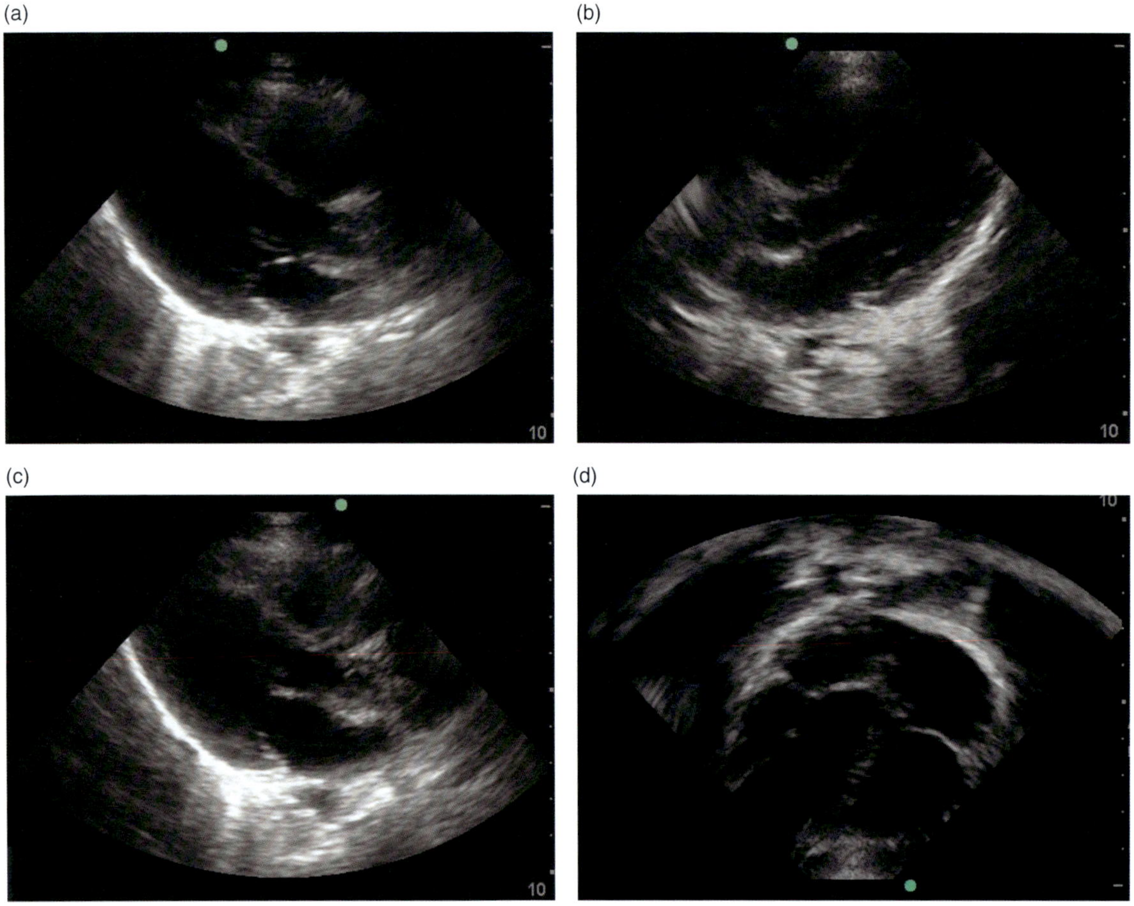

Figure 5.3 (d) Subxiphoid view, pediatric cardiologist's view. The image is flipped both horizontally and vertically, in order to most closely mirror anatomic orientation in the body. This is the apical four-chamber view.

which is expressed as a percentage, may be calculated by the formula:

$$\mathrm{SF} = \frac{(\textbf{End diastolic dimension} - \textbf{End systolic dimension})}{\textbf{End diastolic dimension}}$$

A normal calculated shortening fraction is greater than 30%. In a review of methods of sonographically determining LV function, McGowan *et al.* reported that visual estimation of cardiac function into normal mild, moderate, or severe dysfunction is as good or better than other more complex, calculated methods.

Parasternal short-axis view

The parasternal short-axis view readily allows evaluation of contractility and valvular function. Once the parasternal long-axis view is obtained, the transducer should be rotated 90°, in order to obtain the parasternal short-axis view. The indicator should be directed towards the patient's right hip, or 7 o'clock (Figure 5.7a). One can sweep the transducer from the base of the heart to the apex in order to visualize various levels of the heart in cross-section, from the level of the mitral valve, papillary muscles, and tricuspid valve. The distinguishing feature of the parasternal short-axis view is that the left ventricle (LV) is circular, with a valve in the middle, resembling a "fish-mouth" or "doughnut" (Figure 5.7b–d).

Apical four-chamber view

The apical four-chamber view is the preferred view for evaluating the relative dimensions of the right and left sides of the heart. The transducer is placed at the cardiac apex, which may be located by palpating the point of maximal impulse (PMI). This is typically located at the T4–5 level, at the fifth intercostal space, just lateral to the nipple. The indicator is typically oriented towards the patient's right side, or 9 o'clock (Figure 5.8a). The patient often needs to be rotated to their left side in order to bring the heart more anterior to the chest wall, and to decrease artifact associated with the left lung. In the apical four-chamber view, all four chambers may be visualized and compared for overall size and function (Figure 5.8b–d).

Ultrasound imaging: M-mode

M-mode, or motion mode, allows for a one-dimensional tracing of structure movement over time. While in the parasternal long-axis view, the cursor may be placed over the walls of the left ventricle, in order to assess for contractility (Figure 5.9a). This is the most effective method for evaluating for asystole (Figure 5.9b). It is important to note that, while performing this assessment to assess for cardiac contractions, compressions and artificial respirations must be held in order to avoid motion from external sources other than from the ventricle.

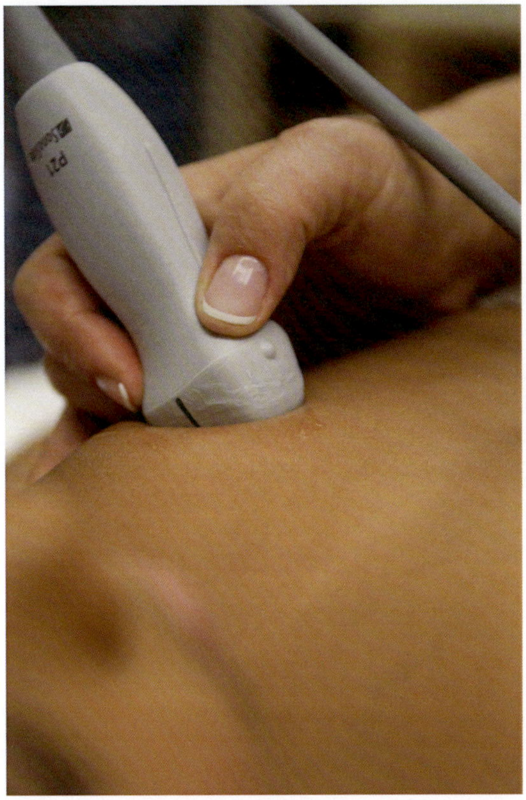

Figure 5.4 Moving the transducer. In order to obtain adequate cardiac windows, it is often necessary to rock and tilt the transducer.

Training and education

In order to grasp focused cardiac ultrasound adequately, it is crucial to become familiar with normal human cardiac anatomy. Jones *et al.* showed that, after a five-hour didactic course followed by one-hour of proctored practical echocardiography training, emergency medicine residents improved in their written and practical examinations regarding image acquisition and interpretation. In addition, commercially available cardiac ultrasound software programs provide simulation in order to recognize particular cardiac pathology (Figure 5.10). Examples of these include Blue Phantom (www.bluephantom.com) and CAE Vimedix^{TM} (www.cae.com).

Pathology

Asystole vs. pulseless electrical activity (PEA)

Pulseless cardiac arrest is the cessation of cardiac activity, and the absence of palpable central pulses. In children, it is especially important to determine whether a pulse is present to initiate early basic and advanced life support in order to improve survival. Unfortunately, pulse palpation is extremely unreliable in diagnosing pediatric cardiac arrest, with an accuracy of only 78%. However, ultrasonography can reliably distinguish cardiac activity from standstill and can be performed in 10 seconds, the time recommended to perform a pulse check. One can rapidly correlate the absence of left ventricular motion and the presence or absence of a pulse. Once the physician determines that the child is pulseless, it is crucial to identify potentially correctable causes of PEA, which include hypovolemia, hypothermia, hypo or hyperkalemia, acidosis, hypoxia, tamponade, tension pneumothorax, toxins, and a thromboembolism. Of these, point-of-care ultrasonography has the potential to rapidly identify tamponade, a tension pneumothorax, thromboembolism, and hypovolemia. It has been shown that in adult patients with PEA or near PEA, emergency physicians can detect pericardial effusions with correctable etiologies and distinguish these from true PEA with ventricular standstill.

Pericardial effusions, tamponade

Pericardial effusions may arise from acute processes, such as trauma or chronic effusions associated with neoplastic diseases, bacterial and fungal infections, or HIV. On sonography, a pericardial effusion appears as an anechoic or dark stripe surrounding the heart. Early effusions appear first at the posterior pericardium and eventually develop anteriorly, ultimately creating a circumferential effusion. An example of an abnormal subxiphoid view is of a child with dilated cardiomyopathy and a circumferential pericardial effusion (Figure 5.11).

Of particular clinical importance is the development of tamponade, which may lead to cardiovascular collapse and, ultimately, death. Cardiac tamponade is defined as the significant compression of the heart by accumulating pericardial contents and fluid. While as little as 150 mL of pericardial fluid may cause tamponade; when developed acutely, a more chronic process may have a much larger volume of fluid without creating tamponade. This development of fluid accumulation leads to increased intrapericardial pressure, progressive limitation of ventricular diastolic filling, and the reduction of stroke volume and cardiac output. Patients may present with nonspecific clinical findings of pulsus paradoxus, hypotension, and tachycardia. On physical examination, tamponade classically presents as Beck's triad, which consists of jugular venous distension, muffled heart tones, and hypotension. However, only one-third of patients with tamponade will have all three features of Beck's triad, and 10% of patients will not have any of them.

Cardiac ultrasonography is the most sensitive and specific means of detecting tamponade, and has the potential to detect early signs of tamponade before the patient becomes unstable. Features of sonographic tamponade include a circumferential pericardial effusion, with a hyperdynamic heart that may exhibit right atrial compression during late diastole and right ventricular collapse during early diastole, also known as "scalloping." Other sonographic findings may include abnormal mitral valve motion, a dilated IVC with lack of inspiratory collapse, and a "swinging heart." A swinging heart is the counterclockwise rotational movement of the heart, and appears late in tamponade.

Pericardiocentesis

Tamponade is the indication for emergent pericardiocentesis (see Chapter 21). "Few medical situations exist in which a

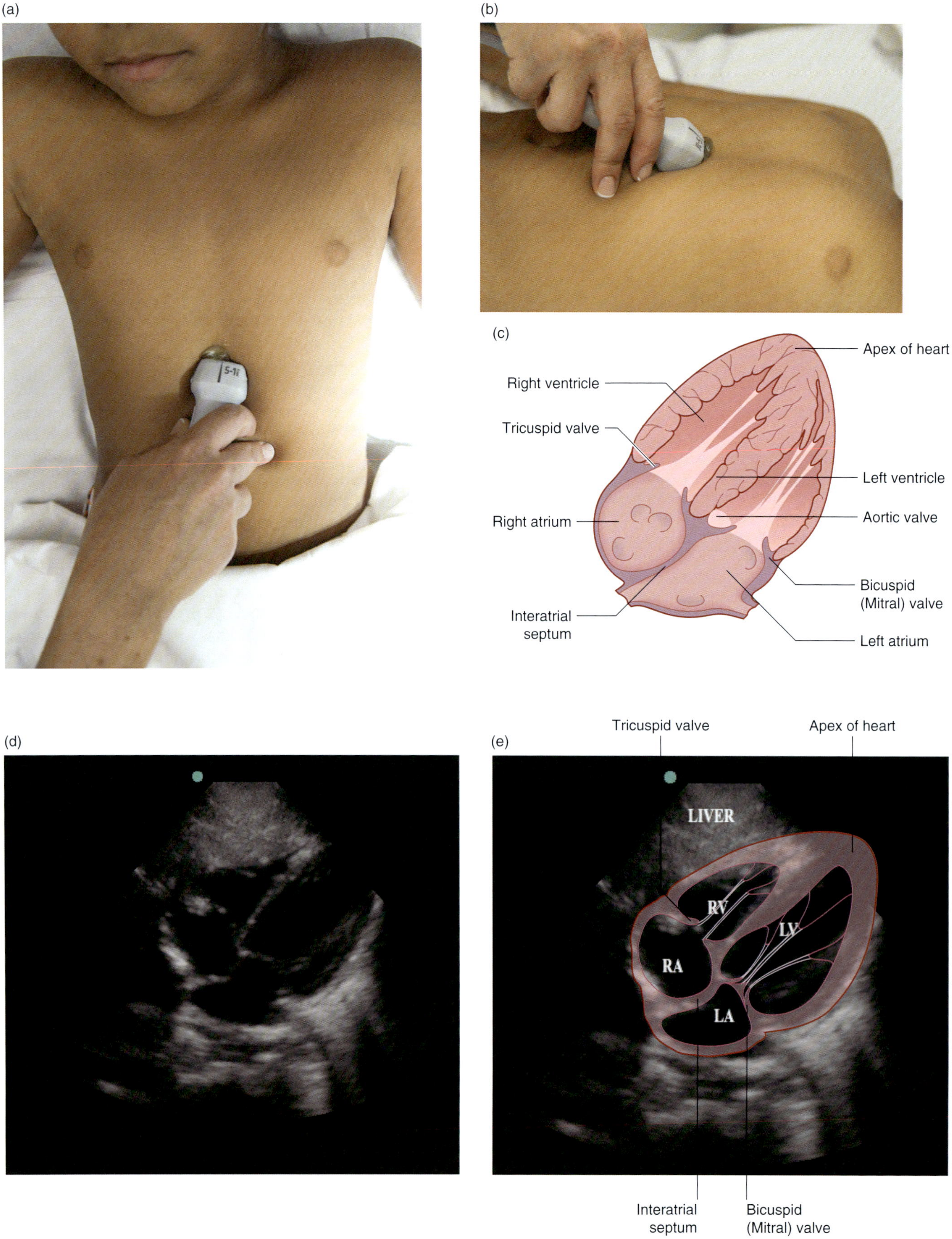

Figure 5.5 Cardiac imaging, subxiphoid view. (a) The transducer is oriented with the indicator towards the patient's right, slightly angled towards the patient's left shoulder. (b) The transducer is placed relatively flat against the patient, at approximately a 15° angle to the patient's body. (d) Ultrasound image of the subxiphoid view. (e) The liver is shown anteriorly. The most anterior structure is the right ventricle (RV). The left ventricle (LV), right atrium (RA), and left atrium (LA) are easily visualized. *Artwork created by Emily Evans © Cambridge University Press.*

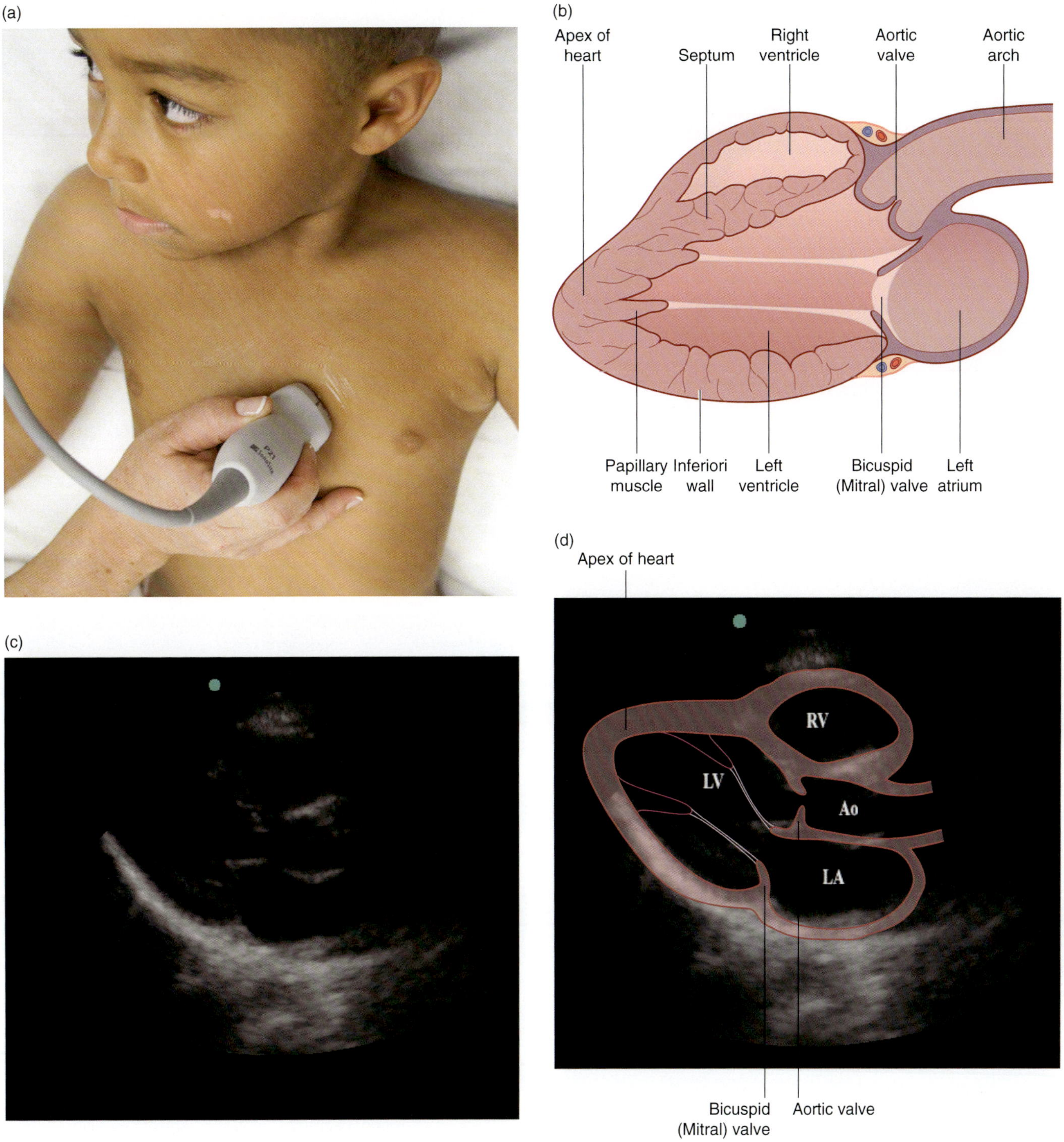

Figure 5.6 Cardiac imaging, parasternal long-axis view. (a) The transducer is placed just lateral to the sternum and is oriented with the indicator oriented towards the patient's left hip, or 4 o'clock and perpendicular to the patient's chest wall (b) Illustration demonstrating the corresponding anatomy. Right ventricular outflow tract (RVOT); left ventricular outflow tract (LVOT); aortic valve (AV); mitral valve (MV). (c) Ultrasound image of the parasternal long-axis view. (d) Left ventricle (LV), right ventricle (RV), aortic outflow tract (Ao), and left atrium (LA). Note that, in the parasternal long-axis view, the right atrium is not visualized. *Artwork created by Emily Evans © Cambridge University Press.*

simple, quickly performed medical procedure can result in immediate life-saving results."

The routine use of ultrasound for pericardiocentesis is strongly encouraged, as it is the most effective means of reducing complications. Prior to the advent of ultrasonography for pericardiocentesis, the complication rate associated with the blind approach was approximately 7–50%. Sonographically, the parasternal long-axis view, in particular, provides a more direct anatomic approach, with direct visualization of the needle. This approach is associated with fewer of the cardiac

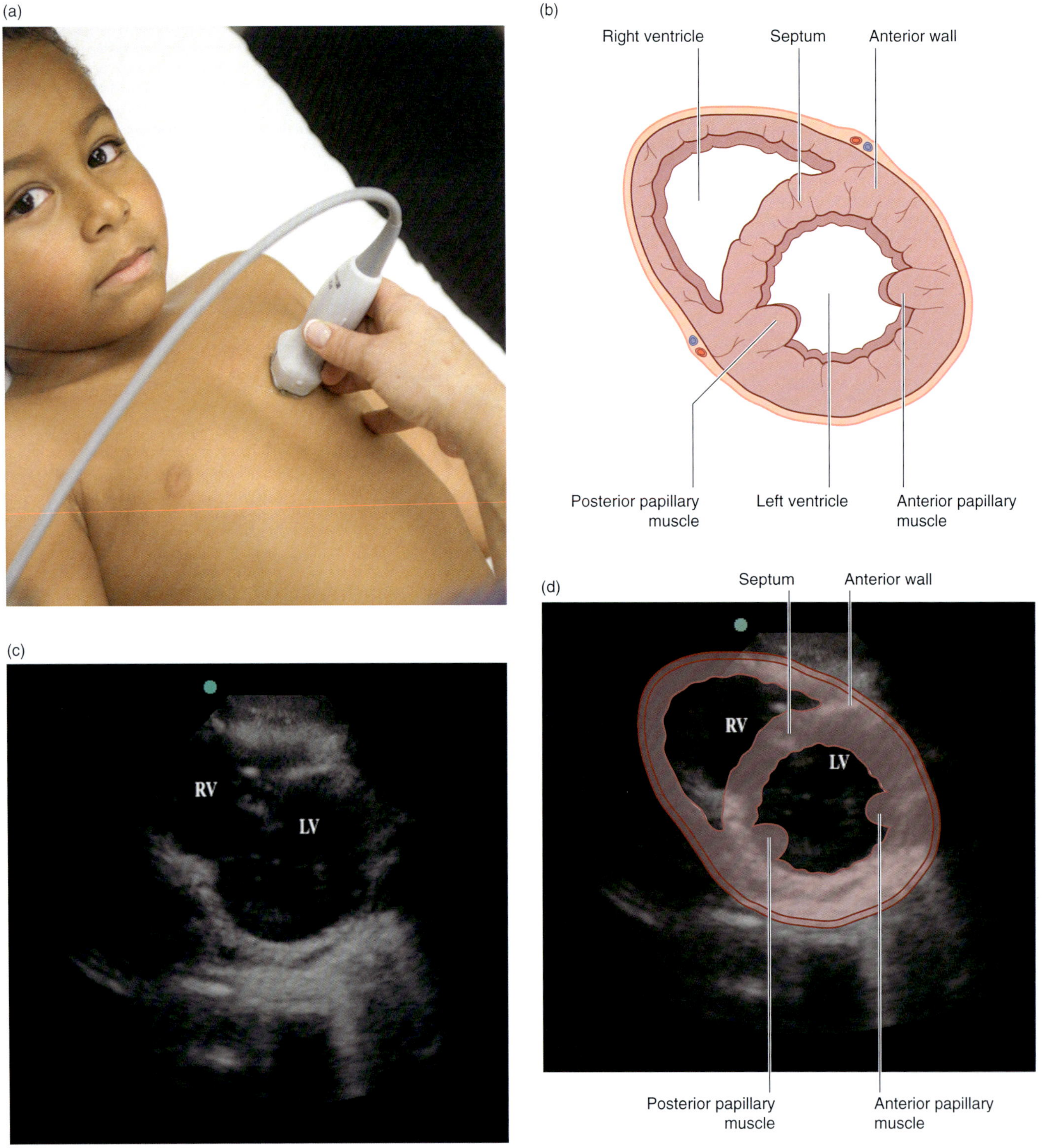

Figure 5.7 The parasternal short-axis view. (a) The transducer is oriented with the indicator towards the patient's right hip, or 7 o'clock. This is a 90° rotation from the parasternal long-axis view. (b) Illustration depicting the anatomy seen in the parasternal short-axis view. (c) Ultrasound image of the parasternal short-axis view, which is also known as the "doughnut" or "fish-mouth" view. (d) Illustration demonstrating the corresponding anatomy. *Artwork created by Emily Evans © Cambridge University Press.*

lacerations, pneumothoraces, pneumoperitoneum, and liver lacerations often associated with pericardiocentesis. A study of ultrasound-guided pericardiocentesis in pediatric patients showed a 99% success rate, with 93% on the first attempt, and 1% major complication and 3% minor complication rate.

Undifferentiated shock, hypotension

A common presenting problem in the emergency department is dehydration. This is especially common in pediatrics, with approximately 9% of children presenting with varying degrees

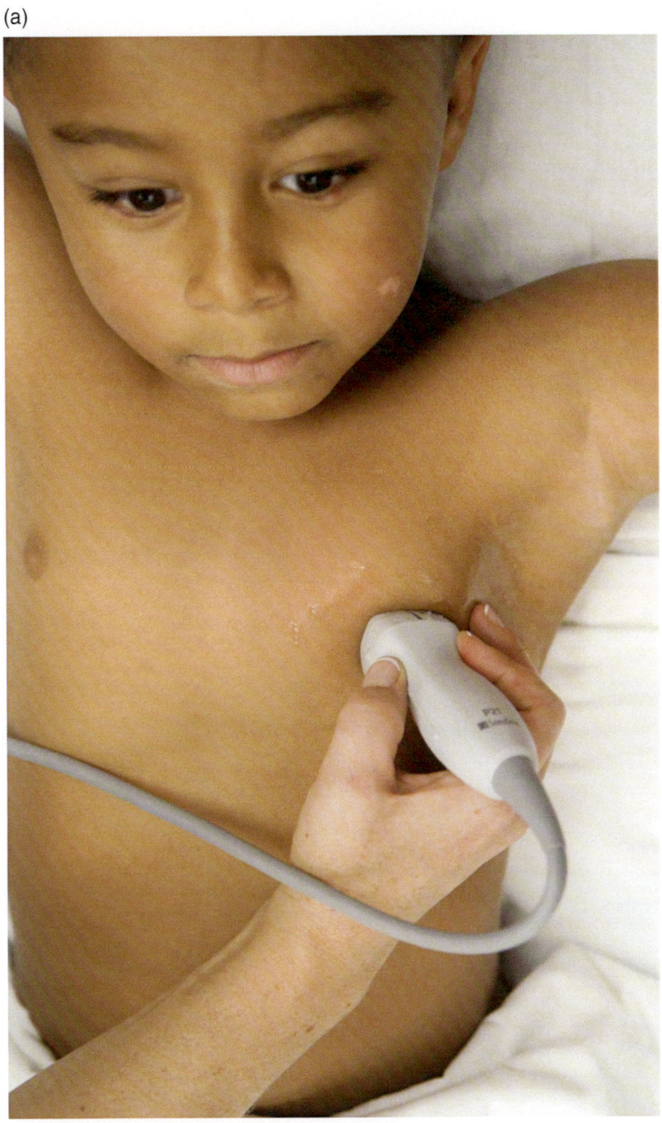

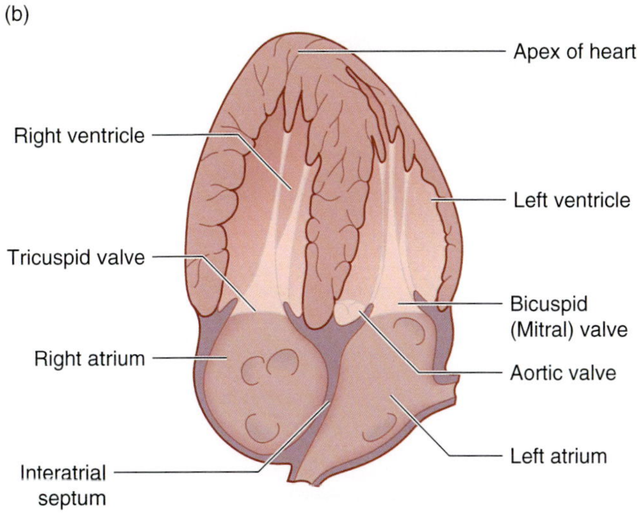

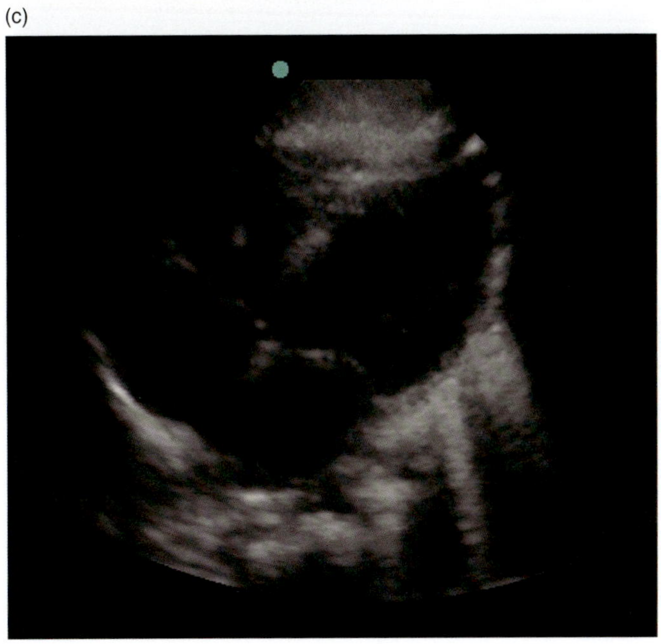

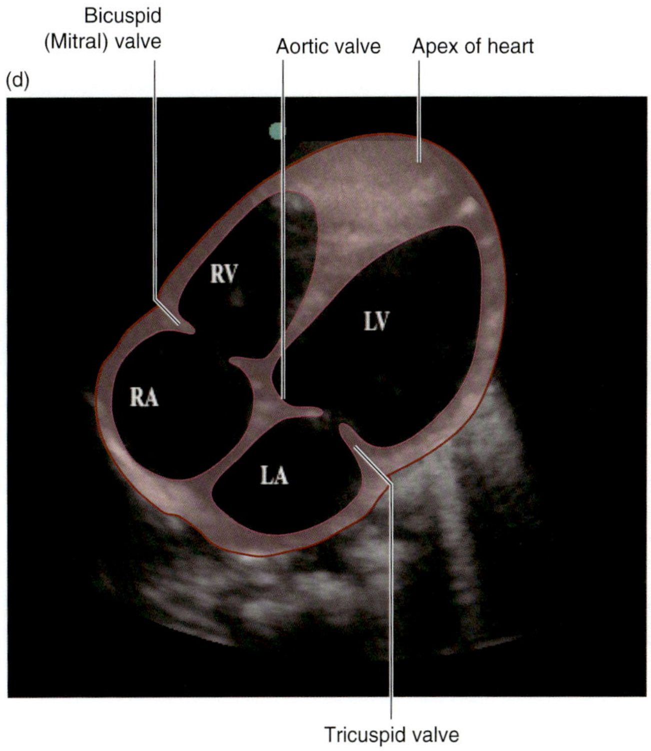

Figure 5.8 The apical four-chamber view. (a) The transducer is placed lateral to the sternum, oriented with the indicator towards the patient's right side. In teenage and adult patients, the apical four-chamber view is usually located more laterally at the nipple line. (b) Illustration depicting the anatomical structures seen in the apical four-chamber view. (c) Ultrasound image of the apical four-chamber view. (d) Illustration demonstrating the corresponding anatomy: right ventricle (RV), left ventricle (LV), right atrium (RA), and left atrium (LA). *Artwork created by Emily Evans © Cambridge University Press.*

(a) (b)

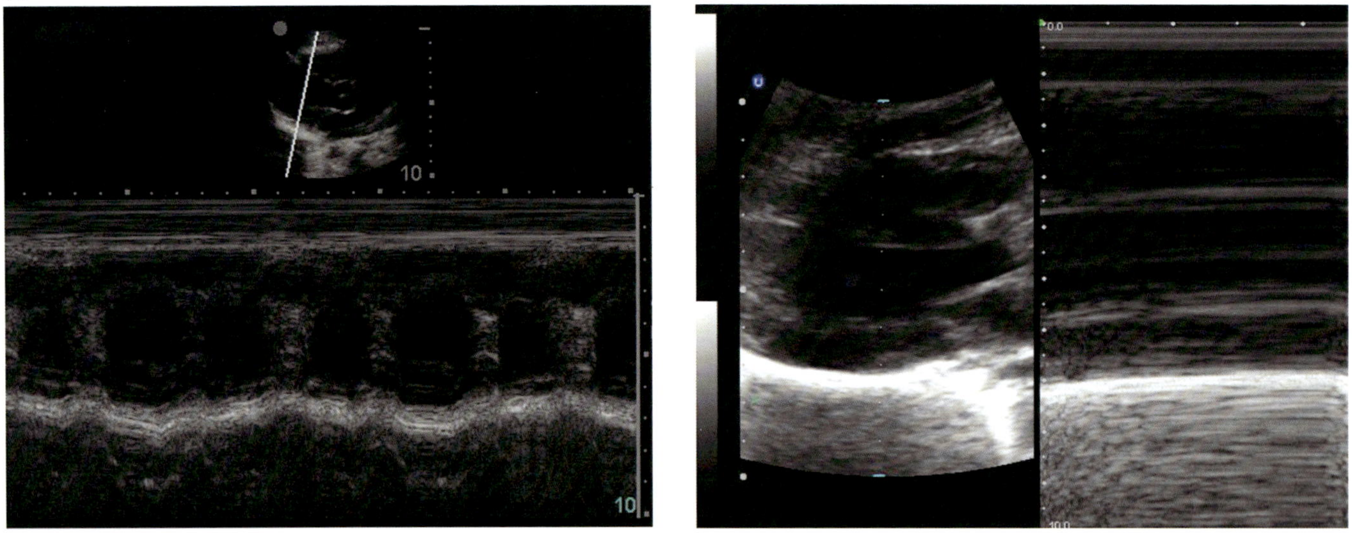

Figure 5.9 M-mode. When the cursor is placed over the left ventricular walls, cardiac contractions are plotted on the one-dimensional representation of motion. (a) Normal cardiac activity on M-mode. (b) The absence of cardiac contractions, or asystole, on M-mode.

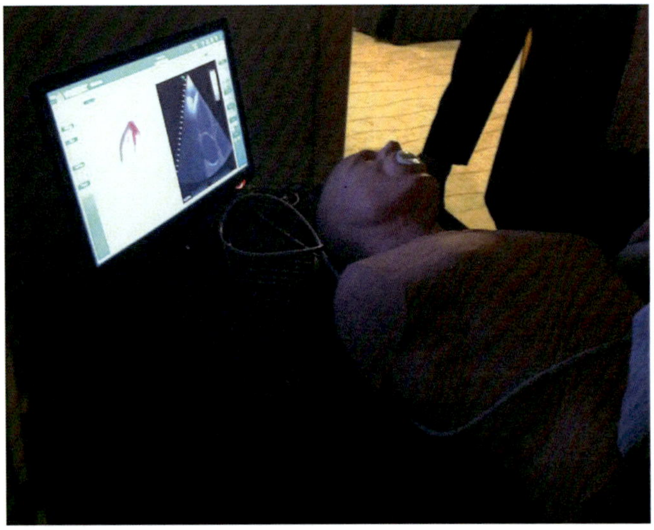

Figure 5.10 Cardiac simulator.

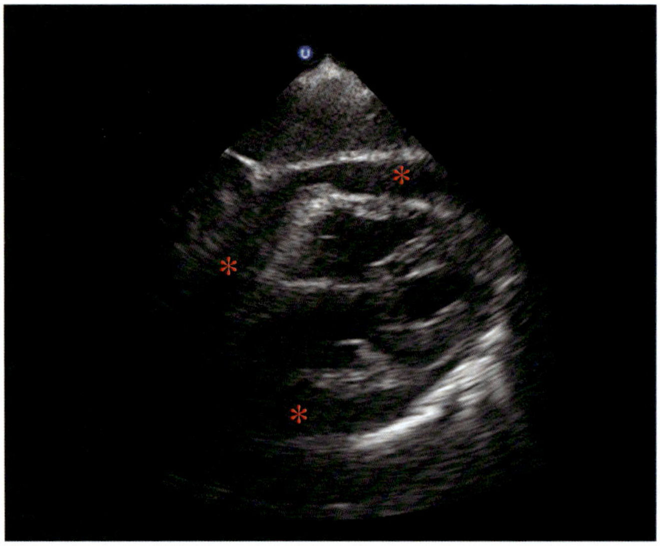

Figure 5.11 Subxiphoid view of a large circumferential pericardial effusion (*).

of dehydration. Unfortunately, hydration status is often difficult to assess since physical examination findings and laboratory studies are often inconsistent and unreliable. As dehydration progresses, shock may develop, which is defined as the failure of the circulatory system to provide adequate oxygen delivery to vital organs. The types of shock may be categorized as hypovolemic, distributive, and cardiogenic. It is often difficult to distinguish between the different etiologies of shock, but this is important in being able to treat appropriately.

The sonographic assessment of left ventricular function, or ejection fraction, may be useful in patients presenting with undifferentiated hypotension or shock. This may expeditiously narrow the differential diagnosis (i.e. distinguishing cardiogenic from hypovolemic shock) to begin early aggressive and appropriate resuscitation. Another means by which ultrasound can aid in evaluating shock and hydration status is the estimation of CVP by performing measurements of the IVC (see Chapter 7).

Congenital heart disease

The incidence of congenital heart disease in the United States is approximately 8–10 cases per 1,000 live births. The age at presentation can vary according to the specific type of lesion. Further, while cardiac emergencies are uncommon in children and the majority of children do not present with ischemic heart disease, the majority of cardiac pathology encompasses congenital heart disease. Such anatomic lesions include tetralogy of Fallot, Hypoplastic Left Heart Syndrome, Atrial Septal Defects (ASDs), and Ventricular Septal Defects (VSDs), to name just a

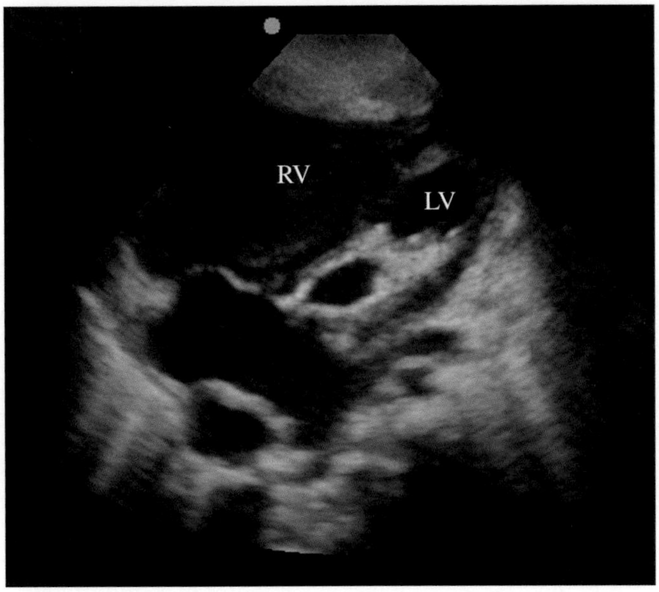

Figure 5.12 The apical four-chamber view of a five-year-old child with repaired hypoplastic left heart syndrome. Note the extremely small size of the left ventricle (LV) in relation to the right ventricle (RV).

few. While the identification of particular congenital heart lesions is complex and beyond the scope of point-of-care echocardiography, patients may present with associated pathology that immediately affects cardiac care. An example of an abnormal apical four-chamber is a child with repaired Hypoplastic Left Heart Syndrome (Figure 5.12). Other acquired disorders, such as dilated cardiomyopathy, may also be identified (see Figure 5.13).

Of particular concern is the infant who presents with shock and in whom it is difficult to distinguish between primary respiratory pathology and congenital heart disease associated with ductal closure. Further cardiac presentations include adolescents who may be evaluated for "sentinel events" and are at risk of sudden cardiac death. Other pathologies include infective endocarditis, hypoxemic attacks (congenital heart disease with reduced pulmonary blood flow), and acute Rheumatic Fever. Point-of-care echocardiography can promptly and easily address specific questions, and identify ventricular dysfunction and pericardial effusions. This may be especially important where there are no pediatric subspecialists readily available. There remains much research to be conducted in determining the utility of point-of-care ultrasound to assess for congenital heart diseases and to facilitate the care of the children who present with them.

Scanning tips

Pitfalls

- There are various methods for performing point-of-care ultrasound for focused cardiac ultrasound. This can often be confusing to the novice sonographer.

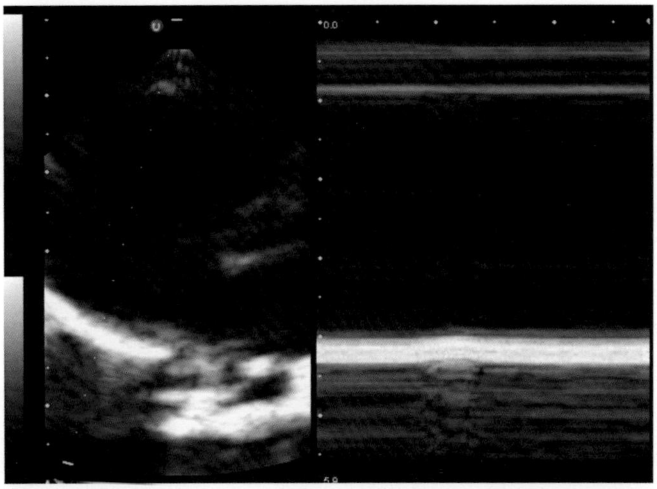

Figure 5.13 Case 1. M-mode of asystole shows the absence of contractions over time. It is important to correctly position the M-mode cursor over the walls of the left ventricle, rather than the valves, in order to correctly assess whether there is the presence of contractions.

- Obtaining the subxiphoid view may be especially difficult in patients presenting with abdominal pain, nausea, or a large body habitus.
- Scanning windows in smaller children tend to be extremely close to the sternum, and superficial (depth needs to be changed significantly).
- An epicardial fat pad may be confused for a pericardial effusion.
- Avoid utilizing point-of-care ultrasonography to identify complex cardiac lesions, such as those present with congenital heart disease

Tips to improve scanning

✓ Choose one method of scanning the heart in order to maintain consistency and avoid confusion.

✓ Use smallest possible footprint, especially in small children, in order to be able to facilitate scanning through the ribs. A higher-frequency transducer may be necessary.

✓ In order to obtain adequate cardiac views, it is often necessary to scan close to the sternum in smaller children and infants.

✓ For the subxiphoid view, use the liver as an acoustic window. Be sure to have the transducer flat against the abdominal wall, with the indicator directed towards the patient's left shoulder.

✓ In order to improve cardiac windows, patient positioning may help: when supine, have the patient bend his/her knees. Alternatively, place the patient on his/her left side, with the left arm above the head.

✓ Consult with pediatric cardiologists and obtain formal echocardiography whenever a finding is in question, or when a more comprehensive examination is necessary.

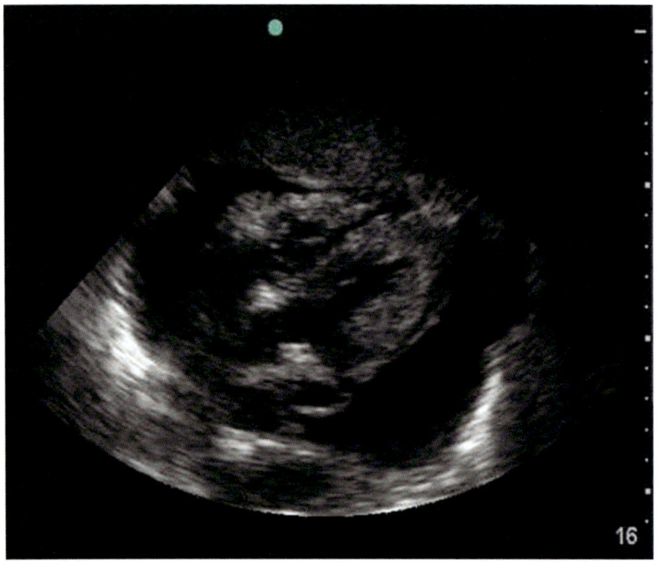

Figure 5.14 **Case 2**. Subxiphoid view of pericardial tamponade, with a large circumferential pericardial effusion and right ventricular scalloping.

Cases

1. A one-month-old baby is brought in by EMS after being found apneic and pulseless at home. Mother had awakened in the morning to find her infant "blue and lifeless" after an unknown period of time. The baby had been well when she put him to sleep a few hours prior. In the field, the child is intubated, and an intraosseous line is placed. Compressions are performed, and multiple doses of epinephrine and atropine are administered. The child arrives at the emergency department with active cardiopulmonary resuscitation (CPR) and compressions in progress. On physical examination, it is difficult to determine whether there are palpable central pulses. A point-of-care cardiac ultrasound is performed in order to evaluate for contractility and asystole. There is no cardiac motion, which is confirmed on M-mode (Figure 5.13). As a result, resuscitative efforts are discontinued.

   In this case, a baby presents after an unknown but presumably prolonged "down time." Cardiopulmonary resuscitation and the administration of several doses of resuscitative medications were unsuccessful in restoring cardiac activity. It is often difficult to reliably determine whether there are palpable pulses in a code situation. Several studies have shown that the pulse evaluation is extremely unreliable. Point-of-care ultrasonography can be extremely helpful in confirming the presence or absence of cardiac activity both by visual estimation and by M-mode. This further helps the clinician, resuscitative team, and family members objectively see that there are no cardiac contractions, and that further resuscitative efforts would be futile.
2. A seven-year-old male presents with a flu-like illness for the past few days. He has developed persistent, profuse vomiting over the past few days, with the inability to tolerate liquids. His triage vital signs are: T 41.3 °C, HR 167 bpm, RR 42/min, BP 70/40 mmHg, pulse oximetry 92% on room air. Immediately after being brought into an examination room, he becomes apneic and unresponsive. He is brought into a resuscitation room where he is intubated, his airway secured, and vascular access is obtained. Pulses are unable to be palpated, so compressions are initiated. The rhythm on the monitor is sinus bradycardia, with a heart rate of 67 bpm. Due to the presentation of PEA, a point-of-care ultrasound is performed in order to evaluate for reversible causes of PEA. Immediately, a large pericardial effusion is appreciated (Figure 5.14). As a result, an emergent pericardiocentesis is performed successfully with real-time ultrasound guidance. The patient is stabilized and is brought to the operating room, where the cardiothoracic surgeons perform a pericardial window procedure.

   In this case, ultrasonography was able to identify a reversible cause of PEA, which was a pericardial effusion. Ultrasound can further assist in performing an emergent pericardiocentesis, with improved safety and decreased complications associated with performing the procedure. In this case, pericardial effusion was likely associated with an infectious process, such as influenza. While extremely rare in children, their presentation can be acutely life threatening. The prompt recognition of a pericardial effusion is especially crucial in a critically ill patient, where a pericardiocentesis can be life saving.
3. A five-year-old boy presents with intermittent chest pain and dyspnea for the past week. It has become much worse over the past day, and the child has become diaphoretic with occasional grunting. The patient's vital signs are: T 38.0 °C, HR 132 bpm, RR 42/min, BP 82/38 mmHg, pulse oximetry 92% on room air. He is uncomfortable and ill appearing. He is sitting upright to breathe more easily. He is placed on oxygen with improvement in his saturations. On examination, the patient is tachypneic and only able to take shallow inspirations. He has coarse breath sounds throughout all lung fields. On cardiac examination, there are no murmurs, gallops, or rubs appreciated, with strong central pulses. A chest radiograph is obtained, which shows pleural effusions and cardiomegaly (Figure 5.15a). As a result, a point-of-care ultrasound examination is performed. In order to evaluate the pleural effusions, the ultrasound is performed at the right upper quadrant (Figure 5.15b) and the left upper quadrant (Figure 5.15c), which shows bilateral pleural effusions. Finally, four views of the heart are obtained. The parasternal long-axis view shows an anechoic pericardial effusion that does not extend past the descending thoracic aorta. This is a moderate organized circumferential pericardial effusion (Figure 5.15d). Since the patient is stable, pediatric cardiology is consulted and drainage is performed in the operating room. The patient actually returns to the

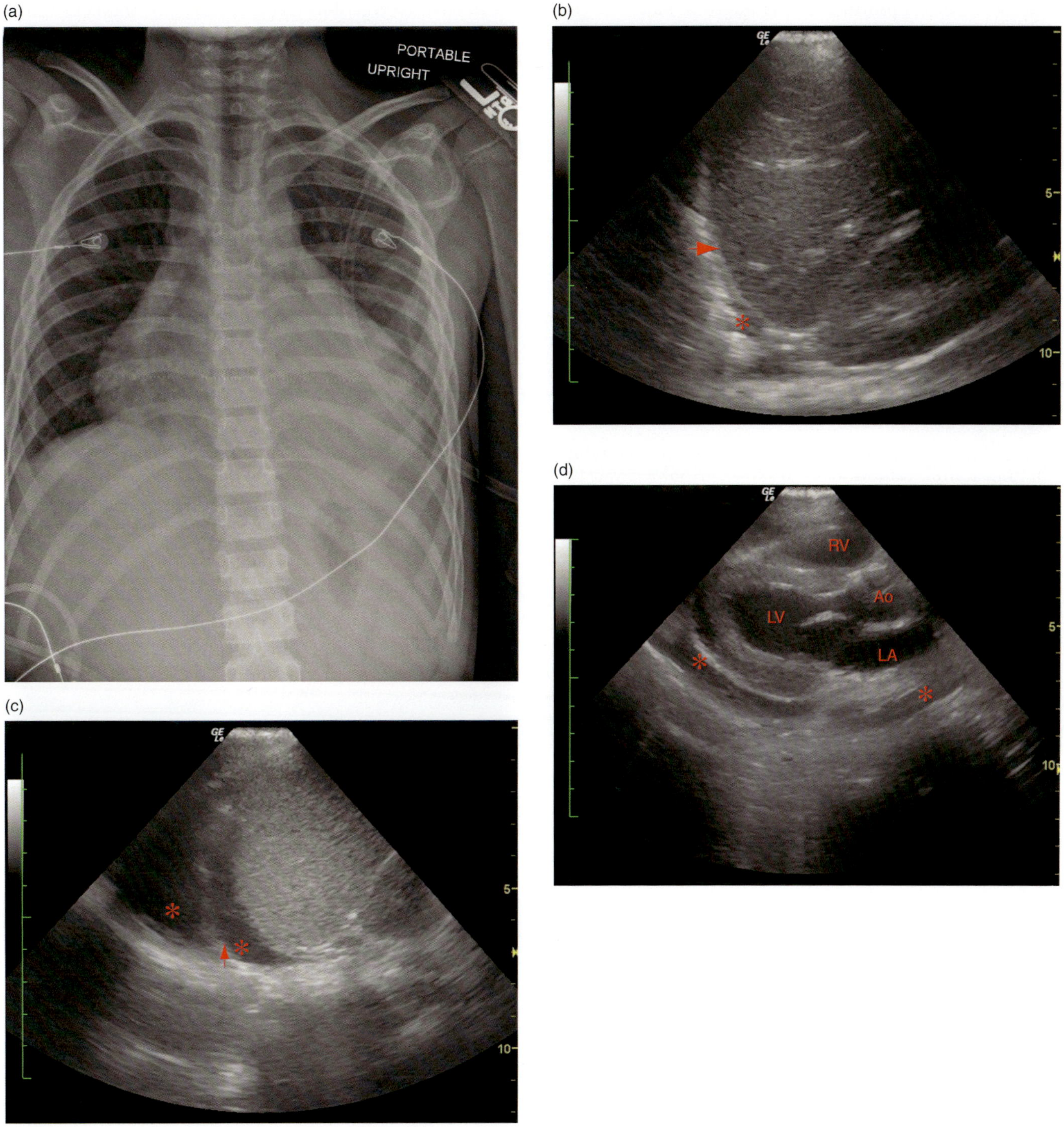

Figure 5.15 Case 3: pericardial effusion and pleural effusions. (a) Chest radiograph, showing pleural effusions and cardiomegaly. (b) Right upper quadrant view, showing a large pleural effusion (*) above the diaphragm (arrow). (c) Left upper quadrant view, showing a small pleural effusion(*); the arrow again indicates the diaphragm. (d) Parasternal long-axis view, showing a moderate organized circumferential pericardial effusion (*). Other structures visualized are the left ventricle (LV), right ventricle (RV), left atrium (LA), and aortic outflow tract (Ao).

emergency department on several occasions with recurrent pericardial and pleural effusions. Unfortunately, no cause could be identified.

This case highlights the utility of point-of-care ultrasonography in evaluating pleural effusions and pericardial effusions. Though they occur rarely in children, ultrasonography is much more specific and provides more detail than conventional radiographs. One can also distinguish between a pericardial and pleural effusion, since a pericardial effusion will not extend past the descending thoracic aorta. The findings on the point-of-care study, allows for more expeditious consultation of the pediatric cardiologists and pediatric cardiac surgeons. Most importantly, point-of-care ultrasound can be paramount in preventing further decompensation of the patient in the emergency department.

Summary/key points

1. While point-of-care ultrasound has only recently become incorporated into the practice of Pediatric Emergency Medicine, several well-established adult applications may be applied towards the care of pediatric patients.
2. Point-of-care focused cardiac ultrasound can be used for the identification of pericardial effusions and tamponade, the assessment of PEA, and asystole. In addition, assessments can be made regarding global contractility, and IVC evaluation for preload.
3. The cardiac views include the subxiphoid, parasternal long-axis, parasternal short-axis, and apical four-chamber views.
4. More research remains to be performed with the application of point-of-care ultrasonography with regards to the early recognition of congenital heart disease and for other pediatric-specific pathologies.
5. Point-of-care focused cardiac ultrasound should not replace formal echocardiography. For a more comprehensive study or when findings are in question, it is crucial to consult a pediatric cardiologist and obtain formal echocardiography.

Selected references

Blaivas, M., Fox, J. (2001) Outcome in cardiac arrest patients found to have cardiac standstill on the bedside emergency department echocardiogram. *Acad Emerg Med* **8**: 616–21.

Doniger, S.J. (2010) Bedside emergency cardiac ultrasound in children. *J Emerg Trauma Shock* **3**(3): 282–91.

Jones A., Craddock P., Tayal V., *et al.* (2003) Focused training of emergency medicine residents in goal-directed echocardiography: a prospective study. *Acad Emerg Med* **10**: 1054–8.

Labovitz, A.J., Noble, V.E., Bierig, M., *et al.* (2010) Focused cardiac ultrasound in the emergent setting: a consensus statement of the Society of Echocardiography and American College of Emergency Physicians. *J Am Soc Echocardiogr* **23**(12): 1225–30.

Longjohn, M., Wan, J., Joshi, V., *et al.* (2011) Point-of-care echocardiography by pediatric emergency physicians. *Ped Emerg Care* **27**(8): 693–6.

Mandavia, D., Hoffner, R., Mahaney, K., *et al.* (2001) Bedside echocardiography by emergency physicians. *Ann Emerg Med* **38**: 377–82.

Moore, C. (2008) Current issues with emergency cardiac ultrasound probe and image conventions. *Acad Emerg Med* **15**: 278–84.

Pershad, J., Myers, S., Plouman, C., *et al.* (2004) Bedside limited echocardiography by the emergency physician is accurate during evaluation of the critically ill patient. *Pediatrics* **114**: e667–71.

Tayal, V., Kline, J. (2003) Emergency echocardiography to detect pericardial effusion in patients in PEA and near-PEA states. *Resuscitation* **59**: 315–18.

Tsung, J., Blaivas, M. (2008) Feasibility of correlating the pulse check with focused point-of-care echocardiography during pediatric cardiac arrest: a case series. *Resuscitation* **77**: 264–9.

Chapter 6

Pulmonary ultrasound

Fernando Silva and Roberto Copetti

Objectives/indications

Pulmonary ultrasound is without question one of the more exciting and controversial fields of emergency and critical care sonography. It is exciting, because it allows for the immediate bedside diagnosis of conditions that traditionally require logistically complex maneuvers, such as the transport of critically ill patients, the use of expensive and bulky equipment, and the dependence on other specialists' expertise for interpretation. All of the above increase risk, time, and radiation exposure, not to mention expense. Pulmonary ultrasound is also rather controversial. While, at first sight, pulmonary ultrasound seems quite objective and has a steep learning curve, it relies fundamentally on the interpretation of artifacts, rather than anatomical structures, to guide the diagnostic process. Therefore, this leaves room for the oversimplification, and the potential for the misunderstanding, of a powerful decision tool. The very basic principles of image acquisition must be respected even after one becomes an experienced lung sonographer.

In the early days of lung ultrasound, the skeptical novice sonographer would question even the most basic of applications of lung ultrasound, such as for pneumothorax and pleural effusions. Today, a massive body of literature on adult patients, in conjunction with extensive clinical practice, has made lung ultrasound an important clinical diagnostic tool. Now, the next step is to expand the body of research, and incorporate lung sonography into clinical practice of more complex applications like pneumonia, interstitial syndromes, and pulmonary embolism.

The well-established applications of lung ultrasound may also be integrated in the management of pediatric patients. Lung ultrasound is especially effective and attractive in children, since they generally have thinner chest walls and a smaller thoracic width, which facilitates ultrasound imaging. Lung ultrasound may be useful in identifying not only the basic applications for the detection of pneumothoraces and pleural effusions, but in the diagnosis of pneumonia, and atelectasis. This chapter will describe both the basic and advanced applications of lung sonography, with a special focus on pediatric patients. The first consensus conference in pleural and lung ultrasound created a major document to support these new and advanced applications in both adult and pediatric patients. We use the nomenclature and description of techniques endorsed by this consensus statement in this chapter.

Background

Lung ultrasound, while relatively new, has evolved into being a modality that can easily and rapidly detect pneumothoraces and pleural effusions. Conventional methods of identifying a pneumothorax include auscultation, portable chest radiographs, and tomography. When compared with portable radiographs, point-of-care ultrasonograpy may actually be more sensitive, with a feasibility of 98.1%. Chest radiographs are especially inaccurate in a supine patient, since air layering anteriorly is difficult to detect. Blaivas *et al.* showed ultrasound to be superior to chest radiographs in identifying traumatic pneumothoraces, having a sensitivity of 98.1% and specificity of 99.2%, compared with chest radiographs, which have a sensitivity of 75.5% and specificity of 100%. When performing a more comprehensive lung assessment, one may further differentiate between a small, medium, and large pneumothorax. When compared to chest radiographs for a traumatic hemothorax, ultrasonography is comparable, with sensitivities of 96.2%.

Several studies have shown that ultrasound signs of lung and pleural pathology found in in adult patients can also be seen in pediatric patients and neonates. Lung ultrasound has similar diagnostic capabilities to chest radiographs in diagnosing respiratory distress syndrome (RDS), and demonstrates unique findings specific to transient tachypnea of the newborn (TTN) (see Chapter 23). Copetti *et al.* found that lung ultrasound performs similarly to conventional radiographs, in the diagnosis of pneumonias in children. More recently, Caiulo *et al.* compared lung ultrasound to chest X-ray in children with bronchiolitis. While lung ultrasound identified more lung abnormalities not found on chest radiographs, all patients with a normal lung ultrasound examination had a normal chest radiograph. Therefore, there is the potential that, with the further development of lung ultrasound in pediatric patients, the utilization of conventional radiographs may be decreased in a wide variety of clinical scenarios, thereby decreasing radiation exposure in children.

Anatomy

Lung ultrasound, in contrast to most ultrasound examinations, is not based on the anatomic representation of the organ itself (Figure 6.1), but on the artifacts generated by the lung. The same principle by which lung was once excluded as an organ that could be studied by ultrasound, is in fact the basis of all the

Pediatric Emergency and Critical Care Ultrasound, ed. Stephanie J. Doniger. Published by Cambridge University Press.

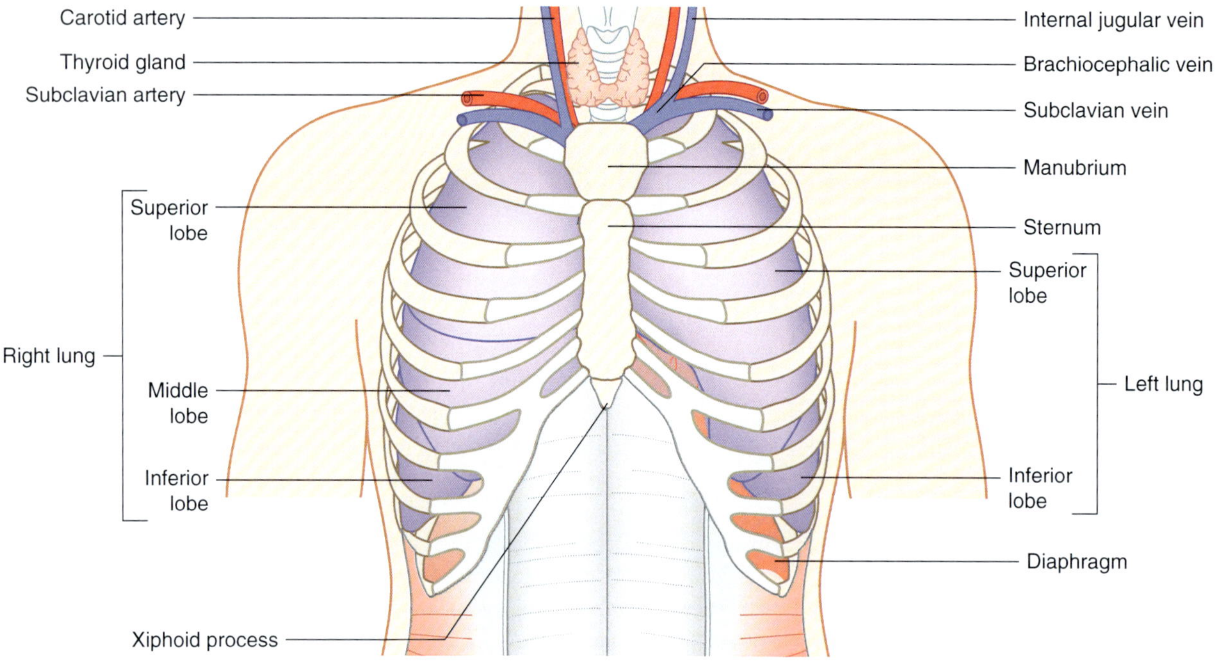

Figure 6.1 Anatomy of the lung. While lung ultrasonography actually does not rely on specific anatomic structures within the lung, it is important to recognize the relationship of the lung with other structures in the thoracic cavity. *Artwork created by Emily Evans © Cambridge University Press.*

technique of pulmonary and pleural sonography: ultrasound is "reflected" by air. Immediately underlying the pleural line, the most prevalent element is air. When a sound wave traverses an interface between two media, the fraction of reflected energy (R) is directly proportional to the difference in acoustic impedance between these media. In the case of chest wall (soft tissue) and lung (air), R is close to 1. Therefore the fraction of energy that is transmitted ($1 - R$) is nil. Therefore, the ultrasound machine renders an image under the pleural line, as generated by the scattering, reflection, and reverberation artifacts (see Chapter 1).

Technique

Point-of-care questions

1. Is a pneumothorax present?
2. Is a pleural effusion present?
3. Are A-lines or B-lines present?
4. Was endotracheal intubation successful?

Transducer selection and orientation

Virtually all types of transducers (Figure 6.2a) have been successfully used in pulmonary ultrasound. The most frequently utilized transducers are the convex 2–5 MHz and linear 5–10 MHz transducers. Convex-array (or abdominal) transducers can also be used, but calcified ribs can be somewhat of an obstacle because of the large footprint. As a general rule, a small-footprint transducer should be used in order to allow for imaging between the ribs. However, the footprint should not be so small that the ribs are not visualized on a longitudinal intercostal scan, since they are the reference to identify the pleural line and lung sliding. This is not a major concern when imaging younger children with non-calcified ribs, where one can image through them and still have their visual reference (Figure 6.5d). Usually a microconvex transducer (Figure 6.2b) offers a small footprint that still allows for visualizing ribs, while maintaining a good image resolution. This transducer can also image other structures like the heart and abdomen, allowing for the quick, complete examination of an unstable patient without changing transducers. If a microconvex transducer is not available, a phased-array transducer offers the same flexibility, but with worse image resolution in the proximal fields. Overall, linear transducers offer the best resolution. Their depth is much more limited, to usually not more than 8 cm. However, this does not seem to be a hindrance in the pediatric population, if the examination is going to be limited to the pleural level. Most of the pediatric literature has described lung ultrasounography with linear transducers.

Paradoxically, modern and advanced ultrasound machines can pose a problem for optimal lung imaging, since these devices excel in eliminating artifacts, which are actually what is needed to image the lung. Usually if a modern machine offers a preset for lung, it will most likely be optimized for pleural effusion, but not for the air artifacts. Older devices with minimal post-processing capabilities tend to generate excellent lung imaging. We encourage the reader to take a look at an older machine prior to programming a lung preset on a modern device. A cardiac preset is usually a good starting point. Make sure to turn off all the post-processing filters, adjust the setting "persistence" to zero, and pick a high-contrast grayscale map.

Patient position and preparation

The pulmonary surface is quite large, and a complete examination would require quite a long time. In most cases, a very focused examination will be much more rapid, and will provide the diagnostic answer to the condition we are looking for.

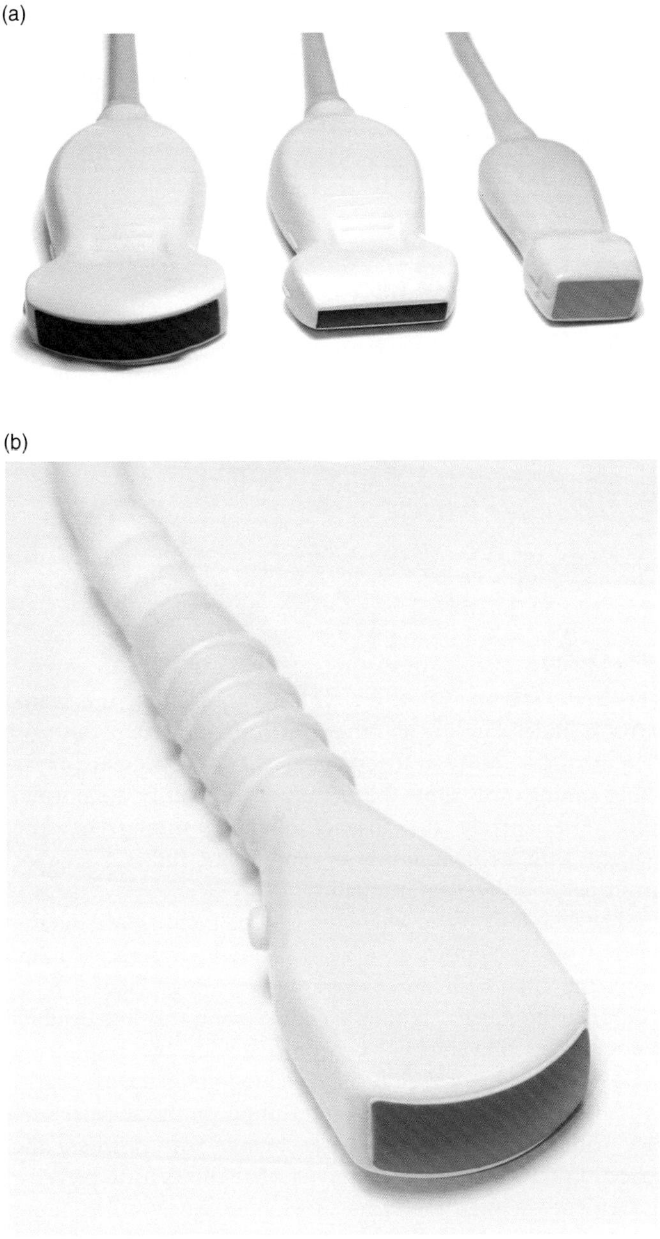

Figure 6.2 Transducers. The most commonly used transducers for lung ultrasonography: (a) curvilinear (left), linear (center), and phased array (right). (b) Microconvex transducer.

Usually a two-phase approach is recommended: initially performing a quick screening scan in the resuscitation phase, followed by a more comprehensive examination. The patient can be examined in a supine or seated position, obviously depending on the clinical condition. In general, pleural effusions are more easily detected in a seated patient, while pneumothoraces are more easily detected in a supine patient. The lateral decubitus positioning can be used to assess the posterior regions on a ventilated patient.

Screening examination

On the initial assessment of an unstable patient, the "A" (airway) and "B" (breathing) of the resuscitation algorithm can be evaluated with examination of two single locations on each side of the chest wall (Figure 6.3). Considering that free air is less dense and fluid is denser than the pulmonary parenchyma, air will behave like a bubble and rise, and fluid will flow to the more dependent regions. The highest spot on each side of the chest, which on the supine patient is approximately at the level of the fourth intercostal space slightly medial to the midclavicular line (Figure 6.3a), will have the highest sensitivity to exclude a pneumothorax. This location can also be used for the indirect assessment of correct placement of an endotracheal tube. A posterolateral scan, in a supine patient (Figure 6.3b), will have high sensitivity for excluding a hemothorax or pleural effusion, particularly at the level of the costophrenic recess. This posterolateral scan is similar to the transducer placement used for the FAST examination, which is a natural transition from the pulmonary examination.

Comprehensive examination

Many techniques have been developed in order to simplify the examination of the entire lung surface, particularly for interstitial syndromes. The method currently recommended by a consensus of experts consists of performing "one spot" scans of 11 regions of the thorax, 6 at each side, with exclusion of the cardiac region on the left (Figure 6.4). With this approach, a very large area of the pulmonary surface is covered within a very short time, while obtaining a good evaluation of the extent of pathology. The regions on each side are the superior and inferior halves of the anterior aspect of the chest, vertically limited by the parasternal, midclavicular, and anterior axillary lines, and superior and inferior halves of the lateral wall between the anterior and posterior axillary lines. The cardiac region (lower medial on left anterior chest) is excluded.

Detailed examination

If we continue to suspect the presence of a small pulmonary consolidation and effusion, a "whole lung" examination can be performed by scanning all intercostal spaces in their entire extent anteriorly, laterally, and posteriorly, from cranial to caudal. In adults and teenagers, this can be more laborious, but in smaller children a large-footprint transducer and the absence of calcified ribs renders this examination quite straightforward. In addition, when we already know there is a focal pathologic process previously found during our screening or comprehensive examinations or by other methods (chest radiograph, CT scans), we can directly examine the region we already know contains the disease.

Ultrasound imaging: artifacts and signs

The normal lung

It is of utmost importance to master the correct identification of the pleural line within the chest wall, while avoiding its confusion with muscle and fascia layers. The pleural line can be identified as a hyperechoic line immediately deep to the ribs. The ribs are the visual reference points to finding the pleural line (Figure 6.5a). Start by imaging the lung at the

(a)

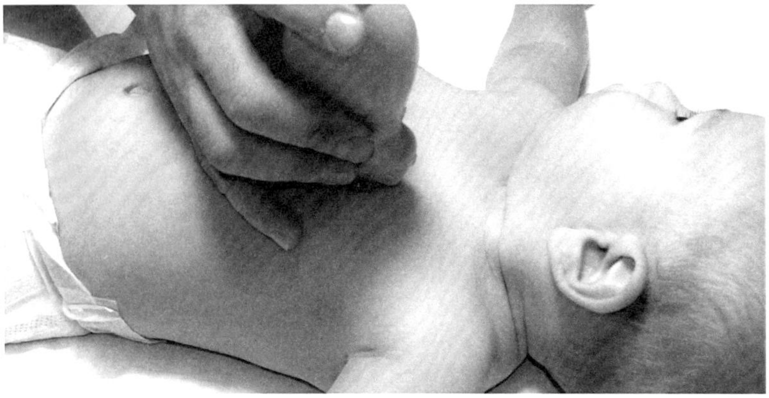

(b)

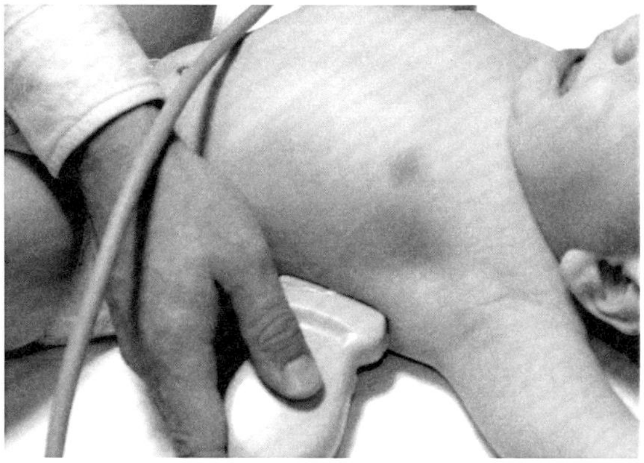

Figure 6.3 Screening examination. (a) Limited lung examination, which is useful post-intubation and for screening for a pneumothorax. The highest spot on the chest is the first scanned. This is usually at the midclavicular line, at the level of the fourth intercostal space. (b) Limited lung examination to identify a hemothorax/pleural effusion. The second scan is at the most posterior spot that can be reached without rotating the patient.

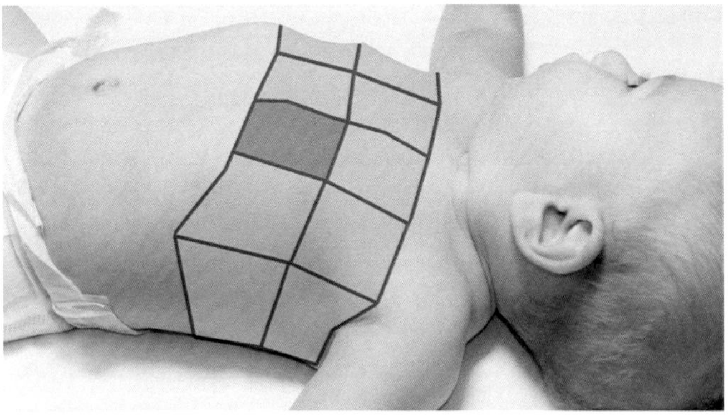

Figure 6.4 Comprehensive examination. The 11 regions of the comprehensive examination. This includes superior and inferior regions of each side, limited by the parasternal, hemiclavicular, anterior axillary, and posterior axillary line. The cardiac region is excluded (shaded).

level of an intercostal space with a longitudinal transducer orientation, with the indicator towards the patient's head. The first step is to identify the ribs with their posterior shadows. These shadows follow the transducer's array: with linear transducers they are vertical and parallel to each other and with phased-array or convex-array transducers they are divergent. The pleural line is then identified immediately below the ribs and should exhibit lung sliding. The typical image formed by two ribs with the pleural line between them is referred to as the "bat sign," resembling a bat with open wings (Figure 6.5b,c). The normal artifact pattern is present underlying the pleural line, where "A-lines" can usually be identified. In many cases, the simple identification of the presence or absence of lung sliding is enough to obtain a diagnosis, but if more detailed pleural visualization is necessary, the transducer can now be rotated 90° to a position parallel to the length of the intercostal space, removing the ribs from the field and increasing the surface of visualized pleura.

Lung sliding

This is the starting point for all lung ultrasound, and is the basis to understanding all other pleuropulmonary pathology. Acquiring the ability to adequately identify the presence of the "lung sliding" will allow the examiner to identify the normal lung. Alternatively, the absence of "lung sliding" may be evident with a pneumothorax, and is an indirect sign of improper endotracheal intubation.

The anatomic plane where the visceral pleura glides on the parietal pleura appears as a nearly straight hyperechoic line along the chest wall on sonographic imaging (Figures 6.6a, 6.7a). During normal ventilatory movement, this line exhibits a to-and-fro movement synchronized with the respiratory cycle. This line has a slightly rough sonographic texture that is caused by the reflection of the ultrasound on the alveolar surface within the pulmonary parenchyma. This is where the reflection occurs, and this texture is what allows us to perceive movement on this line. This moving image is called "lung sliding," and its detection conveys the fact that the visceral pleura is in direct contact with the parietal pleura and that there is lung expansion. The lung sliding is less prominent at the apical regions, where there is less pulmonary expansion, and more prominent on the bases, where there is maximal expansion and pleural gliding. At the costophrenic sinuses the "curtain sign" can be seen, when the aerated lung slides into the image during inspiration, "covering" the image of the subdiaphragmatic structures like a curtain.

M-mode signs: seashore and stratosphere signs, lung pulse

On M-mode, the entire image deep to the pleural line is a reflection artifact; on dynamic imaging, it exhibits a typical "sparkling" pattern synchronized with the pleural movement. In order to capture a still image of this dynamic process and improve the visualization of lung sliding, M-mode can be utilized to generate what is known as the "seashore sign" (Figures 6.6a, 6.7a). This

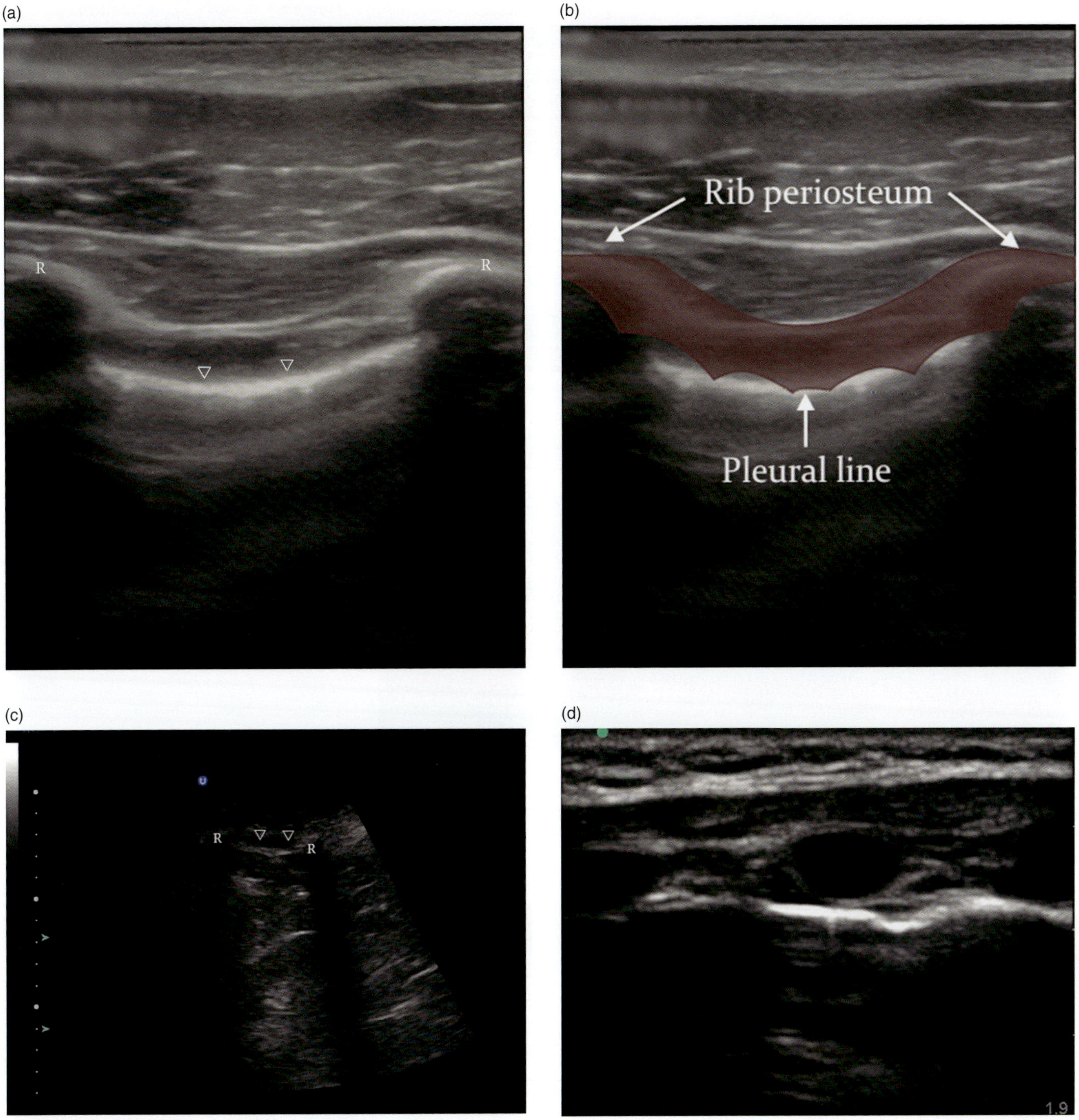

Figure 6.5 Lung imaging, the pleural line. (a) Lung sliding is present at the level of the pleural line (arrowheads), immediately deep to the ribs (R). (b) The landmarks for identifying the pleural line are referred to as the "bat sign," where the wings of the bat represent the ribs and the pleural line is the bat's body. *Illustration by Laura Berg, MD.* (c) The "bat sign" with the curved-array transducer. (d) The pleural line and ribs in a baby; the ribs are non-calcified and the entire pleural line is visible deep to the ribs.

sign is so named because the non-moving chest wall appears as horizontal lines (ocean waves) and the sparkling artifact appears as a grainy pattern (sandy beach) (Figures 6.6a, 6.7a). It demonstrates that the visceral pleura slides directly on the parietal pleura by using one single still image. In contrast, the "stratosphere sign" is the classic sign present in pneumothorax (Figures 6.6b, 6.7b). The ultrasound beam hits the free air directly beneath the parietal pleura after traversing the chest wall, and is immediately reflected back to the transducer without any scatter caused by the underlying alveolar structure. In addition to abolishing lung sliding, the pneumothorax also disrupts the "sparkling" artifact deep to it. All the artifact deep to the pleura line will be static. Therefore M-mode will register only horizontal lines: the "stratosphere sign" (Figures 6.6b, 6.7b). The "seashore sign" and "stratosphere sign" M-mode patterns can also be seen with a linear high-frequency transducer (Figure 6.7a,b).

(a)

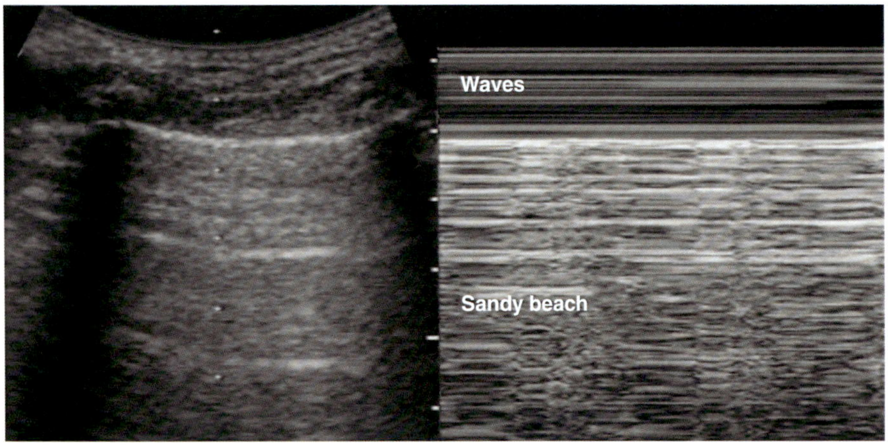

(b)

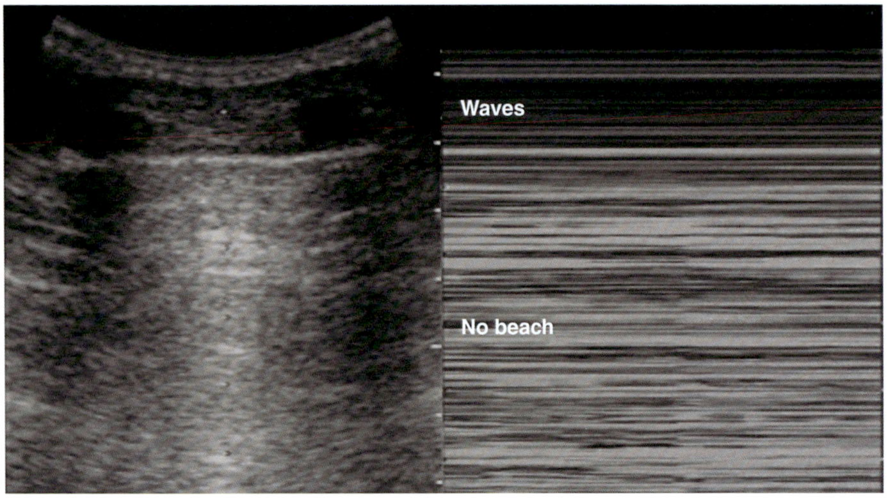

Figure 6.6 M-mode. (a) The "seashore sign" is normal lung sliding in M-mode, which generates a pattern of two different regions: waves and a sandy beach. The horizontal lines (waves) register the absence of movement of the chest wall, and the artifacts deep to the lung sliding on the pleural line generate the grainy pattern (sandy beach). (b) The "stratosphere sign" is the absence of pleural contact; all the artifact is static, as well as the chest wall, generating only horizontal lines in M-mode. This pattern is seen with a pneumothorax.

(a)

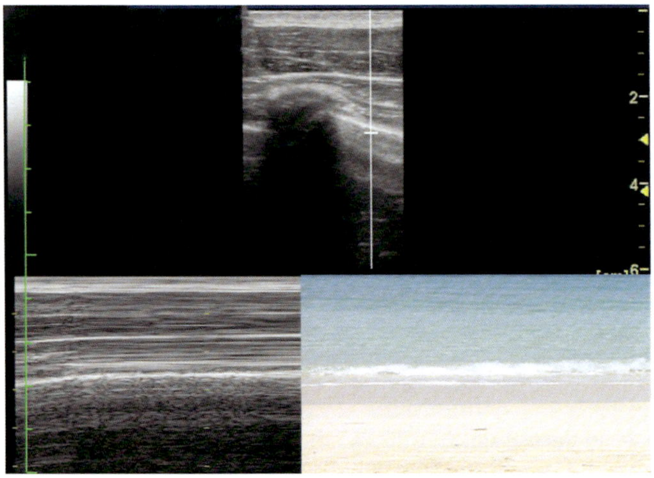

(b)

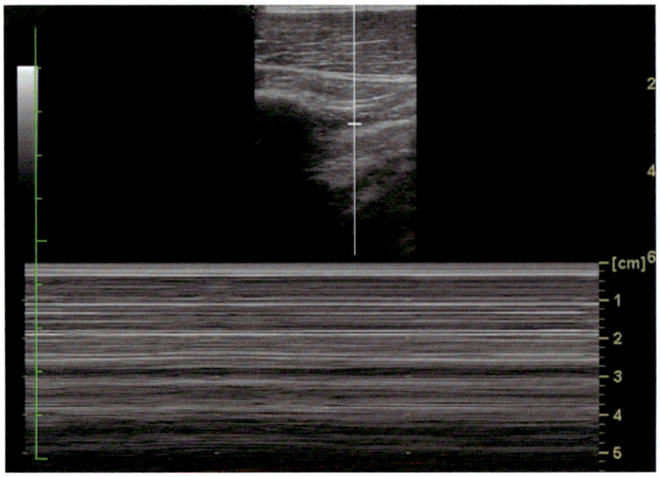

Figure 6.7 M-mode. (a) The "seashore sign" in M-mode, using a linear transducer. (b) The "stratosphere sign" in M-mode, using a linear transducer.

In the non-ventilated lung (i.e. apnea, mainstem intubation, complete atelectasis), the visceral pleura will still present with a tiny rhythmic movement synchronous with the cardiac cycle, caused by the arterial pulse, and by the movement of the heart itself. This can be perceived as minute to-and-fro movements visually identical to the lung sliding, but short and rapid. The presence of this "lung pulse" means that there is pleural contact but there is no pulmonary expansion. M-mode will register

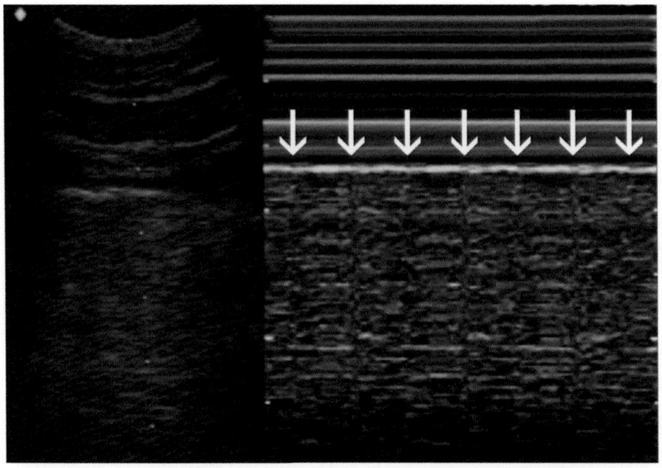

Figure 6.8 Lung pulse. In the absence of lung expansion, the systolic cardiac pulsation can be visualized as a rhythmic movement of the pleural line. This can be seen as regular perturbations in the "seashore sign" (arrows), synchronous with the heartbeat.

rhythmic interferences on a striped seashore pattern (Figure 6.8). This can easily be simulated in the normal individual by holding one's breath.

Water-content artifacts: A-lines and B-lines

"A-lines" (Figure 6.9a,b) are horizontal lines parallel to the pleural line, and are a product of the reverberation of the ultrasound beam between the pleura and the transducer. Since A-lines are generated by the presence of air, as in normal parenchyma, they will also be present in aerated pathologic conditions, such as a pneumothorax or a mainstem intubation. Of note, A-lines are not always seen; their expression depends on the machine's settings and processing filters. The production of A-lines also depends on the transducer's scanning angle; using a perpendicular scanning angle most often generates them.

When the ultrasound waves hit the pulmonary parenchyma, this highly aerated tissue is interpreted as air by the machine. The thin interalveolar and interlobular septa have widths in a range of dimensions inferior to the wavelength of the ultrasound beam, and are therefore below the transducer's resolution. When there is a pathologic process that causes thickening of these septa and/or partial filling of alveoli by fluid, they become large enough to conduct the ultrasound beam. However, since these thickened septa are surrounded by air, they create an intense reverberation artifact. This reverberation appears as a specific kind of ring-down artifact called "B-lines." These artifacts have characteristics that must be identified in order to avoid confusion with other artifacts of different sonographic significance. B-lines arise from the pleural line, move with the pleura during the respiratory cycle, reach the edges of the screen without fading, and are well-defined "laser like" hyperechoic lines. They follow the transducer's array, being parallel to each other with linear-array transducers (Figure 6.10a) and divergent with convex arrays (Figure 6.10b). In fact, B-lines actually "erase" the A-lines. These artifacts have consistently been shown to be highly sensitive for any interstitial process such as acute respiratory distress syndrome (ARDS), infant respiratory distress syndrome (IRDS), Transient Tachypnea of the Newborn (TTN), cardiogenic pulmonary edema, interstitial pneumonias, and pulmonary contusions. Additionally, they are found to respect the anatomic distribution of the process. For example, there are diffuse B-lines in cardiogenic pulmonary edema, focal B-lines in pulmonary contusions, and patchy B-lines in ARDS/IRDS. The finding of a few isolated B-lines is common in the normal lung, particularly at the lung bases. However, the presence of more than three B-line artifacts that are simultaneously visible on an intercostal scan should be considered pathologic. Usually the normal patient will not exhibit more than eight B-lines on the entire pulmonary surface.

As the amount of extravascular lung water increases, the type of artifact generated evolves in a regular pattern (Table 6.1). Of note, the expression "water" refers sonographycally to hypoechoic or anechoic fluid of any origin. Since A-lines and B-lines are primarily reverberation artifacts, the use of high-tech filters and post-processing can eliminate or decrease them, particularly the A-lines.

C-lines: consolidations

Consolidations, also called "*C-lines*" are actually not seen as artifacts, but as soft tissue–like regions in direct contact with the visceral pleura. They usually are of intermediate echogenicity, but occasionally appear hypoechoic, underlie the pleural line, and move with lung sliding during the respiratory cycle. The shape and distribution of the consolidations will vary with the specific etiology. Acute respiratory distress syndrome exhibits multiple, small, subpleural consolidations, more abundant on the more severely affected lung regions. Atelectasis and pneumonia, unless limited by lobar septa, have a gradual transition from aerated to non-aerated parenchyma, which appears as an irregular border surrounded by B-lines. Air bronchograms can be seen within these consolidations. Usually embolic processes appear wedged-shaped, and metastatic cancer appears round-shaped; both are well demarcated.

Training and education

The most widespread use of ultrasound has been for the detection of a pneumothorax. However, there have been challenges in developing reliable training models. Cadaveric models have been described. Most recently, Bloch *et al.* suggested a novel approach in utilizing live porcine models.

Scanning tips

Pitfalls

- Lung ultrasound, as with all sonography, is operator dependent. The recognition of lung sliding can be tricky for the novice examiner.
- The presence of lung sliding excludes a pneumothorax.

Table 6.1 A review of the sonographic artifacts seen with various pathologies. Normal lung has a normal amount of water and therefore has some A-lines with lung sliding.

Pathology	Water	Artifacts
Normal lung	Normal amount	A-lines with lung sliding
Pneumothorax	No water	Pure A-lines
Interstitial syndromes, edema	Increased water content in aerated lung	B-lines
Pneumonia, atelectasis	Water-filled parenchyma	C-lines (consolidation)
Pleural effusion	Water only	No A-lines, B-lines, or C-lines

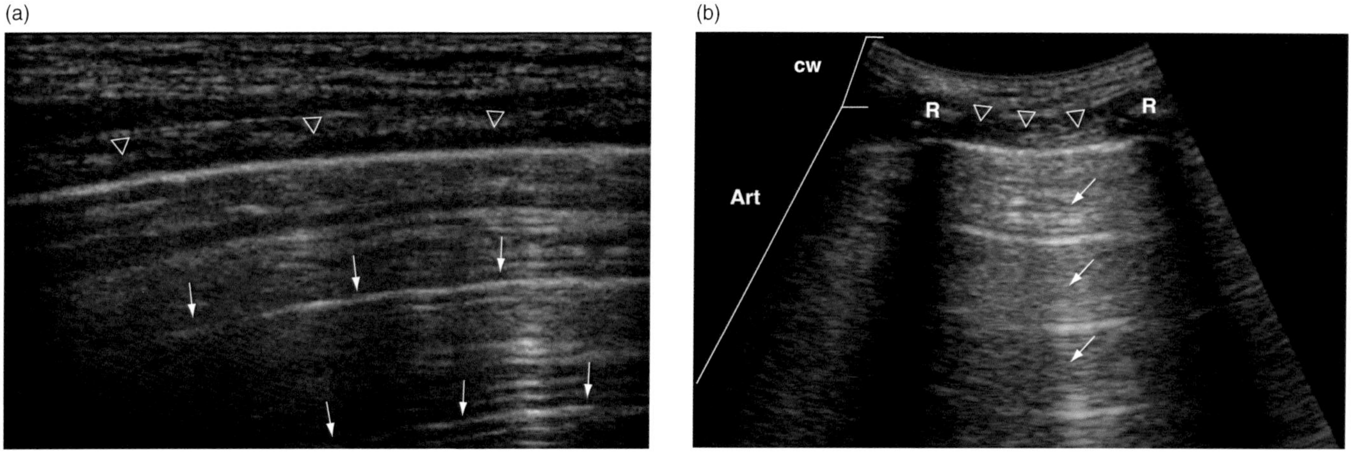

Figure 6.9 A-lines. (a) A-lines (arrows) are reverberation artifacts that reproduce the image of the pleural line (arrowheads). (b) Longitudinal intercostal scan, normal lung: the ribs (R) are seen in the chest wall (CW). All of the image deep to the pleural line is artifactual (Art), composed of the rib shadows and the A-lines (arrows) within the sparkling pattern artifact.

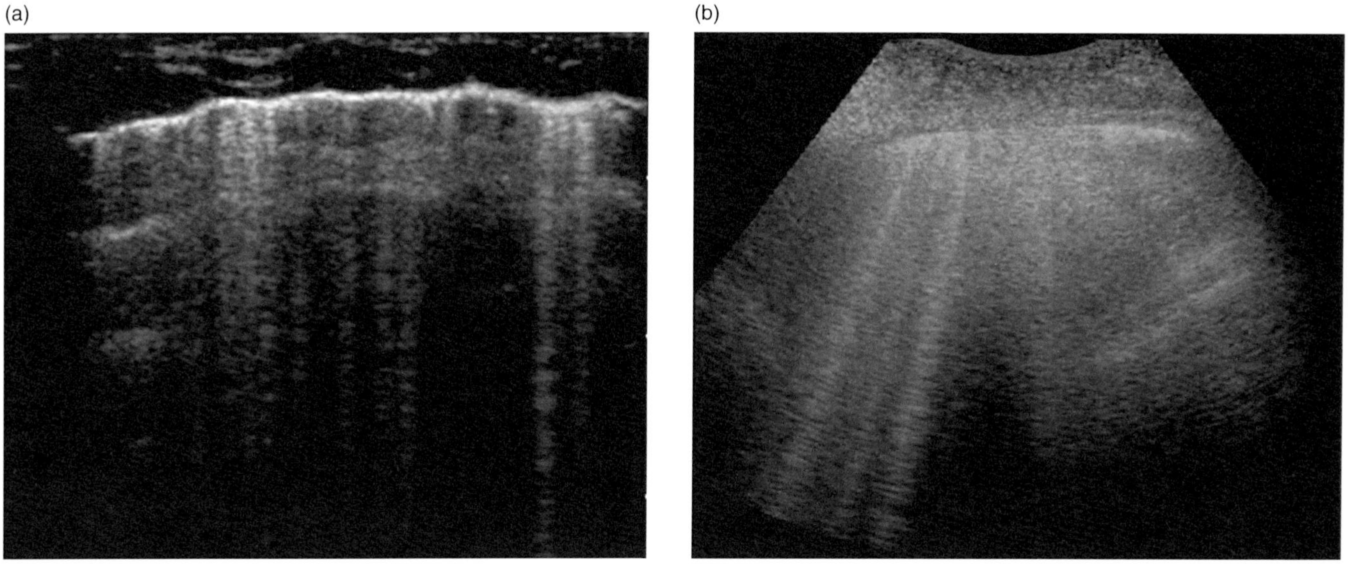

Figure 6.10 B-lines. B-lines are a type of reverberation artifact that arises from the pleural line, and reach the edge of the screen without fading. (a) B-lines are parallel with the linear transducer. (b) B-lines follow the transducer's array and are divergent with the curved-array transducer

- Make sure the vertical artifacts are truly B-lines: B-lines are multiple hyperechoic well-defined vertical lines which start on the pleural line, move with lung sliding, reach the edges of the screen, and erase the A-lines.
- When performing ultrasound on the left lung fields, cardiac movement can be confused for "lung sliding."
- Subcutaneous emphysema presents vertical artifacts (E-lines and W-lines) that are very similar to B-lines, but are

static and are generated in the chest wall, not at the pleural line.

Tips to improve scanning

- ✓ Take a look at how lung sliding and B-lines look with an older machine; use this as your goal to build a preset in your newer portable ultrasound machine.
- ✓ Any transducer should work: the linear, phased-array, or micro-convex. Identify the best setting for each one in your machine.
- ✓ Always use the ribs as a reference to identify the pleural line. The lung sliding can only be identified immediately deep to the ribs. Any hyperechoic lines above the ribs, dynamic or static, are not in the pleural cavity and can represent soft tissue of subcutaneous emphysema.
- ✓ Become familiar with visualizing the normal pleural line.
- ✓ A-lines, B-lines, and C-lines can be identified in characteristic patterns in particular pleuropulmonary pathology.
- ✓ Use M-mode to help visualize lung sliding and to distinguish normal lung from a pneumothorax. Normal lung will exhibit a "seashore sign," while a pneumothorax will have a characteristic "stratosphere sign."

Pathology

Intubation management

In children, traditionally the confirmation of endotracheal placement after an intubation can be achieved by the sonographic visualization of the tube in the trachea; the malpositioned tube in the esophagus can also be visualized. However, this direct technique is currently still in its early stages of clinical research (see Chapter 22). The technique currently more widely accepted is the evaluation of bilateral lung expansion during manual ventilation. This approach still offers the advantage of detecting a mainstem intubation and guiding its correction. Furthermore, it does not add any extra steps to the examination, since it uses the same scanning protocol as for the screening investigation for pneumothorax.

After intubation, the anterior chest is scanned bilaterally. Lung sliding synchronized to the manual ventilations must be seen on both sides. This indirectly confirms adequate tracheal position of the tube by detecting bilateral pulmonary expansion. If lung sliding is seen on the right, but the "lung pulse" is seen on the left, this means the left lung is not being ventilated. The endotracheal tube must then be slowly withdrawn under direct visualization of the left lung until lung sliding is detected. Naturally, care must be taken not to extubate the patient, particularly because the cause of the non-expansion of the left lung can be something other than a mainstem intubation, such as a bronchial foreign body or mucus plugging. More rarely, a left bronchial intubation may occur and there will be "lung sliding" (expansion) on the left, and "lung pulse" (no expansion) on the right. If neither "lung sliding" nor a "lung pulse" is detected, the diagnosis of pneumothorax must be considered.

Pneumothorax

A pneumothorax presents with several sonographic signs: (1) absent lung sliding, (2) the presence of lung points, and (3) the absolute absence of B-lines. Free air is less dense than the lungs and behaves like bubbles in water accumulating in the highest region of the thoracic cavity. The exception is when there are very extensive pleural adhesions, which are quite rare in the pediatric population. Therefore, one single examination of the highest spot on the chest is enough to exclude a pneumothorax: if we find lung sliding in that "spot," a pneumothorax is excluded with sensitivity close to 100%. The visual perception of absent lung sliding vs. present lung sliding can be difficult for the novice user. The use of M-mode ("seashore sign" (Figures 6.6a, 6.7a) *vs.* "stratosphere sign" (Figures 6.6b, 6.7b)) can drastically enhance this detection. The absence of lung sliding, however, is only 60–90% specific. There are multiple processes that can decrease or completely suppress lung sliding. They include all of the causes of non-expansion as described above, but particularly processes that cause pleural adhesions. It can also be a normal variant. The most common cause of absent lung sliding in adults, pulmonary emphysema, can render "lung sliding" virtually imperceptible. This is much less of a concern in the pediatric population.

We can use another artifact to confirm a pneumothorax: it is called the "lung point" which is 100% specific. Its sensitivity is not as high, but as a general rule it will only be absent in clinically evident pneumothoraces, usually tension pneumothoraces. The "lung point" represents the transition line where the collapsed lung loses contact with the chest wall. This line, where visceral pleura detaches from parietal pleura, glides on the chest wall during the respiratory cycle, accompanying residual expansion of the collapsed lung. If the transducer is placed exactly on this line, one may detect an alternation of lung sliding and the absence of lung sliding, synchronous with the respiratory movement. M-mode will record an alternation of "seashore sign" and "stratosphere sign" (Figure 6.11a,b). In order to locate the "lung point" after the absence of "lung sliding" has been detected on the anterior wall, simply proceed with your screening examination, placing the transducer on the posterolateral wall. This is the spot where pleural contact will be detected in a partial pneumothorax, since lung is heavier than free air. If no "lung sliding" is present at this point, there will be no detectable "lung point". Therefore, this is either a complete pneumothorax (no pleural contact) or another process, such as a pleural adhesion. Other methods will be required, in order to confirm or exclude a pneumothorax. If lung sliding is found at the posterolateral wall, slowly slide the transducer back towards the anterior wall looking for the point where lung sliding becomes absent. This is the "lung point". It accurately represents the margin of the pneumothorax, and can be used to monitor the size of a pneumothorax.

A small pneumothorax may be chosen not to be drained in a ventilated patient, and its size can be reliably monitored by ultrasonography. When a chest tube is placed, its efficacy in draining the pneumothorax can also be verified. Lastly, B-lines are rare in the normal individual, but, when present, they can be

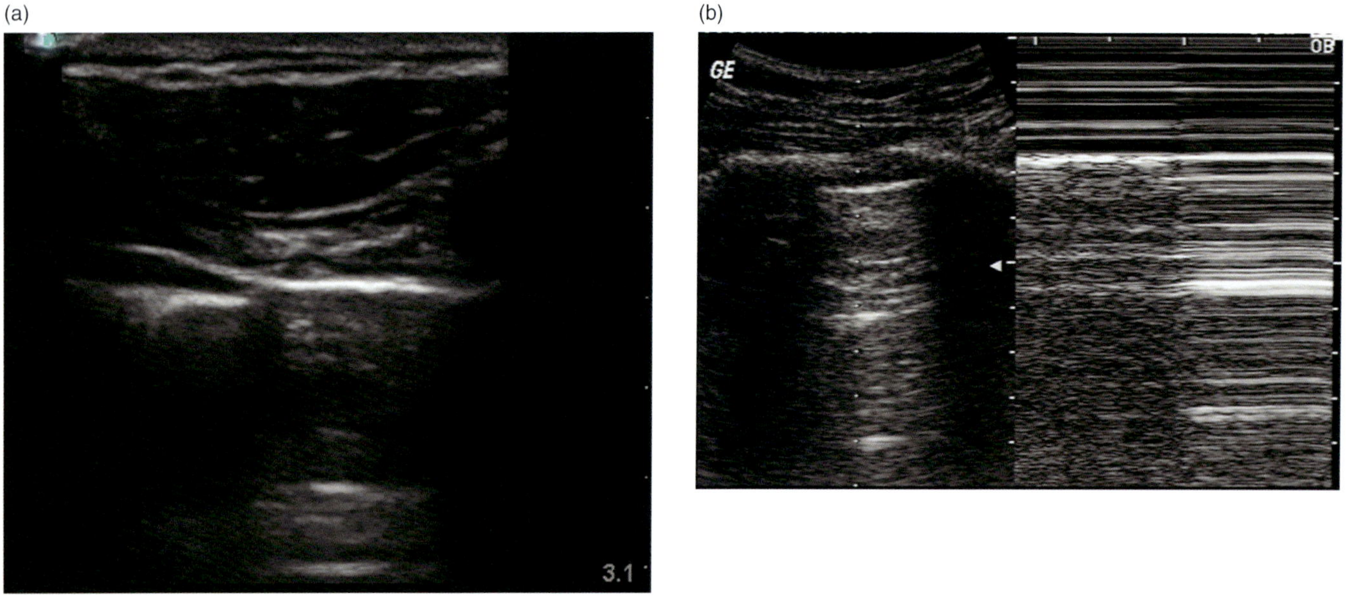

Figure 6.11 Lung point. (a) The lung point is the transition line where the collapsed lung loses contact with the chest wall. (b) If the transducer is placed exactly on this line, one may detect an alternation of lung sliding and the absence of lung sliding in M-mode. On M-mode there will be an alternation of "seashore sign" with "stratosphere sign" synchronous with respirations.

useful in the investigation of pneumothorax. They are generated on the visceral pleura. Therefore, if any B-lines are seen, even in the absence of lung sliding, this means there is direct pleural contact. The sound waves reach the lung without interposed free air, and a pneumothorax is excluded.

Subcutaneous emphysema

As explained in the basic principles section, air reflects ultrasound. If there is free air in the chest wall, we might not be able to see beyond it. Subcutaneous emphysema can be a significant barrier to chest ultrasound. Nevertheless, many times we will be able to "squeeze" the air out of our scanning plane by simply pressing the transducer harder against the chest wall, if it will not inflict pain on a non-sedated patient that may have chest wall tenderness. Subcutaneous emphysema will reveal multiple hyperechoic vertical artifacts originating at multiple levels within the chest wall, when the air is in fat tissue, or at one horizontal level when there is free air between muscle or fascia layers. If we are not able to see clearly beyond these artifacts and identify our anatomic references (ribs and the pleural line deep to them), we cannot trust our pulmonary sonogram and should use other modalities of investigation.

Pleural effusion, thoracentesis

Ultrasound has long been known as being the gold standard for the diagnosis of pleural effusions and for the guidance of thoracentesis. It has been suggested that ultrasound can not only be at least as sensitive as CT scans, but more specific, being able to provide more information regarding the organization/septation of the fluid, volume, and associated pathologic processes (Figure 6.12a). Following basic principles, unless there are extensive pleural adhesions and loculations, fluid will flow to the lowest portions of the pleural cavity, which naturally will vary with patient positioning, but in general the posterior/inferior region (i.e. posterior costophrenic sinus) is the first to accumulate fluid. A pleural effusion will be seen as an anechoic layer overlying pulmonary parenchyma. The lung sliding sign will be absent, and the pulmonary parenchyma will present varying degrees of aeration, depending on the volume of the effusion and the compression caused by it. Atelectatic parenchyma will be seen as soft tissue "floating" in the effusion, and usually an irregular margin of transition to the deeper aerated parenchyma will express B-lines. The fluid can be analyzed regarding its echotexture: purely anechoic fluid has been associated with transudate and hemothorax, which can present organized soft tissue–like clots. Fluid presenting with floating particles, organized fibers and septations has consistently been associated with an empyema (Figure 6.12b). A traumatic hemothorax presents swirling hyperechoic particles (air bubbles) with an associated pneumothorax. Floating fragments within a pleural effusion has been referred to as the "*plankton sign*" (Figure 6.12c).

The safety profile for thoracentesis is drastically improved when performed under ultrasound guidance, allowing for the precise identification of the largest pocket of fluid, for measurement of the chest wall and effusion thickness, and for accurate positioning of the needle at a safe distance from the lung parenchyma (see Chapter 21). Ultrasound guidance is particularly useful for performing thoracentesis on ventilated patients, where the drainage of fluid is beneficial for the ventilatory mechanics, and an iatrogenic pneumothorax could be devastating.

Pneumonia and atelectasis

The diagnostic potential of utilizing ultrasound in the identification of pneumonia remains poorly explored, despite solid

(a)

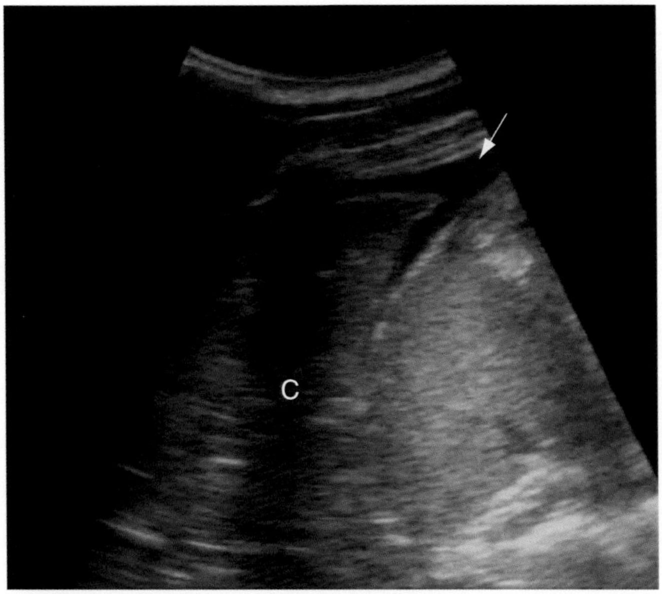

(b)

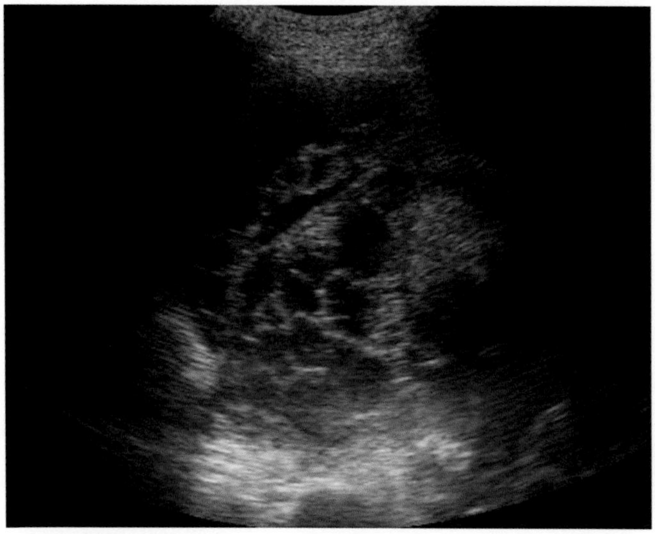

(c)

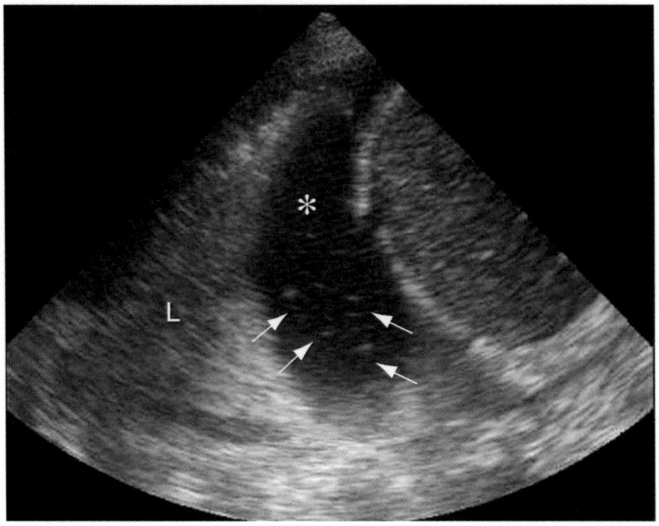

Figure 6.12 Pleural effusions. (a) A very small pleural effusion in the costophrenic sinus (arrow) is seen surrounding a massive consolidation (C). (b) A septated effusion, suggestive of empyema. (c) Air bubbles (arrows) swirling in a hemothorax (*) suggests that there is also an associated pneumothorax. The lung (L) is atelectatic, compressed by the large effusion.

literature in support of it. In adult patients, 98.5% of the pneumonias reach the visceral pleura and over 90% are detectable by ultrasound, as opposed to about 68% by chest radiograph, as compared to CT scan. The pneumonias missed by ultrasound are those unreachable by the transducer, being under the shoulder areas, or in regions limited by wound dressings, and chest tubes.

In the pediatric population, the sensitivity for detecting pneumonias by ultrasound has been found to be even higher than for adults, given the better accessibility of the pediatric lung to the transducer's footprint, non-calcified bones, and the relative larger size of the consolidations reaching the visceral pleura more consistently. A recent study showed an overall sensitivity of 86% and specificity of 89% in diagnosing pneumonia. In the subgroup analysis of those patients with a consolidation of greater than 1 cm, the sensitivity remained at 86% but the specificity increased to 97%.

Pneumonic consolidations appear as a subpleural hypoechoic soft tissue–like mass of variable size and shape. Because of the gradual transition from aerated to non-aerated parenchyma, it has poorly defined borders and is surrounded by a region expressing B-lines. The surrounding B-lines are useful in differentiating pneumonias (and atelectasis) from other consolidative processes. In the very beginning of the infectious process, pneumonia can be visualized as multiple, small (less than one centimeter) C-lines among a region of B-lines, or by a region

(a)

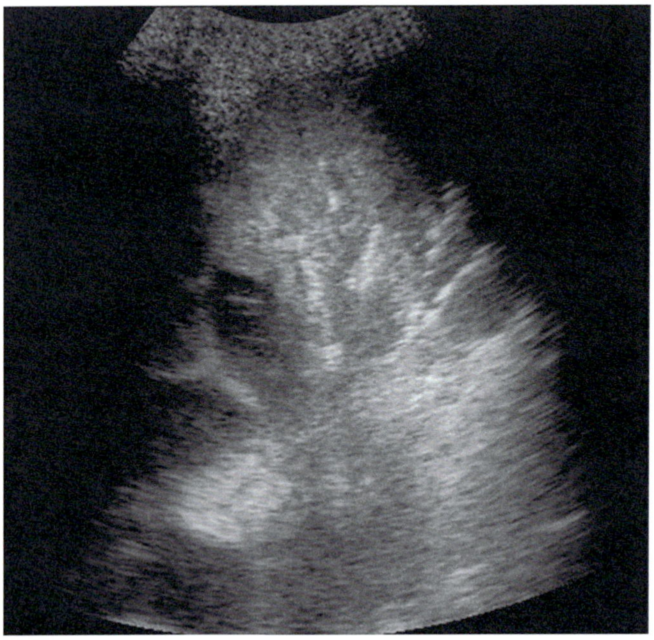

(b)

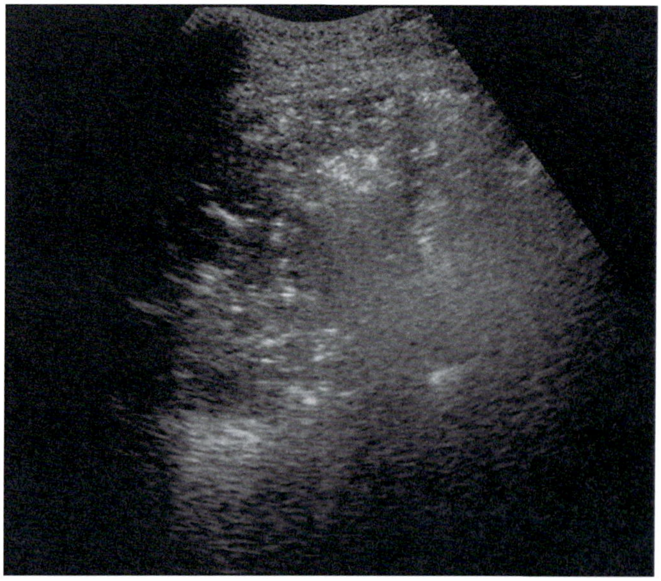

(c)

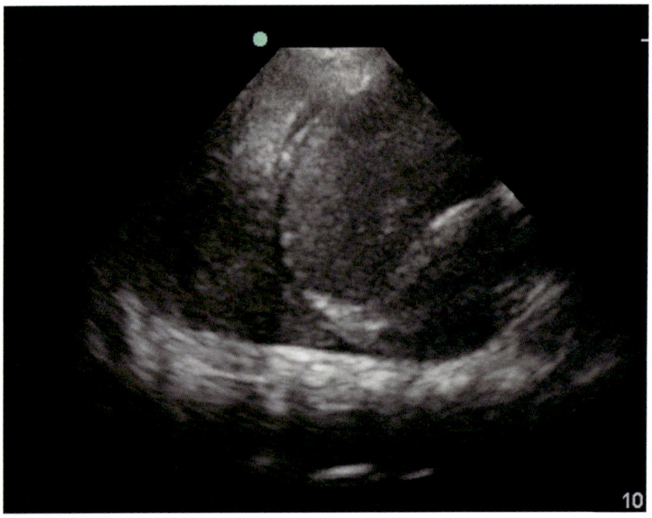

Figure 6.13 Pneumonias. (a) The normal branched pattern of the air bronchograms (hyperechoic lines) can be seen within a consolidation. (b) Air bronchograms seen in transverse section appear as lenticular hyperechoic spots. (c) "Hepatization" of the lung can be seen in consolidations (C).

of confluent B-lines alone. Well-organized pneumonias are excellent conductors of ultrasound waves. They allow for the visualization of deep structures that are contiguous with the consolidation, as well as of details of the pulmonary parenchyma, like vessels and airways (Figure 6.13a). These can be reliably used to confirm the diagnosis of pneumonia and to differentiate pneumonia from atelectasis. Pneumonias are primarily an alveolar process that secondarily floods the larger airways with secretions. There is no initial airway obstruction, and the airflow causes the secretions to move back and forth in the bronchi. This movement of secretions can be seen on ultrasound as the "dynamic air bronchogram" sign, which is pathognomonic for pneumonia. Airways flooded with fluid and without air movement appear quite similar to vessels, but they have hyperechoic walls and do not show a Doppler signal. These are called "fluid bronchograms," which are typical of post-obstructive pneumonias. Multiple lenticular echoes can also be seen within the consolidation, representing air trapped in smaller airways (Figure 6.13b). Furthermore, a dense consolidation above the diaphragm may appear similar to the echotexture of the liver, referred to as the "hepatization" of the lung (Figure 6.13c).

Atelectasis generates the consolidation by reabsorption of the air inside a region that is distal to an occluded airway. This causes not only absence of airflow, but also "static air bronchograms." However, when the lung parenchyma retracts secondarily to the absorption of the trapped air, it causes distortion with volume reduction, bringing the bronchovascular structures closer together tending to a parallel pattern. This is in contrast to the normal, branching, "tree like" pattern seen in pneumonia.

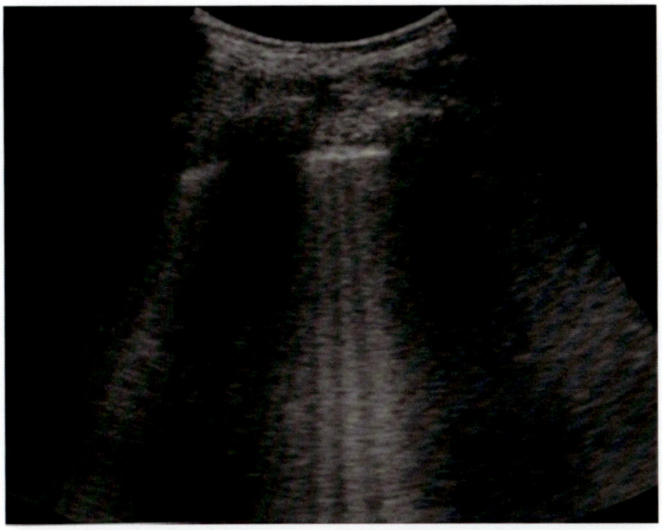

Figure 6.14 Interstitial syndromes. Ultrasound image of a patient with RDS. Interstitial syndromes are characterized by the presence of water and multiple B-lines.

Interstitial syndromes

Pulmonary ultrasound in the neonatal intensive care setting has a promising future as a powerful diagnostic tool and we encourage the reader to become familiar with the emerging research, particularly on TTN and RDS (see Chapter 23). Interstitial syndromes are characterized by an increase in extravascular water, being sonographically expressed by the presence of multiple B-lines. It has been well determined that the presence of a normal sonographic pattern (absent B-lines) excludes the possibility of a cardiogenic pulmonary edema, with a sensitivity of 100%. The clinical impact of this data seems to be crucial in the evaluation of a dyspneic patient.

B-lines are present in all diseases that present with extravascular lung water and/or thickening of the interstitium, with or without alveolar flooding. Their presence is highly sensitive and nonspecific, but the topographic distribution and amount of B-lines varies largely with the baseline pathologic condition, rendering them clinically specific. Cardiogenic pulmonary edema presents initially with B-lines on the dependent regions. As pulmonary edema progresses, the amount of B-lines increases, and they spread all over the pulmonary surface. In severe pulmonary edema, the B-lines can be so numerous that they merge together and generate what is called sonographic "white lung," corresponding to "ground glass" areas seen on CT scan.

The comprehensive examination is used to quantify the severity of interstitial syndromes, assigning a score from 0 to 11, counting the number of positive regions. In the comprehensive lung examination, the 11 regions of the lung are scanned. Each region is then classified as positive or negative, and a score can be obtained by counting the positive regions. A region is considered positive if three or more B-lines are present, no more than 7 mm apart from each other in one scan, and an examination is considered positive for interstitial syndrome if two or more regions are positive, at least one on each side.

Cases

1. A four-year-old male is brought in by EMS after being hit by a car. On primary assessment, he exhibits an open and maintainable airway, and normal heart sounds and pulses. He has an abrasion over his right anterior chest. An E-FAST examination is performed, which reveals fluid above the diaphragm on the right (Figure 6.15a,b). On rapid pulmonary assessment, there is an absence of lung sliding consistent with a pleural effusion (Figure 6.15c). A chest tube is placed which drains 200 mL of bloody fluid.

   This case highlights the utility of the ultrasound examination in trauma, in assessing for traumatic pleural effusions, or a hemothorax. The rapid identification of a hemothorax is crucial in the management of trauma patients, and to expeditiously identify which patients will need a chest tube in order to treat the hemothorax. It is imperative that the clinician evaluate for long pathology both at the anterior chest, and above the diaphragms on the right upper quadrant and left upper quadrant abdominal views. Since fluid develops in the most dependent regions, one is more likely to find a pleural effusion or hemothorax in those locations. There will be a loss of the mirror-image artifact of the liver or spleen.
2. A 16-year-old male presents with the acute onset of left-sided chest pain for the past day. He has had no chest trauma, and no associated fevers. However, he has had significant dyspnea, which worsens when he is in the supine position. He is tachycardic and tachypneic on examination. His lung examination is difficult and limited, secondary to poor effort by the patient, given significant pain on inspiration. A point-of-care ultrasound is immediately performed, which reveals a large, left-sided pneumothorax (Figure 6.16a). These findings are confirmed by portable chest radiography (Figure 6.16b). The patient is placed on oxygen, and the surgery service is consulted for the placement of a pigtail chest tube catheter. After the chest tube is placed, a repeat lung ultrasound is performed, which shows normal lung sliding with the "seashore" sign on M-mode (Figure 6.16c).

   Point-of-care ultrasound can be utilized to rapidly identify a pneumothorax. In this case, the child presents with a spontaneous pneumothorax. When compared with chest radiography, it is often even more sensitive and specific in detecting a pneumothorax. Further, there is often a delay in obtaining radiographic studies, and radiographs are limited in detecting pneumothoraces in supine patients.

Summary/key points

1. The established applications for lung ultrasound include the detection of pneumothoraces and pleural effusions. Newer applications include pneumonias, TTN, RDS, and interstitial syndromes. Lung ultrasound may also indirectly

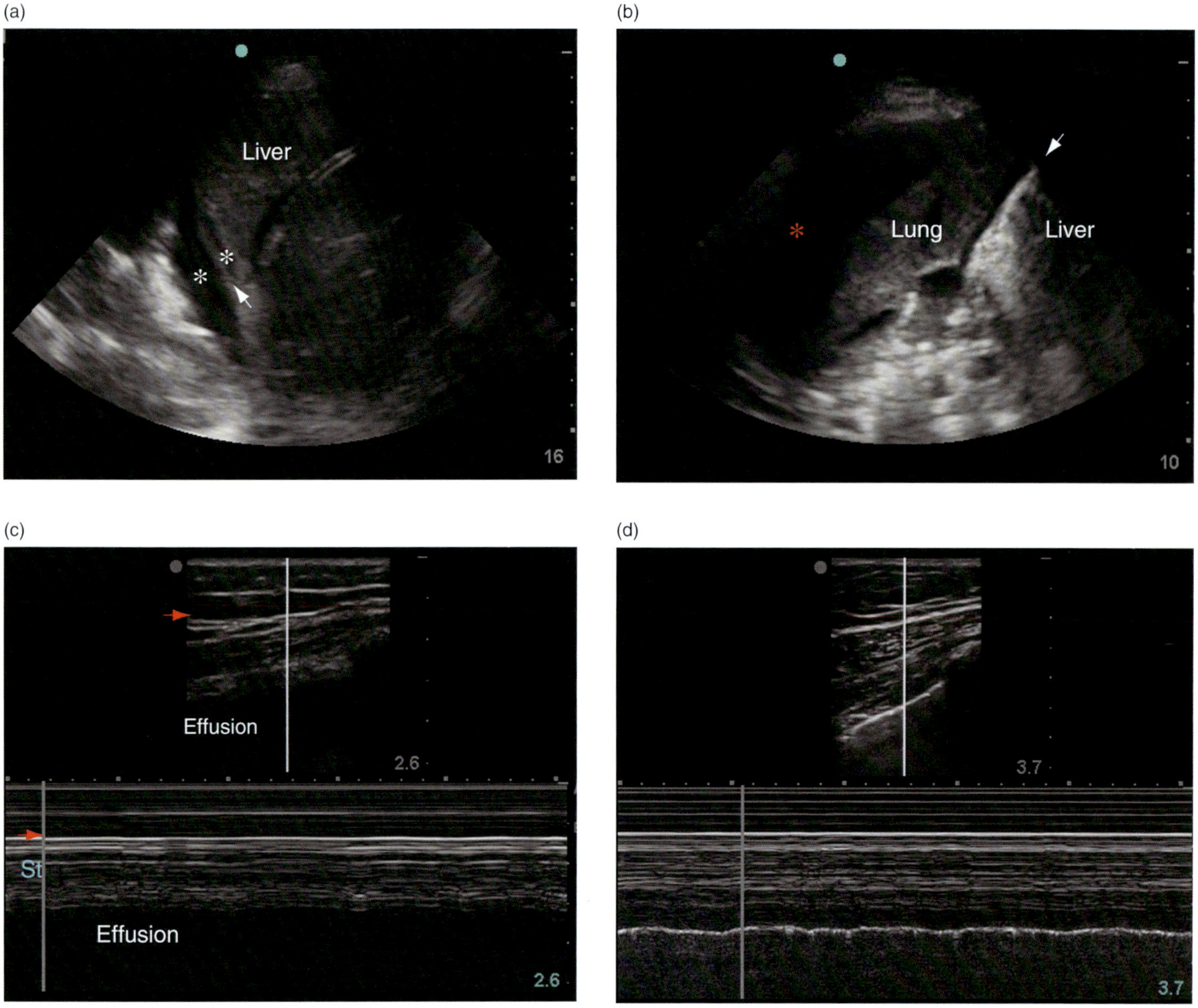

Figure 6.15 Case 1: hemothorax. (a) At the right upper quadrant, fluid (*) below and above the diaphragm (arrow) can be visualized. (b) When moving the transducer superiorly towards the patient's head, a large hemothorax (*) can be appreciated with compressed lung tissue. (c) On M-mode, there is a "stratosphere sign" (St) immediately deep to the pleural line (arrow), and an anechoic area deep to that region, consistent with the effusion. (d) This is in comparison with the normal left lung, which exhibits lung sliding and the "seashore sign."

assess for proper endotracheal tube placement and assist in thoracentesis.

2. An initial lung examination consists of a screening examination performed in one location on the right and left thorax. A comprehensive examination includes a "one spot" scan in each of the 11 regions of the chest. A detailed examination involves scanning the entire lung in the intercostal spaces.
3. The most frequently utilized transducers to perform the lung examination are the convex (2–5 MHz) and linear (5–10 MHz) transducers. As a general rule, smaller-footprint transducers should be utilized, especially in children.
4. A pneumothorax presents with several sonographic signs: (1) absent "lung sliding", (2) the presence of "lung points", and (3) the absolute absence of B-lines.
5. Important signs to become familiar with include lung sliding, A-lines, B-lines, and C-lines. In M-mode, the "seashore sign" represents normal lung sliding, while the "stratosphere sign" represents a pneumothorax.

(a)

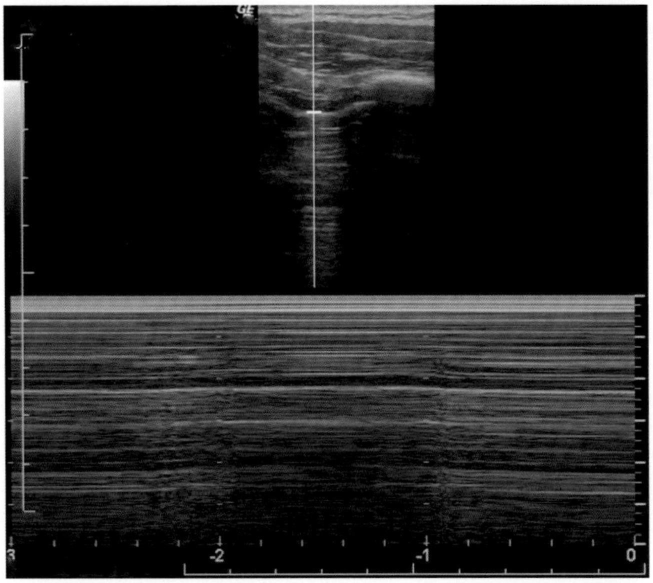

(b)

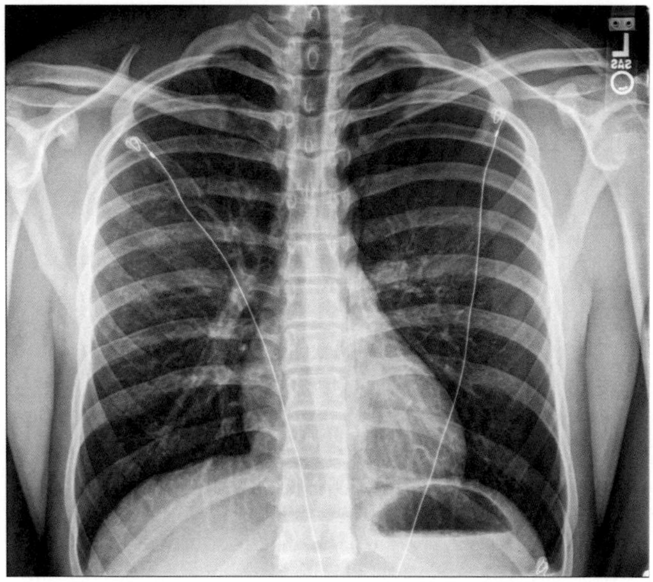

(c)

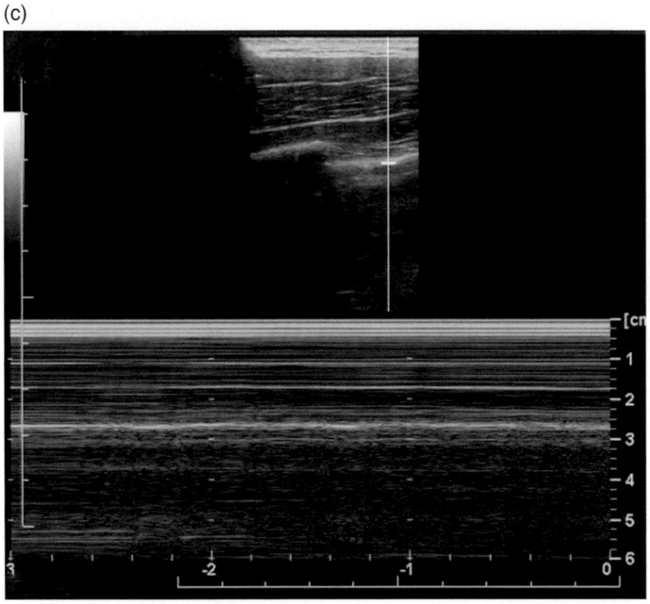

Figure 6.16 Case 2: spontaneous pneumothorax. (a) On M-mode, the characteristic "stratosphere sign" can be visualized. (b) The corresponding chest radiograph was obtained following the point-of-care lung ultrasound examination revealing a large, left-sided pneumothorax. (c) After pigtail catheter placement, the ultrasound was repeated, showing restoration of lung sliding and the "seashore sign."

Selected references

Blaivas, M., Lyon, M., Duggal, S. (2005) A prospective comparison of supine chest radiography and bedside ultrasound for the diagnosis of traumatic pneumothorax. *Ann Emerg Med* **12**(9): 844–9.

Caiulo, V.A., Gargani, L., Caiulo, S., *et al.* (2011) Lung ultrasound in bronchiolitis: comparison with chest X-ray. *Eur J Pediatr* **170**: 1427–33.

Coley, B.D. (2005) Pediatric chest ultrasound. *Radiol Clin North Am* **43**: 405–18.

Copetti, R., Cattarossi, L. (2007) The 'double lung point': an ultrasound sign diagnostic of transient tachypnea of the newborn. *Neonatology* **91**: 203–9.

Khaled, A., Woo, M.Y., Vaillancourt, C. (2012) Test characteristics of ultrasonograpy for the detection of pneumothorax: a systematic review and meta-analysis. *Chest* **141**: 703–8.

Kurian, J., Levin, T.L., Han, B.K., *et al.* (2009) Comparison of ultrasound and CT in the evaluation of pneumonia complicated by parapneumonic effusion in children. *Am J Roentgenol* **193**: 1648–54.

Lichtenstein, D.A. (2009) Ultrasound examination of the lungs in the intensive care unit. *Pediatr Crit Care Med* **10**: 693–8.

Lichtenstein, D.A., Mezière, G.A. (2008) Relevance of lung ultrasound in the diagnosis of acute respiratory failure: the BLUE protocol. *Chest* **134**: 117–25.

Shah, V.P., Tunik, M.G., Tsung, J.W. (2012) Prospective evaluation of point-of-care ultrasonography for the diagnosis of pneumonia in children and young adults. *Arch Pediatr Adolesc Med* December 10: 1–7. doi:10.1001/2013. jamapediatrics.107

Volpicelli, G., Elbarbary, M., Blaivas, M., *et al.* (2012) International evidence-based recommendations for point-of-care lung ultrasound. *Intensive Care Med* **38**: 577–91.

Chapter 7

Inferior vena cava, aorta assessment

Faiza Al Talaq and Vicki E. Noble

Objectives/indications

One of the most common presenting complaints in children is vomiting, diarrhea, and dehydration. The clinician is often faced with the challenge of determining whether a child is dehydrated, which will ultimately guide their treatment management. However, the clinical evaluation of hydration status can be challenging, given the diverse signs and symptoms of the dehydration. The assessment of hypovolemia and dehydration is especially important in critically ill and trauma patients. Methods by which one may evaluate for hypovolemia or dehydration include clinical signs and central venous pressure (CVP) monitoring. Clinical signs of dehydration can be imprecise and inaccurate, so that clinicians are unable to predict the exact degree of dehydration. In one prospective study, a combination of clinical signs including general appearance, absent tears, abnormal respiration, sunken eyes, dry mucus membranes, decreased skin elasticity, capillary refill greater than two seconds, abnormal radial pulse, tachycardia (HR > 150 bpm), and decreased urine output showed a sensitivity of 87% and a specificity of 82%.

Point-of-care ultrasound assessment of the inferior vena cava (IVC) as a marker of hydration status is a novel application in the pediatric population, and has the potential to improve the ability of the clinician to accurately assess for dehydration. It may also serve as a non-invasive method of CVP monitoring in critically ill patients. There are various proposed methods of determining hydration status, including the IVC diameter measurement, the degree of collapsibility on inspiration vs. expiration, and IVC/aorta diameter index. The anteroposterior (AP) diameter of the IVC varies with normal respiration. During inspiration, the negative intrathoracic pressure pulls volume from the intra-abdominal IVC. In contrast, during expiration, the positive intrathoracic pressure pushes fluid back to the low-pressure abdominal venous system. So, the IVC AP diameter reaches its maximum during expiration and minimum during inspiration. Respiratory variation in the AP diameter of the IVC has been investigated as a non-invasive marker of intravascular volume status, correlating its percentage collapse to CVP. This may be visually estimated by the "gestalt method" or by calculating the caval index.

The sonographic assessment of the aorta has largely been utilized in adult populations to diagnose life-threatening abdominal aortic aneurysms (AAAs). Although this entity is not typically present in pediatric patients, the aorta assessment can readily detect the rare occurrence of an aortic dissection. Although most cases of aortic dissection occur in adults, cases have been reported among infants, children, and adolescents. Of a total of 1,085 patients reported in two large series, 3.5% of aortic dissections occurred in persons 19 years of age or younger. Predisposing factors include congenital cardiovascular anomalies, connective tissue disorders, hypertension, and trauma.

This chapter reviews the indications and techniques for both the IVC and aorta evaluations. The objective of the IVC evaluation is to assess for dehydraton/hypovolemia, while the aorta evaluation assesses for the presence of an AAA or aortic dissection.

Background

The use of ultrasound to evaluate the IVC as an objective tool to assess volume status has been studied extensively. The IVC diameter has been shown to correlate with hypovolemia in trauma patients in comparison with controls. In the shock group, the average IVC (7.7 mm) was smaller than the control (13.4 mm; $P < 0.0001$), and there was a significant change in the IVC diameter that was noted after fluid resuscitation. The IVC diameter has also been found to be a better predictor of fluid response than blood pressure, heart rate, or base deficit in trauma patients. The IVC diameter measurement itself has shown a high inter-rater reliability, supporting its reliability and repeatability. In addition to the IVC diameter, the anteroposterior (AP) diameter and its percentage of collapse, otherwise known as the "caval index," has shown a strong correlation with more invasive CVP measurements. Schefold *et al.* showed that absolute IVC diameter measurements correlate with CVP in septic patients. There was a significant correlation of both inspiratory and expiratory IVC diameter with CVP ($P = 0.004$ and $P = 0.001$, respectively). Stawicki *et al.* prospectively compared caval index with CVP in surgical ICU patients and showed that over 60% of patients with a caval index of greater than 60% had a CVP of less than 7 mmHg. They also showed that the caval index correlates best with CVP in the setting of high collapsibility range (>60%). Similarly, Nagdev *et al.* prospectively studied emergency department patients and showed that a caval index of over 50% correlates with low CVP (CVP <8 mmHg), with a positive predictive value (PPV) of 87% and

Pediatric Emergency and Critical Care Ultrasound, ed. Stephanie J. Doniger. Published by Cambridge University Press.

negative predictive value (NPV) of 96%. Therefore the caval index can be used to quickly and reliably evaluate volume status.

The literature investigating the sonographic assessment of the IVC in pediatric patients is small but growing. Krause *et al.* looked at the sonographic assessment of IVC diameter respiratory changes in children on hemodialysis. Those changes were significantly correlated with alterations in body weight following dialysis ($P<0.0001$). Overall, limitations with described IVC measurements include the fact that the IVC changes with age and size or body mass index (BMI). Instead of simply using the IVC diameter measurement or the caval index, Chen *et al.* suggested using the IVC/aorta (IVC/Ao) ratio. It was hypothesized that the IVC/Ao ratio would be easier to obtain in pediatric patients, and that using the ratio would correct for changes in patient size and age. The IVC/Ao ratio was significantly lower in dehydrated children when compared with matched controls. Chen *et al.* performed an additional study that validated that the IVC/Ao ratio correlates with dehydration. They further showed that, with a cut-off ratio of 0.8, the test had a sensitivity of 86% and specificity of 56%. Therefore, this is a marginally accurate measurement which needs further investigation. Most recently, Ng *et al.* called into question the reliability of the IVC measurements when compared to the CVP on children in the pediatric intensive care unit. Further research remains to be carried out to determine further the reliability and utility of the IVC evaluation in children.

Anatomy

The IVC is formed by the union of common iliac veins around the level of the umbilicus. This is also the location where the abdominal aorta bifurcates to form the common iliac arteries. Throughout its course in the abdomen, the IVC runs anterolateral to the spine and to the right of the abdominal aorta. The IVC receives all veins that correspond to the aorta branches, and eventually drains into the right atrium (RA) above the diaphragm (Figure 7.1a). The abdominal aorta starts at the level of the diaphragm and runs caudally, lying anterolateral to the spine and to the left side of the IVC (Figure 7.1b).

Technique

Point-of-care questions

1. Is the patient dehydrated/euvolemic/fluid overloaded?
   a. Is there > **50%** inspiratory collapse?
   b. Is the IVC: aorta < **1:1**?
2. Is an aortic aneurysm (AAA) present?
   a. Is the aorta > **3 cm**?
   b. Are the iliac arteries > **1.5 cm**?
3. Is an aortic dissection present?

Transducer selection and orientation

Depending on the size of the child, different transducer types can be used. Low-frequency (2–5 MHz), curvilinear abdominal transducers are the best for scanning most pediatric abdomens, as they give the highest resolution pictures. It is possible, however, to use phased-array transducers, and, in very small, thin children, linear transducers can also identify the relevant structures.

The transverse view can be obtained by placing the transducer just caudal to the xiphoid process, with the indicator oriented towards the patient's right side (Figure 7.2a). The transducer is oriented perpendicular to the patient's body in order to adequately achieve an accurate cross-section of the IVC. The depth should be deep enough to see the vertebral body shadow. Anterior to the vertebral shadow lie two vascular structures. The IVC is on the patient's right and aorta to the patient's left. The longitudinal view is obtained by rotating the transducer 90° clockwise, with the indicator towards the patient's head (Figure 7.3a). Sliding from side to side, you can move from IVC to aorta. In order to follow the IVC along its long-axis to where it enters into the right atrium, the transducer needs to be angled slightly towards the patient's right (Figure 7.3b).

The transverse and longitudinal views of the aorta are obtained with the same transducer orientation as the views of the IVC. It is important to maintain proper transducer orientation, with the indicator towards the patient's right, in order to appropriately identify the IVC and aorta. In order to thoroughly evaluate the aorta, it should be visualized and measured at the proximal, mid, and distal aorta in addition to the branching of the aorta into the iliac arteries. The scan is generally performed from the xiphoid region down to the umbilicus (Figure 7.4a). Depending on the level of interest you can trace the IVC and aorta caudally by sliding the transducer towards the umbilicus, while maintaining the same orientation. The aorta should also be visualized in its long-axis, or longitudinal view (Figure 7.5a).

Patient position and preparation

The patient should be in a supine position. There is no special preparation for this study. Gentle pressure may be applied to the transducer in order to displace bowel gas, which may obstruct the view of the IVC and aorta.

Ultrasound imaging: IVC

The three most common views for visualizing the IVC include: the subxiphoid transverse view, the subiphoid longitudinal view, and the anterior midaxillary line longitudinal view. A recent study by Saul *et al.* showed that the location which had the highest inter-rater reliability was the anterior midaxillary line longitudinal view, using the liver as an acoustic window. In the transverse view, the IVC lies to the patient's right and the aorta to the patient's left. This corresponds to the left- and right-hand side of the screen, respectively (Figure 7.2b). The IVC and aorta lie anterior to the vertebral body, which exhibits posterior shadowing. The IVC should also be visualized in its long-axis, as it courses through the liver and enters into the right atrium (Figure 7.3c,d).

Sonographically, the IVC may be distinguished from the aorta, since it has thinner walls, does not exhibit pulsations, is

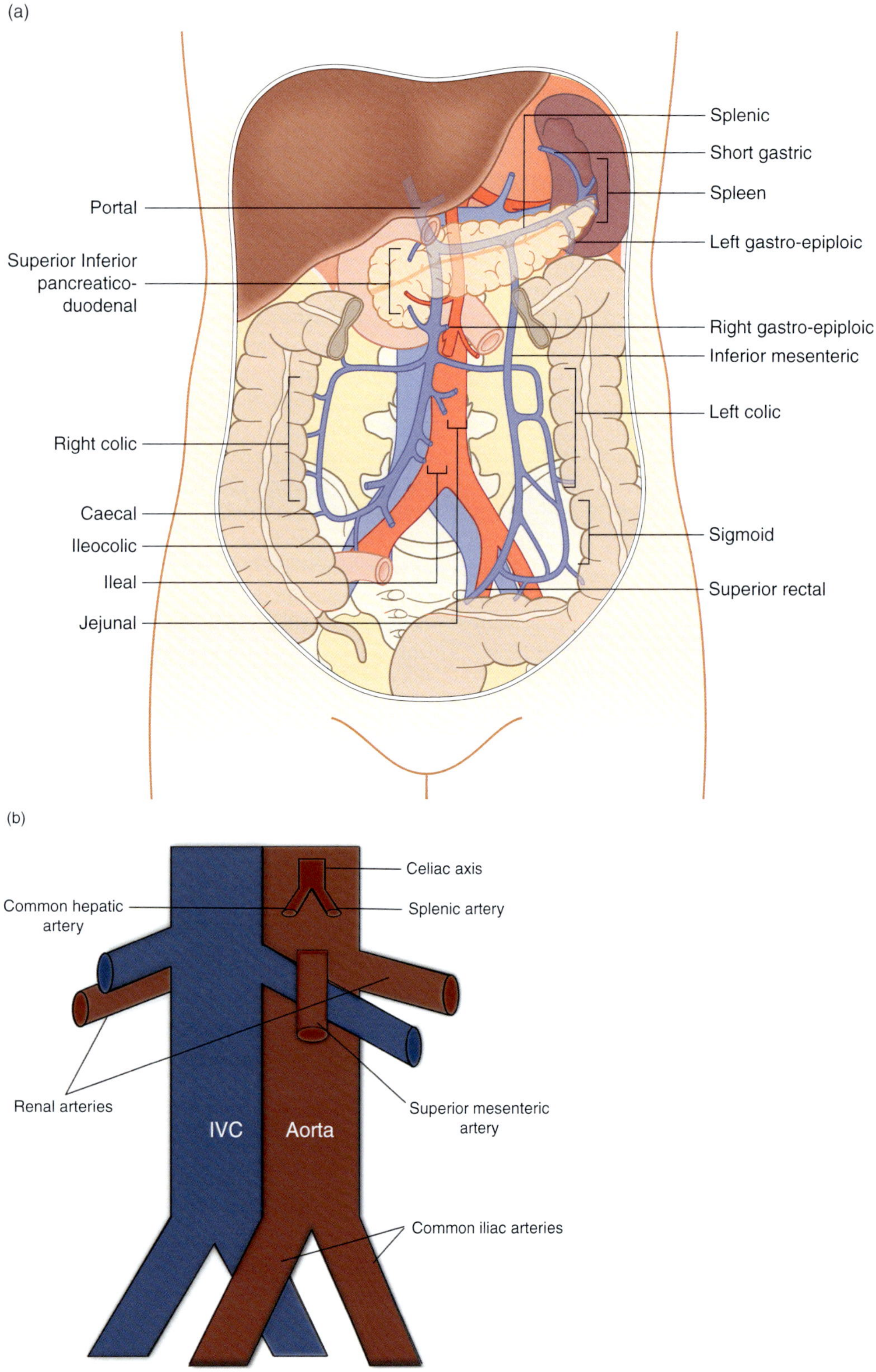

Figure 7.1 **Anatomy**. (a) Relationship of the IVC to the aorta within the abdomen. Note the proximal IVC and aorta course behind the liver. *Artwork created by Emily Evans © Cambridge University Press.* (b) The relationship between the IVC and the aorta and its branches. *Illustration by Laura Berg, MD.*

compressible, exhibits respiratory variation, and courses through the diaphragm in its longitudinal view. It is important to note, however, that the IVC and aorta run close together, and in smaller children aortic pulsations may be transmitted to the IVC, giving the appearance that the IVC has pulsations. In contrast, the aorta has thick echogenic walls, is pulsatile, exhibits high-flow velocity, is not compressible, and does not exhibit respiratory variation.

(a)

(b)

(c)

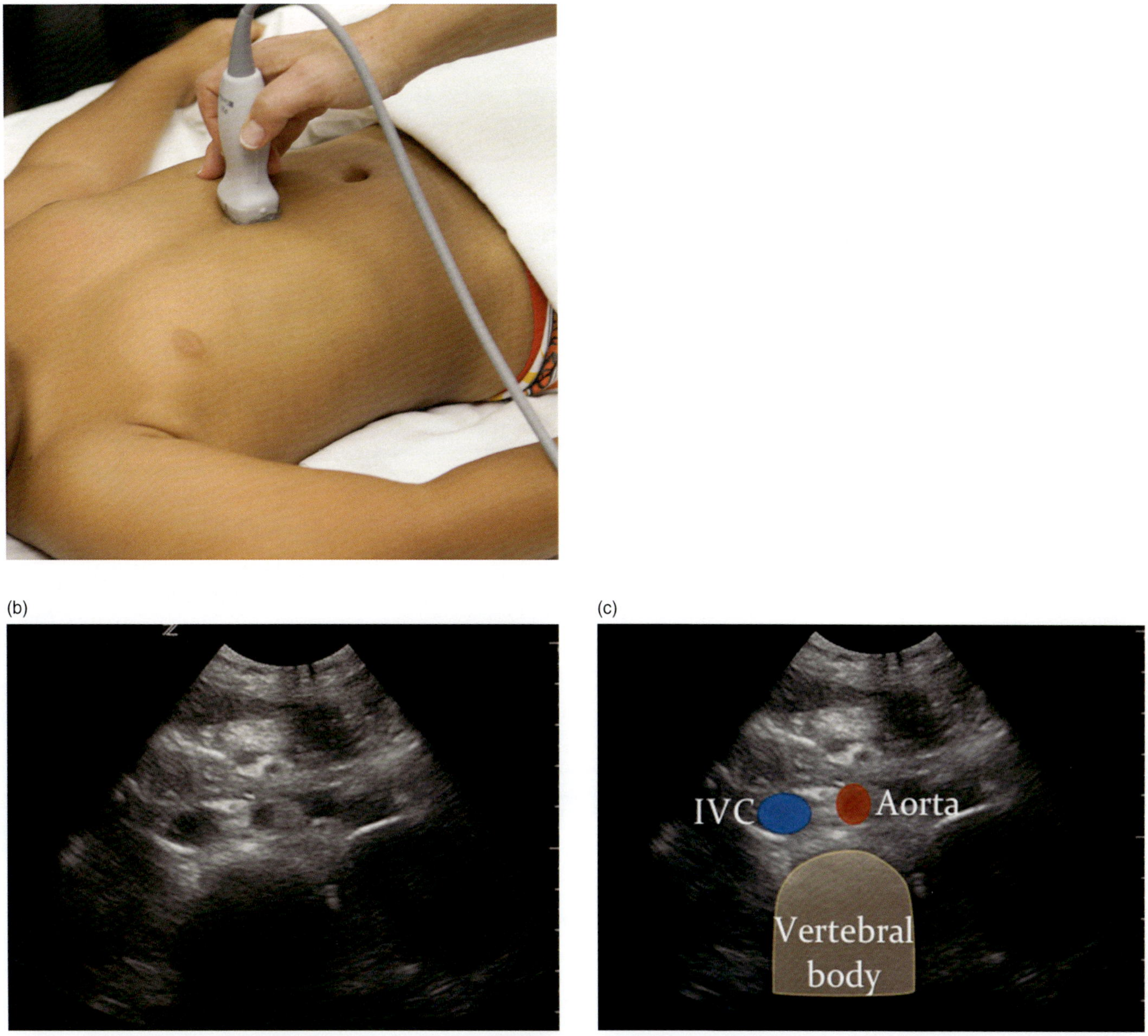

Figure 7.2 IVC imaging, transverse view. (a) Transducer placement, with the indicator oriented towards the patient's right side. (b) Ultrasound image of the transverse view of the aorta and IVC. (c) Illustration indicating important structures visualized on the ultrasound image, with the vertebral body shadow, Aorta, and IVC. *Illustration by Laura Berg, MD.*

IVC/Ao ratio (transverse view)

Obtaining the caval index may be technically difficult and of limited accuracy in young children. It has been hypothesized that there may be a growth curve of the IVC, since presumably the IVC and aorta both grow with age and size or body mass index (BMI). Recent data, that have yet to be validated, suggest that there may be a linear relationship between IVC size and the patient's age in months. Several other studies use the IVC/aorta ratio for this evaluation. This is because the abdominal aorta diameter remains constant despite intravascular volume depletion, and the aorta corrects for size and age of the patient; the IVC/aorta ratio has been suggested to be a more convenient and accurate measurement in the pediatric population. This is a ratio between the AP diameter of the IVC and the AP diameter of the aorta, both being measured in a single still image of the transverse view at the level of the left renal vein. The IVC/Ao ratio is less than 1 in dehydrated children and improves to ≥1 after fluid challenge (Figure 7.4b).

Caval Index (longitudinal view)

The IVC exhibits changes in its size during respiration, due to changes in intrathoracic pressure. During expiration, the IVC expands, while during inspiration it contracts. The caval index may be calculated based on the measurements of the IVC in the

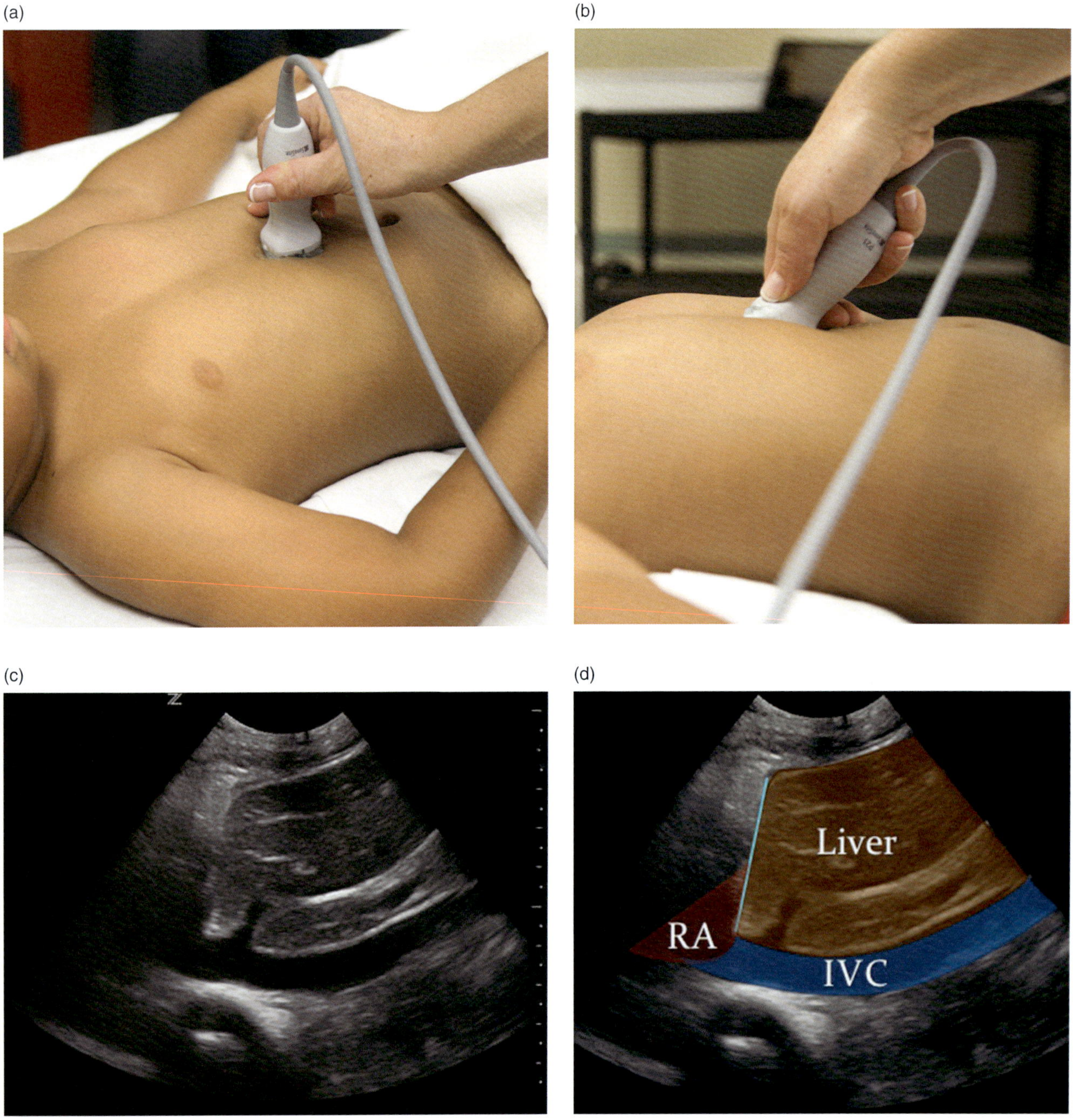

Figure 7.3 IVC imaging, longitudinal view. (a) Transducer placement, with the indicator oriented towards the patient's head. (b). In order to visualize the IVC along its entire length, as it enters the right atrium (RA), it is often necessary to angle the wrist and direct the transducer towards the patient's right side. (c) Ultrasound image of the longitudinal view of the aorta. (d) Illustration indicating important structures visualized on the ultrasound image, including the right atrium (RA), liver, and IVC. *Illustration by Laura Berg, MD.*

longitudinal view (Figure 7.4a,b). Of note, all measurements of the IVC are the AP diameter. A caval index ≥ 50% is strongly associated with a low CVP.

$$\textbf{Caval index} = \frac{\textbf{max (IVC)} - \textbf{min (IVC)}}{\textbf{max (IVC)}} \times \textbf{100}$$

IVC measurements, M-mode (longitudinal view)

Most studies have described the sonographic assessment of the longitudinal IVC diameter, using the calipers on still images of maximal inspiration and expiration (Figure 7.5). The IVC is most commonly measured in the subxiphoid view, where the walls are parallel, which is usually 1 cm before the confluence of the hepatic veins (or 2 cm before the diaphragm). The AP diameter may also be measured using M-mode. By placing the M-mode cursor on the longitudinal view of the IVC at the level of the hepatic veins or approximately 2 cm distal to the diaphragm, you can measure the AP diameter of the vessel over time (Figure 7.5a,b). It is important to note that since the curved abdominal probe creates a pie-shaped image, placing the M-mode cursor on the true AP diameter can be challenging.

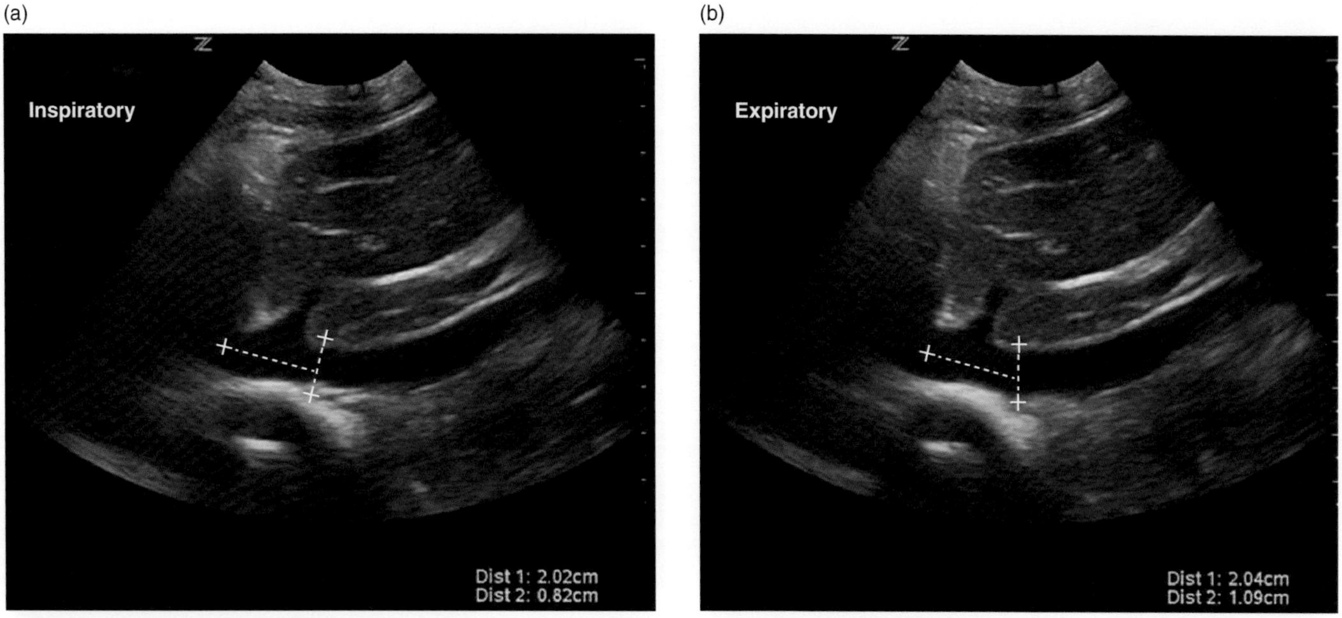

Figure 7.4 IVC respiratory variation, the caval index. (a) In the longitudinal view of the IVC, a measurement can be made of the diameter of the IVC during inspiration 2 cm away from the diaphragm. (b) The longitudinal IVC measurement can be made during expiration. These measurements can be used to calculate the caval index: (1.09 – 0.82) / 1.09 = 0.25 (25%).

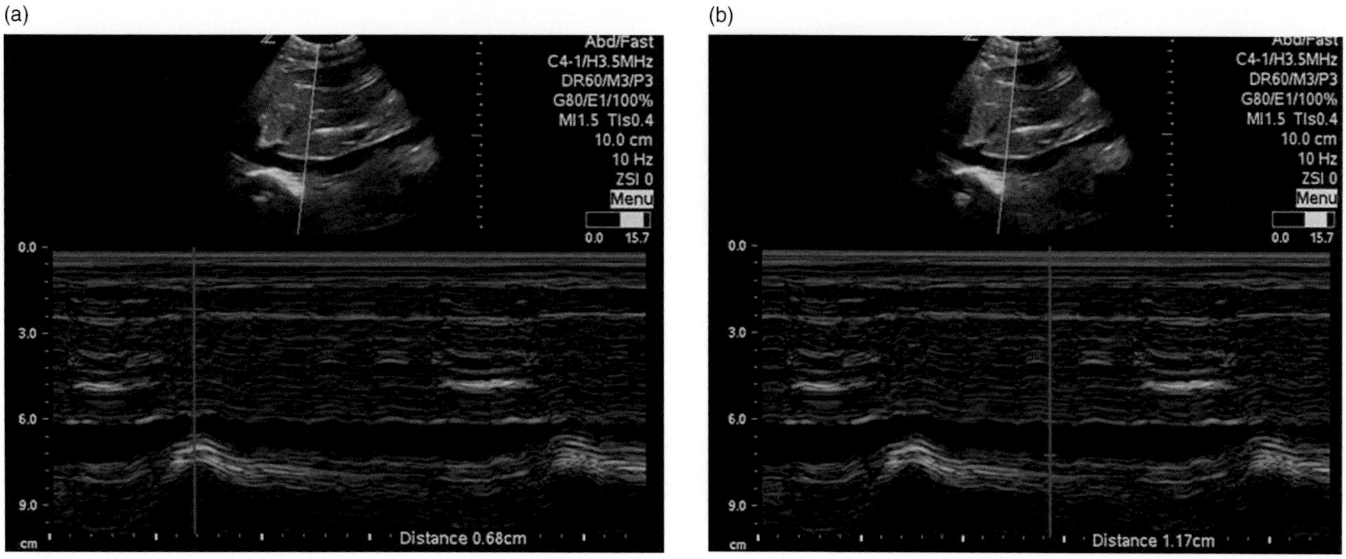

Figure 7.5 M-mode image of IVC. In the longitudinal view of the IVC, measurements can be performed in M-mode during (a) inspiration and (b) expiration.

Ultrasound imaging: aorta

For a complete evaluation of the aorta, it should be evaluated in the transverse view and measured at the proximal aorta (Figure 7.6a), mid aorta (Figure 7.6b), and distal aorta (Figure 7.6c), including the branching into the iliac vessels (Figure 7.6d). The aorta should also be visualized in its long-axis (Figure 7.7). Measurements should be performed from the anterior outer wall to the posterior outer wall. For the transverse view, the aorta is the major vessel lying anterolateral to the vertebral shadow and to the left side of the IVC. The AP diameter of the aorta is measured at the level of proximal, mid, and distal segments. The proximal segment is bounded by the diaphragm and superior mesenteric artery (SMA). The distal segment is the area just proximal to the bifurcation, and the mid-segment is between the proximal and distal segments. The AP diameters of both common iliac arteries are also measured. The purpose of these measurements is to rule out AAA throughout the course of the aorta.

Scanning tips

Pitfalls

- Applying too much pressure during scanning can compress the IVC and would give a false AP diameter measurement.

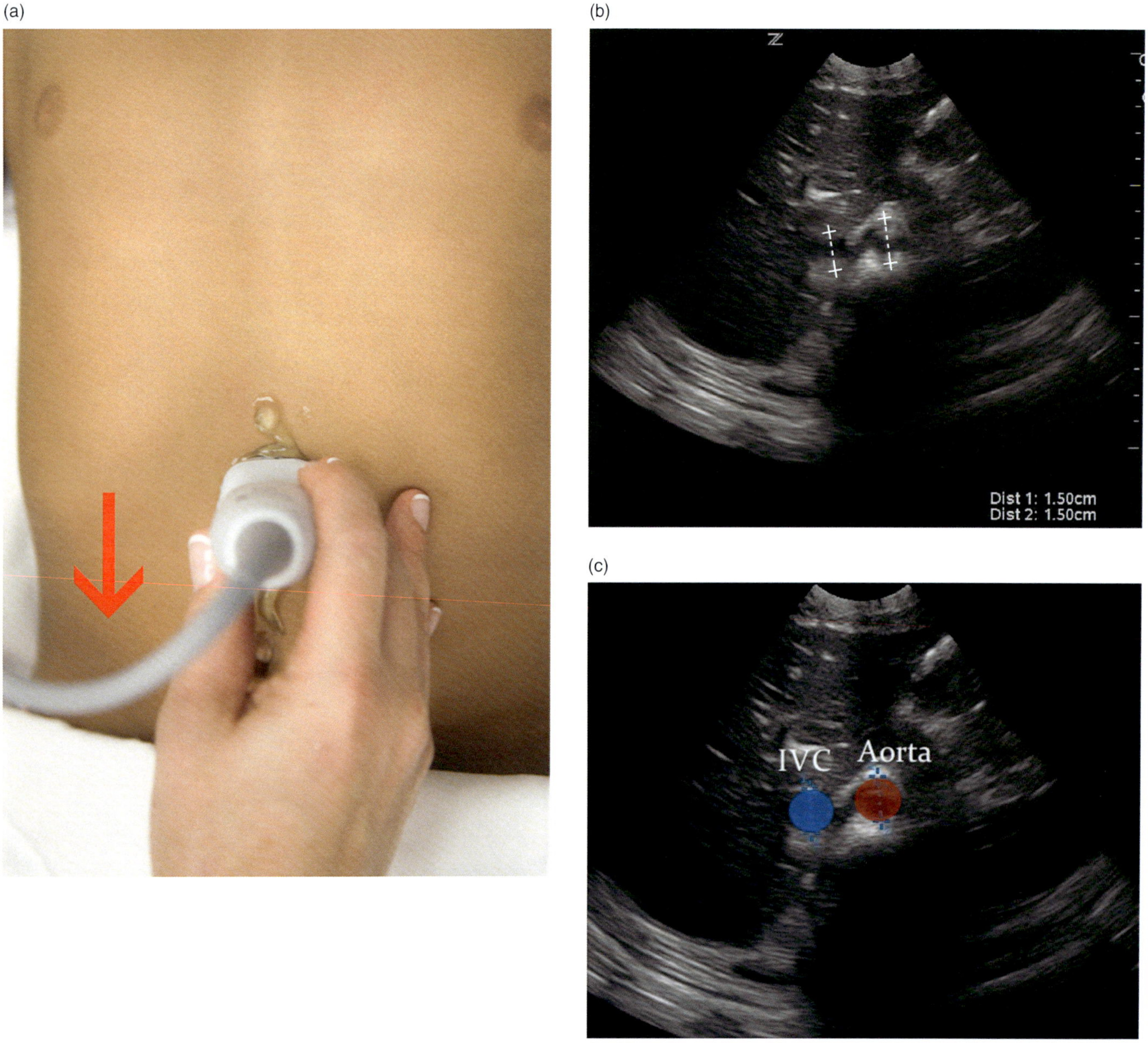

Figure 7.6 Aorta imaging, transverse view. (a) Transducer placement for the evaluation of the aorta is identical to the transducer placement for the IVC. In order to fully evaluate the aorta, it is useful to slide the transducer from the subxiphoid region to the umbilicus, visualizing the aorta along its entirety. (b) The aorta and IVC are visualized in the transverse view. This is a normal IVC/aorta ratio of 1. (c) Illustration indicating important structures visualized on the ultrasound image. *Illustration by Laura Berg, MD.*

Measurements may also be obscured if the transducer is not positioned perpendicular to the patient.

- Scanning superficially, other hollow structures like the gallbladder and other blood vessels in the abdomen can be confused with the IVC and aorta. Always use the vertebral shadow, as the great vessels lie just anterior to the spine. Finding this shadow is the most important imaging landmark to ensure you are scanning correctly.
- Using the size, shape, and pulsation to differentiate the IVC from the aorta can be misleading. Pulsation especially can be transmitted across the thin, low-pressure vena cava wall, especially in small children.
- In the longitudinal view, a false AP diameter can be obtained if the ultrasound beam is not in the mid aorta (Figure 7.9).

Tips to improve scanning

✓ Using the vertebral body as a landmark and right–left orientation is the best way to differentiate the IVC from the aorta.

✓ Aorta AP diameter does not vary with respiration or application of pressure. This can be used to differentiate the aorta from the IVC.

✓ Stomach and bowel lie anterior to the proximal IVC and aorta. Gastrointestinal gas can sometimes make it difficult

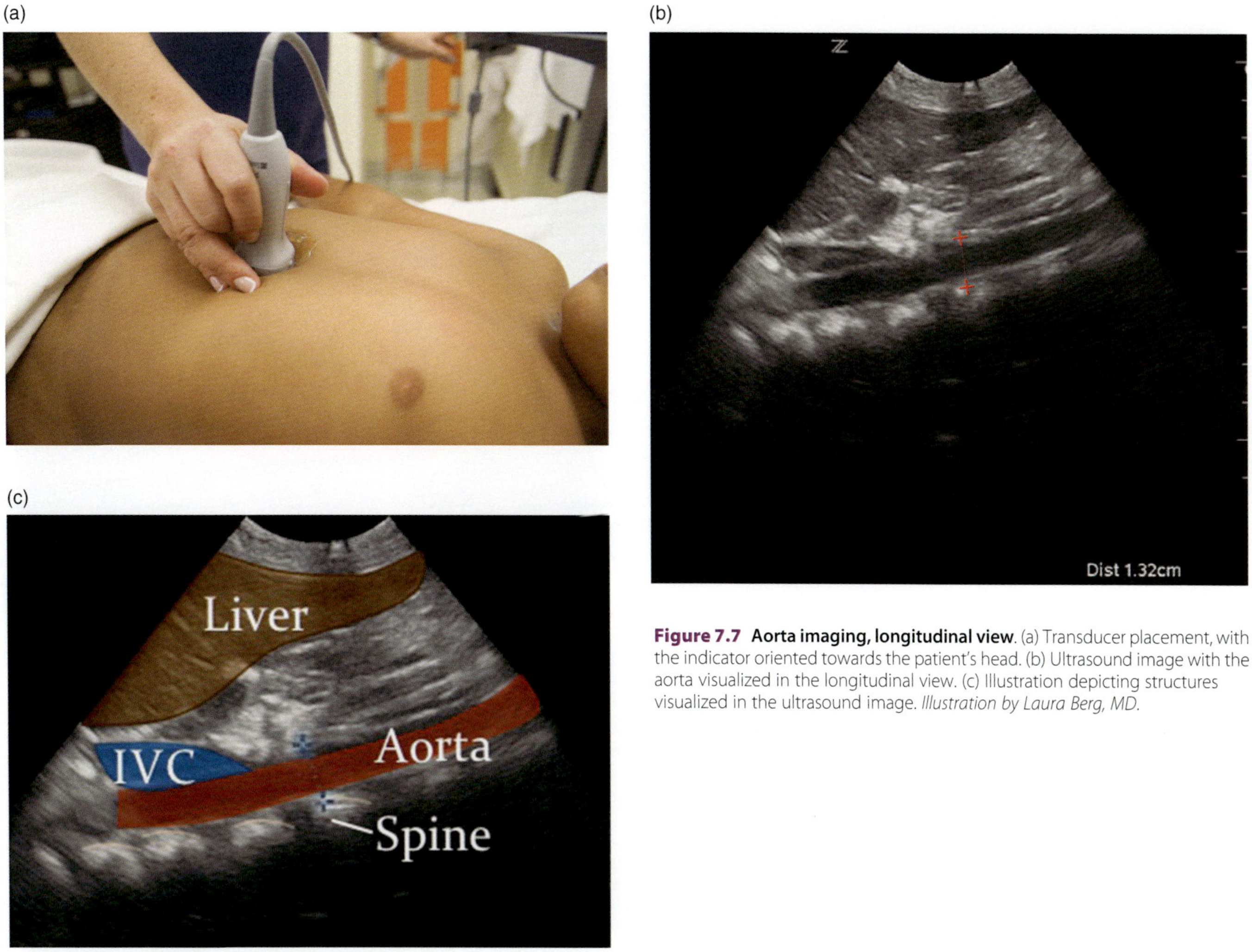

Figure 7.7 Aorta imaging, longitudinal view. (a) Transducer placement, with the indicator oriented towards the patient's head. (b) Ultrasound image with the aorta visualized in the longitudinal view. (c) Illustration depicting structures visualized in the ultrasound image. *Illustration by Laura Berg, MD.*

to visualize the IVC and aorta. Applying gentle pressure or jiggling the transducer can displace the bowel gas and improve the view.

✓ The IVC and aorta can also be viewed from the flanks (coronal plane) and while the patient is in left lateral decubitus to use the liver as an acoustic window (sagittal plane). However, this approach has not been studied as extensively or validated in volume assessment.

✓ In longitudinal view, make sure you fan side to side to get the widest AP diameter.

Pathology

Cases

1. A six-year-old female with a history of a Ventricular Septal Defect (VSD) presents with vomiting, and diarrhea "too numerous times to count" for the past four days. On examination, she is febrile, tachycardic, and irritable. Her mucous membranes are dry and she has a delayed capillary refill time. Her cardiac examination reveals a III/VI systolic ejection murmur heard throughout the precordium. She is given a 20 mL/kg bolus of intravenous fluids but is still tachycardic. A point-of-care ultrasound of the heart reveals a hyperdynamic heart, with good contractility. An ultrasound of the IVC is performed, which shows near complete collapse with respiration. The caval index is calculated to be 60% (Figure 7.10), confirming dehydration.

   This is a commonly encountered clinical scenario that the emergency physician faces. In the setting of congenital heart disease, there is often concern about cardiac function, and overly aggressive fluid rehydration. However, with the utilization of the ultrasound to assess the IVC for dehydration, in conjunction with a focused cardiac ultrasound, the clinician may easily evaluate the function of the heart and hydration status.

2. A two-year-old male presents with vomiting and diarrhea for the past day. According to the parents, he is unable to tolerate any liquids by mouth. On physical examination, the child appears tired and dehydrated. When attempting oral rehydration in the emergency department, he immediately vomits. A point-of-care ultrasound is performed to further evaluate the child's hydration status. Intravenous fluids are administered, and the ultrasound is repeated. The IVC/Ao

(a)

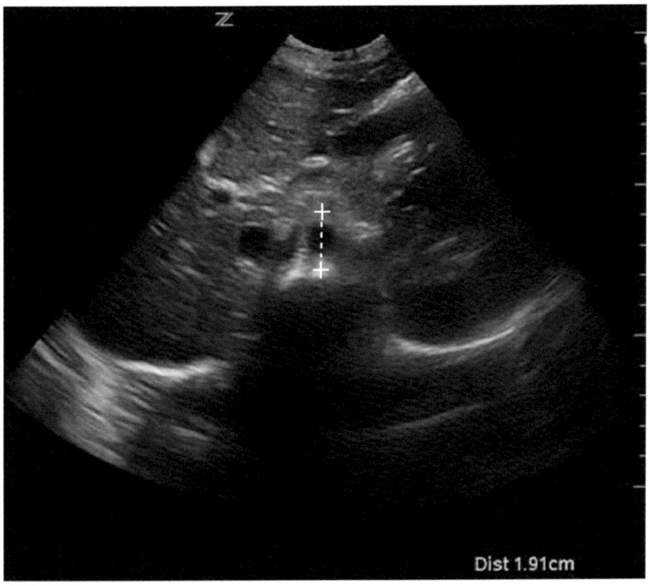

(b)

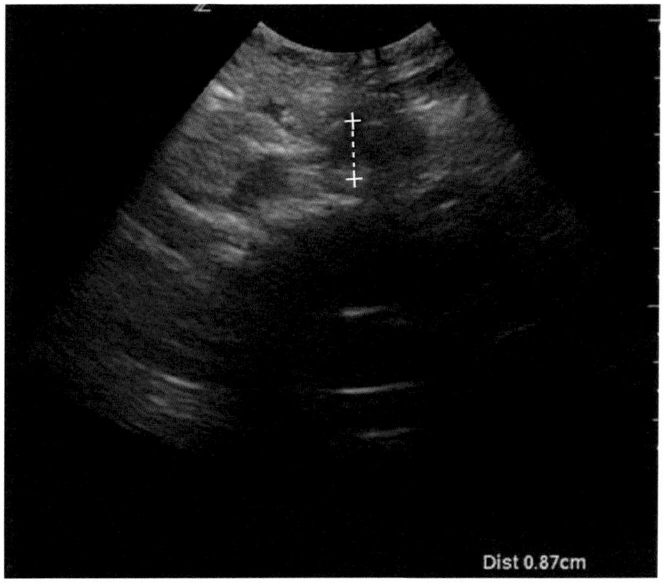

(c)

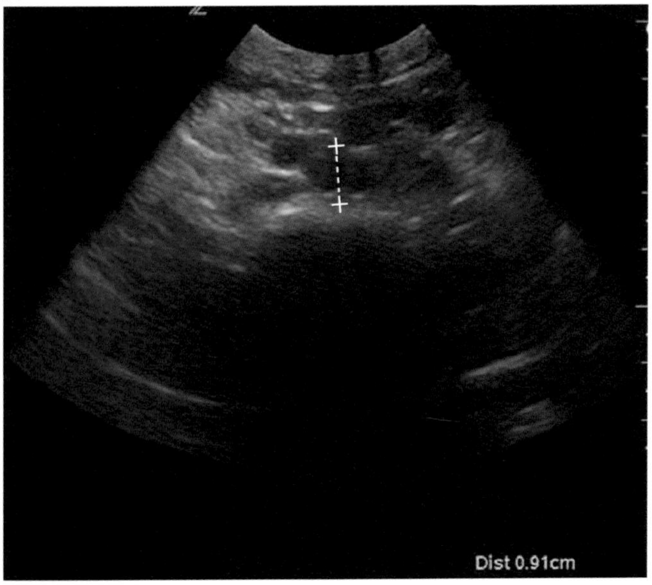

(d)

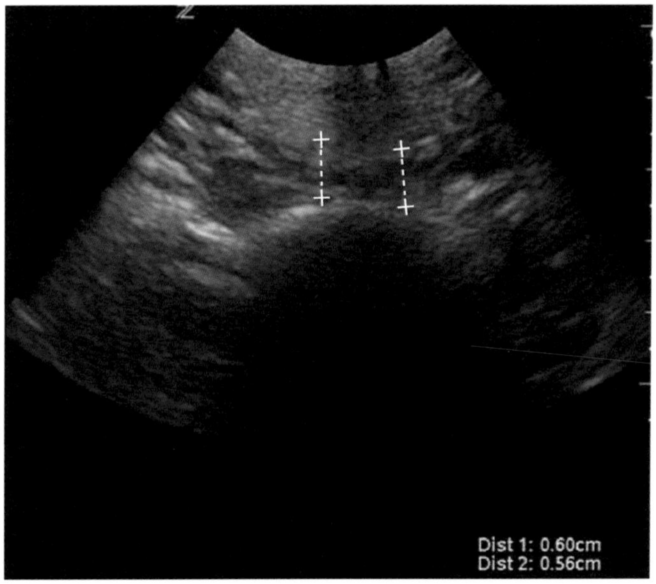

(e)

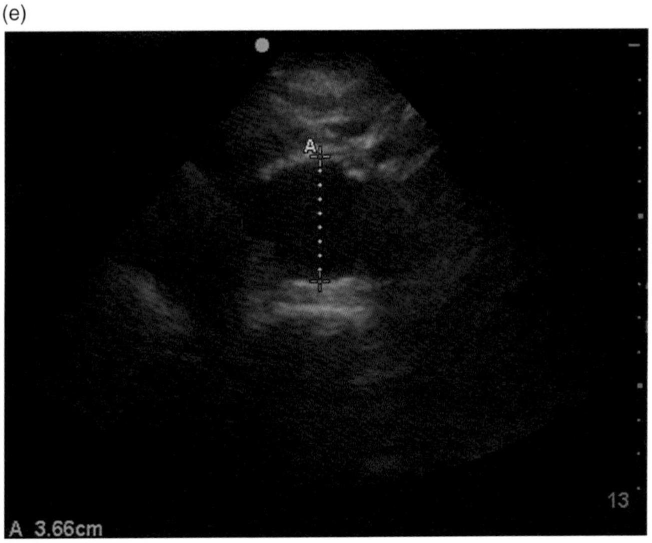

Figure 7.8 Transverse aorta measurements. It is important to perform these measurements anterior–posterior the outer walls at each level. (a) Proximal aorta; note the liver that is visible at this level. (b) Mid aorta. (c) Distal aorta. (d) The iliac arteries.

ratio is calculated both prior to and following intravenous fluid administration (Figure 7.11a,b). The IVC/Ao ratio increases to greater than 1 after fluid administration.

This case highlights the importance of using the IVC/Ao ratio in small children. Since the size of the IVC changes with age and size of the patient, the IVC/Ao ratio allows for a correction factor, since presumably the aorta has the same age and size dependence and does not vary based on hydration status.

3. A 12-year-old male with Marfan syndrome presents with acute chest pain and diffuse abdominal pain. He is unable to describe the pain, but points to the substernal and epigastric regions. On examination, he is acutely ill appearing, diaphoretic, and tachycardic. A point-of-care ultrasound is immediately performed, which shows a dissection flap in the abdominal aorta (Figure 7.12a,b).

Though exceedingly rare, aortic dissection must be considered in children with acute chest pain and predisposing conditions such as Marfan syndrome. Since this entity has a high mortality, the clinician should have a high index of suspicion in the appropriate clinical scenario. While point-of-care ultrasonography may

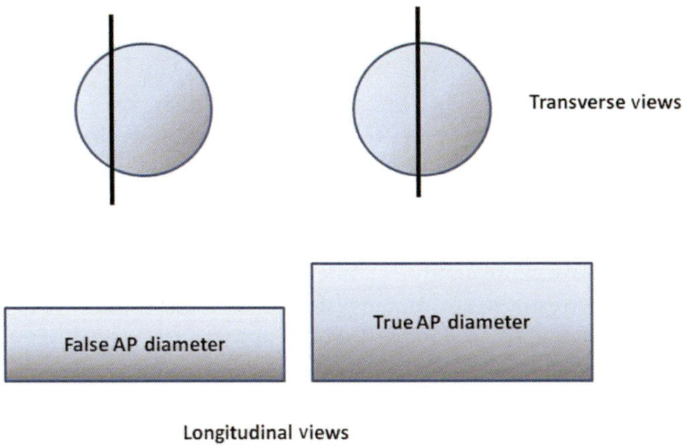

Figure 7.9 True vs. false AP diameter. It is important to maintain proper transducer orientation, especially when performing measurements. Measurements also need to be performed anterior–posteriorly in the center of the vessel. For the aorta, measurements need to be performed from the outer anterior wall to the posterior outer wall.

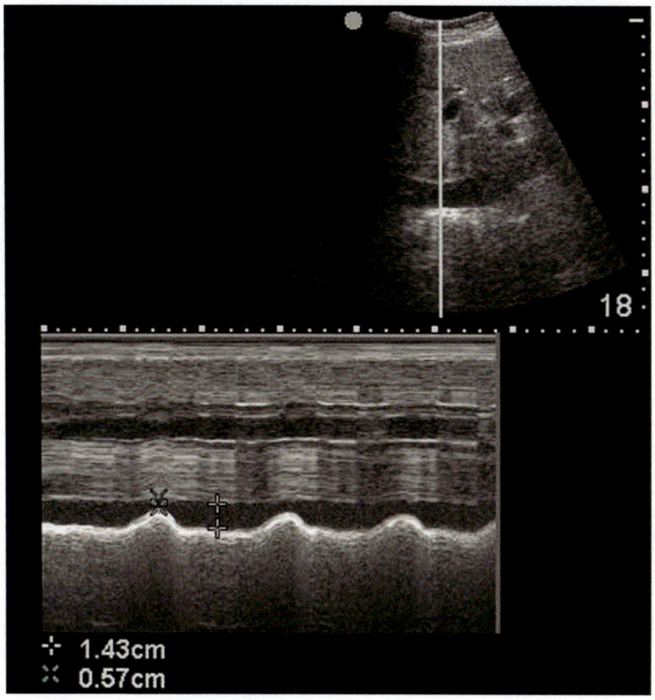

Figure 7.10 Case 1: caval index. In this patient, the caval index is calculated from measurements of the IVC performed in the longitudinal view, in M-mode. The calculated caval index is 60%, which is consistent with dehydration.

(a) (b)

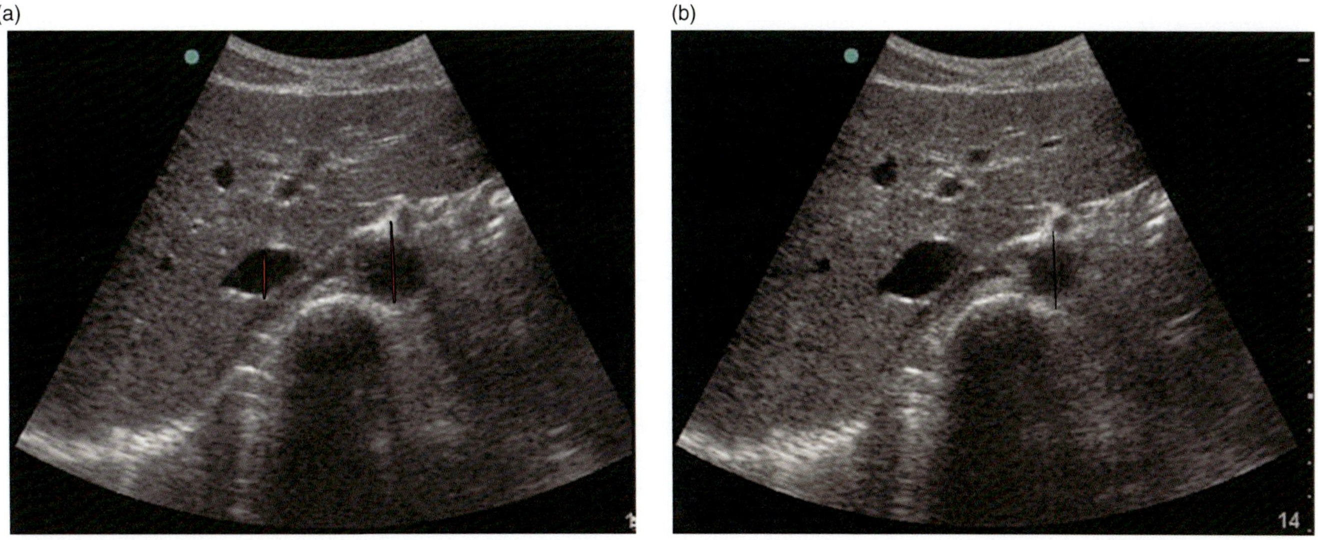

Figure 7.11 Case 2: IVC/Ao ratio. In this dehydrated patient, measurements are performed of the proximal aorta (Ao) and IVC (a) before intravenous fluids, and (b) following intravenous fluids, indicating adequate hydration.

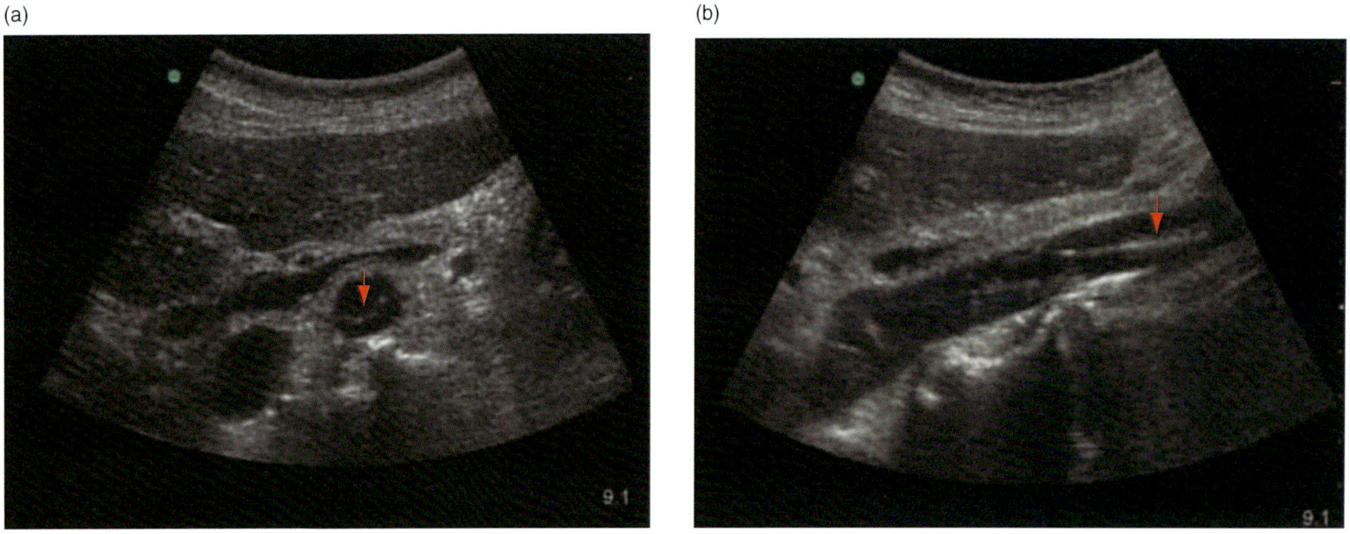

Figure 7.12 Case 3: aortic dissection. The dissection flap (arrow) can be visualized in the (a) transverse aortic view, and the (b) longitudinal aortic view.

be helpful in rapidly identifying this condition, it should not be solely relied upon to diagnose or exclude aortic dissection. Other diagnostic studies to evaluate for the presence of an aortic dissection include MRI and angiography.

Summary/key points

1. Ultrasound assessment of the IVC can be used as an objective tool to evaluate hydration status.
2. A caval index greater than 50% is consistent with a low CVP. A transverse IVC/Ao ratio < 1 is consistent with dehydration in children.
3. The vertebral shadow can be used as a landmark to identify the aorta and IVC, which are anterior to the vertebral shadow. It is important to maintain the correct transducer orientation in order to correctly identify the IVC and aorta.
4. In order to thoroughly evaluate the aorta for the presence of an aneurysm, measurements should be made at the proximal, mid, and distal aorta in addition to the iliac arteries. An aortic measurement of >3 cm and iliac measurement of >1.5 cm is consistent with an aneurysm.
5. Patients may be evaluated for concern of an aortic dissection: a dissection flap can be detected using point-of-care ultrasound.

Selected references

Chen, L., Hsiao, A., Langham, M., *et al.* (2010) Use of bedside ultrasound to assess degree of dehydration in children with gastroenteritis. *Acad Emerg Med* **17**: 1042–7.

Chen, L., Kim, Y., Santucci, K.A. (2007) Use of ultrasound measurement of the inferior vena cava diameter as an objective tool in the assessment of children with clinical dehydration. *Acad Emerg Med* **14**(10): 841–5.

Dipti, A., Soucy, Z., Surana, A., Chandra, S. (2012) Role of inferior vena cava diameter in assessment of volume status: a meta-analysis. *Am J Emerg Med* **30**(8): 1414–19.e1.

Haines, E.J., Chiricolo, G.C., Aralica, K., *et al.* (2012) Derivation of a pediatric growth curve for inferior vena caval diameter in healthy pediatric patients: brief report of initial curve development. *Crit Ultrasound J* **4**(1): 12.

Kosiak., W., Swieton, D., Piskinowicz, M. (2008) Sonographic inferior vena cava/aorta diameter index, a new approach to the body fluid status assessment in children and young adults in emergency ultrasound – preliminary study. *Am J Emerg Med* **26**: 320–5.

Lyon, M., Blaivas, M., Brannam, L. (2005) Sonographic measurement of the inferior vena cava as a marker of blood loss. *Am J Emerg Med* **23**(1): 45–50.

Nagdev, A.D., Merchant, R.C., Tirado-Gonzalez, A., *et al.* (2010) Emergency department bedside ultrasonographic measurement of the caval index for noninvasive determination of low central venous pressure. *Ann Emerg Med* **55**(3): 290–5.

Ng, L., Khine, M., Taragm, B.H., *et al.* (2013) Does bedside sonographic measurement of the inferior vena cava diameter correlate with central renous pressure in the assessment of intravascular volume in children? *Pediatr Emerg Care* **29**(3): 337–41.

Schefold, J.C., Storm, C., Bercker, S., *et al.* (2010) Inferior vena cava diameter correlates with invasive hemodynamic measures in mechanically ventilated intensive care unit patients with sepsis. *Emerg Med* **38**(5): 632–7.

Stawicki, S.P., Braslow, B.M., Panebianco, N.L., *et al.* (2009) Intensivist use of hand-carried ultrasonography to measure IVC collapsibility in estimating intravascular volume status: correlations with CVP. *J Am Coll Surg* **209**(1): 55–61.

Chapter 8

HEENT (head, ears, eyes, nose, throat): ocular, sinus, neck ultrasound

Jennifer R. Marin and Arun Nagdev

Objectives/indications

Children often present to the emergency department with complaints regarding the head and neck. Such pathology affecting the head and neck involves infectious processes, anatomic abnormalities, and trauma. Only recently has point-of-care ultrasound been applied to the diagnosis of pathology affecting the head and neck.

Point-of-care ultrasonography may be applied to various pathologic processes in the head and neck, including ocular, neck masses, peritonsillar abscesses, and sinusitis. Ophthalmologists have utilized ocular ultrasound since the 1950s. With ultrasound, numerous processes can be identified. This includes but is not limited to vitreous hemorrhage, retinal detachment, globe rupture, and foreign bodies. Ocular ultrasound may also be used as an indirect measurement of intracranial pressure.

In addition, children of all ages often present with various neck masses. The identification of the neck mass is integral to the proper management and treatment of these patients. However, it is often clinically difficult to distinguish an enlarged lymph node from an abscess or a congenital anatomic abnormality. Older children may present with signs and symptoms suggestive of a peritonsillar abscess. However, it may be difficult to distinguish an abscess from peritonsillar cellulitis. Further, given the proximity to the vessels, it is imperative to identify a fluid collection prior to incision and drainage. Lastly, there is some role for ultrasonography in identifying sinusitis. In the future, there is potential for point-of-care ultrasound to augment or even eventually replace other diagnostic modalities such as tomography, MRI, or radiographs, which involve radiation and/or extensive cost and resources.

Ultimately, the application of point-of-care ultrasound is still evolving for pathology involving the head and neck. This chapter reviews existing literature for each application, and the technique to perform these examinations.

OCULAR ULTRASOUND

Background

The evaluation of the pediatric eye can be challenging for clinicians, particularly in the setting of trauma. Given the fluid-filled nature of the eye and superficial location, ultrasonography is ideal in detecting both normal anatomy and pathology. Ocular ultrasound offers the unique ability to evaluate all key structures of the eye, with minimal cooperation from the patient. It can be utilized to detect globe rupture, the presence of foreign bodies, and may also be useful in the evaluation of intracranial pressure. Particularly in settings where an ophthalmologist may not be available to evaluate a patient emergently, ocular ultrasound may be used as a screening tool to evaluate those patients that require emergent evaluation versus those patients who can be seen in the next 24 hours.

Ocular ultrasound is a tool that has historically been utilized by ophthalmologists in the diagnosis of ocular pathology and disease processes. The use of ocular ultrasound by emergency physicians was first described in 2000 for the diagnosis of globe rupture and vitreous detachment in adult patients. Since then, several small case series of adult patients have suggested the utility of point-of-care ultrasound for patients with other ocular pathology, including vitreous hemorrhage, retinal detachments, globe rupture, central retinal artery and vein occlusion, lens dislocation, retrobulbar hematomas, and foreign bodies. Blaivas *et al.* studied emergency department patients with a history of eye trauma of acute visual change. Their results showed a sensitivity of 100%, specificity of 97.2%, PPV of 96.2%, and an NPV of 100% in diagnosing ocular pathology. This pathology included penetrating globe injuries, retinal detachments, central retinal artery occlusion, lens dislocation, vitreous hemorrhage, and vitreous detachment. Emergency sonologists were in agreement with the criterion standard in 60 of the 61 cases.

Another use of ocular ultrasound has been optic nerve sheath diameter (ONSD) measurements as a surrogate marker for the diagnosis of elevated intracranial pressure. A positive correlation has been shown between optic nerve sheath diameter and intracranial pressure as measured by an invasive monitoring device. Point-of-care ultrasound may have a role as a screening test for elevated intracranial pressure in patients with traumatic brain injury, as the specificity and negative predictive value were 100% in one study. In another study of patients with suspected elevated intracranial pressure, point-of-care ultrasound demonstrated a high sensitivity and specificity with an enlarged ONSD (>5 mm). There have also been several studies specifically addressing the use of ocular ultrasound in pediatric patients. In a case-control study of symptomatic patients with radiologic confirmation of elevated intracranial pressure (CT or head ultrasound), there was a highly significant difference in the ONSD in the case group compared to the control group. Le *et al.* evaluated patients with

Pediatric Emergency and Critical Care Ultrasound, ed. Stephanie J. Doniger. Published by Cambridge University Press.

suspected increased intracranial pressure in the emergency department and intensive care unit. They used cut-offs as per established norms for ONSD of 4.0 mm in children of less than one year and 4.5 mm in children of one year and older. The gold standard to which the optic nerve measurement was compared was CT scan, ventriculostomy pressure, or lumbar puncture opening pressure. Using the measurements by the ophthalmic sonographers, the study found a sensitivity of 83% and a specificity of 38%. Interestingly, PEM physicians demonstrated the highest sensitivity at 96%, but poor specificity. This difference in sensitivity may be due to the fact that clinicians were not blinded to the signs and symptoms when performing ultrasound examinations. Further studies are needed in patients with blunt head trauma, intraventricular shunts and suspected shunt malfunction, and altered mental status. Point-of-care ultrasound may play a role as a screening tool in the initial assessment of patients presenting with multisystem trauma.

Anatomy

It is important to recognize the anatomic structures of the eye (Figure 8.1). The soft tissue of the eyelid surrounds the globe itself. The cornea, conjunctiva, iris, lens, anterior chamber, and posterior chamber are easily visualized by sonography. The posterior chamber consists of aqueous humor, retina, choroid, and sclera. At the posterior aspect of the globe is the retina, with the optic nerve exiting the eye posteriorly.

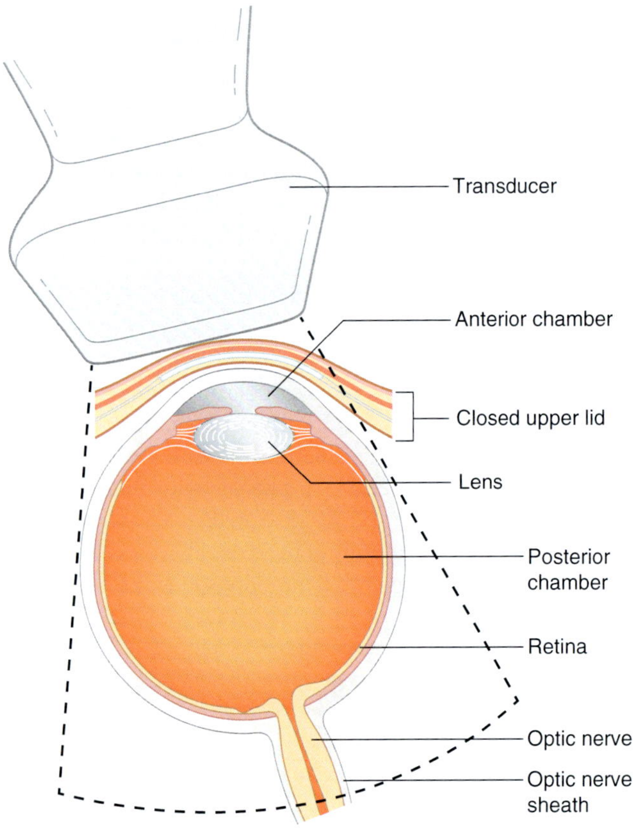

Figure 8.1 Anatomy of the eye. Important structures to become familiar with are the anterior chamber, lens, posterior chamber, retina, and optic nerve. *Artwork created by Emily Evans © Cambridge University Press.*

Technique

Point-of-care questions

1. Is there increased intracranial pressure (optic nerve measurement > 4–5 mm)?
2. Is a ruptured globe present?
3. Is an ocular foreign body present?

Transducer selection and orientation

Ocular ultrasound is best performed with a linear-array, high-frequency transducer (5–10 MHz). The transducer should be applied gently to avoid pressure and trauma to the eye. The indicator should be oriented initially in the transverse plane (towards the patient's right) and then the longitudinal plane (towards the patient's head).

Patient position and preparation

When performing ultrasonography of the eye, particular attention should be paid to patient comfort. In addition, especially when considering a potential globe rupture, very minimal pressure should be placed on the eyelid itself. By resting the operator's hand on the bony orbital rim, more control, and less pressure, will be transmitted to the eye. A copious amount of gel should be placed on the eyelid prior to performing ultrasonography (Figure 8.2a). Alternatively, it is often recommended to place a non-occlusive dressing over the closed eye. Care should be taken to remove all air between the non-occlusive dressing and the eyelid in order to reduce undesired artifacts. Ultrasound gel is then placed over the non-occlusive dressing to form an anechoic window for the sonographic evaluation of the eye.

Ultrasound imaging

Scanning through the entire span of the globe in each plane is important to identify pathology. If the patient is cooperative, it may be helpful to have the patient look up and down and side to side. It is important to optimize the gain settings, as too much gain will create hyperechoic artifacts, particularly in the posterior chamber of the eye. Conversely, too low a gain might lead to a missed vitreous hemorrhage or retinal detachment.

Ultrasound provides images of the eye from the globe anteriorly, extending posteriorly to the optic nerve (Figure 8.2b). The lid and cornea are echogenic structures, and the aqueous humor appears anechoic and fills the anterior chamber. In pathologic conditions, echoes may be seen within the aqueous humor. The anterior chamber is usually a shallow structure and, therefore, may not always be clearly visible by ultrasound. The lens of the eye appears as a hyperechoic, reflective, concave structure and, as such, may demonstrate reverberation artifact. The posterior chamber consists of vitreous humor, which, like the anterior chamber, appears anechoic. In pathologic conditions, internal echoes may be visualized here as well (Figure 8.3). Located most posterior are the retina, choroid, and sclera, which cannot be individually distinguished by ultrasound in a normal eye. In pathologic states, such as with retinal detachment (Figure 8.4), the layers may be distinguished. The optic nerve is located

Table 8.1 Normal optic nerve sheath diameter (ONSD) varies according to age. Measurements greater than these should raise suspicion for increased intracranial pressure.

Age (years)	Measurement (mm)
<1	4.0
1–15	4.5
Adults	5.0

posterior to the globe, and appears as a hypoechoic, tube-like structure surrounded by hyperechoic retrobulbar fat. The vasculature of the eye is located parallel to and within the optic nerve, and can be visualized using color flow.

Pathology

Increased intracranial pressure

The measurement of the optic nerve may be performed in order to indirectly evaluate for suspected increased intracranial pressure. For optic nerve measurements, the optic nerve should be aligned

(a)

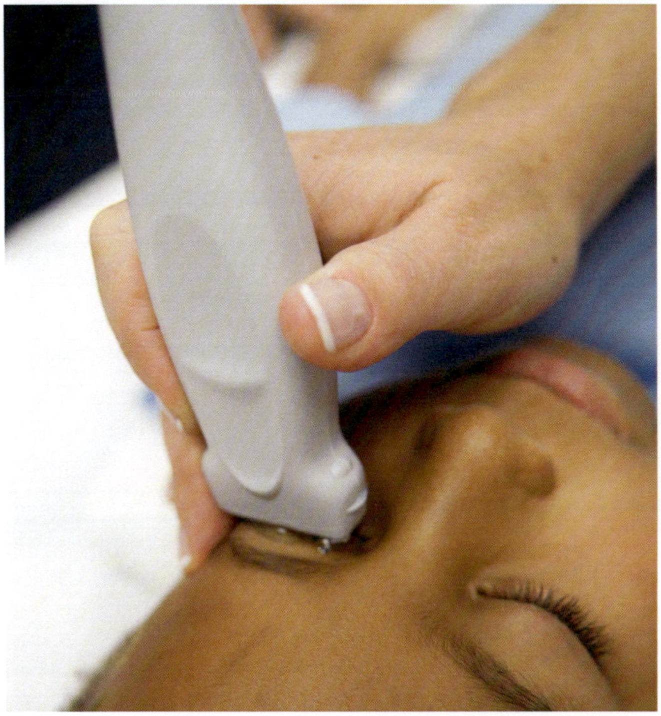

(b)

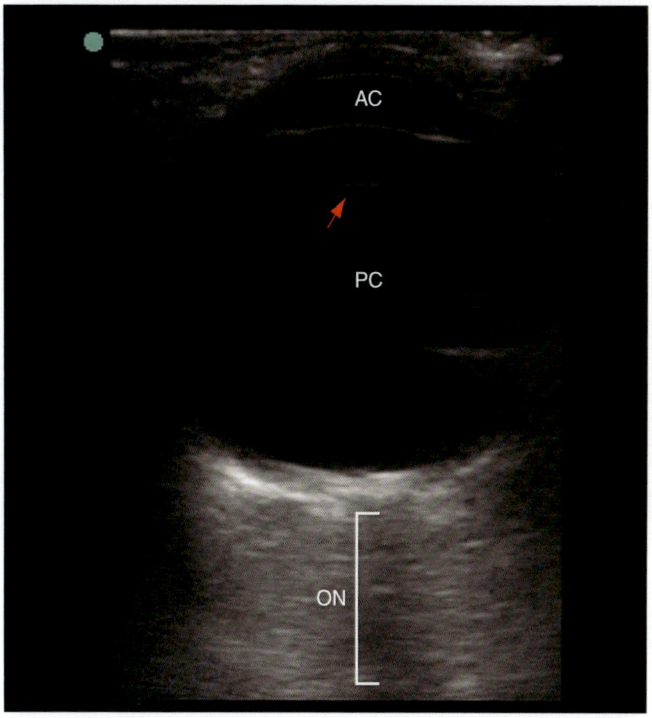

(c)

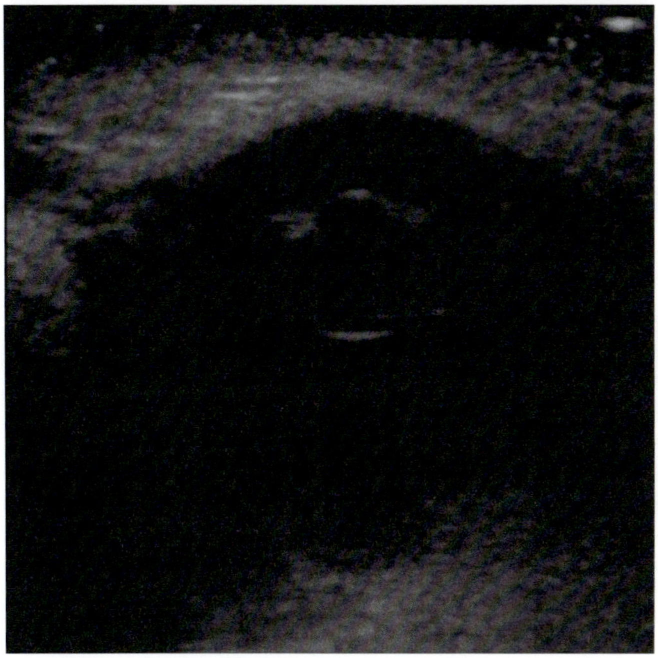

Figure 8.2 Ocular imaging. (a) Transducer placement on a closed eyelid. Note the copious amount of gel, and the clinician resting their hand on the orbital ridge in order to decrease the amount of pressure transmitted to the eye. (b) Ultrasound image of a normal eye, with the anterior chamber (AC), lens (arrow), posterior chamber (PC), optic nerve (ON).

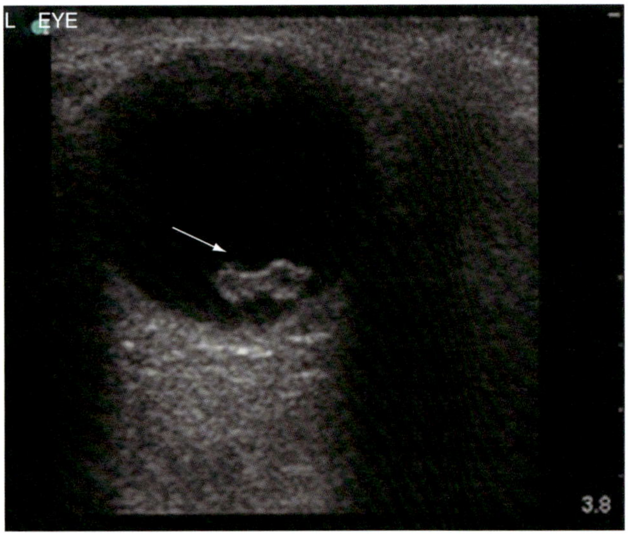

Figure 8.3 **Vitreous hemorrhage** (arrow). *Image courtesy of Dana Sajed, MD.*

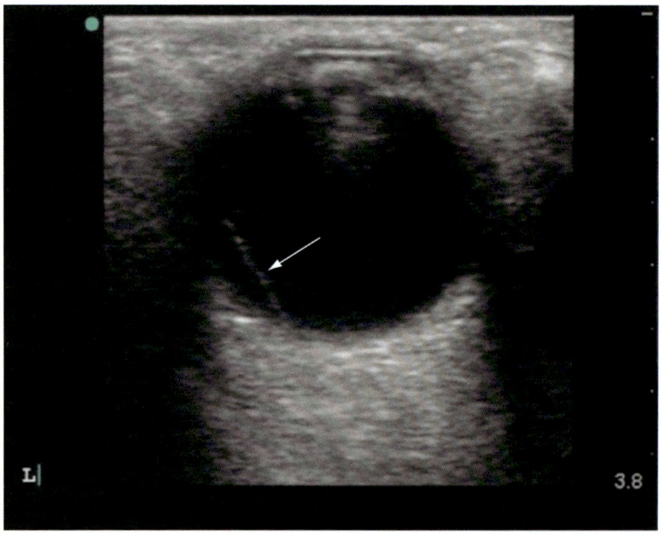

Figure 8.4 **Retinal detachment** (arrow). *Image courtesy of Dana Sajed, MD.*

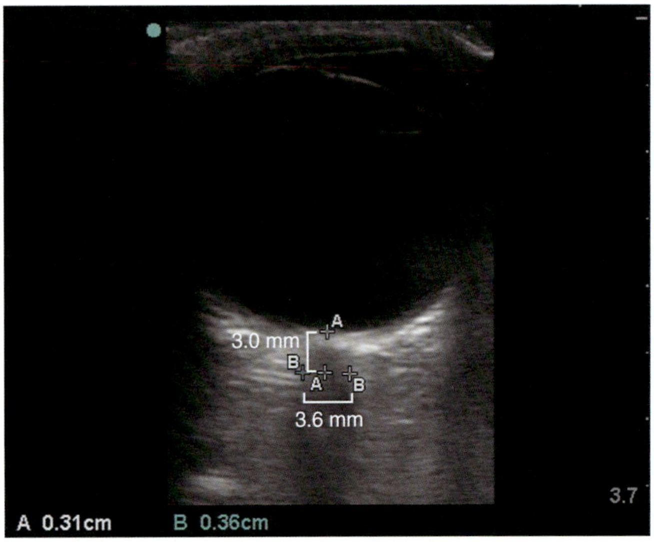

Figure 8.5 **Optic nerve sheath diameter measurement**. The width (B) measures 3.6 mm and is measured 3 mm posterior to the globe (A).

(a)

(b)

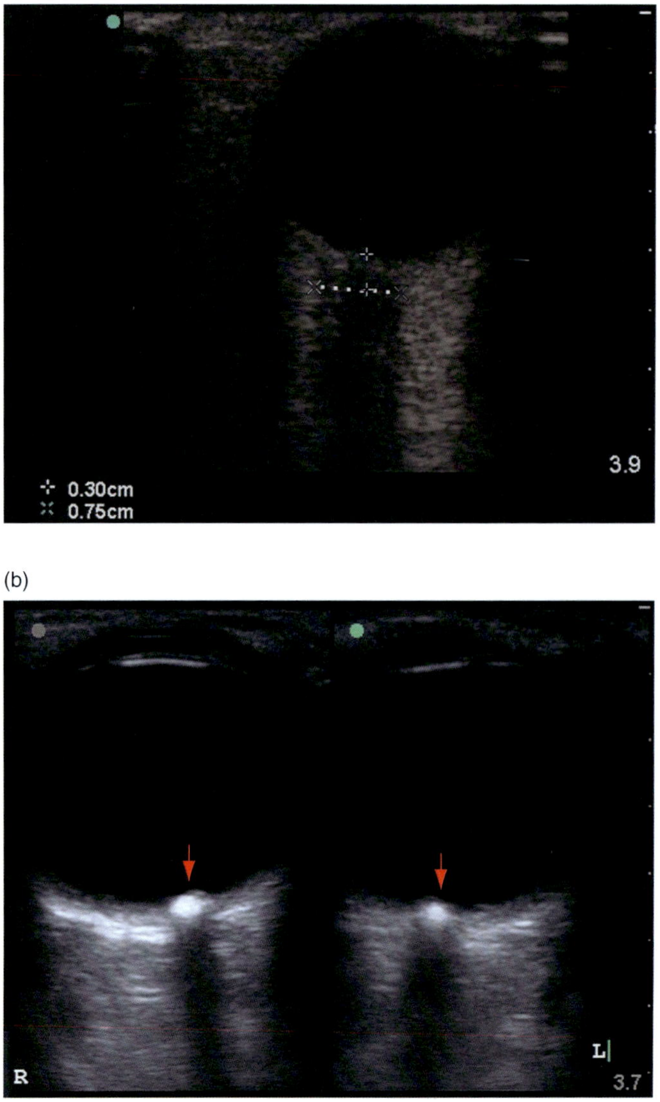

Figure 8.6 **Papilledema**. (a) Optic nerve sheath diameter measuring 7.5 mm, which is consistent with papilledema and increased intracranial pressure. (b) Rare condition mistaken for papilledema, called drusen, in which there is a calcification at the optic nerve.

directly opposite the transducer, with the diameter width perpendicular to the vertical axis of the scanning plane. Measurement of the optic nerve sheath diameter is made 3 mm posterior to the globe (Figure 8.5). Both eyes should be measured, and the mean value used. The upper limit of normal for ONSD varies according to age (Table 8.1). Papilledema is considered when the mean value is greater than the limit for a child's age (Figure 8.6a). A rare condition that may be mistaken for papilledema on both physical examination and ultrasonography is drusen, which involves the deposition of calcium at the optic nerve and creates shadowing posterior to the deposition (Figure 8.6b).

Ruptured globe

Patients with potential globe rupture represent a particular diagnostic dilemma for emergency department physicians. While it is often difficult to diagnose with certainty by clinical examination, it is imperative to diagnose rapidly in order to facilitate operative intervention. The use of point-of-care orbital ultrasonography is

(a)

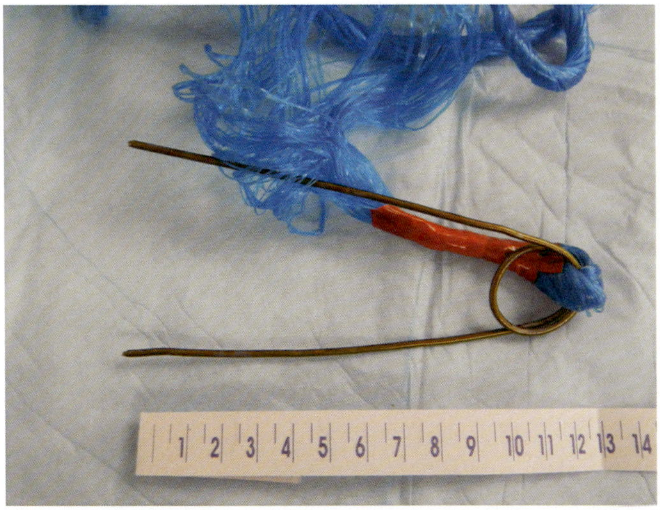

(b)

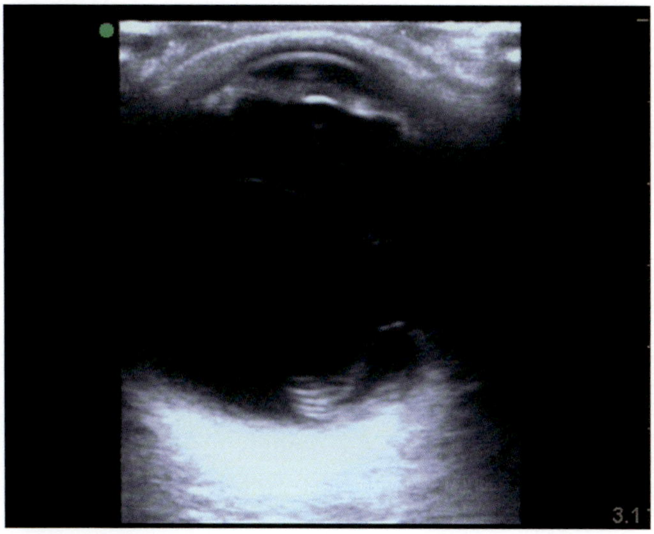

(c)

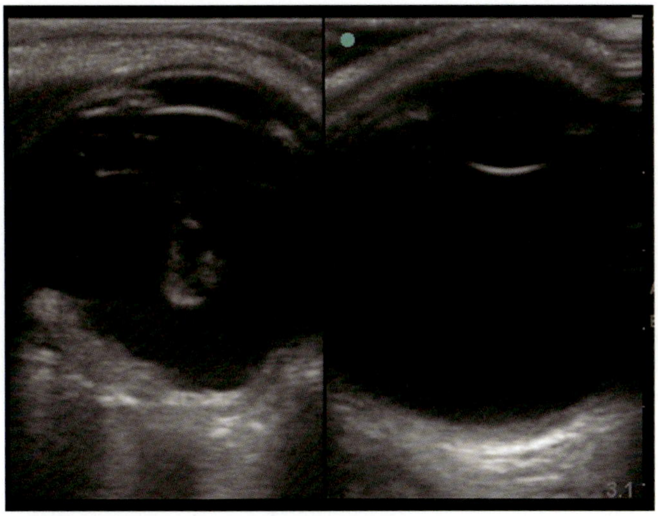

Figure 8.7 Ruptured globe. (a) Object suspected to have punctured a patient's eye. The physical examination was unclear as to whether there was rupture, as the patient had a normal pupil and gross vision was intact. (b) Ultrasound image showing a flattened anterior chambter, hyperechoic regions within the globe, and posterior retinal detachment. (c) Patient with a bullet through his eye. Both eyes are imaged for comparison. The eye on the left side of the image exhibits retinal detachment and globe rupture. Note the decreased overall size, irregularity, and decreased anterior chamber size when compared with the contralateral eye.

an invaluable adjunct to the physical examination in these situations. In ocular trauma, a significant amount of pain, tearing, and orbital and periorbital swelling is often present, further limiting the feasibility of visual inspection. In contrast, orbital ultrasonography is not limited by the degree of soft tissue swelling and edema. Further, it can be performed on a closed eyelid, and can rapidly be performed at the bedside by the emergency physician.

Alternative imaging modalities include plain radiographs, CT scans, and MRI. When compared with ultrasound, each of these methods has significant limitations. Conventional radiographs only allow for the evaluation of major bony injury, and the sensitivity is exceedingly low for other diagnoses of concern as mentioned above. Magnetic resonance imaging is frequently unavailable for emergent cases, is time-consuming, and is contraindicated in the setting of potential metallic foreign bodies. A thin-section helical CT is often considered to be the optimal study, but it also requires patient stabilization and transport outside of the emergency department. Additionally, CT scans expose patients to ionizing radiation, which is of particular concern in pediatric patients. While point-of-care ultrasonography has been used in the diagnosis of globe rupture, controversy remains regarding the safety and theoretical increase in intraocular pressure with placement of the transducer on the eye. Recently, Berg *et al.* measured intraocular pressure during transducer placement in healthy volunteers, showing only a small transient increase in intraocular pressure.

When performing ultrasonography of a patient with a suspected globe rupture, it is imperative that the clinician try to minimize the amount of pressure applied on the eye itself. This may be achieved by resting the operator's hand on the orbital ridge, and applying a copious amount of gel to a closed eyelid. A globe rupture can be visualized as a decreased size of the globe itself, an asymmetric shape, and most notably a collapsed anterior chamber (Figure 8.7). Both the affected and the unaffected eye should be scanned for comparison.

Ocular foreign bodies

Ocular foreign bodies can be metallic, glass, plastic, or wood. They usually become embedded in the conjunctiva or cornea,

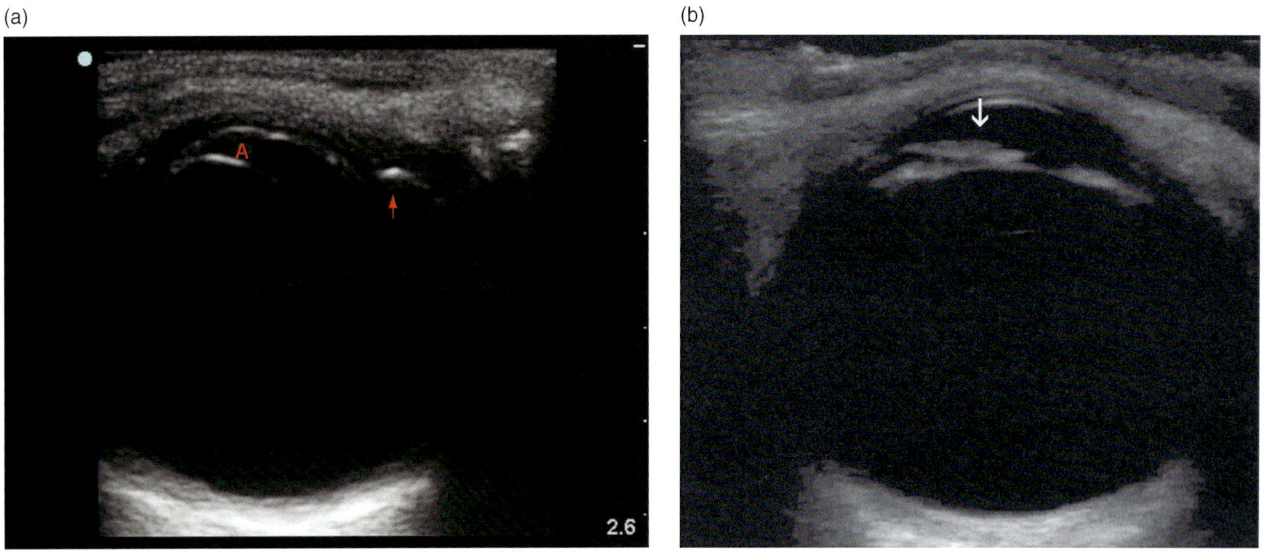

Figure 8.8 Ocular foreign bodies. Glass (arrow) embedded deeply into the cornea, which also led to a globe rupture. Note the small size of the anterior chamber (A).

and are easily appreciated on direct examination. However, occasionally foreign bodies may be small or penetrate deeper through the cornea (Figure 8.8). Ocular foreign bodies can lead to globe rupture, infection, retinal toxicity, and ultimately vision loss. CT scan is the first-line imaging modality of choice. A CT scan can detect metal foreign bodies greater than 1 mm in size. It is also sensitive in detecting glass foreign bodies greater than 1.5 mm in size. However, non-radiopaque materials such as wood are difficult to detect on CT.

Hyphema

A common condition in children is blood in the anterior chamber, or a hyphema. While ultrasound imaging is limited due to the shallow nature of the anterior chamber, a hyphema can be visualized as hyperechoic material within the anterior chamber (Figure 8.8b).

Scanning tips

Pitfalls

- Too little or too much gain can lead to false-negative or false-positive findings.
- Point-of-care ultrasound may not be efficacious in examining the anterior chamber of the eye.
- Controversy exists regarding the application of a transducer on the eye with suspected globe rupture.

Tips to improve scanning

✓ A liberal amount of gel is necessary for optimal imaging and also to minimize pain and further injury to the globe in the case of trauma.

✓ Measurements for optic nerve sheath diameter should be taken 3 mm posterior to the optic disc. Measurements suggesting elevated intracranial pressure: in children of less than 1 year >4.0 mm; children 1–15 years old >4.5 mm; and adults >5.0 mm.

✓ Having the patient move his/her eye in all directions may facilitate scanning through the entire globe.

✓ Be sure to scan the affected eye in two planes, and compare the affected to the unaffected eye.

NECK MASSES

Background

The evaluation of soft tissue neck masses is an important skill in pediatric point-of-care ultrasound, as neck swelling and neck masses are a common complaint, and there are several considerations in the differential diagnosis. Neck masses may be a result of congenital, neoplastic, inflammatory, or infectious conditions. Specifically, it is important to distinguish between surgical and non-surgical diagnoses. In addition to lymphadenopathy and lymphadenitis commonly seen in adult patients, pediatric patients can also present with embryologic remnants previously undiagnosed, which may become acutely enlarged or superinfected. Ultrasound may be used as a first-line modality for the evaluation of these lesions, and in many cases may obviate the need for further imaging.

Ultrasound has been a longstanding first-line imaging tool for radiologists in the evaluation of pediatric neck masses. Radiologists have described the characteristic appearance of inflammatory and non-inflammatory cystic and solid lesions seen in the pediatric neck. Although no studies specific to emergency point-of-care ultrasound for the evaluation of neck masses have been published, there are descriptions in the literature that point-of-care ultrasound is a useful tool for non-radiologists, such as office-based otolaryngologists.

Anatomy

The regions of the neck can be divided into the following scanning areas: the thyroid gland, the paravascular spaces, the anterior and posterior cervical triangles, the supraclavicular fossae, and the major salivary glands. It is important to

(a)

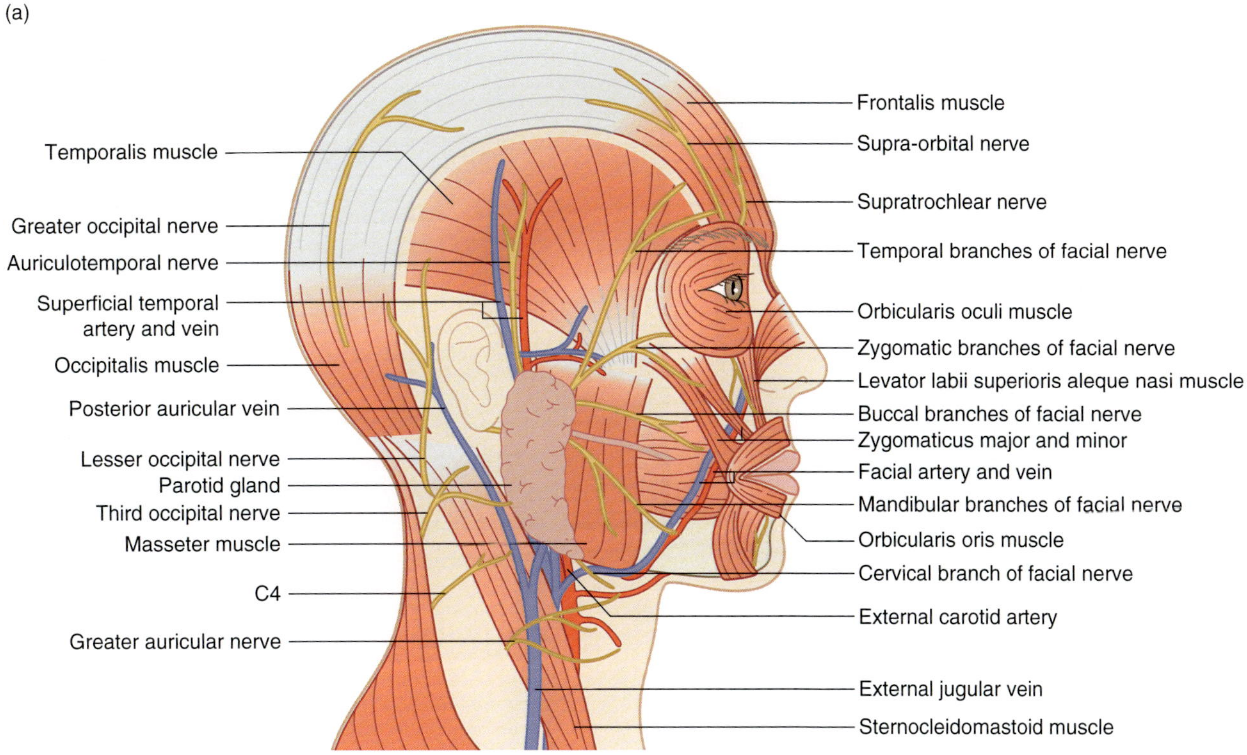

(b)

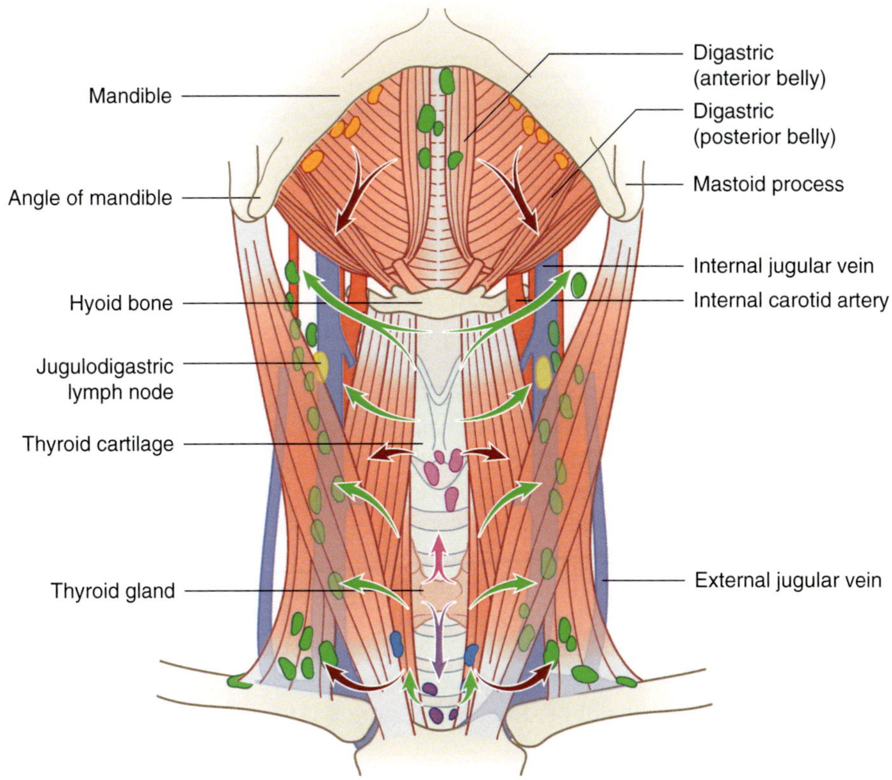

Figure 8.9 Anatomy of the neck. (a) Areas of the neck can be divided into: the thyroid gland, the paravascular spaces, the anterior and posterior cervical triangles, the supraclavicular fossae, and the major salivary glands. (b) Distribution of lymph nodes and lymphatic drainage of the head and neck. *Artwork created by Emily Evans © Cambridge University Press.*

(a)

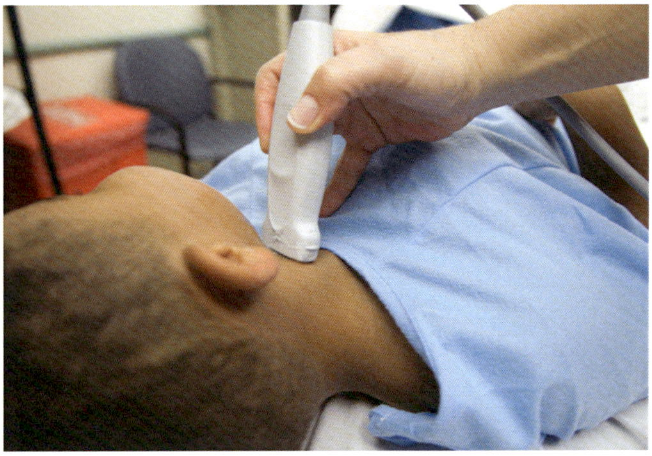

(b)

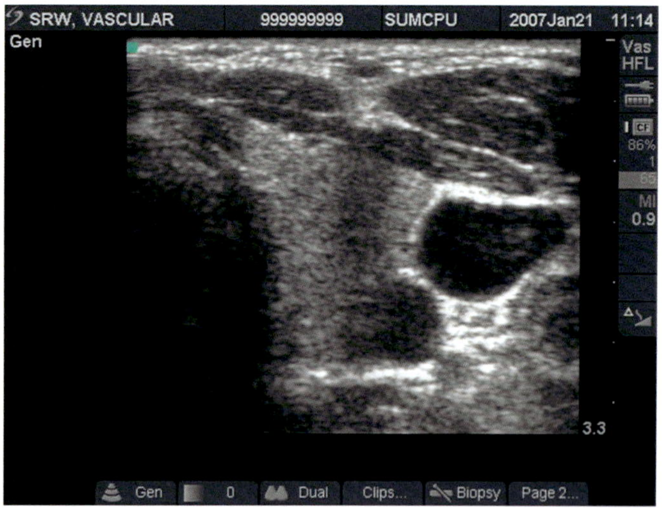

(c)

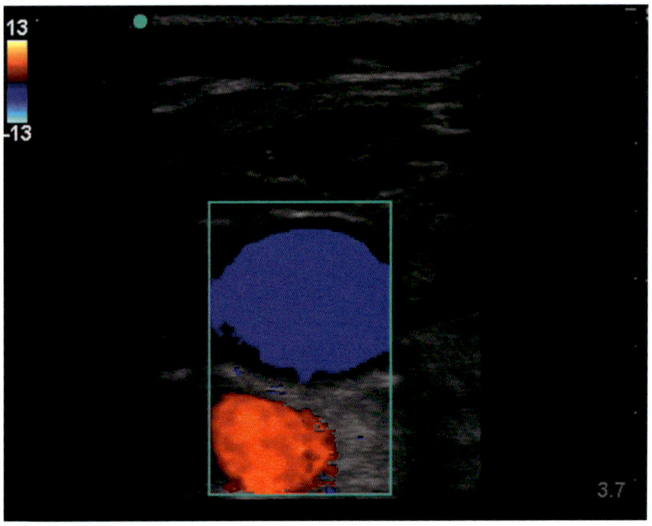

Figure 8.10 **Neck imaging, transverse views.** (a) Transducer placement, with the child in hyperextension and turned to the side. (b) Ultrasound appearance of internal jugular vein (IJ) and carotid artery (C) adjacent to the thyroid gland (Th) and trachea (arrow). (c) Color Doppler flow applied, highlighting the vessels. The blue color represents the blood flow in the direction away from the transducer, seen here in the IJ; the red color represents flow towards the transducer which is seen in the carotid artery.

understand the normal anatomy of the neck before recognizing pathology that may arise in these areas (Figure 8.9a,b).

Technique

Point-of-care questions

1. Is an abscess present? Is an enlarged lymph node present?
2. Is a superinfected congenital anomaly that is causing neck swelling present?

Transducer selection and orientation

A high-frequency, linear transducer (5–10MHz) will allow for the optimal evaluation of the superficial soft tissue structures. If a large lesion is being imaged, however, a curvilinear transducer may be required.

Patient position and preparation

The child should be placed in the supine position with the neck held in hyperextension and turned to the side (Figure 8.10a). It may be helpful to place a towel roll under the shoulders in order to optimize positioning. In the case of tender, painful lesions, a large amount of gel should be used in order to minimize pain.

Ultrasound imaging

It is important to image the contralateral side of the neck, in order to obtain comparison views. As with other ultrasound examinations, lesions should be evaluated in two orthogonal planes, with clips and images recorded in both planes. Color flow imaging may be a useful addition for the more experienced sonographer, allowing for the differentiation between a vasculature structure and a fluid-filled mass. Specifically, color flow evaluation of lymph nodes will demonstrate mixed echogenic masses with low flow in the central aspect. Clinicians should be familiar with the normal appearance of the neck vessels, the internal jugular vein and carotid artery (Figure 8.10b). It is also helpful to be familiar with the neck anatomy, including the thyroid and the trachea, which are midline structures (Figure 8.11).

Pathology

Adenopathy, adenitis, abscesses

Reactive lymph nodes are often seen in the presence of head and neck infections. Sonograpically, they typically appear as discrete, elongated, ovoid lesions with smooth margins, and are located in various regions of lymphatic drainage. They generally appear hypoechoic with a central echogenic hilum (Figure 8.12a). On Color Doppler, reactive lymph nodes exhibit low flow (Figure 8.12b). Normal cervical lymph nodes are rarely seen by ultrasound; however, when seen, they will appear as flattened or oval shaped. A solitary enlarged lymph node, as is seen with adenitis, will appear uniform in echotexture (Figure 8.13a). In the case of a necrotic lymph node, there will be a cystic hypoechoic center (Figure 8.13b).

Distinguishing between reactive and inflammatory lymph nodes by ultrasound can be challenging, and management is often guided by the clinical examination. A key component in the evaluation of lymphadenitis is identifying the presence of an abscess. As with other soft tissue abscesses, ultrasound will demonstrate a hypoechoic or anechoic lesion with irregular margins (Figure 8.14). There may be regions of echogenic debris that may move with gentle pressure. Enlarged salivary glands can also be encountered, as is seen with parotitis (Figure 8.15).

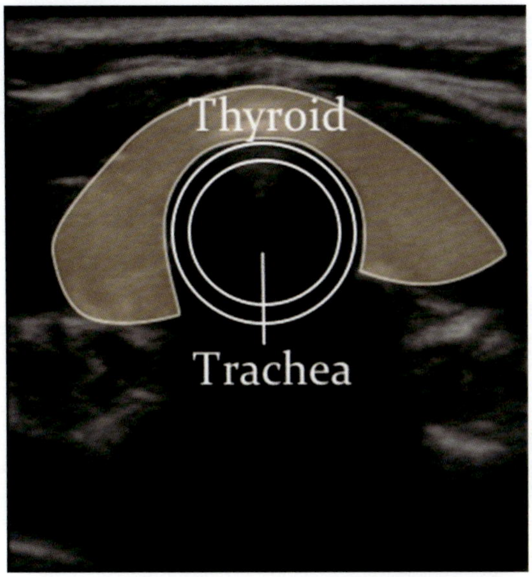

Figure 8.11 Ultrasound anatomy of the neck, midline. Thyroid tissue is outlined and surrounds the trachea. *Illustration by Laura Berg, MD.*

Branchial cleft and thyroglossal duct cysts

Branchial cleft cysts usually arise from the second branchial cleft anterior to the sternocleidomastoid muscle and near the angle of the mandible, but may originate from the first branchial cleft (Figure 8.16a). Sonographically, branchial cleft cysts appear as well-defined, anechoic masses with posterior acoustic enhancement (Figure 8.16c). As with other infected lesions, the mass may appear heterogeneous with echogenic debris, and applying gentle pressure to the lesion may result in movement of the echoes.

Thyroglossal duct cysts are midline structures that arise from a remnant of the thyroglossal duct, which extends from the foramen cecum at the base of the tongue down to the pyramidal lobe of the thyroid gland (Figure 8.17a,b). Since they are cystic structures, thyroglossal duct cysts appear as well-defined, anechoic lesions by ultrasound, with posterior acoustic enhancement. Patients often present with acutely superinfected thyroglossal duct cysts (Figure 8.17c). Sonographically, there may be debris within the cyst, with hypoechoic regions, and heterogeneous, hypoechoic or isoechoic particles (Figure 8.17c,d).

Cystic hygromas

Cystic hygromas are congenital lymphatic malformations due to blocked lymphatic channels. Most lesions present prior to two years of age, with the majority being present at birth. They are located posterior to the sternocleidomastoid muscle. A cystic hygroma characteristically appears as a multiloculated cystic mass. There are septae with variable echogenicities, containing solid components arising from the cyst wall or the septa. Larger lesions have ill-defined boundaries, with cystic components dissecting between normal tissue planes (Figure 8.18). Cystic hygromas can be complicated by infection or hemorrhage, which can lead to increased echogenicity or fluid–fluid levels.

(a)

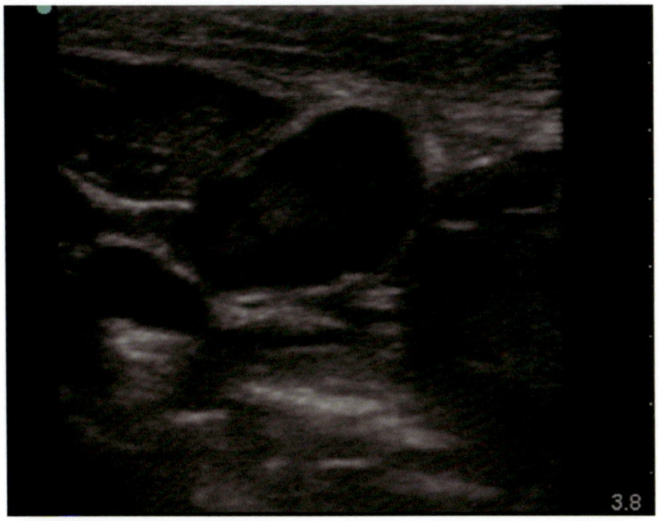

(b)

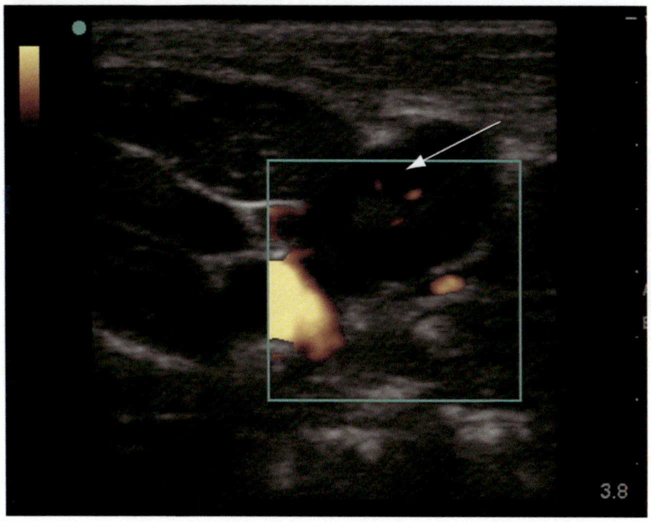

Figure 8.12 Lymph nodes. (a) Multiple enlarged lymph nodes in a patient with unilateral neck swelling. (b) Color Doppler applied. Flow can be seen in the central hilum of the node (arrow).

(a) (b)

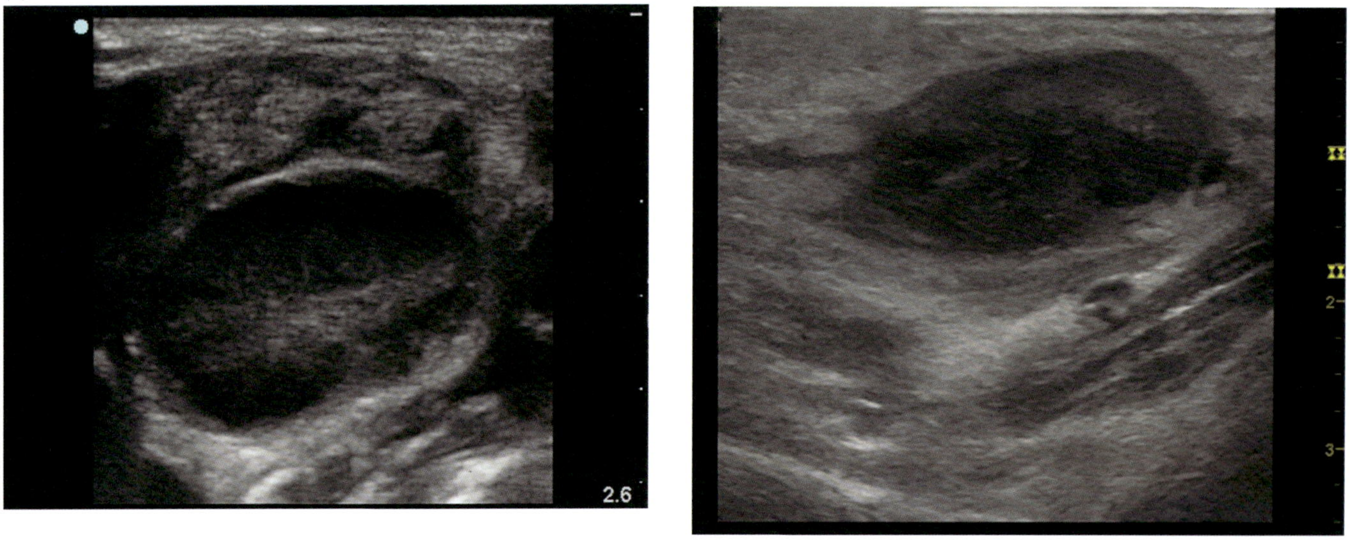

Figure 8.13 Adenitis. (a) An enlarged lymph node exhibits homogeneous echotexture. (b) A necrotic lymph node appears more irregular, with hypoechoic or anechoic regions in the center.

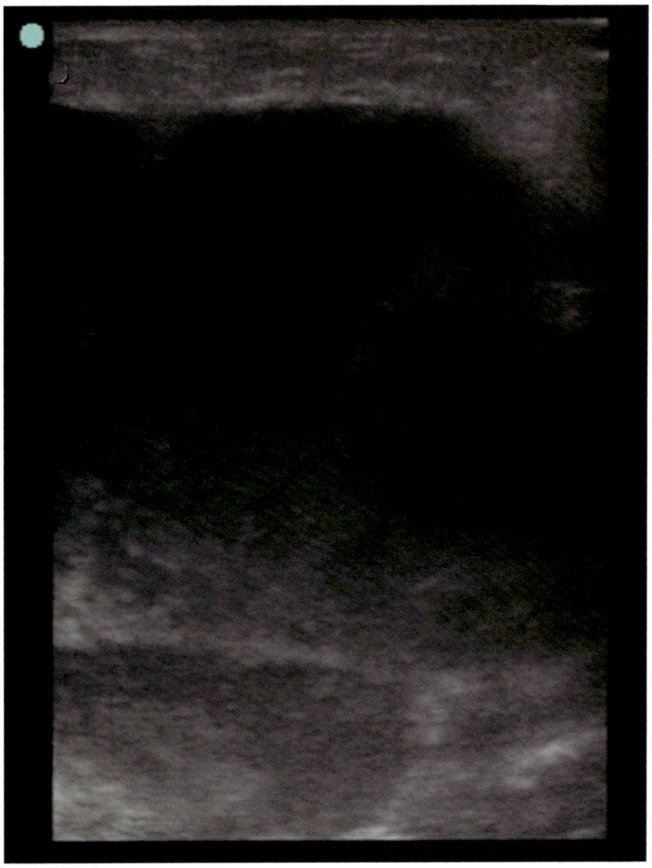

Figure 8.14 Neck abscess. Neck abscesses exhibit an irregular shape containing hypoechoic or anechoic regions in the center.

Fibromatosis coli

Fibromatosis coli is also known as a "sternocleidomastoid tumor of infancy," and is a benign, self-resolving lesion presenting in the neonatal period. Its pathogenesis is largely unknown, but it is likely secondary to birth trauma, which causes secondary pressure necrosis and fibrosis within the muscle. In the initial stages, the mass may enlarge rapidly. After about one to two years of age, it begins to regress, with two-thirds spontaneously resolving.

The lesion is located within the sternocleidomastoid muscle (Figure 8.19a) and consists of dense fibrous tissue. Ultrasound demonstrates a uniformly isoechoic or hypoechoic mass (Figure 8.19c). Clips are helpful to demonstrate the mass moving with the muscle in real time.

Scanning tips

Pitfalls

- The majority of research involving neck masses is in the radiology literature. Further research needs to be performed in order to evaluate the utility and efficacy of point-of-care ultrasound for these applications.
- It is important to distinguish adenitis from an abscess. An abscess will appear as an irregular hypoechoic or anechoic structure.
- Proper patient positioning and analgesia are important in obtaining an adequate scan.

Tips to improve scanning

✓ Perform contralateral imaging in order to image the "normal" anatomy.

✓ Central color flow can help distinguish lymph nodes from other lesions in the neck.

✓ Identification of a superinfected lesion (i.e. abscess) may indicate the need for immediate surgical intervention.

✓ Thyroglossal duct cysts are midline lesions found anywhere along the path of the embryologic thyroglossal duct.

(a)

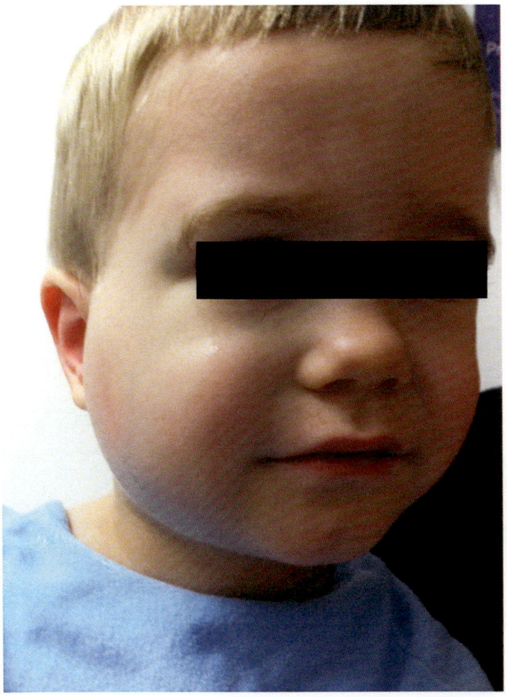

(b)

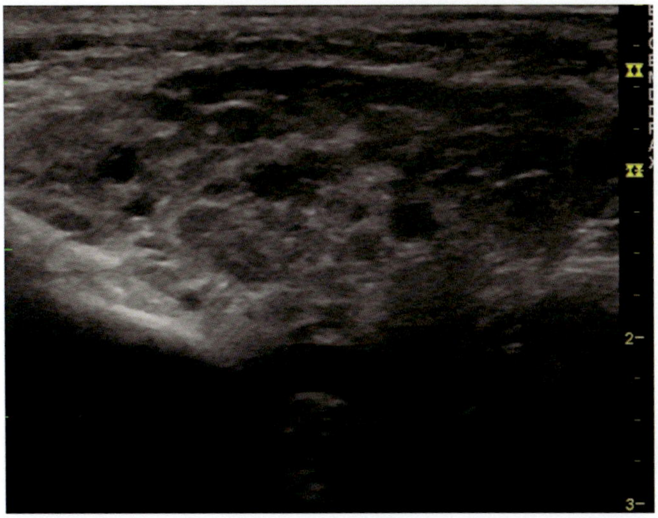

Figure 8.15 **Parotitis.** (a) This child presented with facial and submandibular swelling. (b) On ultrasonography, the mass has a characteristic appearance of parotitis, with multiple hypoechoic round structures.

✓ The most common location for a branchial cleft cyst is anterior to the sternocleidomastoid, just under the angle of the mandible.

PERITONSILLAR ABSCESSES

Background

A peritonsillar abscess (PTA) is the most common deep-space infection of the head and neck region. PTAs are thought to be an extension of an adjacent acute tonsillitis or obstruction of Webers gland at the superior tonsillar pole. The incidence is approximately 30 cases per 100,000 in the United States, and thought to be increasing in the era of judicious antibiotic use. PTAs more often occur in children over 10 years of age, but there are many reported cases in younger children.

Classical signs and symptoms include fever, sore throat, odynophagia, muffled voice, and an inferior medial displacement of the tonsil with contralateral deviation of the uvula. Unfortunately, simple clinical differentiation between a peritonsillar abscess and peritonsillar cellulitis can be inaccurate, with sensitivities of around 75% for even highly trained specialists. In cases of indecision, repeated blind needle aspiration is often recommended in the otolaryngology (ENT) literature. However, blind needle aspiration may not be tolerated even in older children, and is associated with complications. Alternatively, CT scan of the head and neck may be performed in order to diagnose a PTA. However, CT scans expose children to large doses of radation, involving particularly radiosensitive organs such as the thyroid gland. Point-of-care ultrasound, in conjunction with clinical acumen (in a cooperative patient), may offer an alternative diagnostic modality. A few case series in the adult emergency medicine literature have demonstrated the utility of intraoral ultrasonography, demonstrating a sensitivity of 95.2%. Currently, there are no emergency medicine studies that define the efficacy of ultrasound in differentiating peritonsillar cellulitis from abscess in the pediatric population.

Anatomy

The palatine tonsils lie in the depression between the palatoglossal and palatopharyngeal arches, covered by a capsule formed by the intrapharyngeal aponeurosis (Figure 8.20). Peritonsillar abscesses form in the space between the palatine tonsil and its capsule. The infection can spread in this pharyngeal potential space and into muscles and adjacent vascular structures, which may lead to a life-threatening airway obstruction.

Technique

Point-of-care questions

1. Is a peritonsillar abscess present?
2. Where are the surrounding vascular structures? Can an incision and drainage be safely performed?

Transducer selection and orientation

The endocavitary, high-frequency (5–9 MHz) transducer allows for the transducer tip to be placed immediately adjacent to the peritonsillar region. The transducer should be cleaned and covered with a disposable, internally lubricated cover (Figure 8.21a). Care should be taken to remove air and fluid from the contact area between the transducer tip and the cover lining. It is not recommended to place gel on the external surface of the covered transducer, since most patients will have a moist mucosal surface, and lubricant can cause patient discomfort. Place the ultrasound system in the line of sight to allow ease of viewing (Figure 8.21b). The ultrasound transducer should be rotated with the indicator

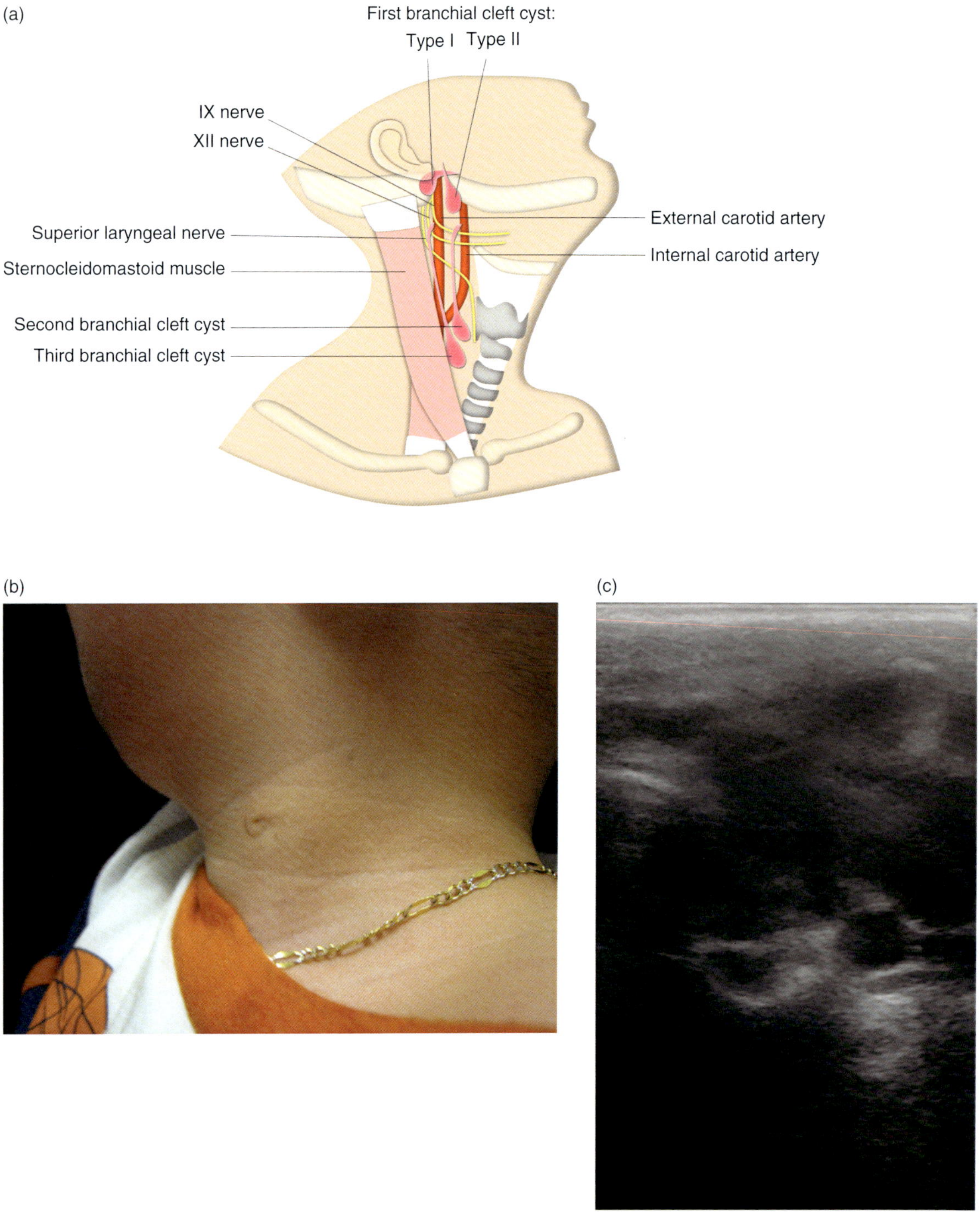

Figure 8.16 Branchial cleft cysts. (a) Locations of branchial cleft cysts. (b) Photograph of a child with a branchial cleft cyst draining saliva. (c) Ultrasound image of a recurrent branchial cleft cyst, with a thyroid abscess. *Illustration by Laura Berg, MD.*

oriented towards the patient's right side to facilitate easy entry into the mouth (Figure 8.21c). For the examination of the left paratonsillar region, it is often helpful to enter the oral cavity from the contralateral/right side and slowly advance the transducer until there is contact with the posterior oropharynx. For the evaluation of the right paratonsillar region, perform a similar method of entering via the contralateral side.

If the patient cannot tolerate the intraoral transducer due to trismus, a high-frequency (5–10MHz), linear transducer may be utilized to evaluate the peritonsillar region from the external neck. Place a linear, high-frequency transducer under the mandible with the indicator oriented towards the patient's right side.

Patient position and preparation

Patients should be seated upright. Nebulized lidocaine 2% via a non-rebreather mask can be administered (children 0.8–2.5 mg/kg per dose, in 5 mL normal saline) along with analgesia

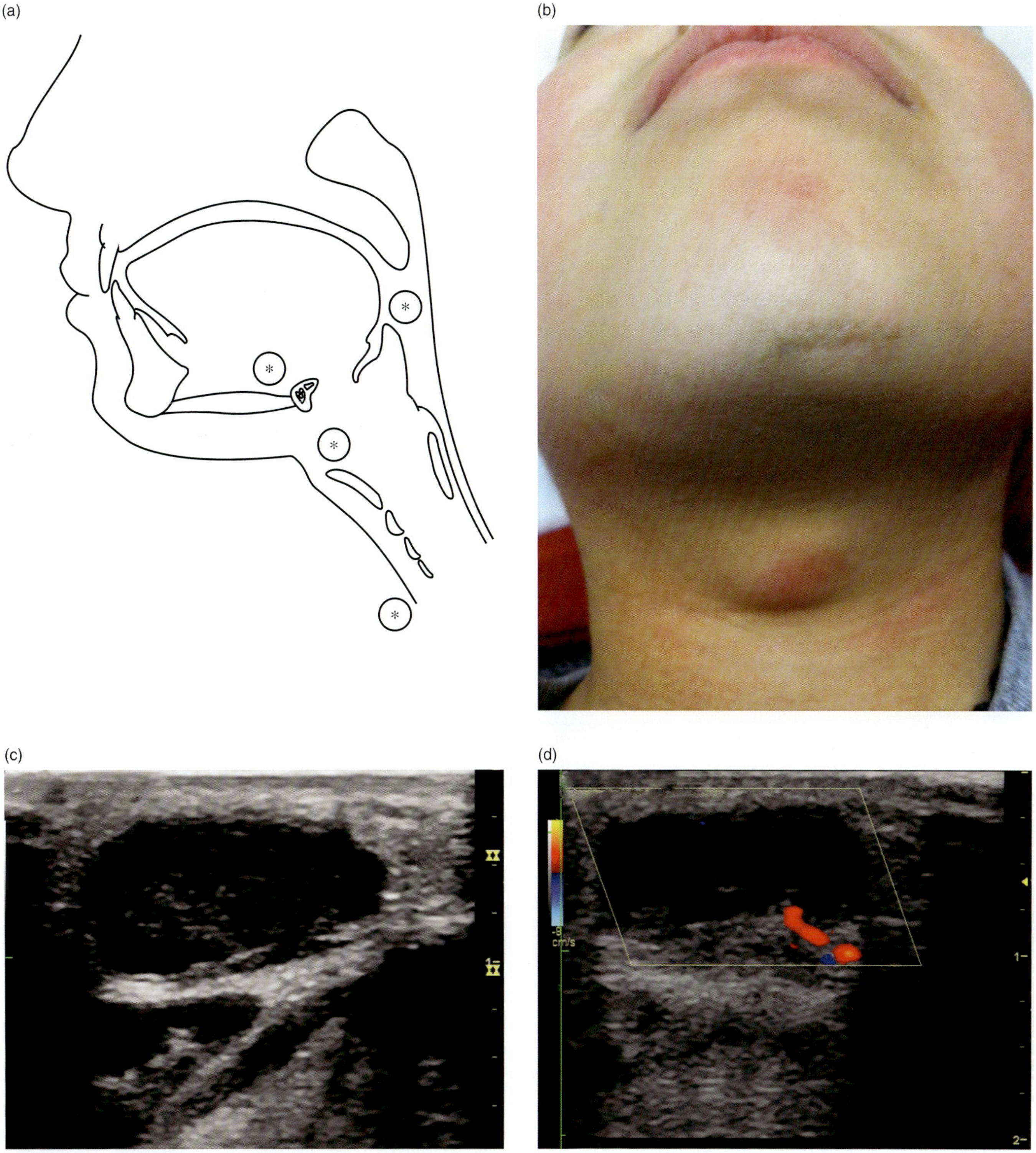

Figure 8.17 Thyroglossal duct cysts. (a) Potential locations of a thyroglossal duct cyst. (b) Photo of a child presenting with an acutely painful, superinfected thyroglossal duct cyst. (c) Ultrasound image of thyroglossal duct cyst. (d) Color Doppler of thyroglossal duct cyst.

(either an opioid or non-steroidal anti-inflammatory agent), to reduce trismus and allow for a thorough ultrasound examination. Alternatively, topical benzocaine spray (Hurricaine®) may be administered to suppress the gag reflex and provide topical anesthesia to the posterior pharynx.

Ultrasound imaging

Visualization of the pharyngeal tonsil and the paratonsillar region will not be achieved if contact between the transducer tip and the posterior pharyngeal area does not occur. Because a PTA causes medial displacement of the pharyngeal tonsil, locate

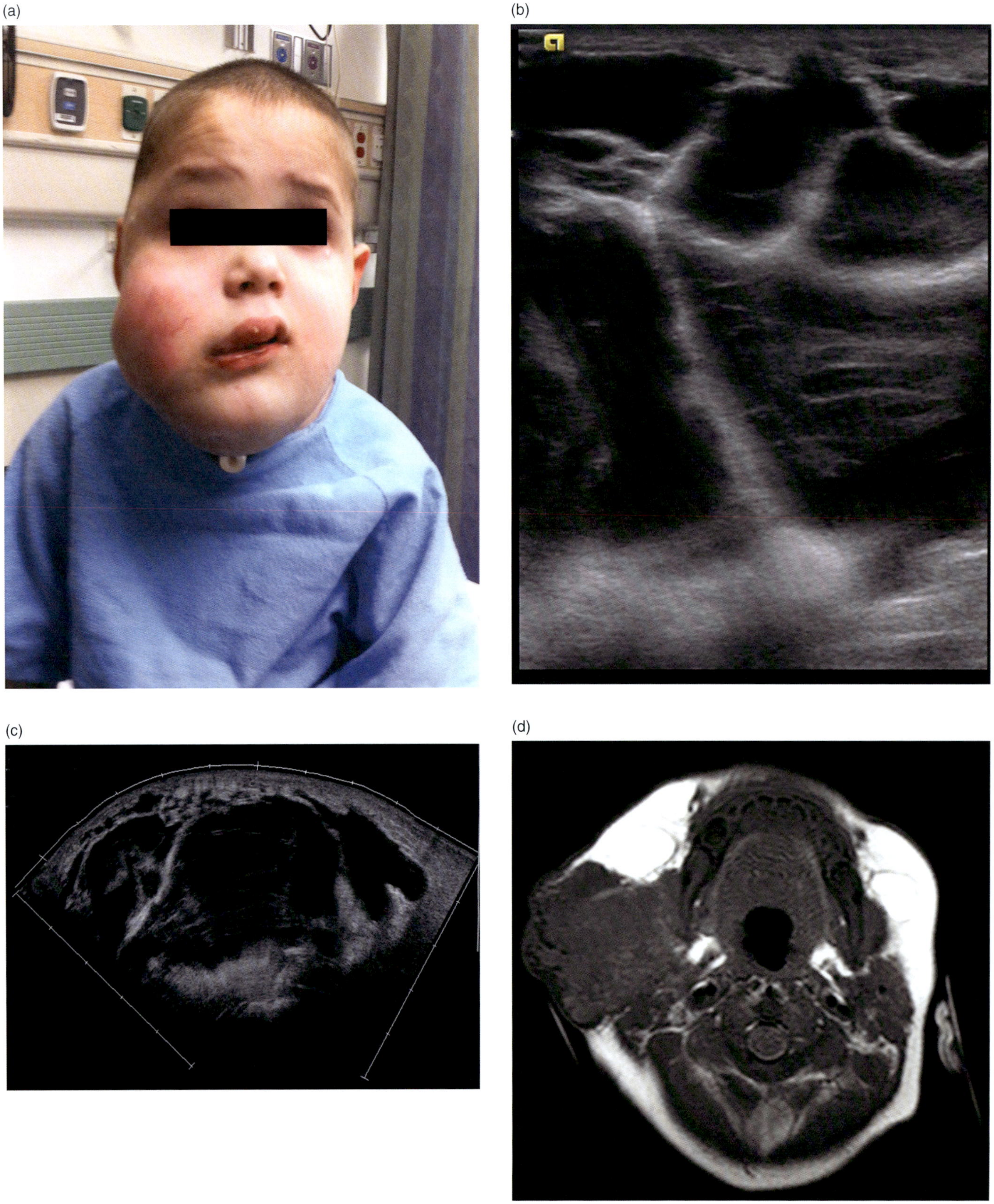

Figure 8.18 Cystic hygromas. (a) Photo of a child with a large cystic hygroma. (b) Corresponding ultrasound image of a cystic hygroma, showing irregularity and a multicystic structure. (c,d) MRI showing the extensive nature of the cystic hygroma.

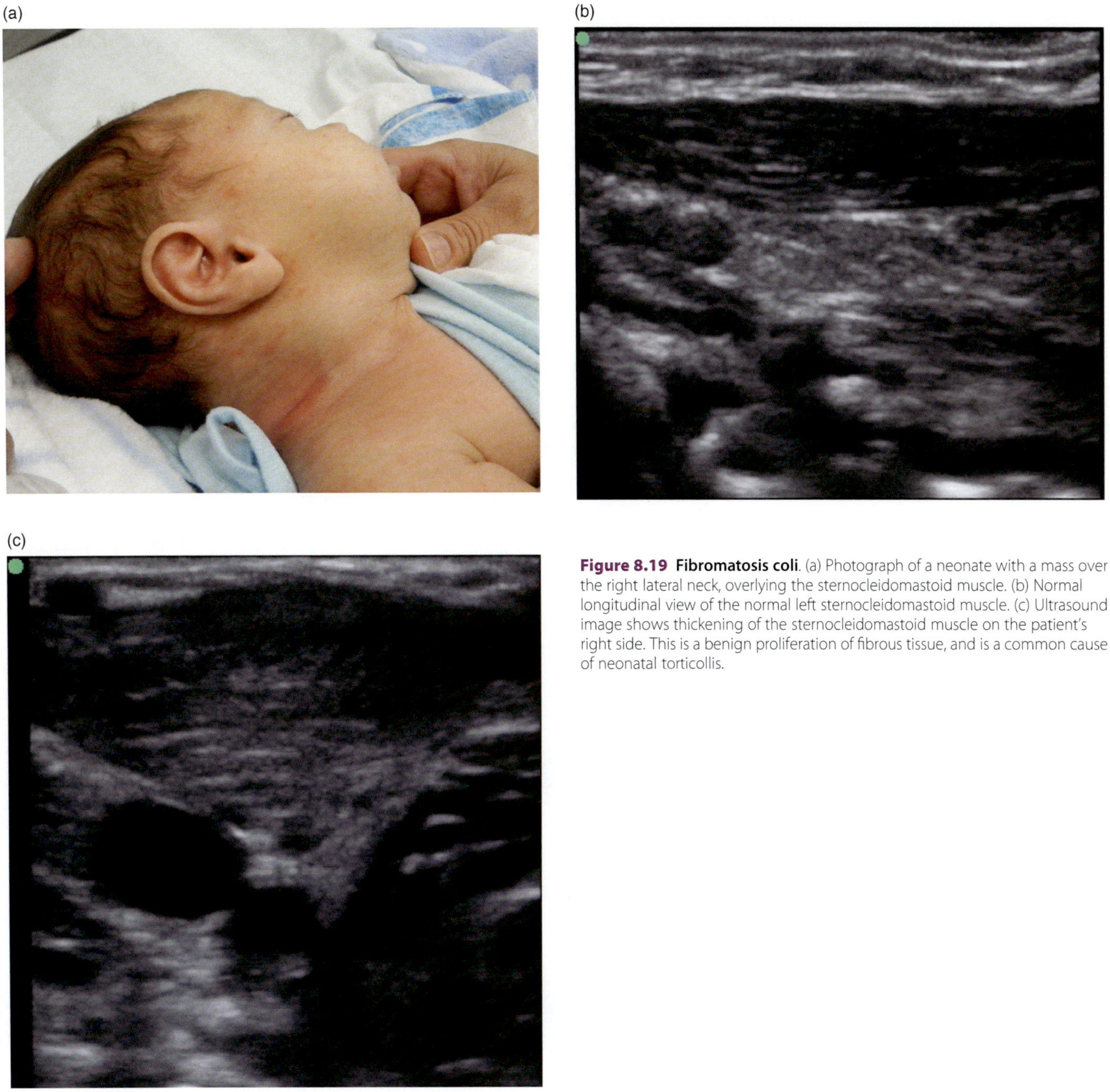

Figure 8.19 Fibromatosis coli. (a) Photograph of a neonate with a mass over the right lateral neck, overlying the sternocleidomastoid muscle. (b) Normal longitudinal view of the normal left sternocleidomastoid muscle. (c) Ultrasound image shows thickening of the sternocleidomastoid muscle on the patient's right side. This is a benign proliferation of fibrous tissue, and is a common cause of neonatal torticollis.

the tonsil and then scan laterally in order to ensure adequate evaluation of the peritonsillar space. Misidentification of the pharyngeal tonsil as a peritonsillar abscess is a common mistake made by novice clinicians. Alternatively, a linear transducer may be utilized to scan the external neck. For novice sonographers, we recommend locating the internal jugular vein and carotid artery, and then fanning cephalad until the pharyngeal tonsil is located. Similarly to the intraoral examination, the transducer should be moved laterally after identifying the pharyngeal tonsil.

There are no clear described standards in the differentiation between peritonsillar cellulitis and a peritonsillar abscess. Clinicians should be aware of the appearance of a normal pharyngeal tonsil (Figure 8.21c) as compared to an abscess. Classically, pharyngeal tonsils are circular with an echogenic center. Conversely, a peritonsillar abscess (Figure 8.22) will be anechoic in the center with an irregular, but well-defined circumference. We recommend the identification of the pharyngeal tonsil prior to looking for a peritonsillar abscess. False-positive identifications are not uncommon in the non-experienced sonographer, and clear localization of a fluid-filled structure lateral to the visualized pharyngeal tonsil may be prudent. Once a peritonsillar abscess has been identified, ultrasound-guidance for incision and drainage may be performed.

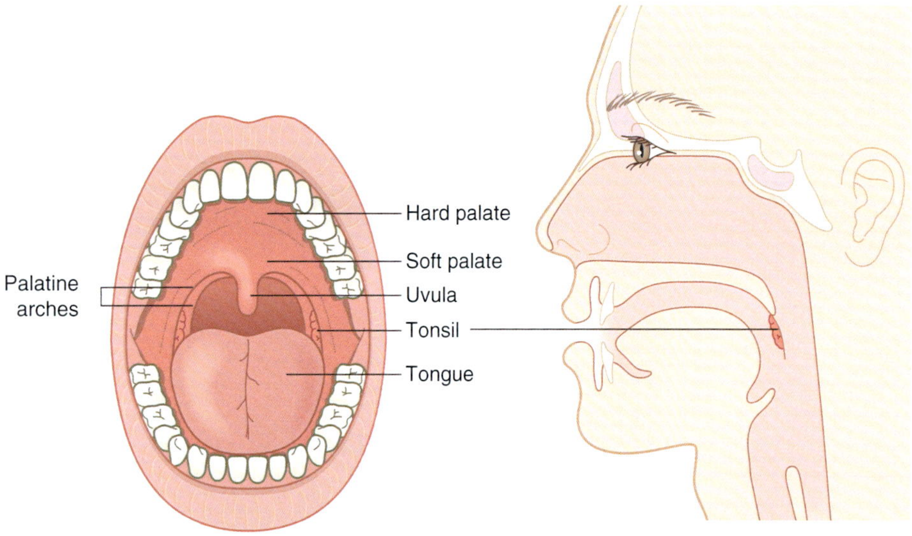

Figure 8.20 Anatomy of the tonsils. Important structures are the hard and soft palate, the tonsils, the palatine fossa, and the uvula. *Artwork created by Emily Evans © Cambridge University Press.*

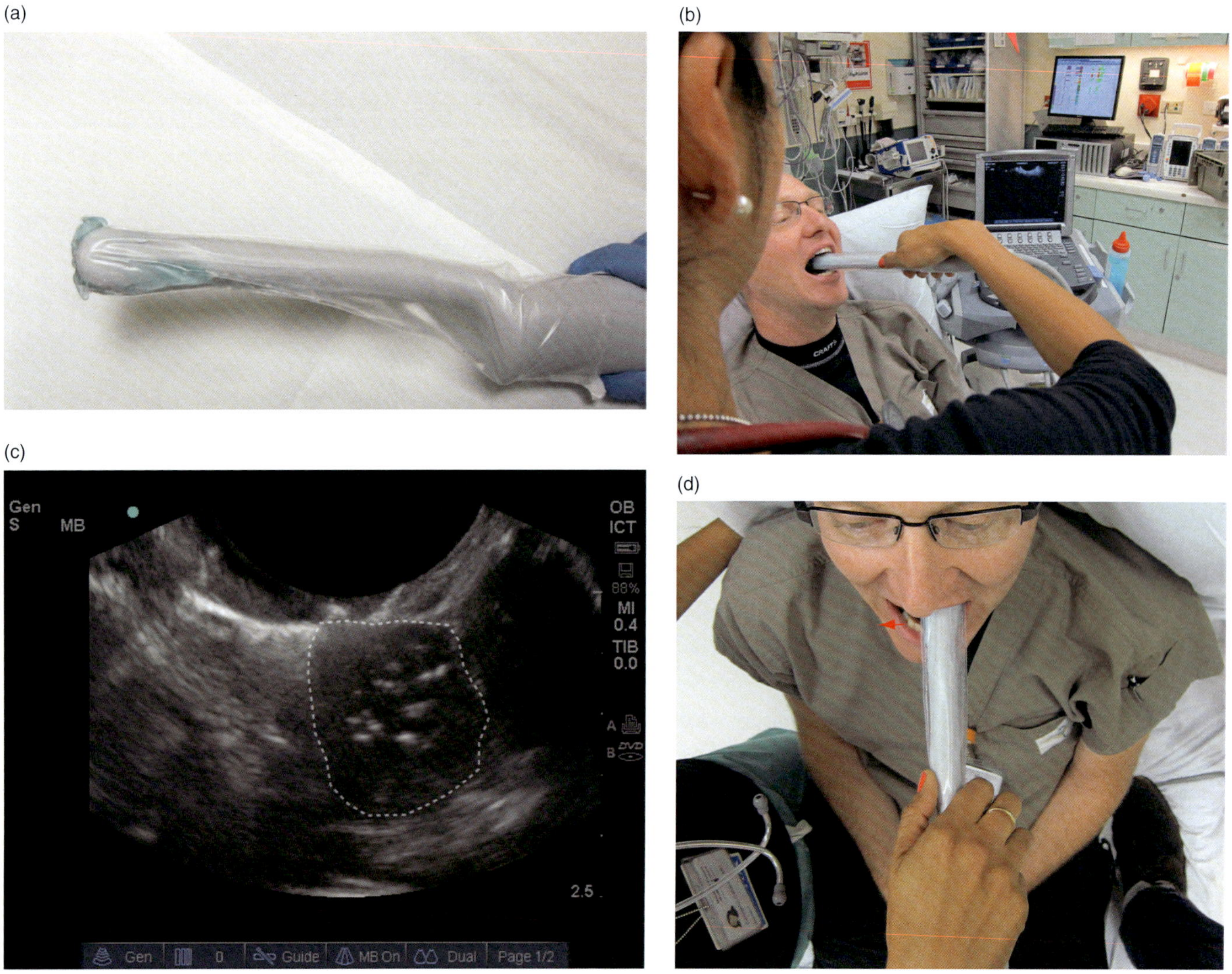

Figure 8.21 Transducer preparation. (a) Make sure to remove all air from the tip of the transducer. Gel is not needed on the external aspect of the probe cover. (b) Ensure that the ultrasound screen is in clear line of sight of the provider. (c) The transducer indicated is oriented towards the patient's right side. (d) Ultrasound image of a normal pharyngeal tonsil outlined with dashed line. Note the hyperechoic center with lack of adjacent/paratonsillar anechoic fluid.

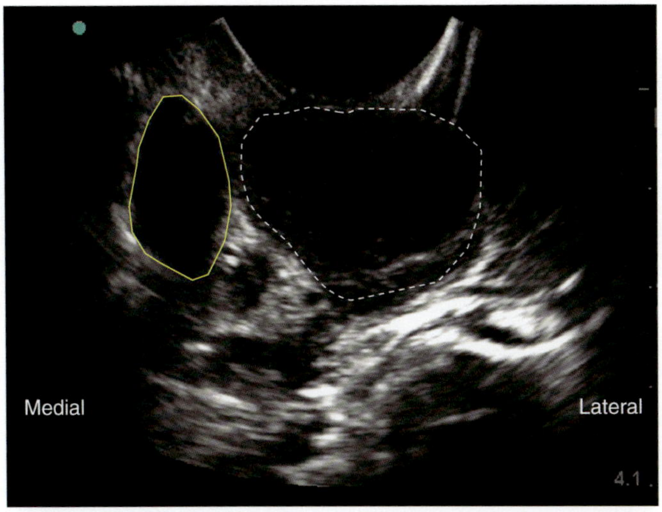

Figure 8.22 Peritonsillar abscess. The peritonsillar abscess is an anechoic fluid collection (dashed white line) located lateral to the displaced palatine tonsil (solid yellow line).

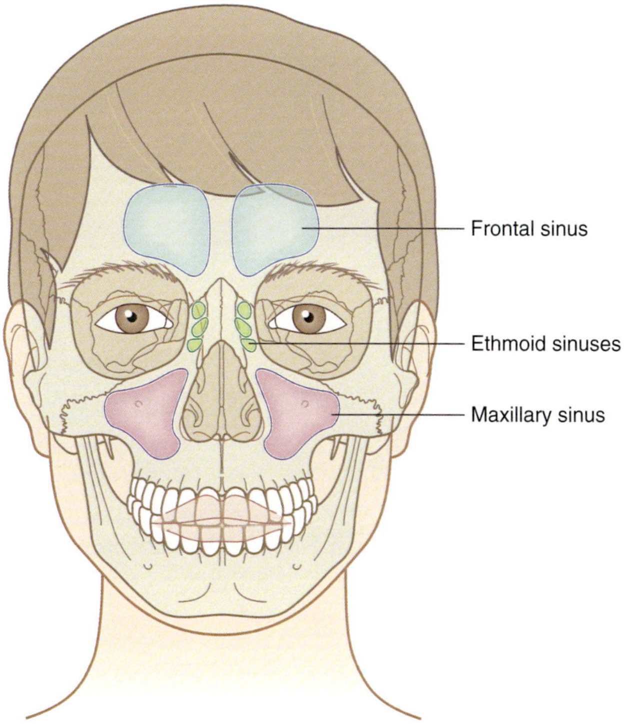

Figure 8.23 Anatomy. The frontal, ethmoid, and maxillary sinuses can be evaluated with ultrasonography. *Artwork created by Emily Evans © Cambridge University Press.*

Scanning tips

Pitfalls

- Misidentification of the pharyngeal tonsil as a peritonsillar abscess is a common mistake in novice clinicians.
- Some patients cannot tolerate the endocavitary probe due to trismus. An alternative method of scanning involves the linear high-frequency transducer placed under the mandible in the region of the pharyngeal tonsil.

Tips to improve scanning

✓ Administering an adequate analgesia and anti-inflammatory medicine prior to performing the ultrasound evaluation will allow for optimal interrogation without patient discomfort.

✓ The patient should be seated with the head supported, to prevent patient movement during the examination.

✓ Cover the endocavitary probe with a disposable sheath and rotate the transducer with the indicator oriented towards the patient's right side to allow for easy entry into the oral cavity.

✓ Locate the pharyngeal tonsil and then move the transducer laterally to identify the fluid-filled anechoic peritonsillar abscess.

SINUSITIS

Background

The differentiation between viral and other (bacterial, fungal, etc.) etiologies of maxillary rhinosinusitis is often difficult in both pediatrics and adult patients, leaving clinicians to over-prescribe unnecessary antibiotics. Ionizing diagnostic imaging (radiographs and CT) has been shown to be nonspecific, with direct sinus puncture invasive and impractical. Ultrasonographic evaluation of the maxillary sinus for presence of a fluid-filled cavity may be a useful adjunct in the clinical evaluation of a patient with suspected sinusitis. Especially in the critically ill and extremely young children, symptoms are often not present, thereby making ultrasound a desirable tool for the clinician.

The initial reports detailing the utility of ultrasound in the detection of maxillary sinusitis in intubated adult ICU patients demonstrated a high sensitivity and specificity: 100% and 96.7%, respectively. Further research using various gold standards (CT and sinus puncture) has demonstrated a lower sensitivity and specificity, but indicates that ultrasound may be a useful test in detecting fluid in the maxillary sinus. The only pediatric study to date demonstrated concordant results between ultrasound and plain radiographs in 83.5% of maxillary sinuses evaluated. The high correlation was specific in determining the presence of a fluid-filled maxillary sinus as compared to an occipitomental-view radiograph. Compared to standard radiographs, ultrasonography had a sensitivity and specificity of 94.9% and 98.4% respectively.

Anatomy

Embryologically, the maxillary sinus begins developing at three to four months of gestation, and it reaches a maximal size of approximately 15 mL by the teenage years. These air-filled cavities drain directly into the nares, specifically into the medial meatus (Figure 8.23). Inhibition of unidirectional flow (from sinus to nares) can lead to inflammation and infection. Most cases of sinusitis are viral in etiology, with a small proportion

(a) (b)

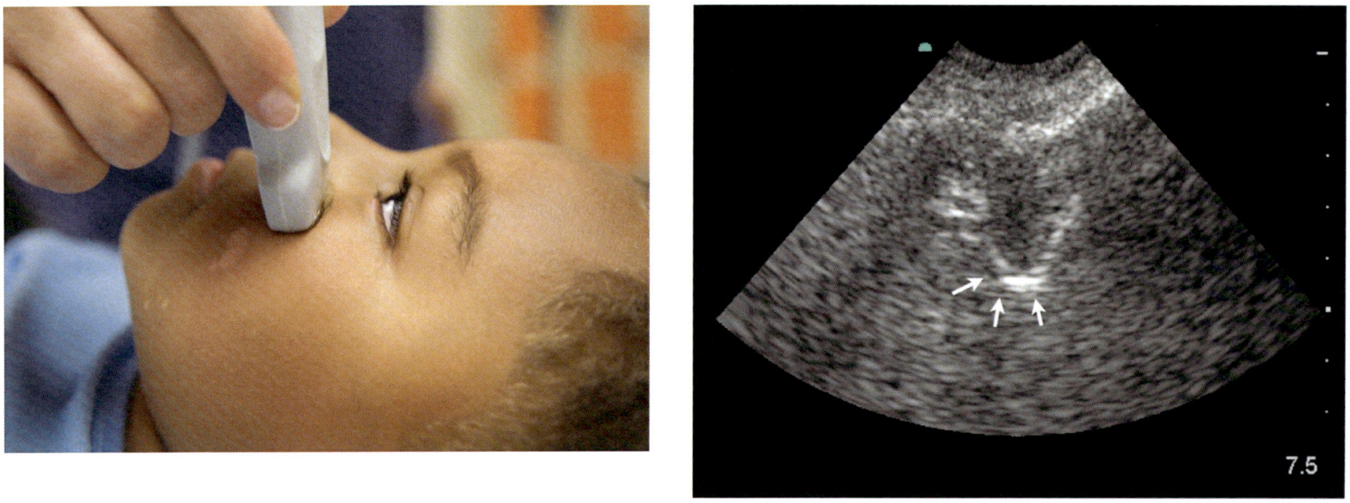

Figure 8.24 Sinus imaging. (a) Small-footprint transducer parallel to the floor with the indicator oriented towards the patient's right side. (b) The posterior hyperechoic wall (arrows) indicates the presence of a fluid-filled sinus.

progressing to a superinfection with either a bacterial or fungal pathogen. The differentiation between viral and other pathogens is difficult without obtaining cavity samples. Therefore, most expert sources recommend treatment in only those patients with persistent signs and symptoms of sinus inflammation.

Technique

Point-of-care questions

1. Is fluid present in the sinuses?

Transducer selection and orientation

A small-footprint, curvilinear transducer (2–5 MHz) is ideal, but any low-frequency transducer can also be used. Alternatively, a high-frequency, linear transducer may be utilized The transducer is placed parallel to the floor, with the indicator oriented towards the patient's right side (Figure 8.24a).

Patient position and preparation

The patient should be kept in an upright position with the head slightly bent forward. The ultrasound monitor should be placed on the contralateral side of the patient, in order to allow for the direct visualization of the ultrasound image. A small amount of ultrasound gel is needed to ensure contact between the gel and facial skin.

Ultrasound imaging

A shallow depth will be required for the scan, since the goal is to image the posterior and lateral walls of the maxillary sinus. Fanning the transducer in the cephalad to caudal direction will allow for the interrogation of the entire maxillary sinus in a standardized manner.

A normal maxillary sinus should be filled with air, causing dispersion of the ultrasound beam, and thereby preventing the visualization of the lateral and posterior walls of the maxillary sinus. In a normal state, the operator should not be able to visualize either the lateral or posterior walls. When scanning a maxillary sinus that is completely filled with fluid, the operator will be able to visualize the posterior and lateral walls (Figure 8.24b). If there is an air–fluid level or just mucosal thickening without a completely fluid-filled sinus, both the lateral and the posterior walls may not be visualized. The clinical relevance of a partially fluid-filled maxillary sinus is unclear.

Scanning tips

Pitfalls

- Ultrasound may be comparable to plain radiographs in determining the presence of a fluid-filled maxillary sinus. However, it is insensitive in the detection of mucosal wall thickening.
- Improper depth may prevent the visualization of the posterior wall of the maxillary sinus.

Tips to improve scanning

✓ Ultrasound evaluation of the maxillary sinus may be a useful tool in conjunction with clinical evaluation in determining the presence of maxillary sinusitis.

✓ The presence of fluid in the maxillary sinus allows for the sonographic visualization of the posterior and lateral walls.

✓ Fanning the curvilinear transducer in a cephalad to caudal direction, with the patient seated upright, will allow for a thorough examination of the maxillary sinus.

Cases

1. An eight-year-old male is playing with a bullet he finds in the park. He decides to see what would happen if he sets it on fire. The bullet explodes and hits him in the face. He

(a) (b)

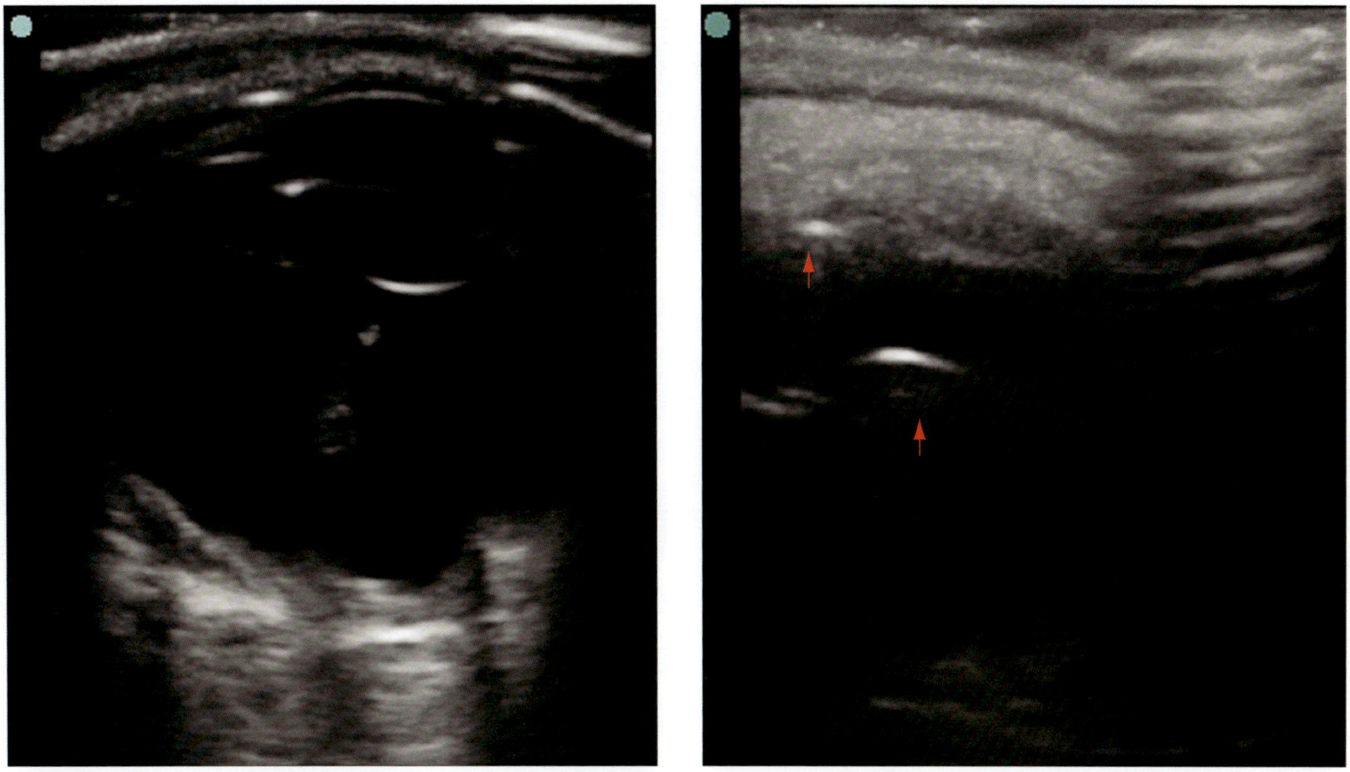

Figure 8.25 Case 1: bullet. This ultrasound was performed after a CT scan showed a bullet that appeared to be lodged in the orbit. (a) On ultrasonography, there was an obvious ruptured globe. (b) On further scanning, bullet fragments (arrows) were actually lodged in the globe itself, rather than the bony orbit.

doesn't want to "get in trouble," so he goes to a neighbor's house. He is finally brought to the hospital six hours after the initial event. At the outside hospital, a CT scan is performed which reportedly shows the bullet lodged in the bony orbit.

On arrival from the transferring hospital, the child is extremely uncomfortable, exhibiting marked periorbital edema. There is a small, 0.5 cm laceration inferior to the medial canthus of the affected eye. There is serosanguinous discharge from the laceration. Due to the amount of pain and swelling, a direct examination of the eye is limited. Point-of-care ultrasonography is performed with a linear, high-frequency transducer. A copious amount of gel is placed on the eyelid prior to performing the ultrasound examination. The globe is markedly irregular, with hyperechoic material throughout the posterior chamber (Figure 8.25). On further scanning, hyperechoic structures with a ring-down artifact are appreciated, consistent with bullet fragments lodged in the globe itself. Ophthalmology immediately takes the patient to the operating room. Unfortunately, due to the marked delay in seeking medical care, the eye is not salvageable and has to be enucleated.

This case highlights the utility of point-of-care ultrasonography in the evaluation of pediatric eye trauma. Often the initial examination is difficult and limited due to swelling and lack of patient cooperation. Ultrasonography can easily detect both radiopaque and non-radiopaque objects. While controversial, ultrasonography can also allow evaluation for globe rupture, especially in situations where it is unclear whether the globe has been penetrated by a foreign body.

2. A five-month-old male presents with unilateral neck swelling for the past five days. His mother brings him to the emergency department at 4 am, because he has now developed a tactile temperature, irritability, and decreased oral intake. On examination, his vital signs are: T 39.4 °C (axillary), HR 155 bpm, RR 32/min, BP is unable to be obtained, pulse oximetry 98% on room air. He is fussy and difficult to console. He has marked swelling and erythema below the left angle of the mandible. There is no discrete palpable mass. A bedside ultrasound examination is performed with the linear transducer. A large abscess is visualized anterior to an enlarged lymph node (Figure 8.26). These findings are confirmed the following morning by formal ultrasonography. The patient is admitted and placed on intravenous antibiotics. The child recovers uneventfully and does not require surgical intervention.

Children often present with neck masses; it is difficult to distinguish inflammatory conditions such as lymphadenitis from abscesses. Ultrasonography can readily distinguish these conditions, without the use of ionizing radiation. Unfortunately, without the use of ultrasonography, children often require CT scans. In this age group, a CT scan with intravenous contrast often requires sedation, and there is a high dose of radiation to the radiosensitive tissues of the neck, such as the thyroid

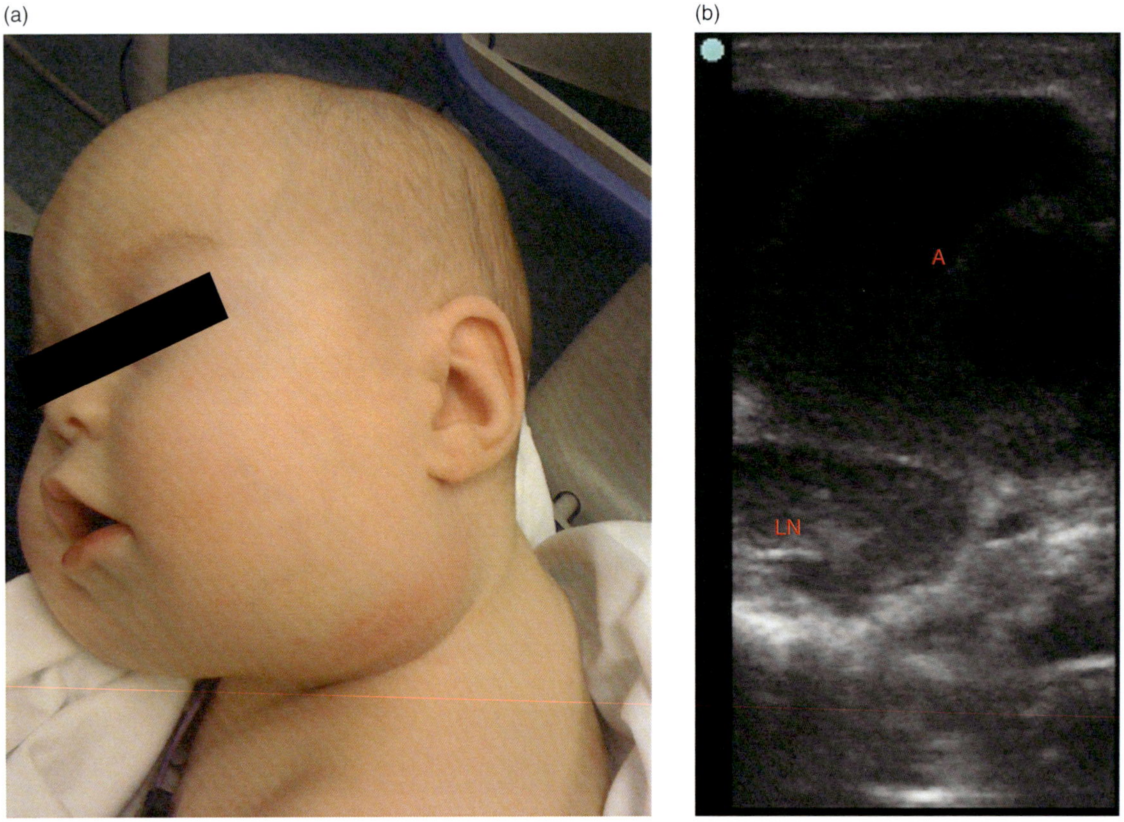

Figure 8.26 **Case 2: mandibular abscess**. (a) This baby presented with neck swelling of unclear etiology. (b) On ultrasonography, a large abscess (A) is visualized anterior to a lymph node (LN).

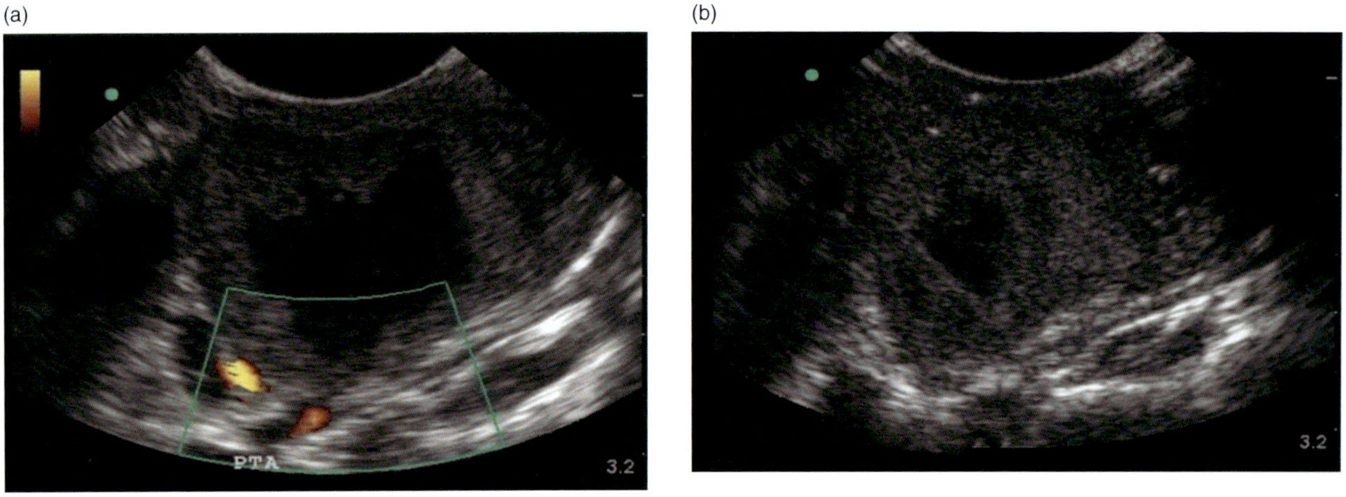

Figure 8.27 **Case 3: Peritonsillar abscess**. (a) Large PTA. (b) Post-incision and drainage ultrasound.

gland. However, since this is a relatively new application for point-of-care ultrasonography, it is important to obtain formal radiologic studies to confirm findings of point-of-care ultrasound studies.

3. A 14-year-old female presents with two days of progressively worsening pharyngitis. She now has developed a hoarse voice, drooling, and difficulty drinking liquids. On examination, she exhibits some trismus. Both tonsils are enlarged, with the right larger than the left side, but no overlying exudate. There is slight uvular deviation and some bulging at the soft palate on the right side. Based on this examination, there is concern for the presence of a peritonsillar abscess. A point-of-care ultrasound examination is performed with the endocavitary probe, revealing a fluid pocket amenable to incision and drainage (Figure 8.27a). Incision and drainage is performed with ultrasound guidance in order to avoid puncturing adjacent vessels. Following incision and drainage, the ultrasound is

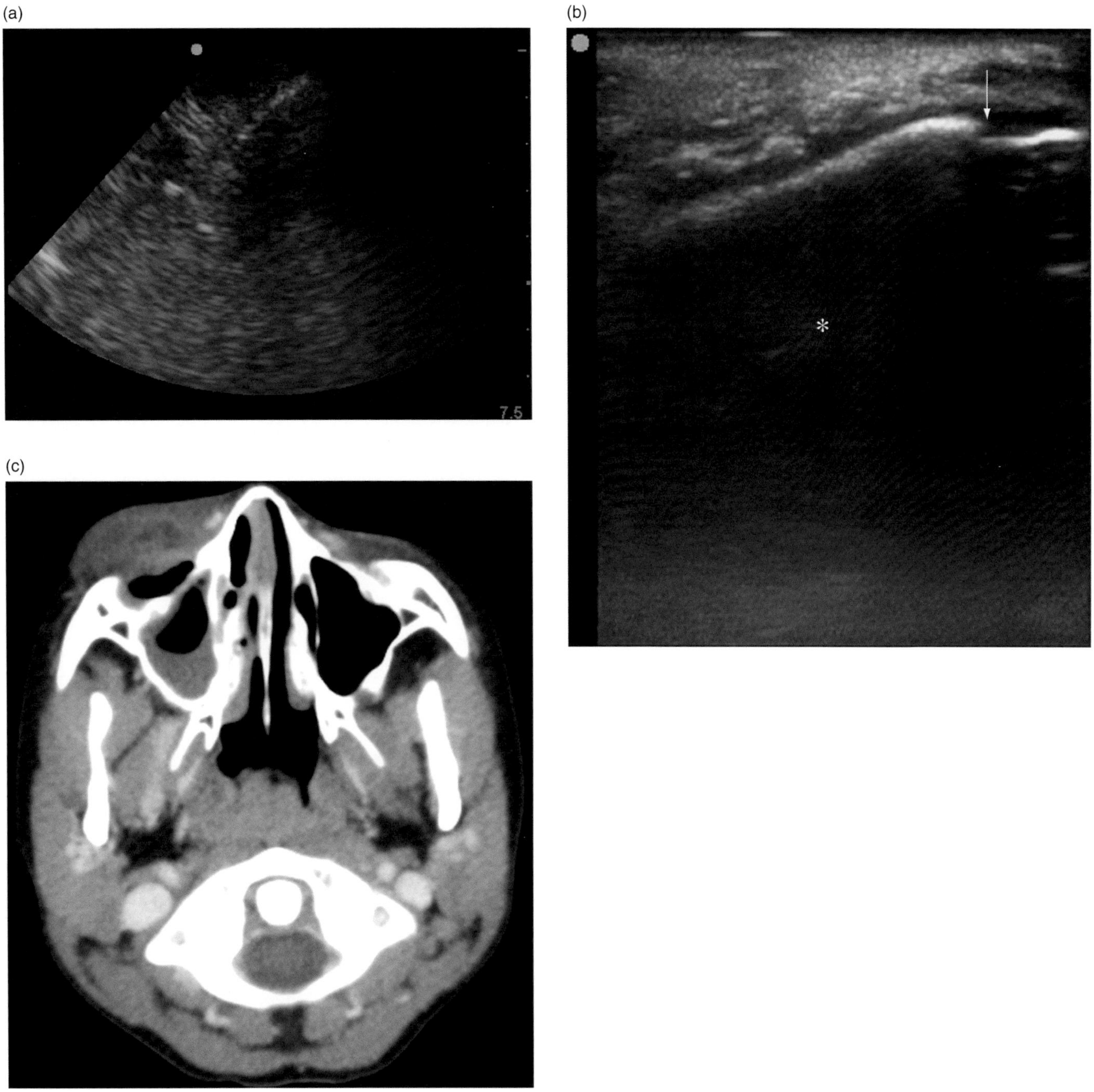

Figure 8.28 **Case 4: sinusitis with periorbital cellulitis**. (a) Sinus ultrasound performed with a phased-array transducer. (b) A linear, high-frequency transducer is used, and shows a fluid collection (*) and bone fracture (arrow). (c) The CT scan shows extensive sinusitis and orbital cellulitis.

repeated, showing a marked decrease in the amount of pus visualized (Figure 8.27b).

Ultrasonography is useful in the identification of a peritonsillar abscess, especially in situations where it is not entirely clear by physical examination. In addition, it can be helpful in decreasing complications associated with the incision and drainage of peritonsillar abscesses.

4. An eight-year-old boy is transferred from an outside hospital, with retro-orbital headaches, fever, and vomiting for the past day. There is high concern for meningitis, but the family refuses permission for a lumbar puncture to be performed. On presentation, the patient has now developed rapidly progressive eye swelling, which was reportedly not present at the outside hospital. The patient is ill appearing and has marked photophobia and pain with eye movements bilaterally. He also has marked tenderness to palpation over his maxillary and ethmoid sinuses. He exhibits no meningismus and an otherwise non-focal neurologic examination.

A point-of-care ultrasound examination is performed, initially with a low-frequency, phased-array transducer. Bilateral fluid collections are appreciated (Figure 8.28a), consistent with sinusitis. A linear, high-frequency transducer is also used, which shows this fluid collection, and a small fracture of the bone (Figure 8.28b). A CT scan is performed which shows extensive sinusitis, with erosion of the orbit and development of an orbital cellulitis (Figure 8.28c). The patient is admitted with intravenous antibiotics and is closely followed by the infectious disease and ophthalmology services.

While it is a relatively new application, point-of-care ultrasonography may be useful in diagnosing sinusitis. Especially in an era of trying to decrease the use of antibiotics, it is often helpful to be able to diagnose sinusitis, rather than to empirically treat with antibiotics. It is particularly helpful in cases that are chronic. Alternative diagnostic modalities include CT scan, which involves radiation, and MRI, which is costly and often unavailable.

Summary/key points

1. Ocular ultrasonography may be utilized in situations of acute trauma of visual loss. With a linear, high-frequency transducer, one may detect ocular foreign bodies, globe rupture, and indirectly assess for increased intracranial pressure.
2. Neck masses may be readily evaluated by point-of-care ultrasonography. Ultrasound can distinguish between congenital/anatomic, neoplastic, inflammatory, and infectious pathologies.
3. The high-frequency endocavitary probe may be utilized to diagnose a peritonsillar abscess, and serve as an adjunct for incision and drainage. In patients who cannot tolerate the endocavitary probe, an alternative technique may be utilized, which involves the linear, high-frequency transducer placed at the lateral neck.
4. Ultrasound may be comparable to plain radiographs in the diagnosis of maxillary sinusitis. The examination is performed with the lower-frequency, curvilinear transducer.
5. While being relatively new applications for point-of-care ultrasonography, ocular, sinus, and neck ultrasound are useful in pediatric patients. Further research needs to be performed for these applications in particular. It is recommended to obtain subspecialty consultation in conjunction with formal ultrasonography, whenever available.

Selected references

Berg, C.K., Zaia, B., Doniger, S.J., Williams, S. (2011) Determining the change in intraocular pressure during bedside orbital ultrasonography [abstract]. *Annals Emerg Med* **58**(4 Suppl): S205.

Blaivas, M., Theodoro, D., Duggal, S. (2003) Ultrasound-guided drainage of peritonsillar abscess by the emergency physician. *Am J Emerg Med* **21**(2): 155–8.

Blaivas, M., Theodoro, D., Sierzenski, P.R. (2002) A study of bedside ocular ultrasonography in the emergency department. *Acad Emerg Med* **9**: 791–9.

Fufezan, O., Asavoaie, C., Cherecheş Panta, P., *et al.* (2010) The role of ultrasonography in the evaluation of maxillary sinusitis in pediatrics. *Med Ultrason* **12**(1): 4–11.

Gritzmann, N., Hollerweger, A., Macheiner, P., *et al.* (2002) Sonography of soft tissue masses of the neck. *J Clin Ultrasound* **30** (6): 356–73.

Hilbert, G., Vargas, F., Valentino, R., *et al.* (2001) Comparison of B-mode ultrasound and computed tomography in the diagnosis of maxillary sinusitis in mechanically ventilated patients. *Crit Care Med* **29** (7): 1337–42.

Le, A., Hoehn, M.E., Smith, M.E., *et al.* (2009) Bedside sonographic measurement of optic nerve sheath diameter as a predictor of increased intracranial pressure in children. *Ann Emerg Med* **53**: 785–91.

Lyon, M., Blaivas, M. (2005) Intraoral ultrasound in the diagnosis and treatment of suspected peritonsillar abscess in the emergency department. *Acad Emerg Med* **12**(1): 85–8.

Malayeri, A.A., Bavarian, S., Mehdizadeh, M. (2005) Sonographic evaluation of optic nerve diameter in children with raised intracranial pressure. *J Ultrasound Med* **24**: 143–7.

Varonen, H., Mäkelä, M., Savolainen, S., *et al.* (2000) Comparison of ultrasound, radiography, and clinical examination in the diagnosis of acute maxillary sinusitis: a systematic review. *J Clin Epidemiol* **53**(9): 940–8.

Chapter 9

Renal, bladder

David Kessler

Objectives/indications

Ultrasound can be a helpful adjunct in diagnosing renal or bladder pathology in the emergency department setting. The majority of point-of-care renal ultrasound involves the identification of hydronephrosis. Hydronephrosis refers to dilation in the collecting system of the kidney and is caused by elevated hydrostatic pressure, usually from partial or complete obstruction of urine egress. Obstruction may occur at any level, from the urethral opening to the renal pelvis itself, and may occur internally or externally to the urinary system. In children, common causes of hydronephrosis include vesicoureter reflux from a uretopelvic junction obstruction or posterior uretheral valves. Less common causes include renal or ureteral calculi and abdominopelvic tumors. Hydronephrosis may also occur secondary to neurologic problems that affect the bladder, or congenital malformations of the urinary tract. Some genetic conditions may mimic true hydronephrosis, such as megaureter, in which dilated ureters and hydronephrosis are present in the absence of an obstruction causing increased pressure.

The most common application of renal ultrasound in adults is to evaluate the patient with flank pain and suspected urolithiasis. The incidence of urolithiasis in industrialized countries may be as high as 5%. While the incidence of urolithiasis in children is approximately one-tenth of that in adults, recent reports suggest that rates may be on the rise in the United States. During the last 10 years, there has been a fourfold increase in the number of children evaluated for nephrolithiasis and, of those, a sevenfold increase in stone disease. Computerized tomography is the gold standard for the evaluation of renal stones. While renal ultrasound is much less sensitive and specific than CT, a CT scan might be avoided in a patient who has sonographic unilateral hydronephrosis in the setting of renal colic.

Other applications of renal ultrasound in the emergency department and critical care settings include renal failure, pyelonephritis, and urinary retention. Ultrasound may be used in the initial evaluation of a patient with a new diagnosis of kidney failure. Large kidneys may indicate an acute cause such as renovascular thrombus or transplant rejection, while smaller kidneys usually suggest a more chronic problem. In addition, while pyelonephritis is usually a clinical diagnosis, there are sonographic features that may be useful in cases of diagnostic uncertainty. Ultrasound is also useful in evaluating for complications of pyelonephritis, such as perinephric abscesses. Finally, bladder volume determination is useful in determining post-void residuals, identifying obstructive pathology, and improving successful urethral catheterization in infants and small children.

This chapter reviews techniques and applications for scanning the bladder and kidneys in the emergency department setting. Normal and pathologic states are discussed, including: hydronephrosis, nephrolithiasis, multicystic kidneys, and childhood renal tumors. The determination and calculation of bladder volume is discussed in further detail in Chapter 16.

Background

Several studies have investigated the use of point-of-care ultrasound by emergency physicians in evaluating adult patients with flank pain. While CT remains the gold standard in the detection of urolithiasis, ultrasound still plays a role in the evaluation of a patient with suspected urolithiasis. One review of the literature revealed that ultrasonography has a pooled sensitivity and specificity of 45% and 88%, respectively, for the detection of renal calculi, and 45% and 94% for detection of ureteric stones. While ultrasound may detect hydronephrosis as a result of obstruction, it has poor sensitivity and specificity in actually detecting a stone. However, obstructing stones will lead to hydronephrosis on the affected side, leading some to advocate simply looking for hydronephrosis on ultrasound as a marker for clinically significant disease. It has been shown that emergency physicians can accurately identify hydronephrosis. Those emergency physicians who were already experienced in ultrasound could detect hydronephrosis with accuracy that is comparable to CT scan, with sensitivity of 87% and specificity of 82%. Ultrasound may also play a role in determining which patients with renal colic can be safely discharged. Using ultrasound as part of a diagnostic algorithm, Rosen *et al.* were able to safely discharge 50% of patients with acute flank pain after a normal urinalysis and point-of-care renal ultrasound.

Pediatric Emergency and Critical Care Ultrasound, ed. Stephanie J. Doniger. Published by Cambridge University Press.

Limited studies have been performed in pediatric patients. Palmer *et al.* retrospectively studied 75 pediatric patients with urolithiasis. They found that ultrasound had a high detection rate for renal calculi (90%) but a low rate for ureteral calculi (38%), compared with the CT detection rates of 90% and 100% respectively. Overall, ultrasound failed to detect urolithiasis in 41% of the patients with urolithiasis symptoms. Another study investigated a secondary sign of urolithiasis: the absence of ureteral jets in children. The presence of normal ureteral jets can be used as a sign that there is no ureteral obstruction on the side with pain. De Bessa *et al.* investigated 51 children less than 14 years old, and showed that ureteral jet frequency that was less than 25% of the normal side over five minutes had a sensitivity of 87% and a specificity of 96% for obstruction.

Additional applications of point-of-care renal ultrasound in children are still evolving. The radiology literature is robust in the detection of cysts, tumors, and obstructive uropathy, but it is unknown what role point-of-care ultrasound will play in evaluating for this additional pathology.

Anatomy

The renal system is comprised of the kidneys, ureters, and bladder (Figure 9.1a). The kidneys normally rest in the retroperitoneal space below the liver and spleen, on the right and left side of the body respectively. The kidneys are bordered by peritoneum anteriorly, transversalis fascia posteriorly, and are encapsulated by a layer of fascia referred to as Gerota's fascia. Beneath Gerota's fascia is another layer of perinephric fat, which may vary in size between individuals. The kidney itself is divided into the cortex and the medulla (Figure 9.1b). In the cortex, renal tubules and blood vessels organize to perform ultrafiltration of the body's liquid waste. The medulla is divided into sections known as renal pyramids, which represent parallel nephrons that collect urine and ultimately empty into the ureters via the renal pelvis.

The ureters course from the renal hilum, descend along the posterior aspect of the lateral pelvic walls, and cross into the pelvic brim at the bifurcation of the iliac arteries. After crossing the pelviureteric junction, they turn anteriorly and medially towards the trigone of the bladder, where they enter. The bladder lies posterior to the pubic bone and anterior to the

(a)

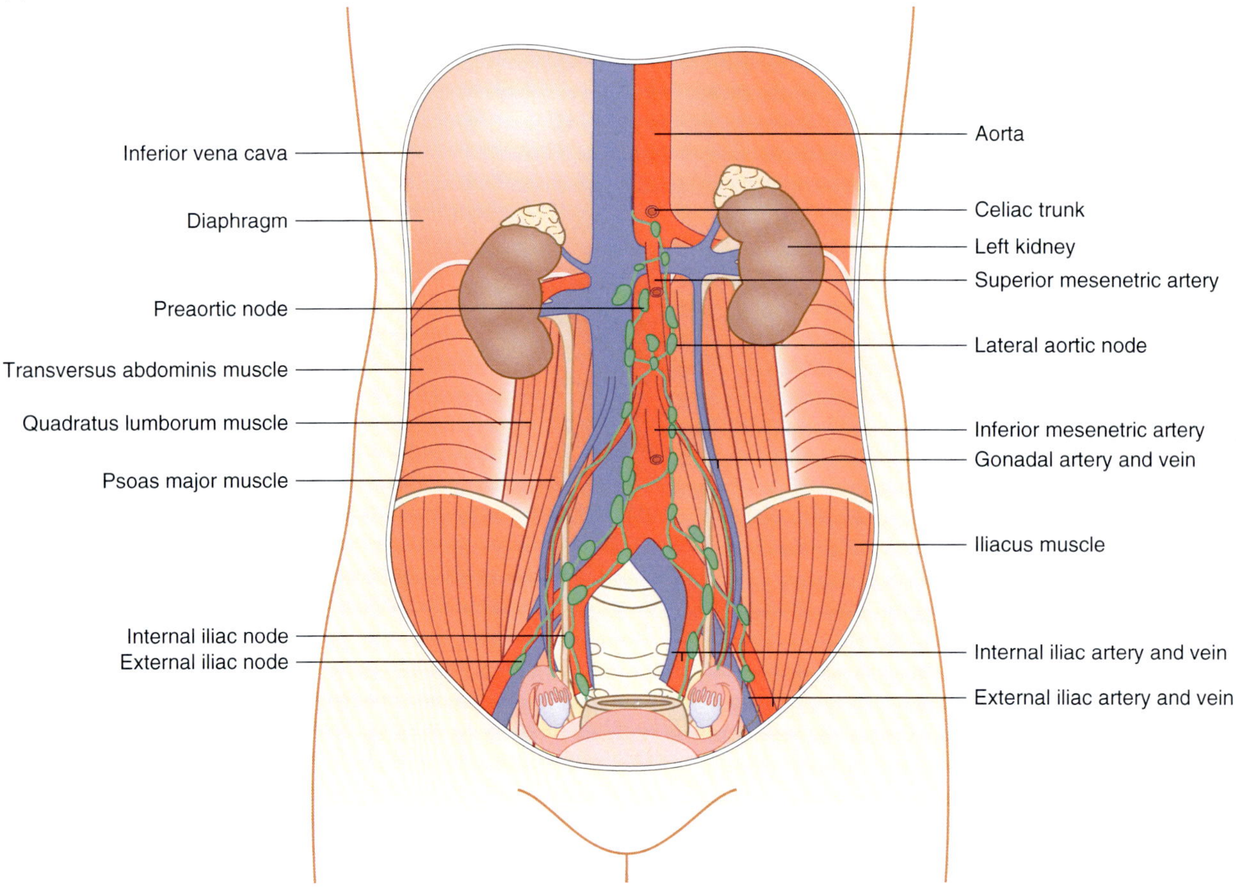

Figure 9.1 **Anatomy**. (a) The kidneys, ureter, and bladder. (b) The structure of the kidney itself, including the cortex and medulla. *Artwork created by Emily Evans © Cambridge University Press.*

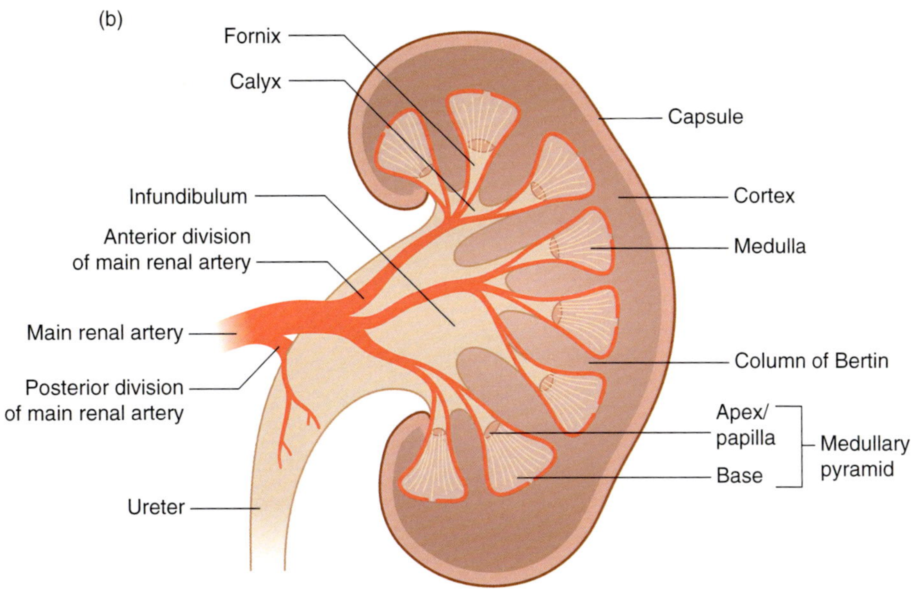

Figure 9.1 (cont.)

uterus and rectum in females. It is considered a pelvic organ, but the superior surface, or the dome of the bladder, is intraperitoneal. However, in young children the entire bladder may still be located in the abdomen.

Technique

Point-of-care questions

1. Is hydronephrosis present?
2. Is the bladder distended?
3. What is the bladder volume? (See Chapter 16.)

Transducer selection and orientation

The transducer selection for visualizing the kidney depends on the age of the patient. For the most part, the lower-frequency (2–5 MHz) transducers are utilized; either the curvilinear or phased-array transducers. The phased-array transducer offers a smaller footprint, and is ideal for smaller children. In infants, a higher-frequency, linear transducer may be utilized, offering the greatest resolution without sacrificing the field of view.

For imaging of the kidneys, the transducer is placed at the right upper and left upper quadrants. The kidney lies directly next to the liver on the right side, and next to the spleen on the left side of the body. The indicator is oriented towards the patient's head, along the midaxillary line. Due to the oblique positioning of the kidneys, it is important to rotate the transducer indicator approximately 10° posteriorly, in order to allow for the adequate visualization along the long-axis of the kidney (Figure 9.2a). Alternatively, for a more direct approach of imaging the kidney, the patient may be rolled on his/her side and the transducer placed on the back (Figure 9.2c). It is important to note that, in relation to the right kidney, the left kidney is located more superior and more posterior. On the patient's left side, the kidney is often 1–2 cm more superior than on the right side (Figure 9.2b). The transducer may even come close to touching the patient's bed in order to get the ideal view of the left kidney. After viewing the kidney along its longitudinal axis, the transducer is then rotated 90° in order to obtain the transverse or short-axis view (Figure 9.3a).

Finally, in order to evaluate the bladder, start by identifying the pubic symphysis. The transducer should be positioned in a transverse orientation (with indicator to the patient's right side) directly caudad to the pubic symphysis and angled slightly towards the patient's feet (Figure 9.4a). Then, in order to obtain the sagittal bladder view, the indicator should be rotated towards the patient's head (Figure 9.5a).

Patient position and preparation

Begin the ultrasound examination with the patient in a supine position. Alternatively, patients may be seated upright or in a left lateral decubitus position (Figure 9.2c) in order to displace bowel gas and improve image acquisition. There is no special patient preparation. Proper draping may enhance patient comfort and maintain modesty during the examination of the bladder.

Ultrasound imaging

The renal ultrasound examination consists of both right and left kidneys in two views (longitudinal and transverse), and the bladder in two views (transverse and sagittal). Additionally, color Doppler may be utilized in order to identify ureteral jets in the bladder.

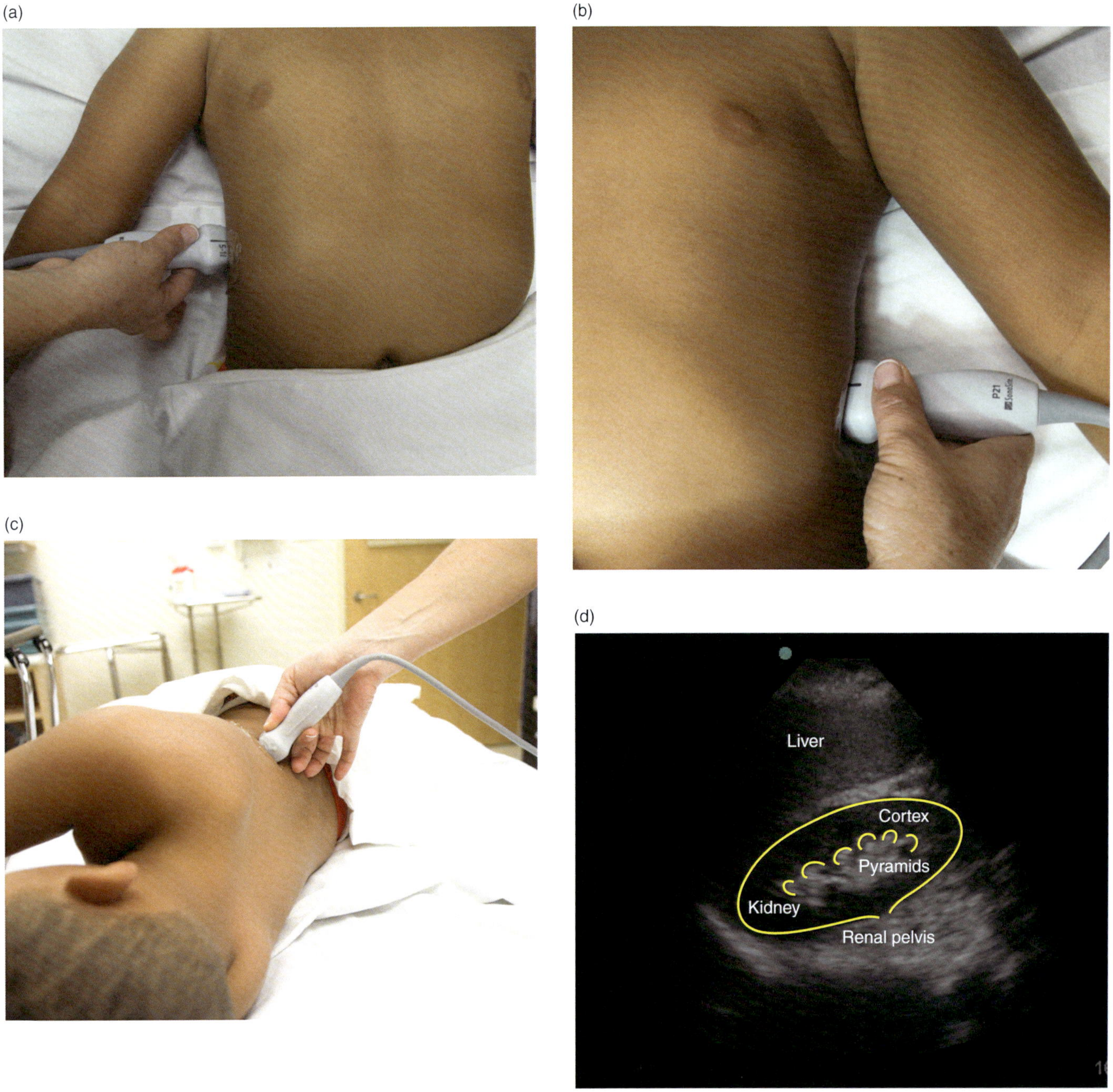

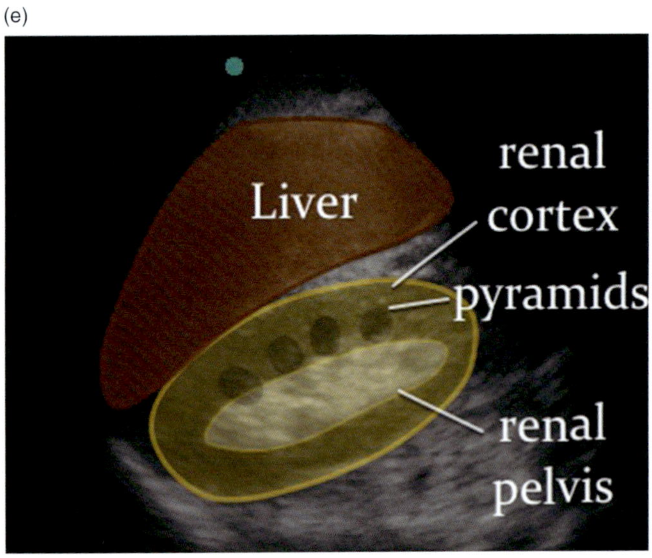

Figure 9.2 Renal imaging, longitudinal view. (a) Right transducer placement, with the indicator oriented towards the patient's head, at a slightly posterior oblique angle, to be in the plane of the kidney. (b) Left transducer placement. Note that the left kidney is located superior and posterior when compared with the right kidney. (c) Alternatively, the transducer may be placed at the back for a more direct approach to scanning the kidneys. (d) Ultrasound image of the longitudinal kidney. (e) Illustration highlighting important structures visualized on the ultrasound image. *Illustration by Laura Berg, MD.*

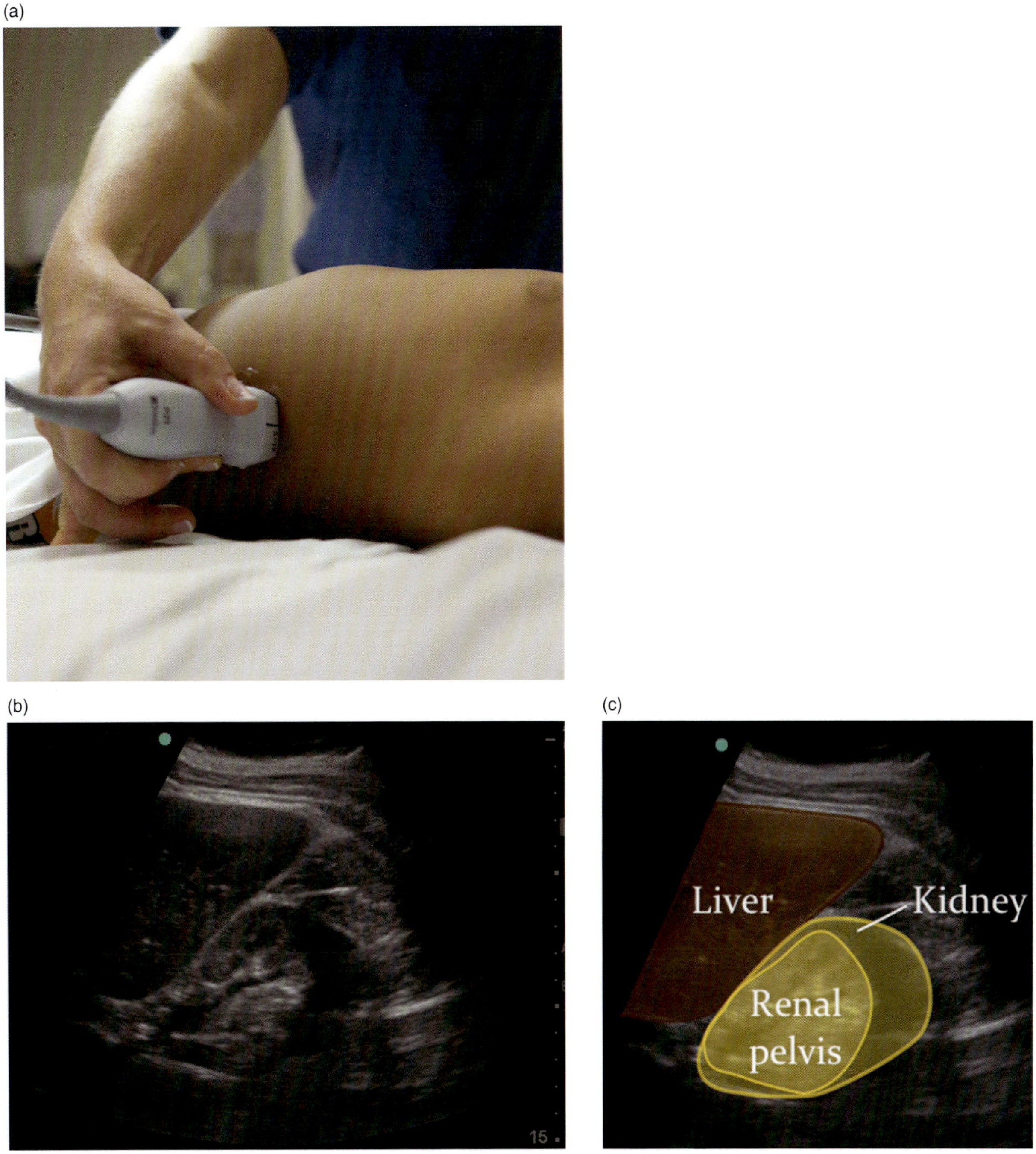

Figure 9.3 Renal imaging, transverse view. (a) Transducer placement, with the indicator oriented 90° from the longitudinal view, with the indicator oriented posteriorly. (b) Ultrasound image of the transverse kidney. (c) Illustration highlighting important structures visualized on the ultrasound image. *Illustration by Laura Berg, MD.*

Kidneys

The kidney should be viewed in both the transverse (short-axis) and longitudinal (long-axis) orientations, fanning completely through the kidney in both planes. The sonographic appearance of a normal kidney, in its long-axis, is a kidney-bean-shaped structure, measuring around 5 cm wide and 10 cm long in adults (Figure 9.2c,d). Normal kidneys are usually within 2 cm of each other in size. In the transverse view, the kidney appears in a cross-section, as a "c"-shaped organ surrounding an echo-dense center that represents the collecting system and hilum (Figure 9.3b,c).

The right kidney typically rests in a more inferior position than the left kidney due to displacement by the liver on that side. On the right side of the body, the liver will provide an acoustic window and can serve as a landmark in locating the kidney, which should lie adjacent to and inferior to the liver. On the left side, the spleen provides an acoustic window to view

(a)

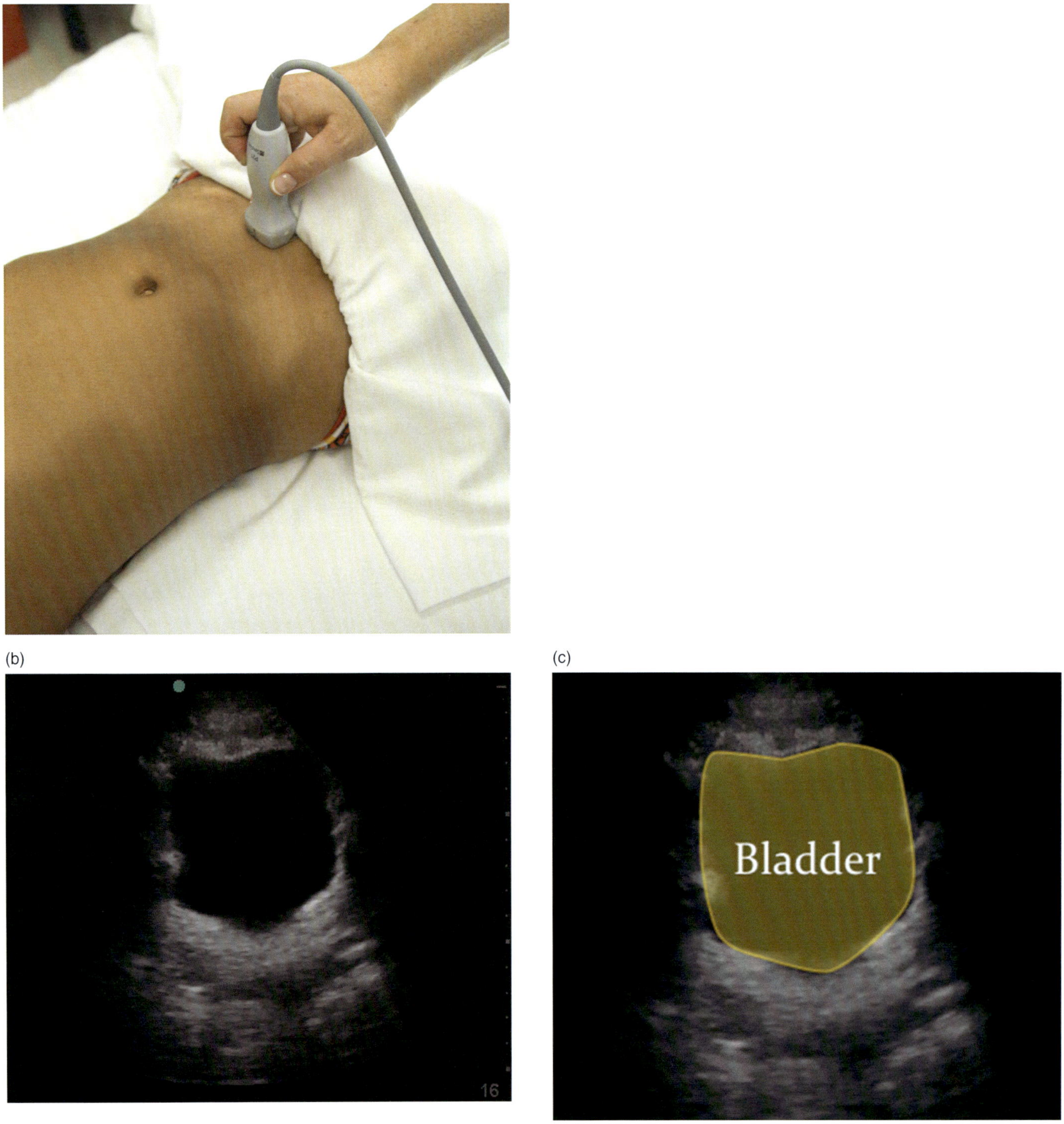

Figure 9.4 Bladder imaging, transverse view. (a) Transducer placement, with the indicator oriented towards the patient's right side. (b) Ultrasound image of the transverse view of the bladder. (c) Illustration highlighting important structures visualized on the ultrasound image. *Illustration by Laura Berg, MD.*

the kidney. It is, however, more challenging to scan the left kidney, since stomach, bowel gas, and rib shadows may interfere with obtaining a clear image. Having the patient take a deep breath and holding it will help displace the kidney inferiorly and out from behind the rib cage in order to create a better image.

The kidney appears hypoechoic, in comparison to the adjacent liver or spleen. Surrounding the kidney is an echogenic capsule called Gerota's fascia. In between the liver/spleen and Gerota's fascia is a layer of perinephric fat, which appears hyperechoic, but is less echogenic than Gerota's fascia. Within the structure of the kidney itself, the renal pyramids in the

(a)

(b)

(c)

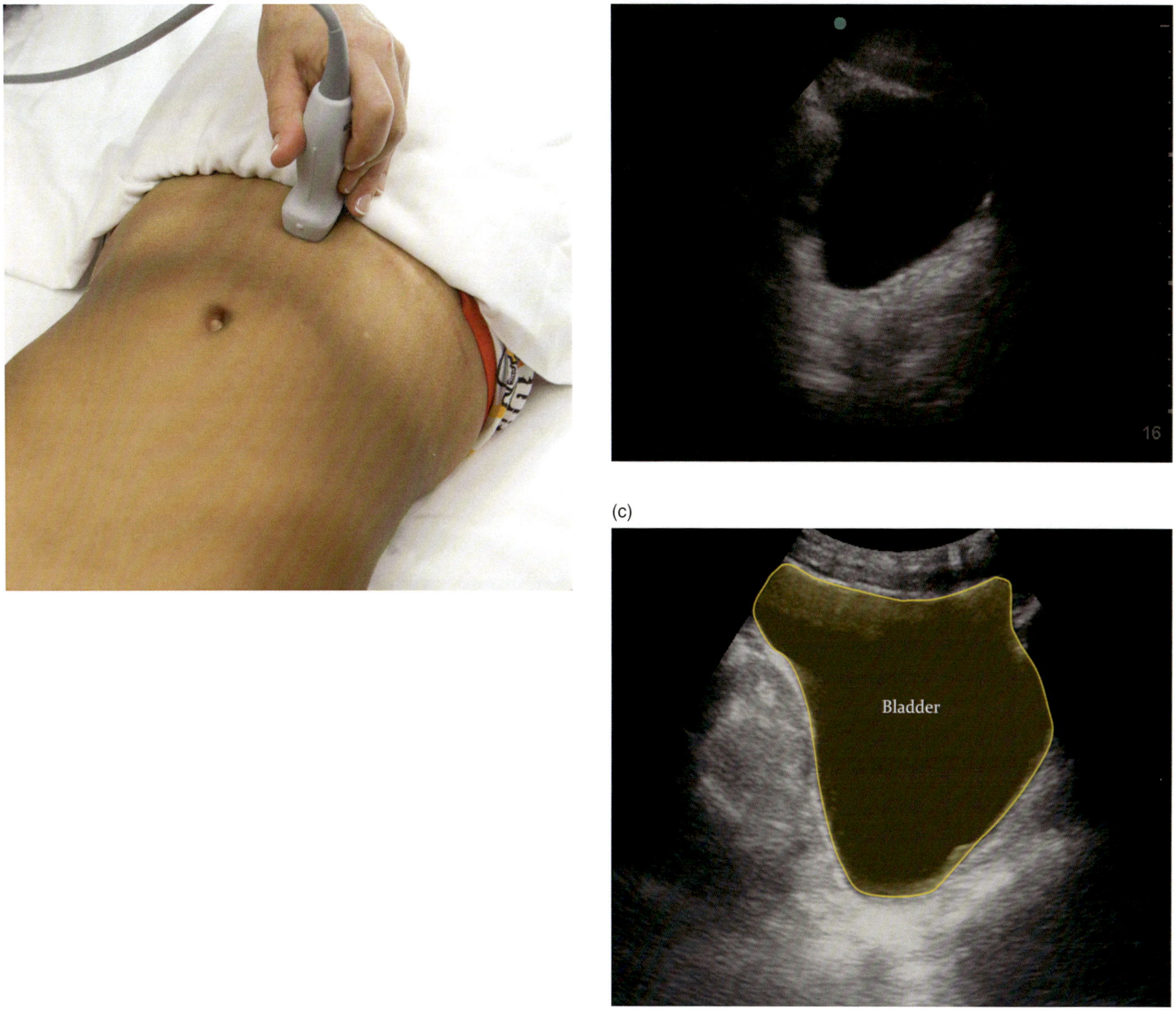

Figure 9.5 Bladder imaging, sagittal view. (a) Transducer placement, with the indicator oriented towards the patient's head. (b) Ultrasound image of the sagittal view of the bladder. (c) Illustration highlighting important structures visualized on the ultrasound image. *Illustration by Laura Berg, MD.*

medulla appear hypoechoic. The calyces appear echodense and converge medially into the echodense renal pelvis. Finally, color Doppler may further elucidate the renal vessels located in the hilum (Figure 9.6).

There are certain sonographic features that are unique to pediatric patients. In the first few months of life, the renal parenchyma may appear isoechoic, or even hyperechoic in comparison to the liver. Outside of the newborn period, a hyperechoic renal parenchyma may be a sign of intrinsic disease or renal failure. In addition, children with healthy kidneys may exhibit prominent pyramids, or a pronounced corticomedullary distinction (Figure 9.7). However, this feature is largely dependent on the quality and resolution of the ultrasound imaging; its absence does not signify renal pathology.

Bladder

The bladder should be visualized in both the transverse and sagittal views. In transverse view, the bladder is a centrally located, trapezoidal-shaped, echodense structure surrounded by an echogenic wall (Figure 9.4b,c). In the sagittal view, the bladder appears as a wedge shape (Figure 9.5b,c). Depending on the degree of fullness, the bladder may take on some irregularities in its shape, conforming to the fluid within and pressure from other organs in the pelvis and abdomen.

Ureters

Normal ureters are difficult to visualize throughout their entire course with ultrasound. However, they can easily be visualized as they exit the kidneys. While evaluating the bladder in the transverse orientation, color flow Doppler may be utilized in order to

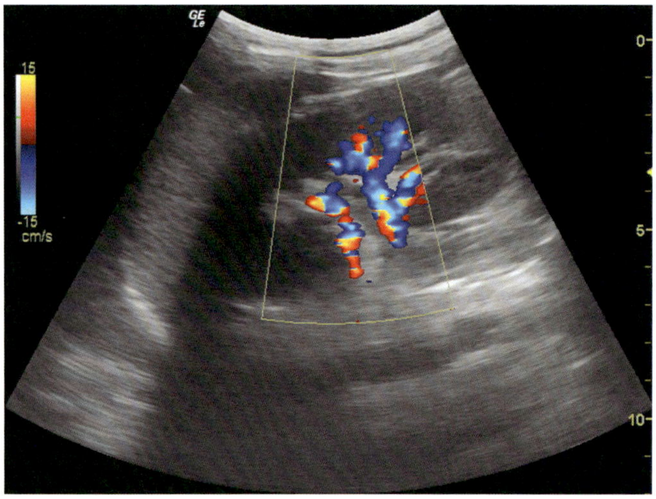

Figure 9.6 Color Doppler of the kidney. Longitudinal view of the kidney, with renal vessels in the hilum illuminated with Doppler color flow.

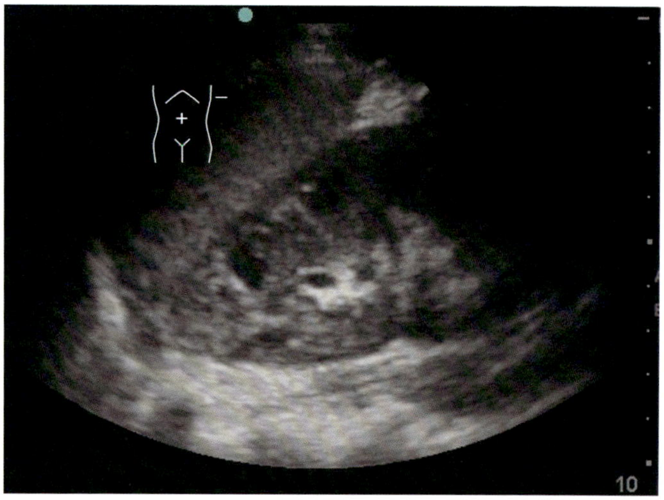

Figure 9.7 Pyramids. Prominent pyramids (P) are especially prevalent in pediatric patients. These may often be mistaken for cysts. The distinguishing feature between pyramids and cysts is that cysts are eccentrically located and often solitary.

(a) (b)

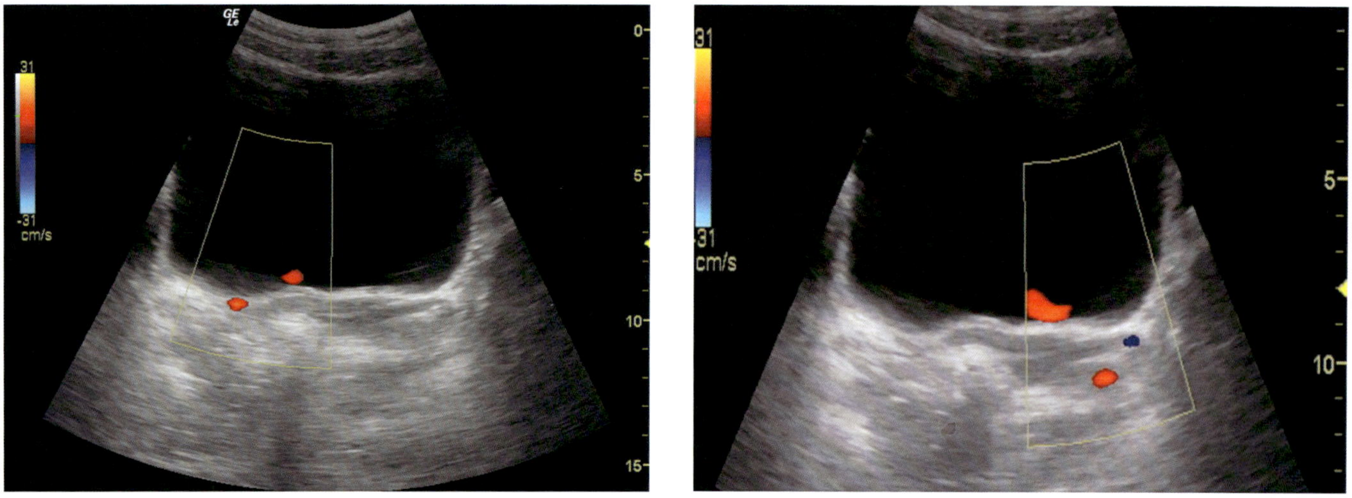

Figure 9.8 Color Doppler: ureteral jets. The ureteral jets are most commonly located at the inferomedial portion of the bladder, and are highlighted in red. (a) Right ureteral jet. (b) Left ureteral jet. Both sides are compared to evaluate for symmetry.

evaluate the ureteral jets for symmetry. Ureteral jets are most commonly located at the inferomedial portion of the bladder (Figure 9.8a,b).

Scanning tips

Pitfalls

- An overhydrated patient or a full bladder may give a false appearance of hydronephrosis, when no obstruction is actually present.
- Dehydration may falsely mask the presence of hydronephrosis.
- Sometimes renal cysts, which are anechoic, may be confused for hydronephrosis. However, cysts are usually eccentrically located, whereas hydronephrosis occurs more centrally at the renal pelvis.
- Medullary pyramids are typically more hypoechoic in infancy and when prominent may also be mistaken for dilated calyces or hydronephrosis.
- One should be aware of normal variants, such as duplicated collecting system, horseshoe kidney, ectopically placed or aplastic kidneys.

Tips to improve scanning

✓ If having difficulty obtaining adequate images of a patient in the supine position, an upright seated or lateral decubitus position may help to displace bowel gas that may be obscuring a good image.

- ✓ Hydronephrosis may become more visible after patients have been hydrated.
- ✓ If bilateral hydronephrosis is present with an overdistended bladder, have the patient urinate and repeat the renal scan.
- ✓ The liver and the spleen may serve as acoustic windows, allowing for better visualization of the right and left kidneys, respectively.
- ✓ Having the patient take a deep breath and hold it will help displace the kidney inferiorly and out from behind the rib cage, to provide a better image.
- ✓ Use Doppler to identify ureteral jets in the transverse bladder view.

Pathology

Hydronephrosis, obstructive uropathy

Hydronephrosis is the dilatation of the collecting system. Sonographically, hydronephrosis is visualized centrally at the renal pelvis. Hydronephrosis may be classified as mild, moderate, or severe, depending on the degree of fluid and obliteration of normal renal architecture (Figure 9.9a–d). It is important to note that hydronephrosis may be underestimated in the setting of dehydration, leading to a false-negative ultrasound interpretation. Alternatively, when the bladder is over-distended, there may be mild hydronephrosis as a result. One may visualize resolution of this hydronephrosis after the patient empties his/her bladder.

In adult patients, obstructive uropathy is primarily caused by an impacted renal stone. However, obstruction in children is more commonly seen with anatomical mechanical obstructions, such as a ureteropelvic junction obstruction or posterior urethral valves. Increased pressures within the system cause distension of the ureter on the obstructed side (hydroureter) and dilatation at the renal pelvis (hydronephrosis). Ultimately, the loss of renal function is directly related to the degree and amount of time of obstruction and increased pressure backing up into the renal parenchyma.

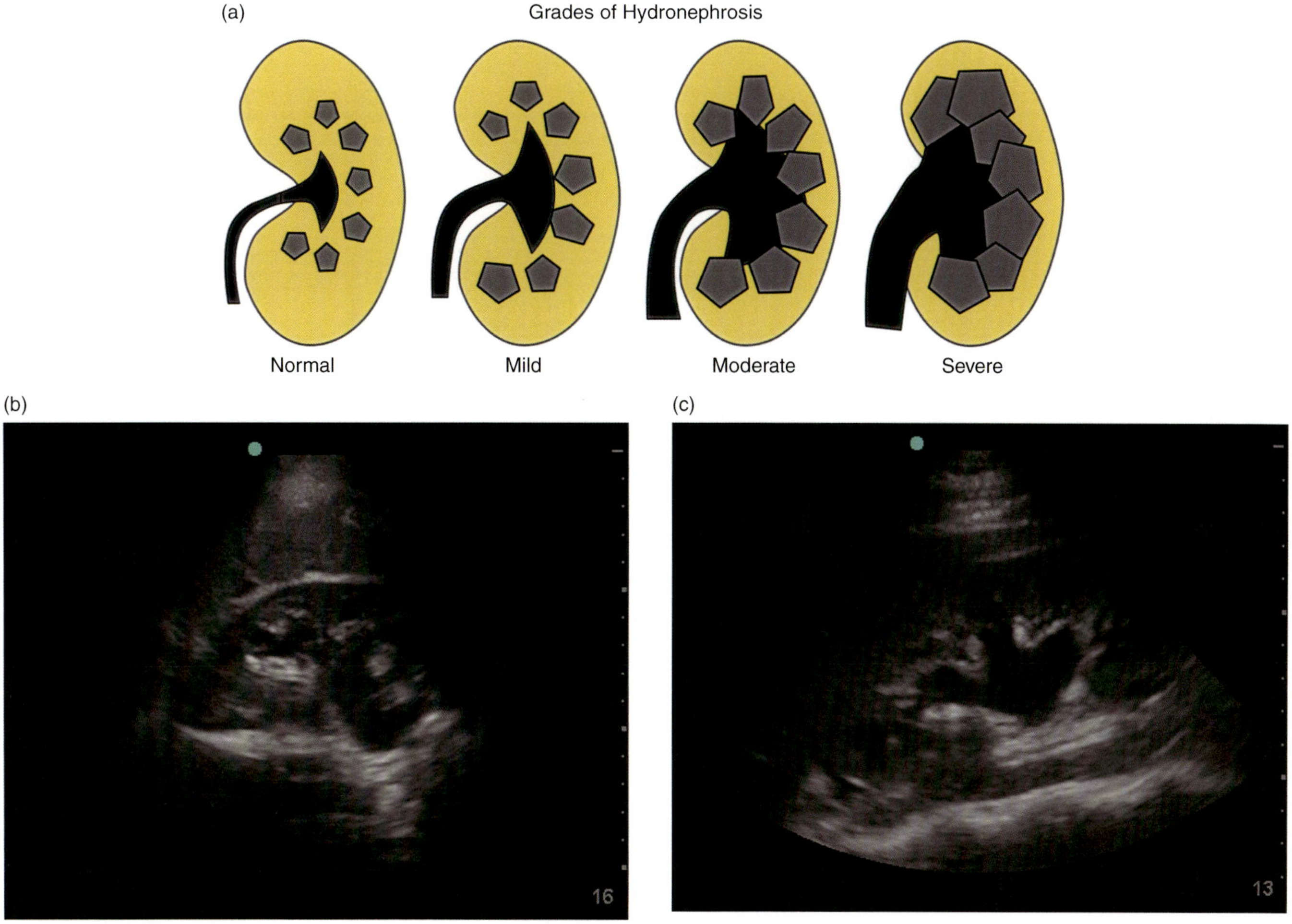

Figure 9.9 Hydronephrosis (a) Illustration of the degrees of hydronephrosis. *Illustration by Laura Berg, MD.* (b) Ultrasound image of mild hydronephrosis. (c) Ultrasound image longitudinal view, of moderate hydronephrosis. (d) Ultrasound image longitudinal view, of severe hydronephrosis. Of note, this patient also has a large cyst present in the adjacent spleen. (e) Transverse view of severe hydronephrosis. (f) Nephrostomy tube visualized within a kidney with severe hydronephrosis.

(d)

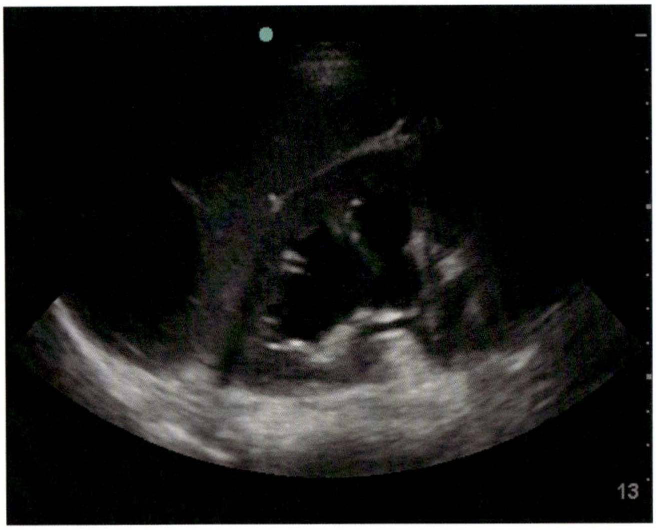

(e)

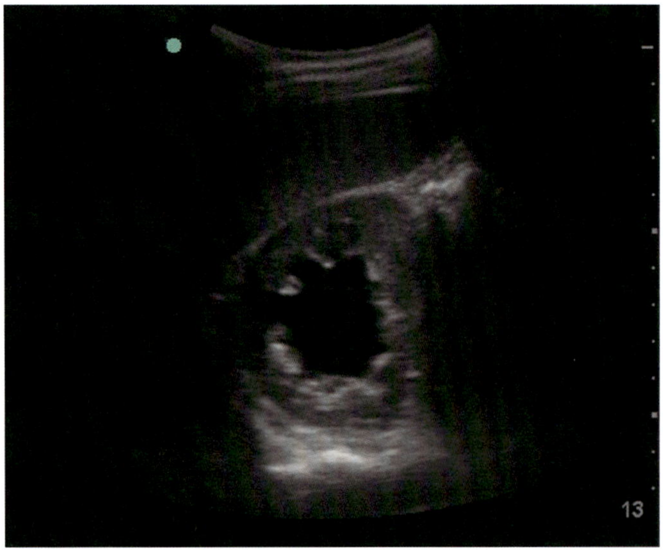

(f)

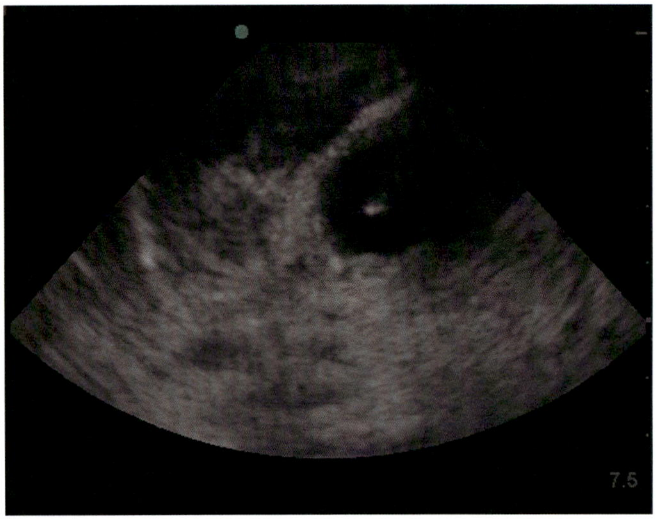

Figure 9.9 (cont.)

Urolithiasis, nephrolithiasis

Kidney stones may be difficult to visualize once they have entered into the ureters. Regardless of their location, whether in the renal pelvis, ureter, or bladder, the appearance on ultrasound is similar, as a brightly echogenic structure with a posterior shadow artifact (Figure 9.10). Once a stone is identified, measurements should be calculated in at least two planes, for the most accurate assessment of its true size.

Bladder with Foley catheter

The emergency sonographer should be aware of the appearance of a Foley catheter within the bladder (Figure 9.11), so as not to confuse it with an alternative diagnosis. A normally functioning Foley catheter should have a bladder decompressed around it. As a result, it may be difficult to visualize the catheter. In order to best visualize the bladder, the catheter may be clamped and/or saline infused through the catheter.

Cystitis, pyelonephritis

The role of ultrasound in evaluating a patient with cystitis is mainly to rule out other causes or complications of infection such as an obstructive pathology or renal stones. Ultrasound can also be used in the evaluation for pyelonephritis. However, pyelonephritis is largely a clinical diagnosis. Ultrasound may reveal a hypoechoic cortex, increased blood flow, or perinephric fluid or abscess collection with renal infections. Cystitis may reveal a thickened bladder wall (Figure 9.12).

(a) (b)

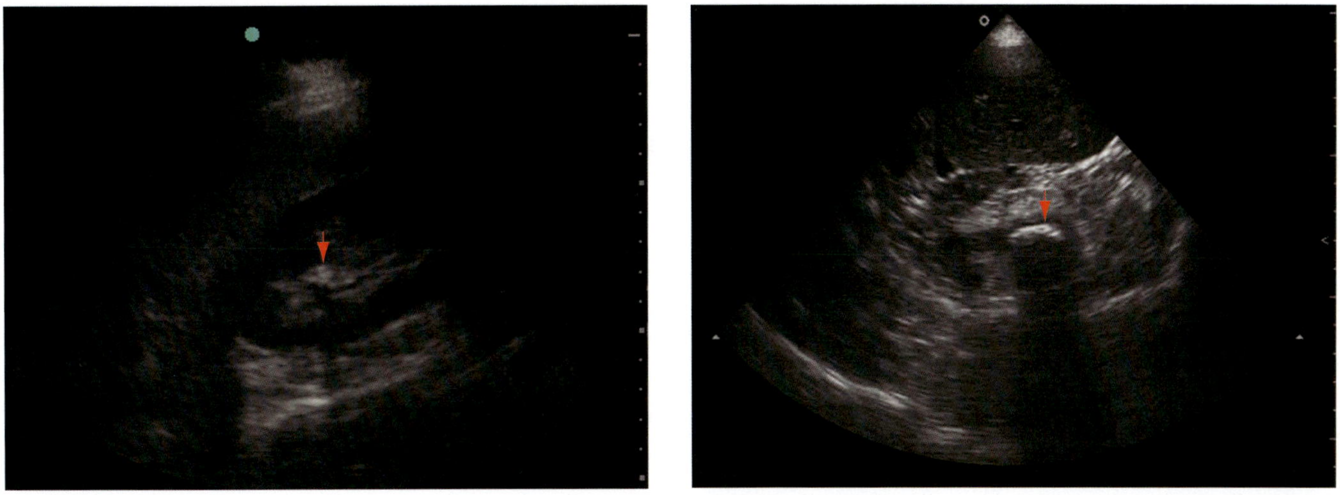

Figure 9.10 Nephrolithiasis. Stones may be visualized if they are located proximally at the renal parenchyma or distally where the ureters enter the bladder. For those stones not visualized, secondary obstruction may be visualized as hydronephrosis. (a) Longitudinal view of a hyperechoic small stone (arrow) within the renal parenchyma, with posterior shadowing. (b) Longitudinal view of a large renal stone (arrow) with posterior shadowing.

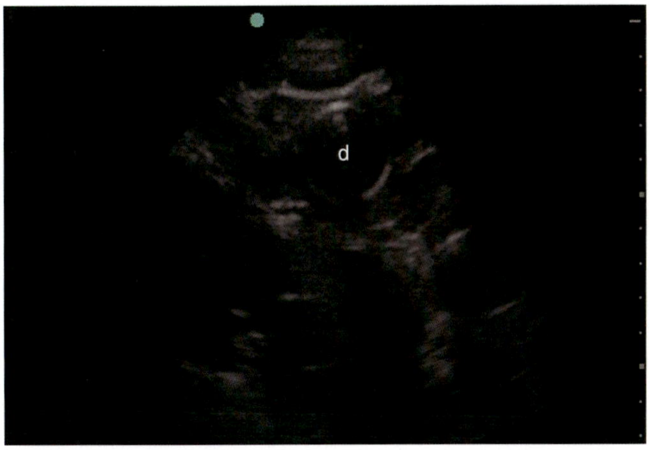

Figure 9.11 Bladder with Foley catheter. When a Foley catheter is present, the bladder is usually compressed around it.

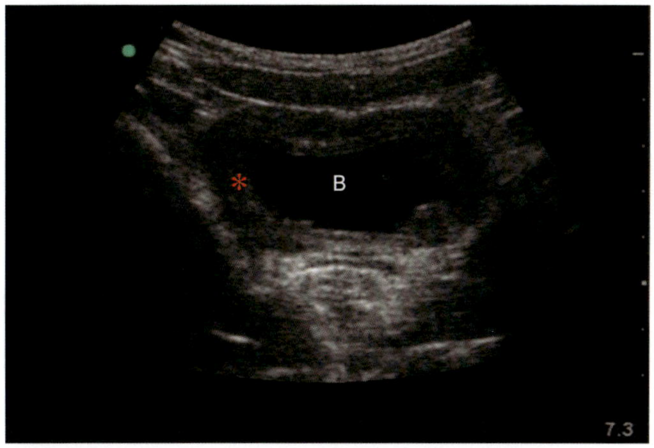

Figure 9.12 Cystitis. Transverse view of the bladder (B) with a thickened bladder wall (*). Debris within the bladder can also be visualized.

Renal cysts, polycystic, and multicystic kidneys

Renal cysts may be congenital or acquired. Cysts are uncommon in children but appear in up to half of adults over the age of 50. Ultrasound is a good starting point for evaluating and diagnosing cystic diseases of the kidney. Sonographically, an isolated cyst appears as an oval or round structure with an anechoic center (Figure 9.13). Cysts as small as 1 mm may be visualized using ultrasound. Size may vary and, in some cases, can be quite large.

Multiple cysts, especially when bilateral, should prompt investigation for congenital polycystic kidney disease (Figure 9.14). Autosomal-dominant polycystic kidney disease (ADPKD) is the most common type of cystic malformation seen in children, with an incidence of 1 in 800. The cysts' appearance increases in size and number with each decade of life, but in many cases they may not be present before the second decade. Extrarenal manifestations may include cysts in the liver, spleen, or pancreas.

Congenital anatomic abnormalities

When performing ultrasonograpy of the kidneys and bladder, the clinician may often encounter congenital anatomic abnormalities, especially in children. These include, but are not limited to, a duplicated collecting system (Figure 9.15a), horseshoe kidney (Figure 9.15b), and pelvic kidney (Figure 9.15c). There may even be an incidental finding of a congenital abscess on one of the kidneys.

One particular type of congenital abnormality that can cause an obstructive uropathy is a ureterocele. A ureterocele is

(a)

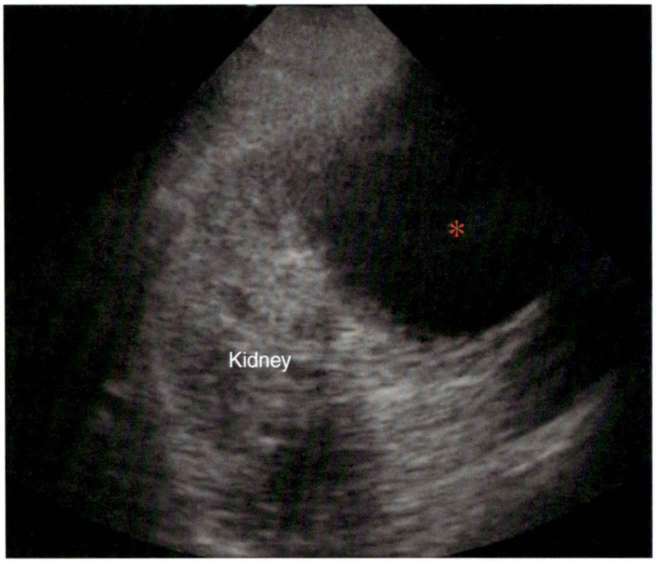

(b)

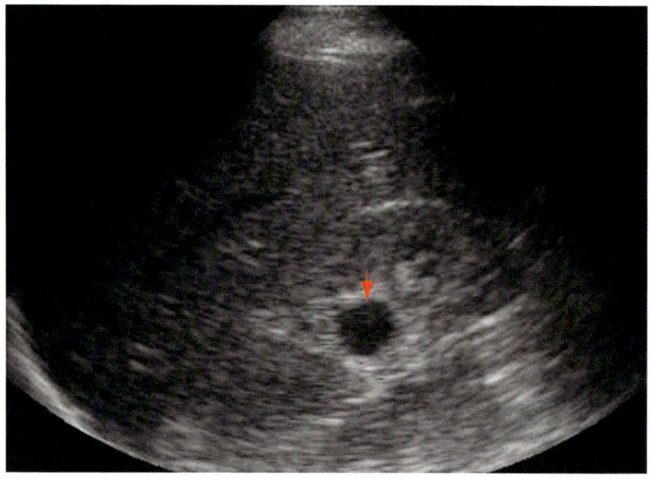

Figure 9.13 Renal cysts. Cysts are anechoic and eccentrically located. (a) Large cyst (*) visualized on the transverse view of the kidney. (b) Small, simple renal cyst (arrow).

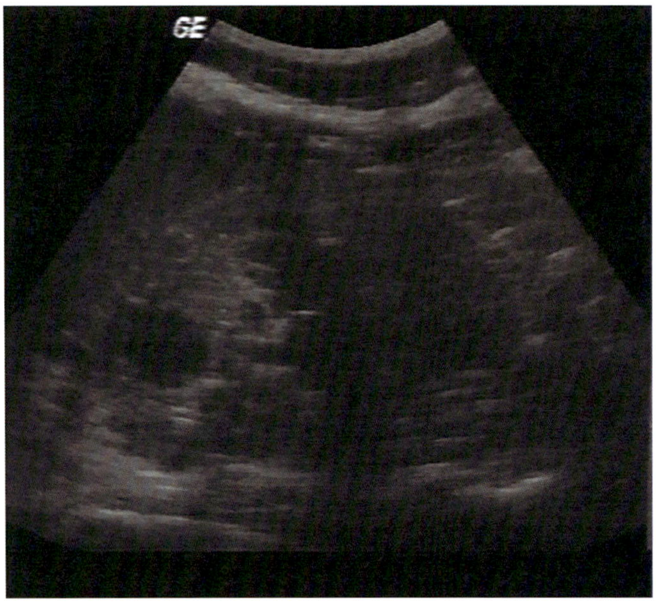

Figure 9.14 Polycystic kidney disease (PCKD). An autosomal dominant condition, in which multiple cysts of different sizes are present throughout the kidneys.

a cystic outpouching that arises from the part of the ureter that inserts into the bladder. It is a congenital anatomic defect of the ureter that occurs in 1 in 5000 infants; it is three times more prevalent in females, and may be associated with a duplicated collecting system or an ectopic ureteral insertion. Ureteroceles may be unilateral or bilateral. Due to its location, a ureterocele can cause obstruction of urine flow into the bladder on that side. On ultrasound, a ureterocele (Figure 9.16a) appears as a thin-walled cystic outpouching within the bladder and is commonly associated with hydroureter (Figure 9.16b) and hydronephrosis on that side (Figure 9.16c).

Renal tumors

An abnormal appearance of the renal parenchyma or a mass should raise suspicion for a renal tumor. The most common tumors to affect the kidneys in children are Wilms tumor and neuroblastoma. It is less important to identify the particular tumor, but to identify an abnormality that will warrant further investigation.

Wilms tumors may appear as a solitary or multiple, solid or cystic parenchymal mass with increased vascular flow. Often the tumor is compressing or obliterating the normal renal structure (Figure 9.17). Similarly, neuroblastomas that originate from the adrenal tissue may have a similar solid or cystic appearance. However, neuroblastomas are more likely to have foci of echogenic calcifications (Figure 9.18).

Cases

1. A four-year-old male with a history of urinary tract infections presents with dysuria and the inability to urinate. Evaluation reveals an irritable child in diapers, who is febrile and exhibits diffuse abdominal tenderness. The mother is resistant to urinary catheterizations due to the associated “emotional stress.” A bladder ultrasound is performed to improve success of catheterization. Ultrasonography demonstrates severe bilateral hydronephrosis (Figure 9.19a,b) and bilateral hydroureter (Figure 9.19c,d). Due to this obstruction,

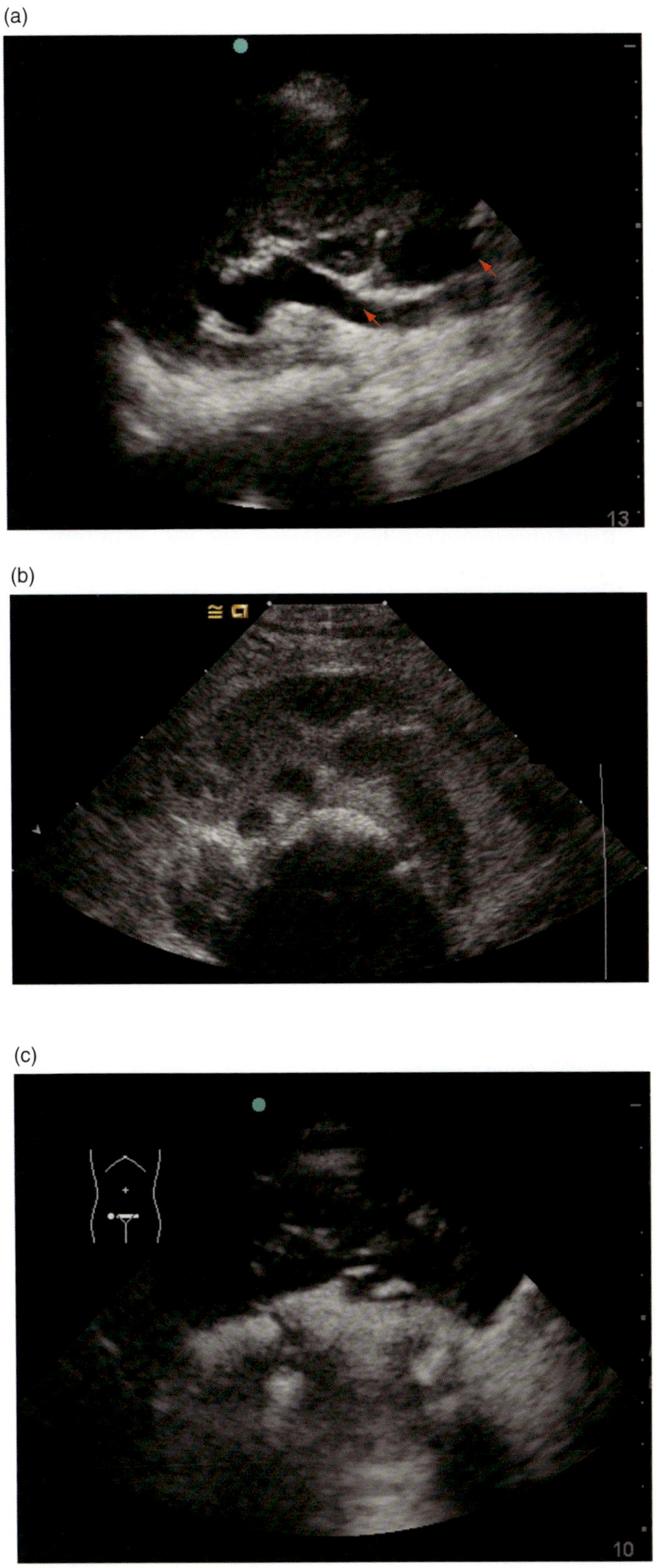

Figure 9.15 Congenital abnormalities. (a) Duplicated collecting system. On this right upper quadrant view is a duplicated kidney; the left-hand side of the kidney exhibits hydronephrosis and hydroureter. Two renal pelvises with ureters (arrows) are visualized. (b) Horseshoe kidney. (c) Pelvic kidney – note the transducer is placed at the suprapubic region.

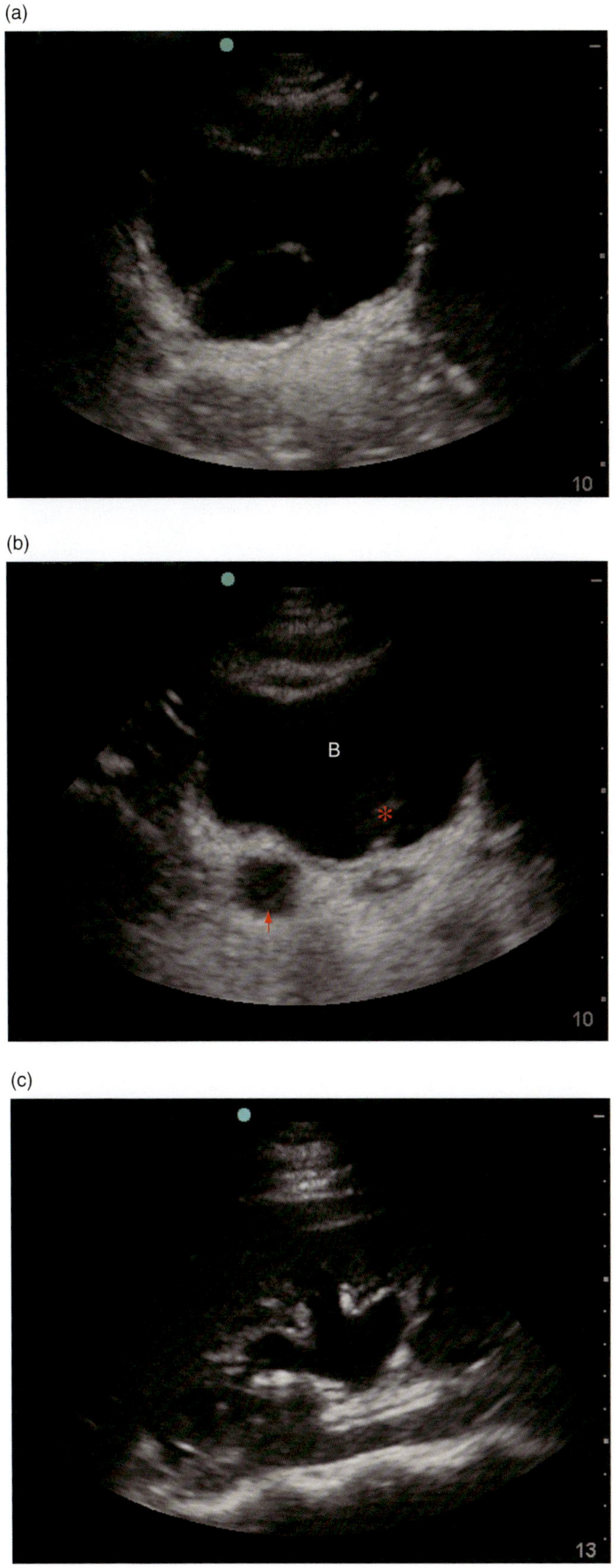

Figure 9.16 Ureterocele. (a) A ureterocele (*) is a congenital condition in which there is an outpouching of the ureter as it enters the bladder (B), and often causes obstruction. There may be associated obstruction with (b) hydroureter (arrow) and (c) hydronephrosis.

a Foley catheter is placed, with immediate complete resolution of his abdominal pain. Laboratory studies reveals a leukocytosis, anemia, abnormal electrolytes, and renal insufficiency (BUN 73 mg/dL, Cr 4 mg/dL). Catheterized urinalysis is positive for infection.

Hydronephrosis is the dilatation of the renal pelvis and calyces; while hydroureter is the dilatation of the ureter. Hydronephrosis and hydroureter are seen when there is an interruption in the flow of urine, often as a result of an obstructive process. Etiologies include congenital lesions, the most common of which is uteteropelvic junction obstruction from posterior urethral valves. Renal functional impairment may develop slowly and progressively and ultimately lead to renal failure (13–44%). More than 30% of all chronic and end-stage renal disease (ESRD) in children is due to obstructive uropathy. Other complications include pain, stones, hypertension, and infection. Prompt bladder decompression helps prevent further complications, and point-of-care ultrasonography has been shown to improve success rates of bladder catheterization.

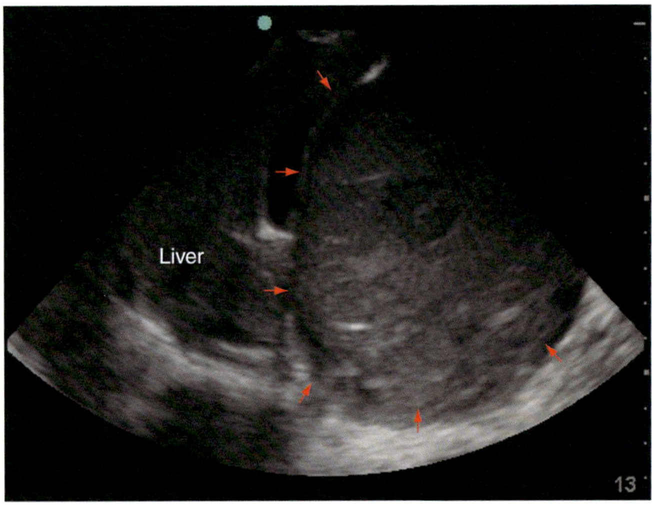

Figure 9.17 Wilms tumor. Wilms tumors (arrows) may appear as a cystic or solid mass with increased vascular flow, and obliterate normal renal architecture.

Summary/key points

1. Renal ultrasound involves scanning each kidney in two views (longitudinal and transverse), and the bladder in two views (transverse and sagittal). Additionally, color Doppler may be used to assess ureteral jets.
2. The most common application of renal/bladder ultrasound is the assessment for hydronephrosis.
3. Disadvantages to renal sonography include the limited evaluation for renal stones. Therefore, patients may still require definitive radiologic tests.
4. In a normally hydrated patient, renal sonography is generally sensitive for detecting hydronephrosis.
5. Pediatric-specific applications are evolving. It is important to identify normal kidneys and distinguish them from pathology or anatomic variants.

(a) (b)

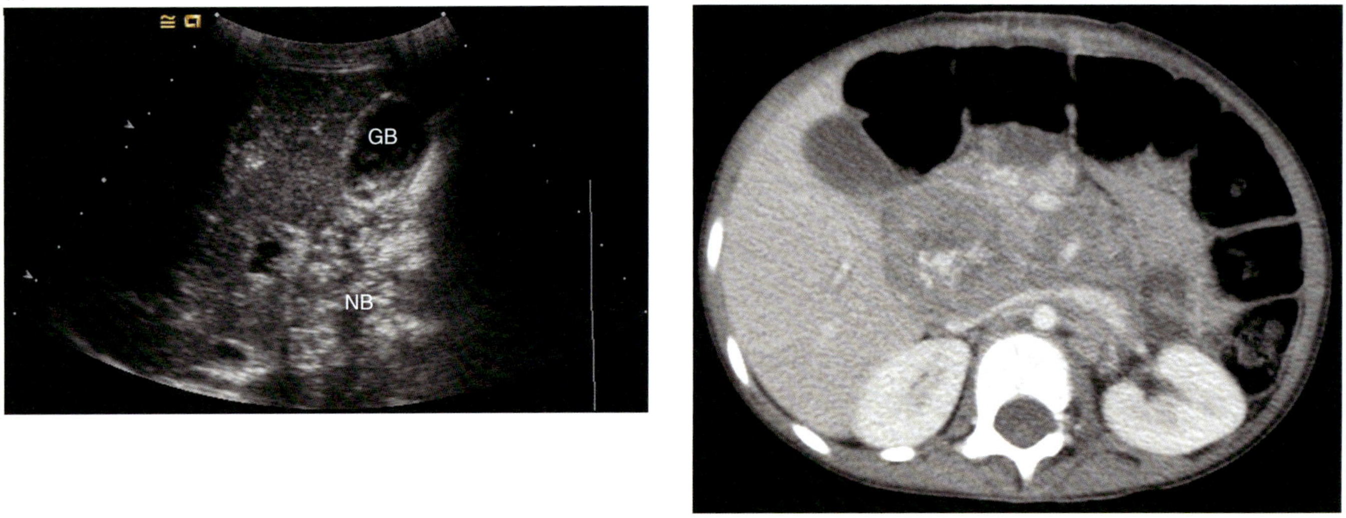

Figure 9.18 Neuroblastoma. (a) Ultrasound of metastatic neuroblastoma. The majority of the tumor is retroperitoneal, and cannot be visualized by the ultrasound. However, a portion of the tumor (NB) can be visualized adjacent to the gallbladder (GB). There are also abnormal, hyperechoic regions within the liver. (b) A CT scan of the neuroblastoma tumor. *Images courtesy of Alanna Braun, MD.*

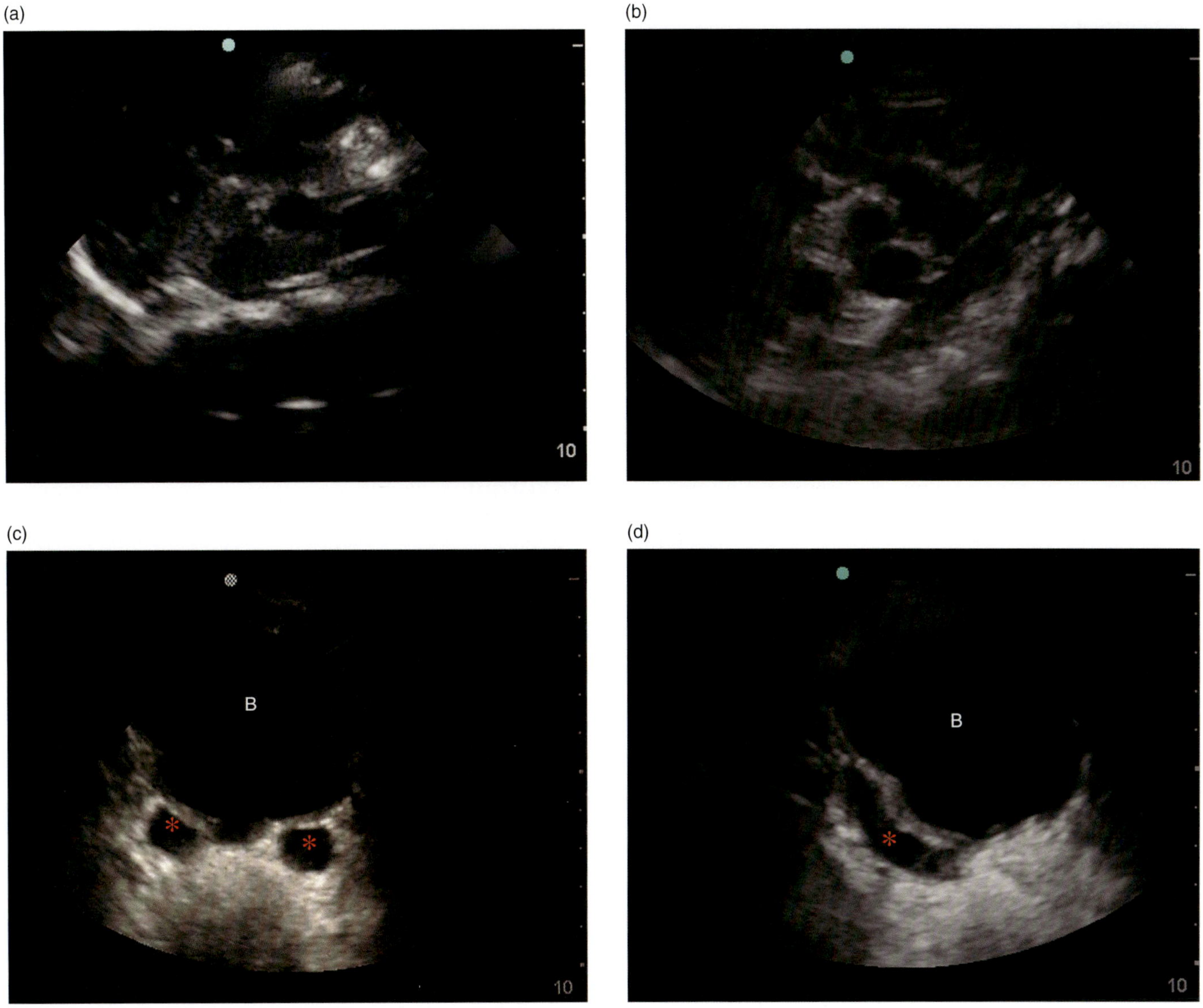

Figure 9.19 Case 1: obstructive uropathy. (a,b) Bilateral hydronephrosis. (c) Transverse suprapubic view. Note the dilated ureters (*) posterior to the bladder (B). (d) Sagittal suprapubic view, slightly off center. The dilated ureter (*) may be visualized longitudinally. Normal ureters are unable to be visualized. This patient also had corresponding bilateral hydronephrosis.

Selected references

Dalziel, P. J., Noble, V. E. (2013) Bedside ultrasound and the assessment of renal colic: a review. *Emerg Med J* **30**(1): 3–8.

de Bessa, J. Jr, Dénes, F.T., Chammas, M.C., *et al.* (2008) Diagnostic accuracy of color Doppler sonographic study of the ureteric jets in evaluation of hydronephrosis. *Pediatr Urol* **4**(2): 113–17.

Gaspari, R.J., Horst, K. (2003) Emergency ultrasound and urinalysis in the evaluation of flank pain. *Acad Emerg Med* **12**(12): 1180–4.

Hoppe, B., Kemper, M.J. (2010) Diagnostic evaluation of the child with urolithiasis or nephrocalcinosis. *Pediatr Nephrol* **25**(3): 403–13.

Noble, V.E., Brown, D.F. (2004) Renal ultrasound. *Emerg Med Clin North Am* **22**(3): 641–59.

Palmer, J.S., Donaher, E.R., O'Riordan, M. A., *et al.* (2005) Diagnosis of pediatric urolithiasis: role of ultrasound and computerized tomography. *J Urol* **174** (4 Pt 1): 1413–16.

Ricabonna, M. (2003) Imaging of renal tumours in infancy and childhood. *Eur Radiol* **13**: L116–29.

Rosen, C.L., Brown, D.F., Sagarin, M.J., *et al.* (1998) Ultrasonography by emergency physicians in patients with suspected ureteral colic. *J Emerg Med* **16** (6): 865–70.

Schissel, B.L., Johnson, B.K. (2011) Renal stones: evolving epidemiology and management. *Pediatr Emerg Care* **27**(7): 676–81.

Vester, U., Kranz, B., Hoyer, P.F. (2010) The diagnostic value of ultrasound in cystic kidney diseases. *Pediatr Nephrol* **25**: 231–40.

Chapter 10

The pediatric abdomen

Adam B. Sivitz

Objectives/indications

Children frequently present to the pediatric emergency department with symptoms of abdominal pain, vomiting, and diarrhea. While these symptoms are most often related to self-limiting illnesses, they may be presenting signs for more serious conditions. A thorough history and meticulous examination may still be insufficient to differentiate the common malady from the more serious diseases. Moreover, it is often difficult to obtain an accurate history and reliably localize pain in young children, and nearly impossible in non-verbal children. The treating physician is then left to decide on a route of possible laboratory investigations and imaging modalities. Ideally, this route would include non-invasive, accurate, and readily available tests.

Abdominal ultrasound is one such modality, which is valuable, rapid, and it has an excellent accuracy in children presenting with abdominal complaints. While there are many advantages, abdominal ultrasonography can be a challenging exercise for various reasons. Intestinal peristalsis and intraluminal bowel gas may obscure target structures, or create artifacts that mimic other findings. Imaging a child presents other specific challenges related to the patient's age and emotional maturity. Intants have a rapid physiologic respiratory rate in infants, which, when compounded by irritability and crying, makes abdominal structures move rapidly in and out of the sonographer's viewing field. Moreover, a child in pain, or who is anxious, may not cooperate with the examination. It is of utmost importance to make the examination as comfortable as possible for the patient. This may be accomplished by using sucrose water solutions and warmed gel for infants, utilizing child-life specialists to explain the examination to younger children, having a caregiver at the bedside, and always paying particular attention to pain management.

While the majority of studies on utilizing ultrasonography for abdominal pathology have been performed in the radiology suite, there is a rapidly growing body of evidence that shows that point-of-care ultrasound can be rapidly used at the bedside as an effective screening and diagnostic tool. Point-of-care ultrasonography may be utilized to identify important abdominal pathology that causes bowel obstruction. The most common causes of bowel obstruction in children that are discussed in this chapter are: intussusception, acute appendicitis, and pyloric stenosis.

INTUSSUSCEPTION

Background

Intussusception is the most common cause of intestinal obstruction in young children worldwide. Intussusception describes the process whereby one segment of bowel telescopes into the immediate distal segment. The proximal segment of bowel, the intussusceptum, telescopes into a distal segment, the intussuscipiens. The attached mesentery gets pulled along with the loop of bowel, resulting in constriction of venous outflow and impaired arterial perfusion. If left untreated, intussusception leads to bowel wall necrosis, perforation, and, rarely, death. This may occur throughout the lower gastrointestinal tract; however, the most common location is ileocolic. It occurs most often between three months and six years of age, with a peak presentation late in the first year of life. Incidence is 1–4 / 1000 live births, with males having a fourfold risk. The etiology of most cases of intussusception is unknown. Intussusception presenting outside the typical age range carries suspicion for an anatomic lead point. Up to 10% of cases have an identifiable lead point, such as a Meckel's diverticulum, an inverted appendiceal stump, an intestinal polyp, lymphoma, or intestinal duplication. Patients with cystic fibrosis and Henoch–Schönlein purpura are predisposed to developing intussusception.

The typical clinical presentation is a previously healthy child who has developed sudden severe bouts of colicky pain or irritability interspersed with periods of lethargy. These symptoms are classically accompanied by vomiting, and guaiac-positive or grossly bloody stools. The classic finding of "currant jelly" stool represents a late finding (Figure 10.1). The triad of colicky abdominal pain, bloody stool, and vomiting is seen in less than 40% of patients, and 20% will present without pain. On physical examination, more than half of patients will have a palpable "sausage-shaped" mass in the right upper quadrant. Making the correct diagnosis is dependent on a high index of clinical suspicion. The initial imaging study is often abdominal

Pediatric Emergency and Critical Care Ultrasound, ed. Stephanie J. Doniger. Published by Cambridge University Press.

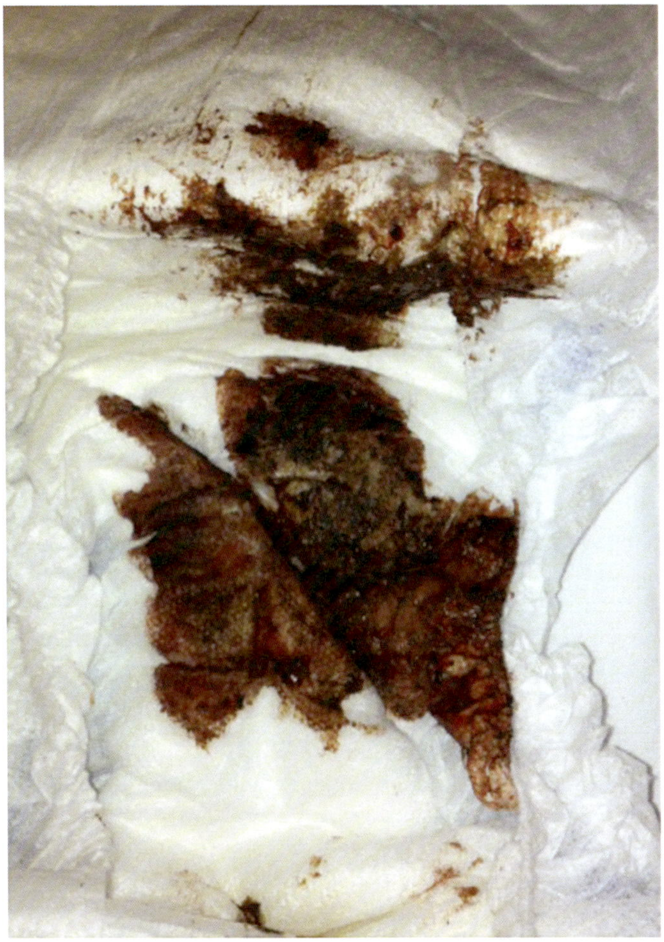

Figure 10.1 Currant-jelly stool, which is a classic finding in intussusception, but is rarely seen.

radiography which may reveal a small-bowel obstruction (Figure 10.2a), a right upper quadrant soft tissue mass, a "target" or "crescent" sign (Figure 10.2b), where the terminal end of the intussusceptus meets with colonic air. Radiography can be normal in up to 45% of patients with proven intussusception, diagnostic in only 20–30%, and clinically unhelpful in 50% of cases. The most important finding on a plain film is the presence of free air, which indicates bowel wall necrosis and perforation and is an absolute contraindication to non-surgical reduction. Ultimately, the study of choice is an air or contrast enema, which is both diagnostic and therapeutic. In order to reduce the telescoped segment and restore perfusion, an air or contrast enema is performed. High pressure is administered through a tube in the rectum, which creates a pressure gradient until free passage of contrast or air is seen in the ileum. In cases where contrast or air enema is unsuccessful, surgical reduction is required and involves manual reduction or bowel resection. It is important to note that there is a 10% recurrence rate with enema-reduced intussusception, vs. 3–5% with surgical reduction. For this reason, children are generally admitted to the hospital for observation following reduction. However, it is important to note, almost half of the recurrences occur greater than 48 hours later.

Ultrasonography has become increasingly utilized as a useful screening modality in the workup of intussusception. Several studies have been performed investigating formal ultrasonography, with a sensitivity of 98–100% and specificity of 88–100%. A recent study of 640 patients in Vietnam showed a sensitivity of 97.5% and specificity of 99%. It is suggested that utilizing ultrasound as a first-line diagnostic modality would decrease radiation-induced malignancy by 79.3 and 59.7 cases per 100,000 male and female children,

(a)

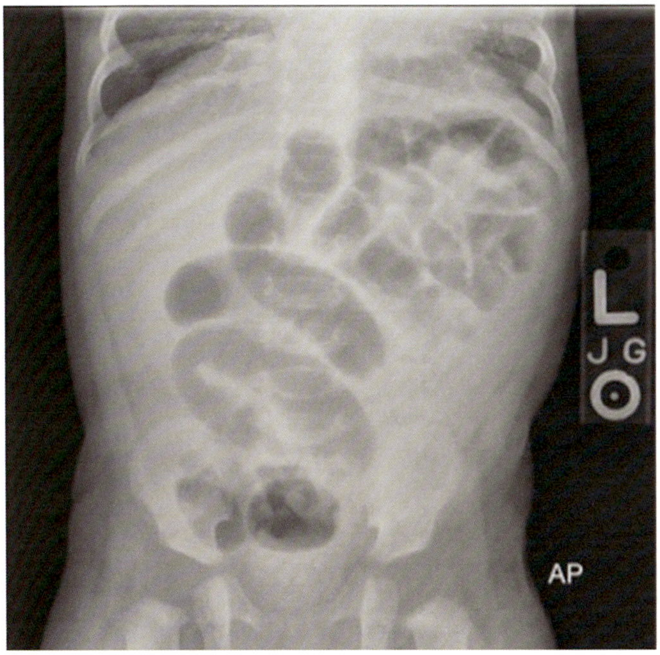

(b)

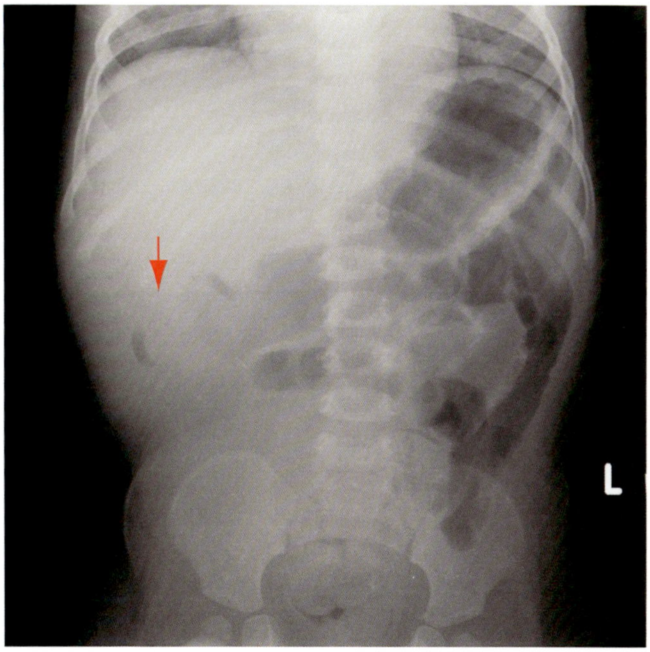

Figure 10.2 Radiographs in intussusception. Often, plain radiographs are nonspecific or normal. (a) Signs of obstruction may also be seen. (b) A classic finding is the "crescent" sign (arrow) at the location of the intussusception.

respectively. Since the sensitivity and specificity of ultrasonography are both approaching 100%, it serves as an ideal screening tool, amenable to use in the emergency department. Riera *et al.* recently prospectively studied point-of-care ultrasound performed by pediatric emergency physicians with limited training. Point-of-care ultrasound had a sensitivity of 85%, specificity of 97%, NPV of 97%, and PPV of 85%.

Anatomy

When imaging the gastrointestinal (GI) tract, it is important to be familiar with the four histologic layers: (1) the luminal mucosa, (2) submucosa (including the muscularis mucosa), (3) muscularis propria, and (4) serosa (Figure 10.3). Intussusception in the typical pediatric age range involves the invagination of the ileum into the cecum, termed an ileocolic intussusception (Figure 10.4). Sometimes this process starts as ileoileal and then ileocolic, when there is first a small-bowel intussusception which then invaginates.

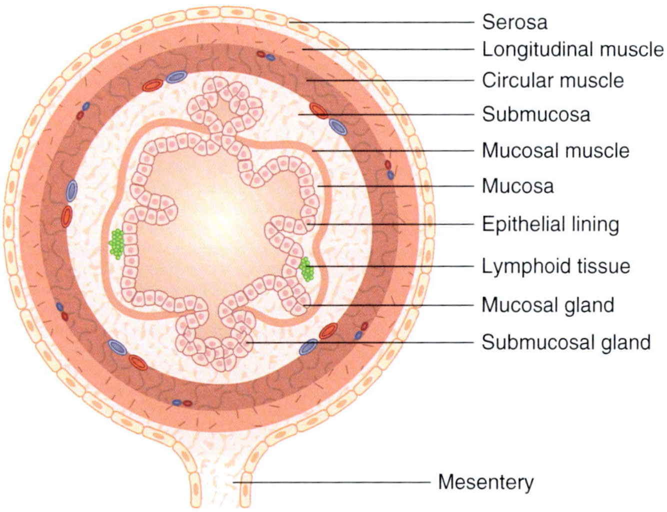

Figure 10.3 Bowel wall layers. (1) The luminal mucosa (small area of columnar cells noted secondary to mucosal destruction), (2) submucosa (including the muscularis mucosa), (3) muscularis propria, and (4) serosa. *Artwork created by Emily Evans © Cambridge University Press.*

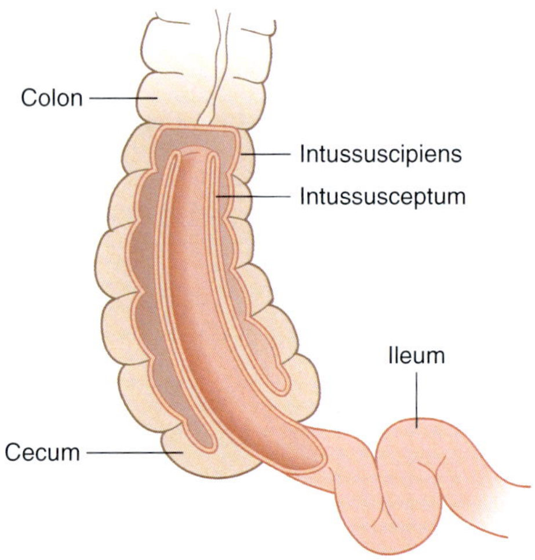

Figure 10.4 Intussusception. Intussusception involves the invagination of bowel layers: the intussusceptum into the intusscipiens. *Artwork created by Emily Evans © Cambridge University Press.*

Technique

Point-of-care questions

1. Is an intussusception present?
2. Is there surrounding free fluid and edema?

Transducer selection and orientation

Using a linear, high-frequency (5–10 MHz) transducer, the examiner should start in a transverse view at the level of the hepatic flexure (Figure 10.5a). From this position, identify the transverse and ascending colon, then trace down the ascending colon to the cecum and the level of the ileocecal valve.

Patient position and preparation

The ultrasound examination begins with the patient in a supine position. Using pre-warmed gel and distraction techniques will help alleviate the anxiety and discomfort in the young patient. The scan can be attempted with the child in a parent's lap if need be.

Ultrasound imaging

The ascending colon can be identified as the most lateral bowel structure on the right side of the abdomen. Visualization of a normal colon may be obscured by gas or fecal material. In the fluid-filled colon, haustral markings may be noted. Sonographically, normal bowel has alternating hyperechoic and hypoechoic structures. In cross-section, this creates a "target" or "bull's eye" appearance with, potentially, five distinct layers representing the mucosa, muscularis mucosa, submucosa, outer circular muscularis, and serosa. The number of visible layers depends on the degrees of inflammation or distention present. Normal bowel wall thickness ranges from 3 to 5 mm in diameter. Sonographically, other anatomic features of normal bowel include gastric rugae, small-bowel valvulae conniventes, or colonic haustra (Figure 10.5b,c).

The visualization of an empty ileocecal valve can help to rule out an ileocecal intussusception. The identification of an intussusception consists of visualizing an oval, target-shaped mass typically seen at the hepatic flexure that was initially described in 1977 by Burke. The "target" or "doughnut" appearance is accentuated by the redundant alternating appearance of hyperechoic–hypoechoic bowel wall, stacked within one another with trapped mesentery inside (Figure 10.6a,b). Moving the transducer into a long-

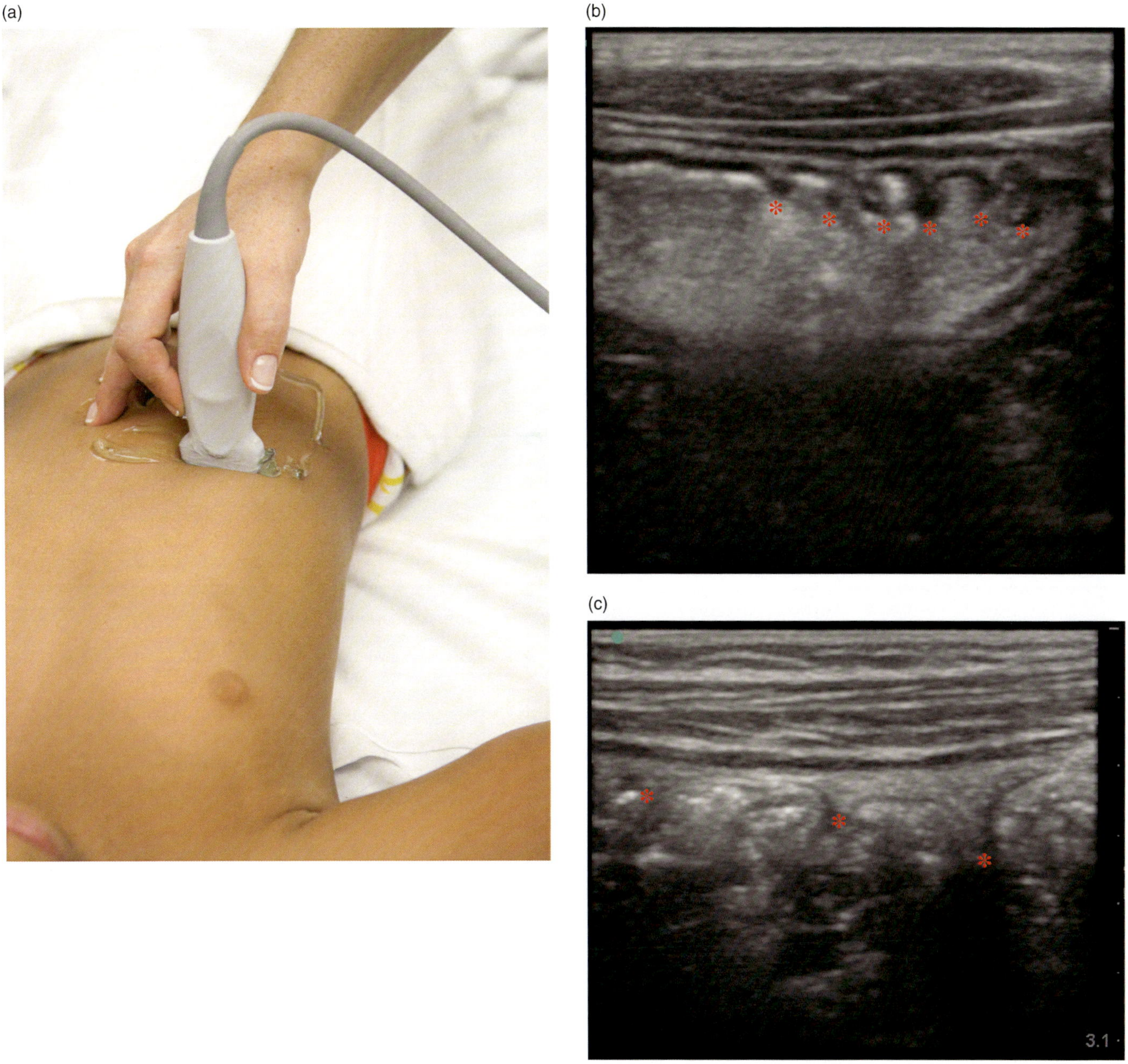

Figure 10.5 The evaluation for intussusception. (a) Transducer placement, transverse view with the indicator oriented towards the patient's right side. Scanning is performed from the transverse to ascending colon, down to the cecum. (b) Ultrasound image, transverse view of the stomach showing hyperechoic gastric contents and the undulating gastric rugae (*). (c) Sagittal view of the ascending colon visualizing colonic haustra (*).

axis view produces the "hayfork" (Figure 10.6c,d) or "pseudokidney" sign (Figure 10.6e), which describes the invagination of the intussusceptum into the intussuscipiens. Mesenteric lymph nodes (Figure 10.7a) and fluid within or around the intussusception may also be seen (Figure 10.7b). There may also be secondary signs of small-bowel obstruction (Figure 10.7c,d). In addition, there are several signs seen on ultrasound that may predict failure of non-operative management. These include: large amounts of trapped fluid within the intussusception, poor or no blood flow on color Doppler imaging, multiple lymph nodes greater than 1 cm in diameter within the intussusceptum, or an outer wall thickness of greater than 1 cm (Figure 10.7e).

Ultrasound imaging: measurements

Measurements of the bowel wall or overall diameter are an important part of the abdominal examination. Transducer

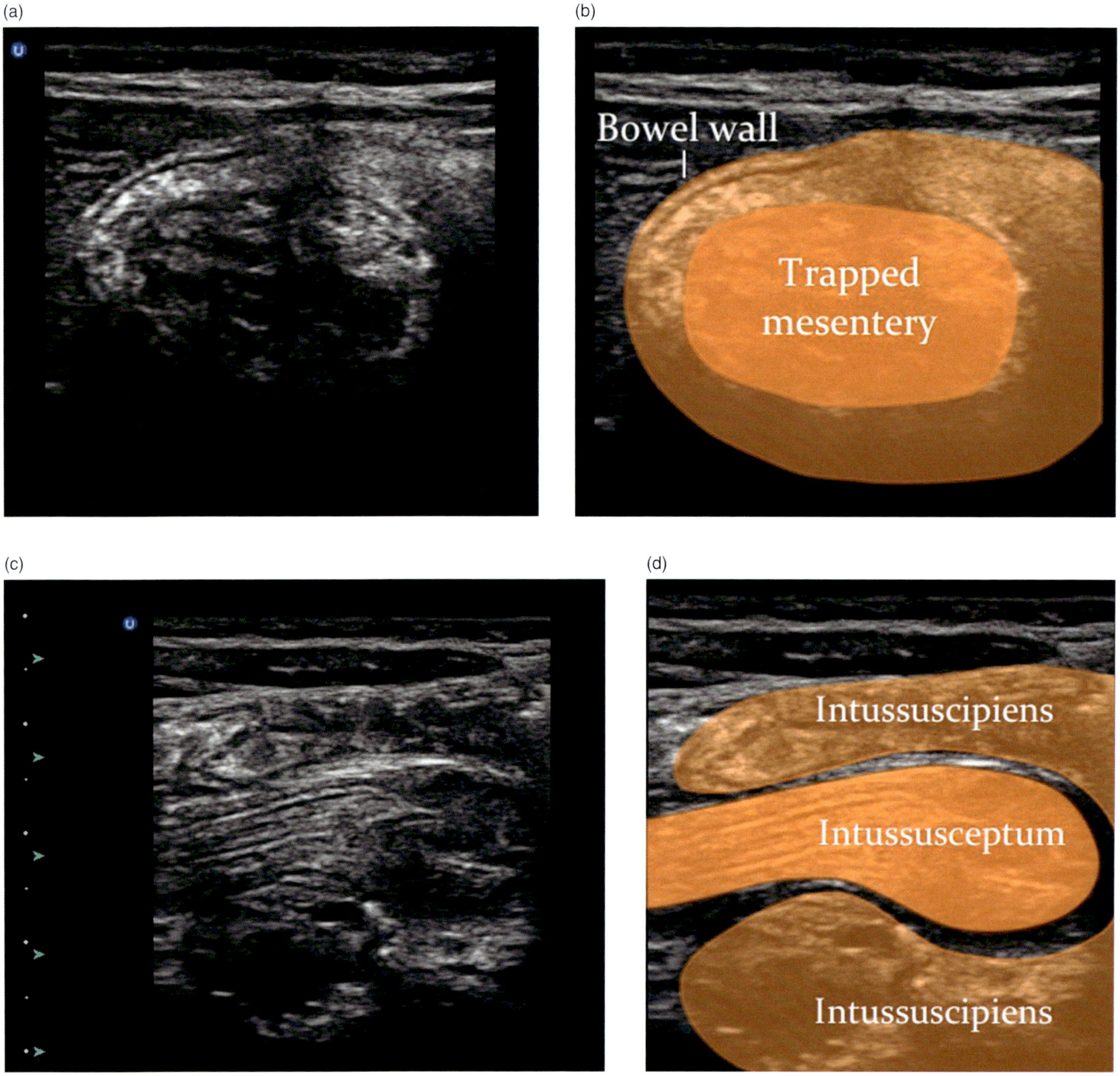

Figure 10.6 Intussusception. (a) Transverse view of an intussuception has layers of bowel around trapped hyperechoic mesentery in the center. (b) The transverse view is referred to as the "target" sign. (c) The longitudinal view of an intussusception shows the invagination of the intussusceptum into the intussuscipiens. (d) The longitudinal view is referred to as the "hayfork" sign. (e) The longitudinal view is also referred to as the "pseudokidney" sign. *Illustrations by Laura Berg, MD.*

positioning should be in the ideal plane to avoid incorrect measurements giving falsely positive or negative findings depending on the planes of view. When the difference between positive and negative findings is measured in millimeters, correct positing is imperative. With intussusception, though there are size measurements that can be made (2.5–5 cm), the diagnosis is based on sonographic appearance alone.

Scanning tips

Pitfalls

- Ultrasound examinations are largely operator dependent. Despite this, studies have shown that junior radiology residents have a similar accuracy when compared with their radiology attendings in identifying intussusception by ultrasound.

(e)

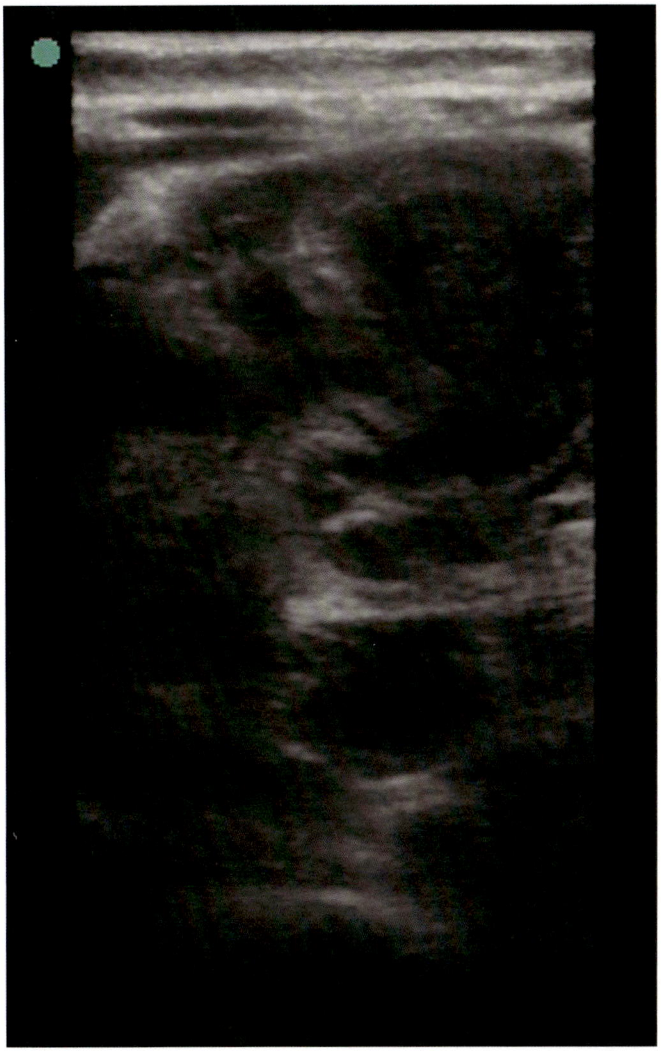

Figure 10.6 (cont.)

- False-positive studies may arise from other etiologies of bowel wall thickening that may give a "pseudokidney" sign, including enterocolitis, inflammatory bowel disease, and an intramural hematoma.
- Stool may be mistaken for an intussusception. However, stool does not exhibit circumferential layering of the bowel wall, as is seen with intussusception.
- False-positive or false-negative studies may be found in a child with intermittent self-reducing intussusception.
- When the depth is not properly adjusted, the intussusception may be missed. It is important to increase the depth enough to visualize the anterior and posterior walls of the intussusception.
- There may be misidentification of the position of the intussusception; finding it within the small bowel instead of the typical ileocolic position.
- Ileoileal intussusceptions may be missed by ultrasonography.

Tips to improve scanning

✓ Using pre-warmed gel and distraction techniques will help alleviate the anxiety and discomfort in the young patient.

(a)

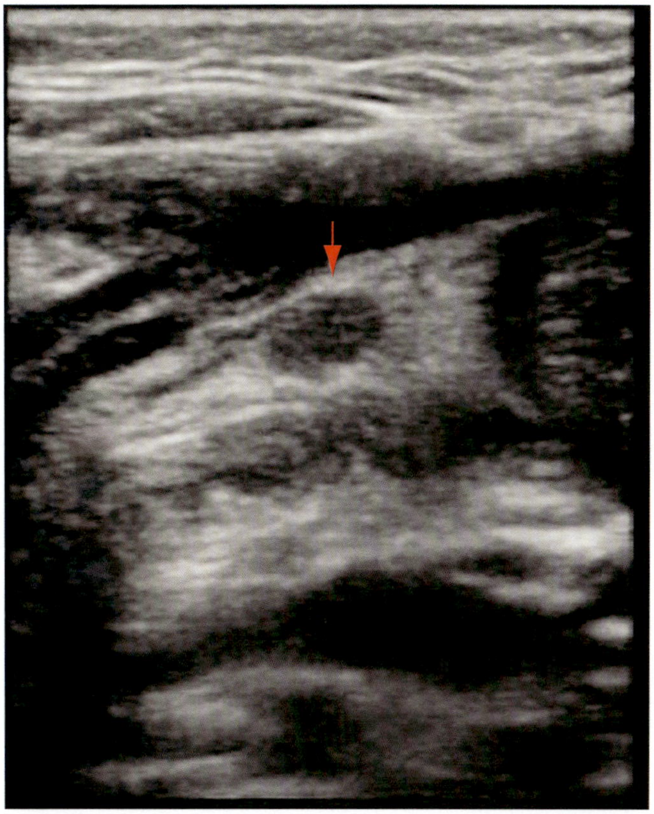

(b)

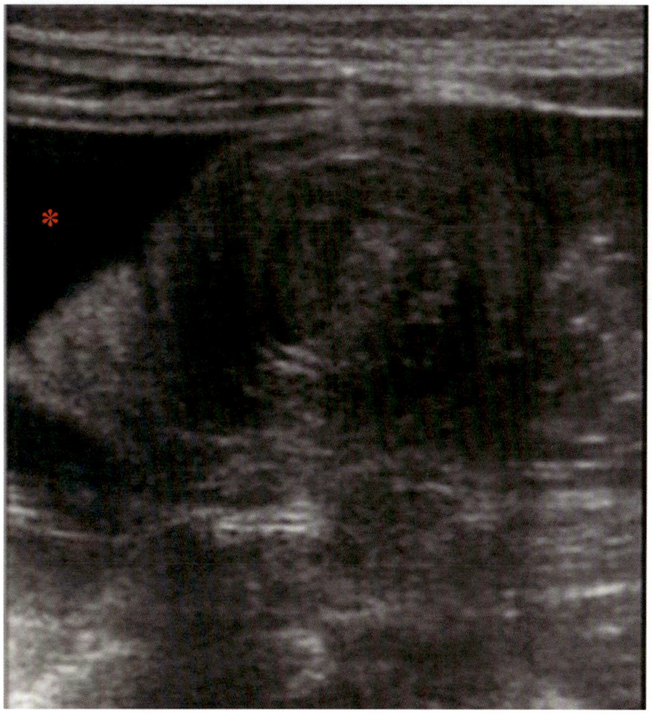

Figure 10.7 Additional findings in intussusception. (a) Mesenteric lymph nodes (arrow). (b) Fluid (*) surrounding the intussusception. (c) Dilated loops of small bowel associated with a small-bowel obstruction. (d) Dilated loops of bowel (*) anterior to an ileocolic intussusception (arrows). (e) Normal color Doppler of the bowel wall in an intussusception. The absence of flow may indicate a reduced chance of non-operative reduction.

(c)

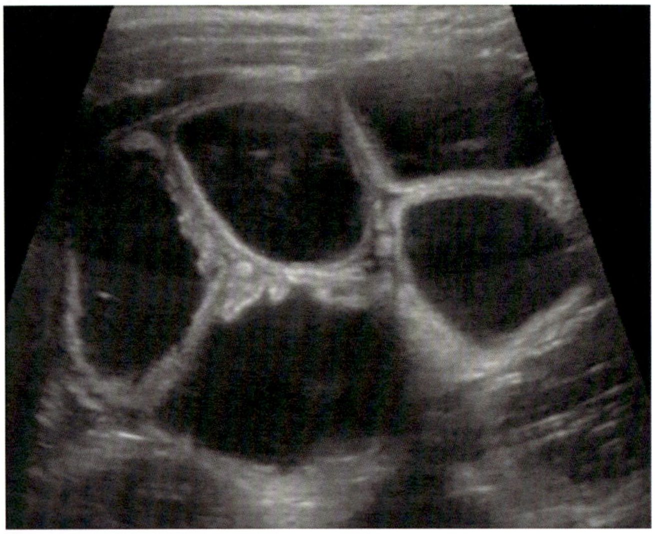

(d)

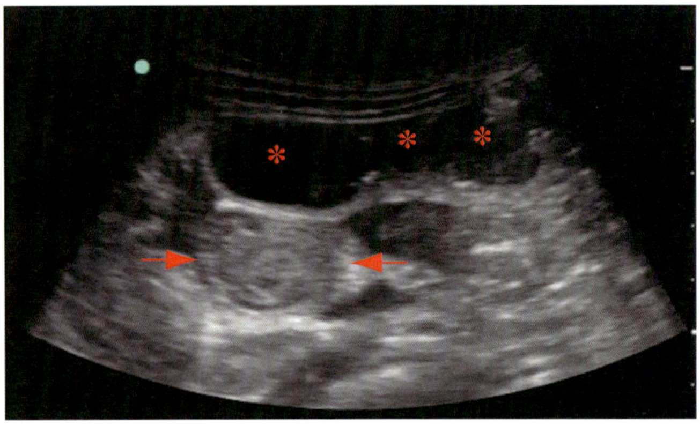

(e)

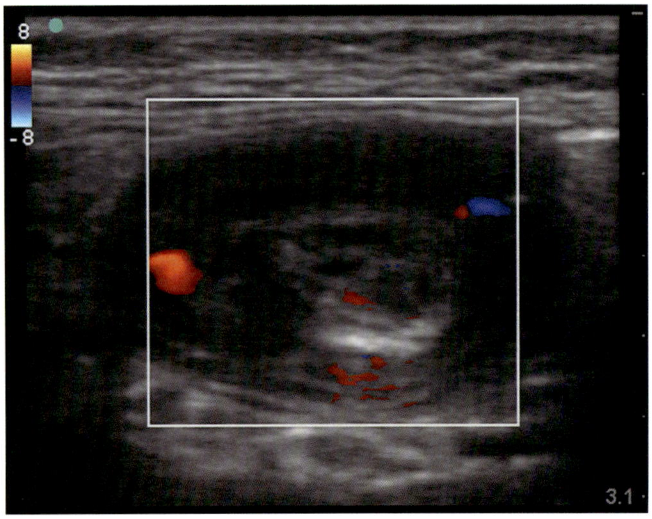

Figure 10.7 (cont.)

The scan can be attempted with the child in a parent's lap if need be.

✓ Keep a high index of suspicion when patients with pre-existing risk factors such as cystic fibrosis or Henoch–Schonlein purpura (HSP) present with colicky abdominal pain. With HSP, the location of their intussusception may be at an atypical location.

✓ Be sure to visualize the intussusception in two views. In cross-section it will appear as a "target" or "doughnut" shape. In the long-axis, it will appear as a "hayfork" or "pseudokidney."

✓ Sonographic signs suggestive of difficulty reducing the intussusception by air or contrast enema include trapped or surrounding fluid, edematous bowel wall, and decreased Doppler blood flow to the bowel wall.

✓ With high clinical suspicion for intussusception, patients may be observed and then the ultrasound repeated.

APPENDICITIS

Background

Appendicitis is the most common abdominal emergency requiring surgery in children, with an incidence of about 80,000 cases per year in the United States. Its peak presentation is in the second decade of life, with males being affected more often than females. Acute appendicitis results from obstruction of the appendiceal lumen, promoting distal inflammation and distention (Figure 10.8). This process compromises perfusion, facilitating microbial invasion into the appendiceal wall, ultimately leading to perforation, peritonitis, and abscess formation. Rates of ruptured appendicitis range from 10–20% in adolescents, to as high as 100% in patients less than four years of age. This difference is attributed to both earlier and more typical presentations in the adolescent age group, compared to the younger, non-verbal children.

The classic presentation of appendicitis begins with vague periumbillical abdominal pain that worsens over time and localizes to the right lower quadrant. There is associated vomiting, anorexia, and fever. The symptoms typically evolve over a period of 24–48 hours, with delays in diagnosis greater than 48 hours associated with an increased risk of perforation. Unfortunately, only about 50% of patients present with the classic features of appendicitis. Other signs or symptoms may also be present. Abdominal inflammation may cause irritation of nearby structures such as the bladder or sigmoid colon, causing dysuria or diarrhea, respectively. Ultimately, the localization of pain to the right lower quadrant arises secondary to local irritation of the overlaying peritoneum, while a retrocecal appendicitis may localize pain to the hip, mimicking a septic arthritis. While late findings of peritonitis are typically unmistakable, treating physicians can miss the diagnosis with earlier presentations. The diagnosis is further complicated in children who are poor historians, and in adolescent females who may have presentations that overlap with potential gynecologic pathology. Several clinical scoring systems have been developed, such as the Alvarado score and the Pediatric Appendicitis score, which take into

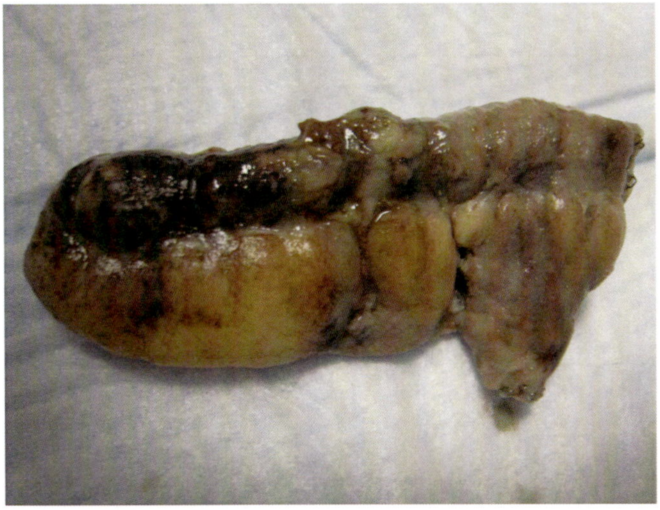

Figure 10.8 Appendicitis. Pathology specimen in an inflamed appendix with a necrotic tip, consistent with acute appendicitis.

consideration a patient's clinical presentation and laboratory studies. While these scoring systems may help guide the clinician, they cannot be solely relied upon in the diagnosis or exclusion of appendicitis. Laboratory investigations are often used to aid in diagnosis, and may include but are not limited to a complete blood count, C-reactive protein (CRP), and urine analysis. While an elevation in the white blood cells or absolute neutrophil count suggests appendicitis, patients may not have significantly elevated levels. In addition, the irritation of the ureter or urinary bladder from an acutely inflamed appendix may cause white and red blood cells to appear in the urine, falsely suggesting a urinary tract infection. While unambiguous cases may proceed to the operative suite, equivocal cases often lead to further imaging studies.

In 1986, Puylaert described the technique of graded compression ultrasonography for the evaluation of acute appendicitis. The author based the diagnosis of appendicitis only on the presence or absence of a visible appendix. In a study of healthy patients without any abdominal complaints, Rettenbacher *et al.* showed that 23% of subjects had an appendiceal diameter greater than 6 mm, and 9% were greater than 7 mm. Therefore, a measurement greater than 6 mm does not automatically indicate acute appendicitis. In another study, the same group found that a consistently ovoid, as opposed to a completely or distally round, appendix correlated with a normal appendix. In the case of an ovoid-appearing appendix, the relevant measurement should be made at the narrowest part of the oval. The overall sensitivity of an ultrasound examination ranges between 50 and 100%, and specificity is between 88 and 99%. Therefore, a negative study cannot reliably rule out acute disease. Further complicating matters is that visualization of the appendix varies widely from 22 to 98%. Visualization may largely be operator dependent, but also dependent on patient characteristics. Recent studies show that children with a BMI of greater than 85, with a clinical probability of less than 50% of having appendicitis, had a 58.1% probability of having an inaccurate or equivocal ultrasound examination. Most recently, Mittal *et al.* performed a large pediatric cohort study of radiologist-performed ultrasound. Results showed an overall sensitivity and specificity of 72.5% and 97% respectively, which is consistent with prior studies. However, in separating out those cases where the appendix was clearly identified, the sensitivity increased to 97.9%, but with a slightly lower specificity of 91.7%. Despite these drawbacks, institutions looking to reduce radiation exposure have proposed using ultrasonography as the initial diagnostic modality, with CT only in negative or equivocal cases. This staged approach has resulted in acceptable rates of negative appendectomies and significant reductions in CT utilization. With a staged ultrasound protocol, the sensitivity and specificity were shown to be 98.6% and 90.6% respectively, with a negative appendectomy rate of 8.1% and a missed appendicitis rate of less than 0.5%. Further, upon review of recent published evidence, in 2010 the American College of Radiology reaffirmed that ultrasonography should be the first-line imaging study in children under 14 years of age and in pregnant women.

Recently, Fox *et al.* applied this technology to the bedside. Prospectively enrolled patients had a point-of-care ultrasound performed by attending physicians and residents in the emergency department. Sensitivity for the point-of-care ultrasound was 65% and specificity was 90%, with a PPV of 84% and an NPV of 76%. Since point-of-care ultrasound has a low sensitivity, it should only be utilized as a "rule in" modality, but not to rule out disease. Further larger-scale studies need to be performed as clinicians gain further experience in utilizing point-of-care ultrasound for appendicitis.

Anatomy

The vermiform appendix is a blind-ending tubular structure that arises from the cecum, 1–2 cm from the ileocecal valve (Figure 10.9a). In infancy, it has a more conical shape that becomes characteristically tubular by one to two years of life. The length can range from 2 to 20 cm, and the tip may lie in variable positions within the abdominal-pelvic cavity (Figure 10.9b). Blood to the appendix is supplied by the appendicular artery, a branch of the ileocolic artery.

Technique

Point-of-care questions

1. Can the appendix be visualized?
2. Is the appendix a blind-ending, non-compressible, tubular structure **greater than 0.6 cm diameter**?
3. Is appendicitis present?
4. Is there surrounding free fluid, perforation, or an abscess?

Transducer selection and orientation

A high-frequency (5–10 MHz) linear transducer provides the optimal level of detail. The examination should be performed

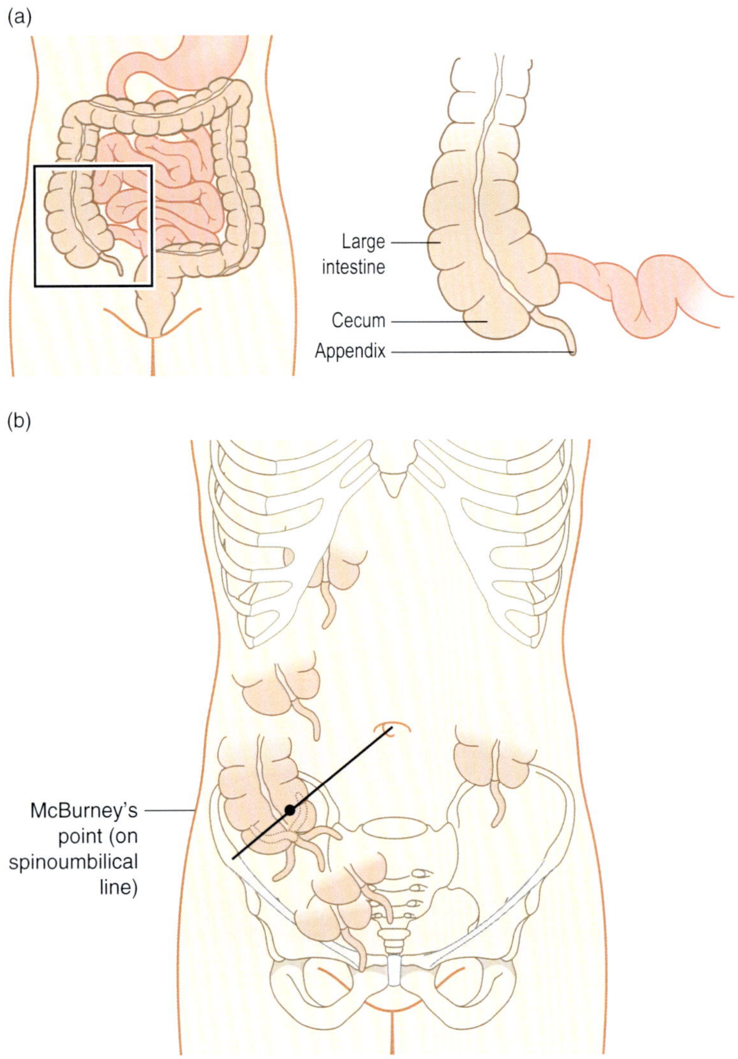

Figure 10.9 **The appendix anatomy**. (a) Illustration of the appendix anatomy. (b) The appendix has various orientations in the body, making it especially challenging to identify. *Artwork created by Emily Evans © Cambridge University Press.*

in both the transverse and longitudinal views, though the appendix may be visible in multiple planes along its course. Older adolescents or obese children may require the increased depth penetration that a lower-frequency (2–5 MHz) curvilinear transducer offers. This improved penetration sacrifices the level of detail necessary for the most accurate observations, so, even in an obese patient, the linear, high-frequency transducer should be utilized whenever possible. Transducer positioning should be in the ideal plane to avoid incorrect measurements giving falsely positive or negative findings depending on the planes of view (Figure 10.10a). When the difference between positive and negative findings is measured in millimeters, correct positioning is imperative.

Patient position and preparation

The patient should be in a supine position. Rotating the patient in an oblique position, with the right hip propped on towels, may be helpful when bowel gas obstructs the view of the appendix. In contrast to other imaging protocols of fixed anatomical structures, finding the appendix does not rely on a single probe position or location. The appendix always originates from the cecum, but the cecum may not always lie in the retrocecal recess. Furthermore, the distal end of the appendix may travel into the pelvis, up to the costal margin, or towards the umbilicus. Inflammation may only appear at the tip, mandating that a complete study not only include identification of a tubular, non-compressible structure, but also that the blind end is visualized. Complete visualization may be difficult for the inexperienced sonographer, and can still be elusive even for the experienced sonographer.

Ultrasound imaging

In an older patient who can localize their abdominal pain to a specific point, the examination may start in this location. If there is poor localization, or if the examiner is unable to visualize the appendix, the examination should then follow a structured approach. In general, the goals of the examination are to identify the cecum and trace its borders to find where the appendix is arising off it, or to sector-search the abdomen for where the appendix is most likely to be found.

(a)

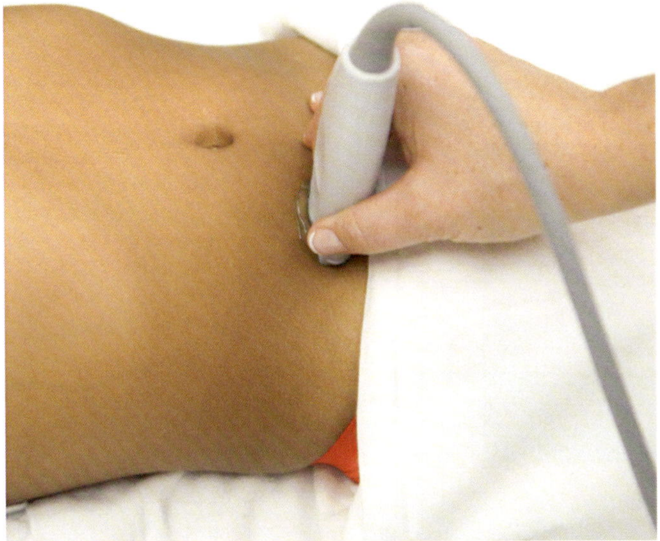

(b)

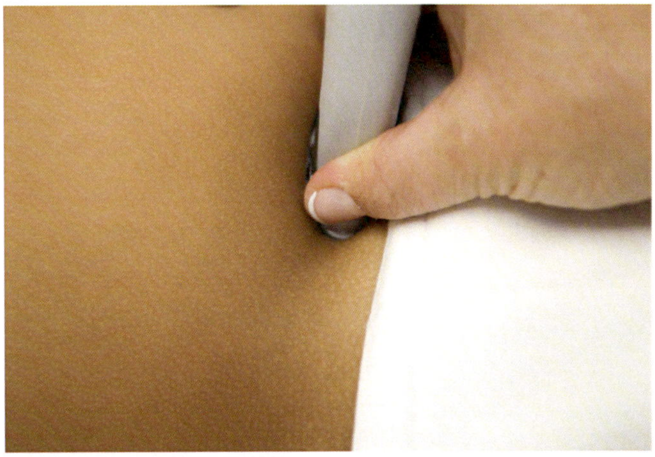

(c)

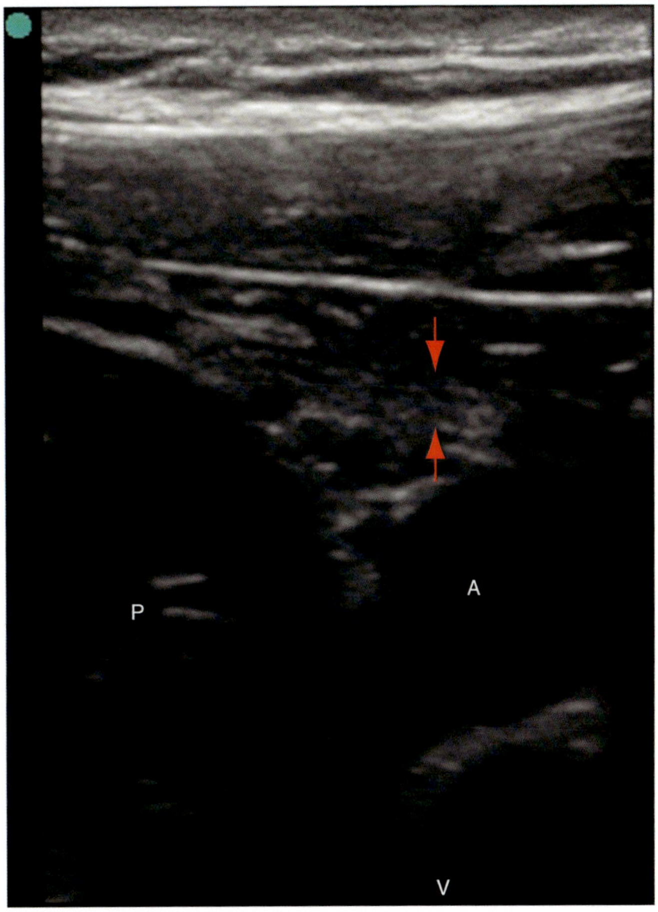

Figure 10.10 The evaluation for appendicitis. (a) Transducer placement at the right lower quadrant, or McBurney's point. (b) Graded compression, or gentle pressure, is utilized to compress the soft tissue and bowel layers. (c) The psoas muscle (P) and iliac artery (A) and vein (V) are used as landmarks to identify the appendix. (d) Illustration depicting graded compression, and its utility in compressing the soft tissue and bowel layers, bringing the appendix into view. *Illustration by Laura Berg, MD*. (e) Longitudinal view of the appendix, prior to graded compression. (f) With graded compression, the appendix is more easily visualized (arrows); A, iliac artery.

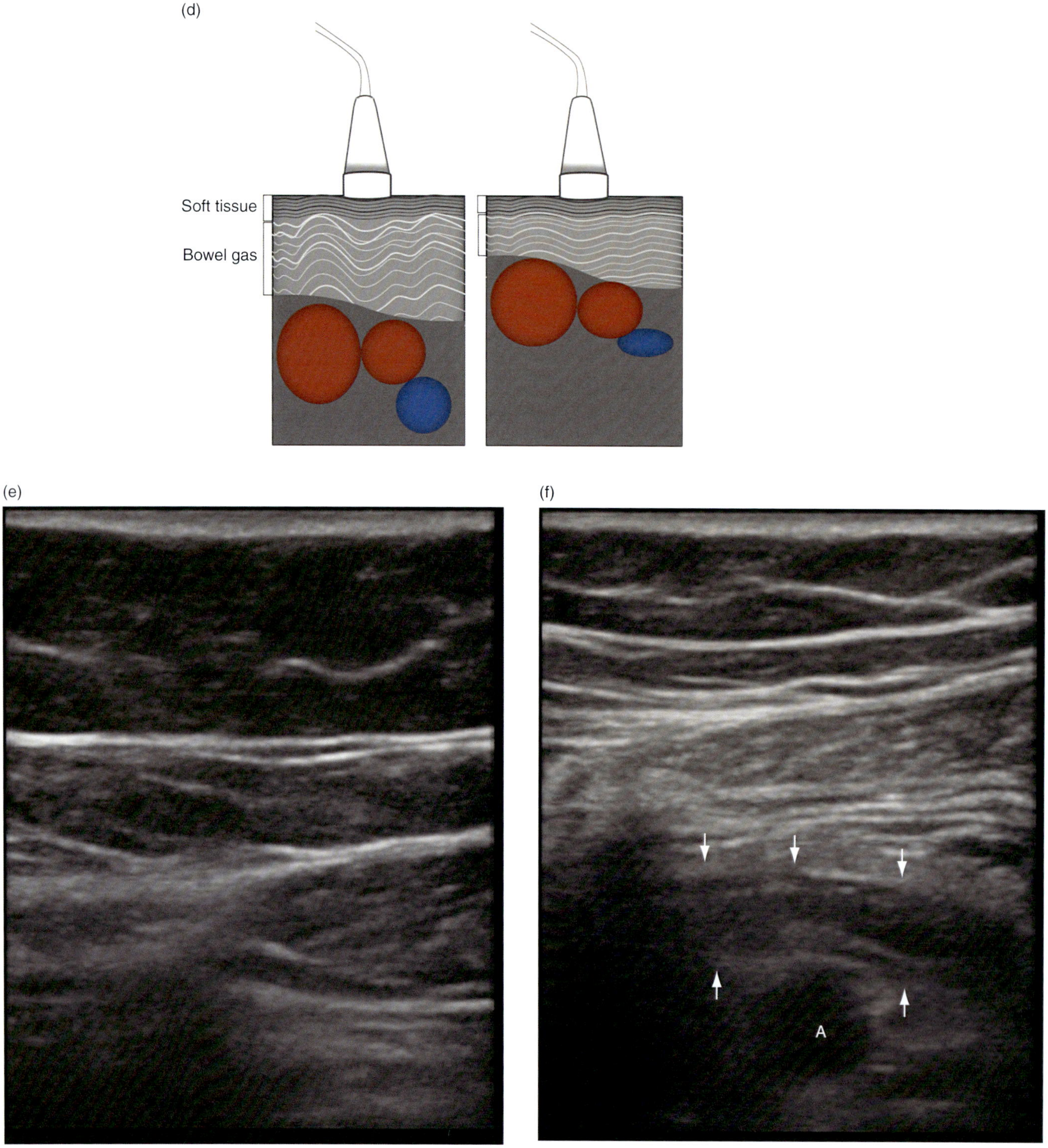

Figure 10.10 (cont.)

In those patients whose pain cannot be localized, the examination should begin with the transducer in the transverse plane at the level of the umbilicus. The graded compression technique delivers a gentle, gradual-to-consistent pressure until the psoas muscle and iliac vessels are visualized (Figure 10.10c). Graded compression uses anterior pressure from the examining hand (Figure 10.10b) to minimize the distance between the transducer and the pathologic process by compressing overlying soft tissues while displacing bowel gas and fluid (Figure 10.10d–f). Trace the lateral border of the aperistaltic ascending colon down the right

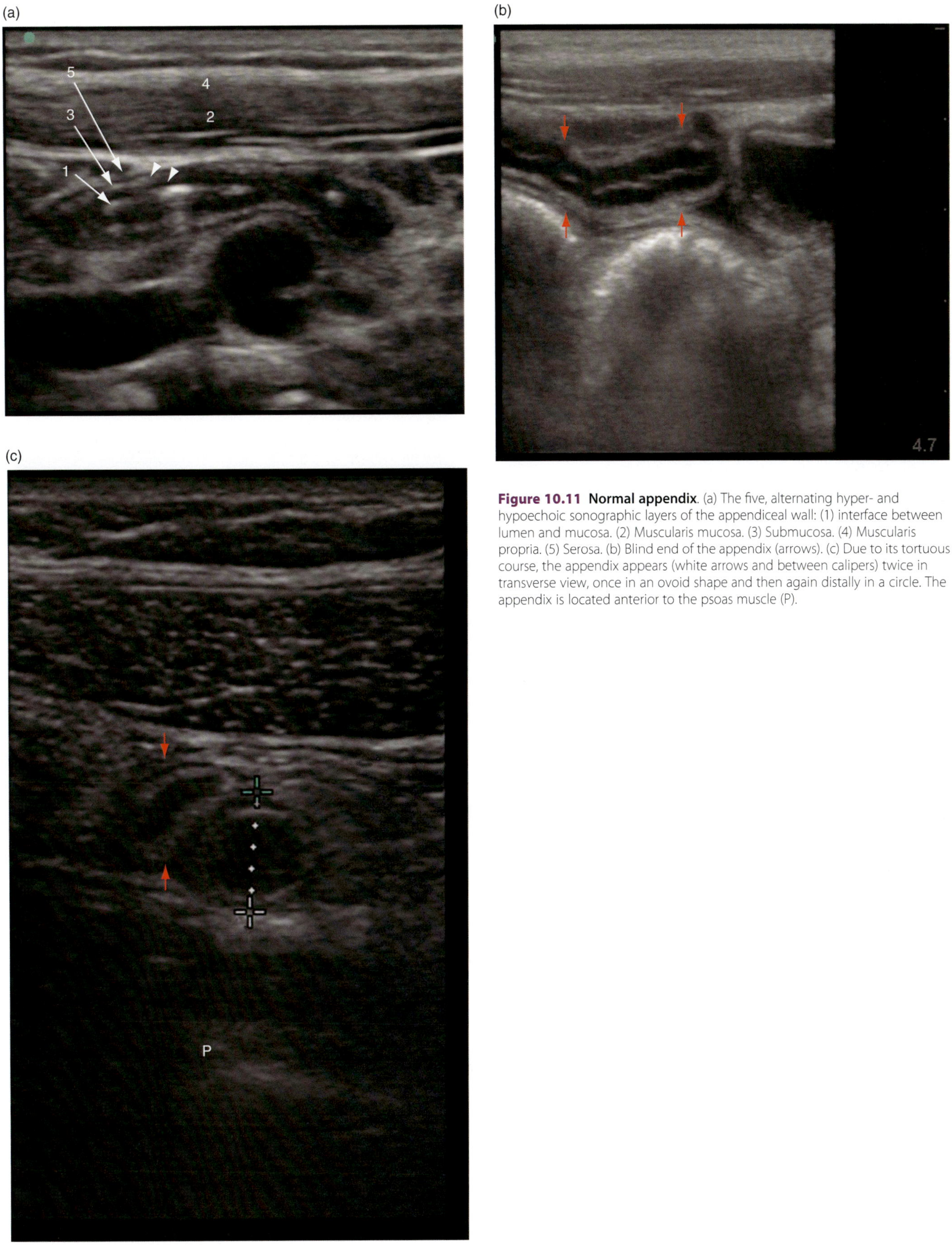

Figure 10.11 Normal appendix. (a) The five, alternating hyper- and hypoechoic sonographic layers of the appendiceal wall: (1) interface between lumen and mucosa. (2) Muscularis mucosa. (3) Submucosa. (4) Muscularis propria. (5) Serosa. (b) Blind end of the appendix (arrows). (c) Due to its tortuous course, the appendix appears (white arrows and between calipers) twice in transverse view, once in an ovoid shape and then again distally in a circle. The appendix is located anterior to the psoas muscle (P).

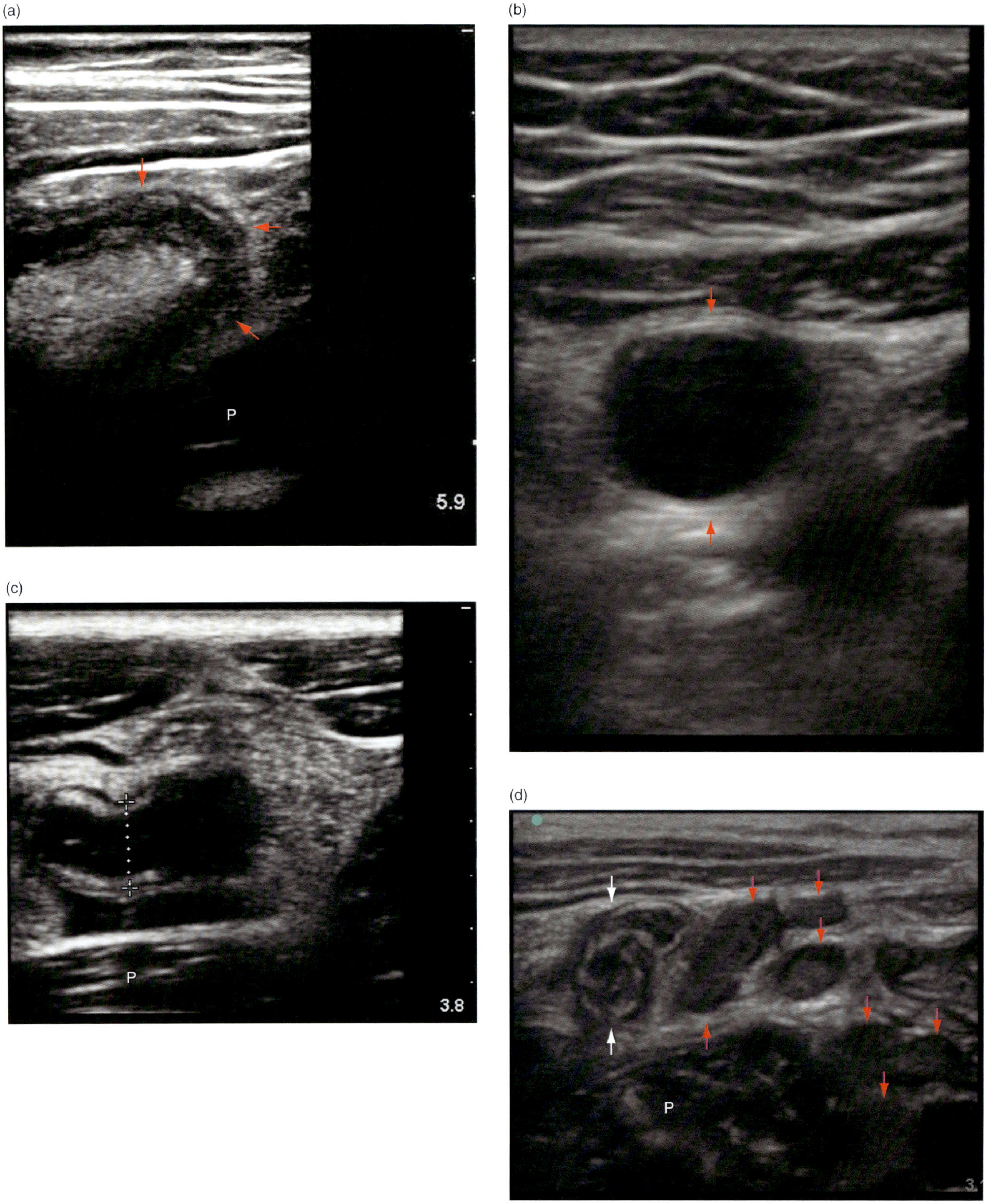

Figure 10.12 **Acute appendicitis**. (a) Longitudinal view of an enlarged appendix (red arrows) over the psoas muscle (P), with associated periappendiceal inflammation. (b) Transverse view of an inflamed appendix measuring 2 cm with no recognizable ultrasonographic wall structure. (c) Longitudinal view of the appendix (between calipers) over the psoas muscle (P). (d) Transverse view of an enlarged appendix curved on itself (white arrows) overlying the psoas muscle (P) and numerous lymph nodes (red arrows).

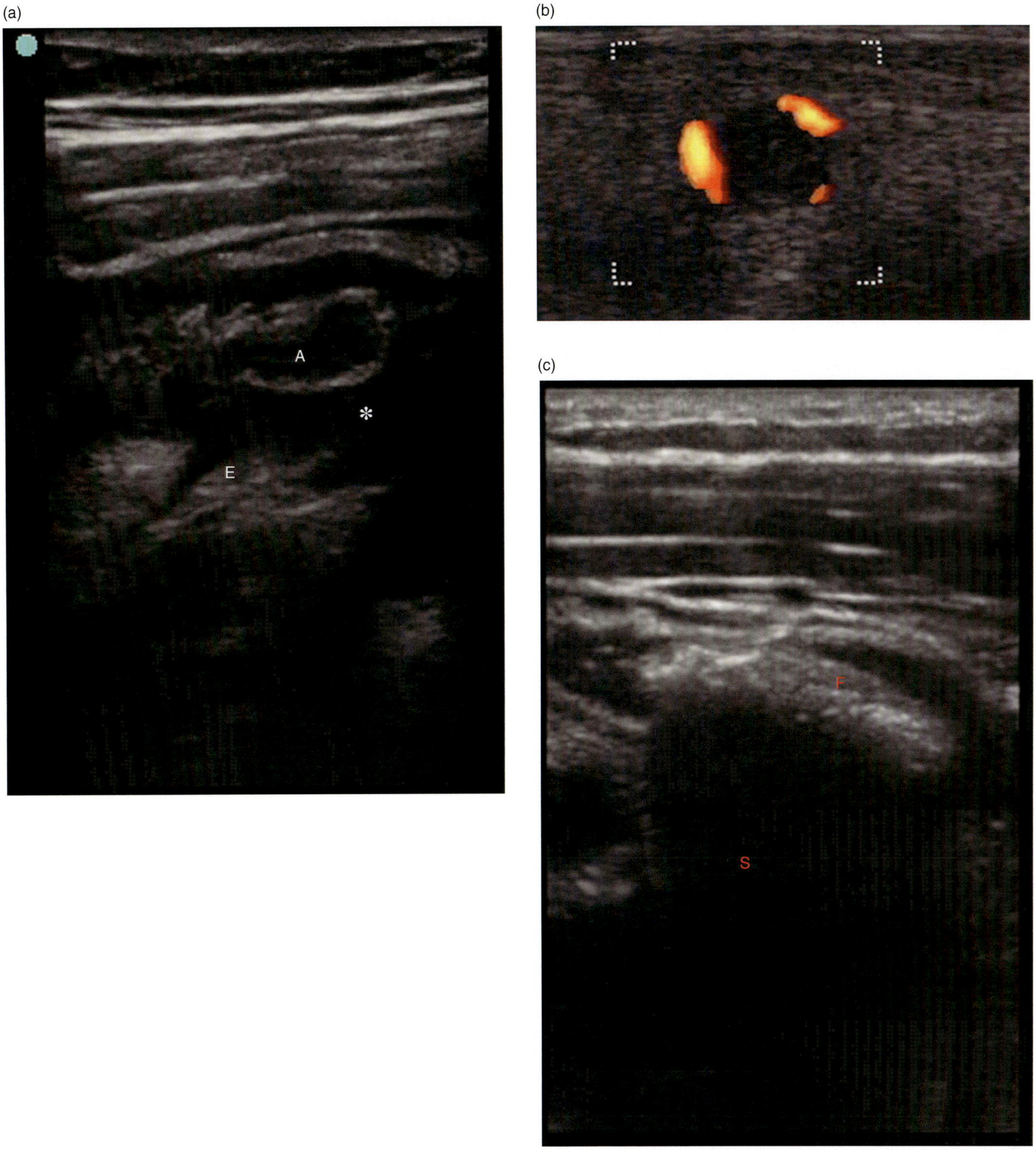

Figure 10.13 **Additional findings in acute appendicitis.** (a) An enlarged, non-compressible appendix (A), with surrounding free fluid (*) and edema (E). (b) Color power Doppler showing increased flow or "ring of fire" surrounding an inflamed appendix. (c) Fecalith (F) in the appendix tip, with associated posterior shadowing (S).

paracolic gutter into the retrocecal fossa, to visualize a potentially laterally oriented appendix and identify the cecum. The appendix originates 1 to 2 cm from the ileocecal valve. From this position, move medially across the cecum and identify the psoas muscle and iliac vessels (Figure 10.10c). The peristalsing terminal ileum lies over these structures, as may the appendix.

The definitive identification of the appendix depends on the size of the appendix if and where it crosses the psoas, and the examiner's ability to adequately compress and displace normal bowel loops. Continued scanning, caudad into the pelvis, medial to the psoas and iliac vessels, then cephalad using the same landmarks, may identify the distal appendix.

The appendix can then be traced to its blind end and back to the cecal origin.

The wall of the appendix is composed of luminal mucosa, submucosa, muscularis, and serosa, which on ultrasound translate to five sonographic layers on longitudinal view (Figure 10.11a,b). A normal appendix appears target-shaped in transverse view, maintaining the characteristic, alternating, hyperechoic–hypoechoic wall pattern (Figure 10.11c). While a normal appendix may measure greater than 6 mm, one can exclude appendicitis with a smaller diameter. The lumen may contain air, fluid, or may be collapsed. Posterior compression may be helpful when a patient does not have a visible appendix, or is obese with a limited field of view. This technique involves application of posterior pressure in combination with anterior graded compression to lift the area of interest into the viewing field. This procedure locates the appendix in 67% of patients where the appendix was not previously visible. It is important to note that, in obese patients, when the appendix is deep, graded compression is unreliable in determining whether the appendix is compressible or not.

A non-compressible, non-peristalsing, tubular structure in the right lower quadrant measuring greater than 6 mm in diameter corresponds to acute appendicitis (Figure 10.12). Additional findings supporting the diagnosis of acute appendicitis include inflamed perienteric fat, free fluid (Figure 10.13a), and hyperemia of the appendiceal wall on color Doppler (Figure 10.13b). In addition, hyperechoic foci with posterior shadowing are seen with an appendicolith (Figure 10.13c).The sonographic appearance of the submucosal layer, ranging from sharply delineated to hazy to absent in advanced disease, has been suggested as a tool to grade acute appendicitis. These findings should be noted on both the transverse and long-axis views. The presence of mesenteric lymph nodes can be noted in both mesenteric adenitis and acute appendicitis. Perforation should be suspected when a focal or loculated fluid collection is visualized even in the absence of direct visualization of the appendix itself (Figure 10.14). In women, an appendix that enters the true pelvis may only be visualized by transvaginal sonography; however, definitive identification of the cecal origin of the appendix is unlikely. Evidence of a perforated appendix, such as free fluid or an abscess, may be indistinguishable from other manifestations of pelvic inflammatory disease.

Ultrasound imaging: measurements

In order to diagnose appendicitis, the appendix must measure **greater than 6 mm** in diameter, regardless of the patient's age and body habitus. However, in some circumstances, a patient may have an entirely normal appendix that measures greater than 6 mm in diameter, but lacks secondary signs of inflammation corresponding to acute appendicitis. While a diameter of less than 6 mm effectively rules out acute appendicitis, a normal appendix may measure greater than 6 mm. The absence of inflammation in a patient with low probability helps differentiate a larger than normal appendix from acute appendicitis.

Scanning tips

Pitfalls

- A false-positive diagnosis of acute appendicitis often occurs when a normal appendix greater than 6 mm in diameter is visualized.
- Secondary causes of periappendiceal inflammation which may be mistaken for acute appendicitis include inflammatory bowel disease or pelvic inflammatory disease.
- False-negative studies arise primarily from the non-visualization of the appendix secondary to obesity, a retrocecal appendix position, or an atypical appendix position.
- In cases of perforated appendicitis, the resultant peritonitis and ileus may not allow for adequate compression and displacement of overlying bowel.
- Inflammation isolated to the appendiceal tip may lead to a false-negative study if a more proximal segment is misidentified as the tip and the remaining length is not interrogated. Thus, additional investigation should be pursued when complete visualization is unsuccessful in patients with a high index of clinical suspicion.
- Be careful in utilizing both formal and point-of-care ultrasonography to rule out appendicitis. A normal appendix must be entirely visualized in order to consider ruling out appendicitis.

Tips to improve scanning

- ✓ In a patient already presenting with acute abdominal pain, consider waiting for adequate analgesia prior to attempting the examination, especially in younger children.
- ✓ The examination can be expedited by asking the patient to point to the area of maximal tenderness, then starting the investigation from this position.
- ✓ Moving the patient in an oblique positioning (with the right hip upwards, propped on towels) may allow for improved visualization of the appendix.
- ✓ Be sure to visualize the entire appendix including the tip, in both transverse and long-axes.
- ✓ While graded compression is a mandatory part of the examination, sometimes releasing pressure helps to differentiate compressed small bowel from what was thought to be the appendix.
- ✓ In patients where the appendix cannot be visualized, posterior compression along with anterior graded compression may bring the appendix into view.
- ✓ For a retrocecal appendix, it may be helpful to scan on the right lateral side of the abdomen.

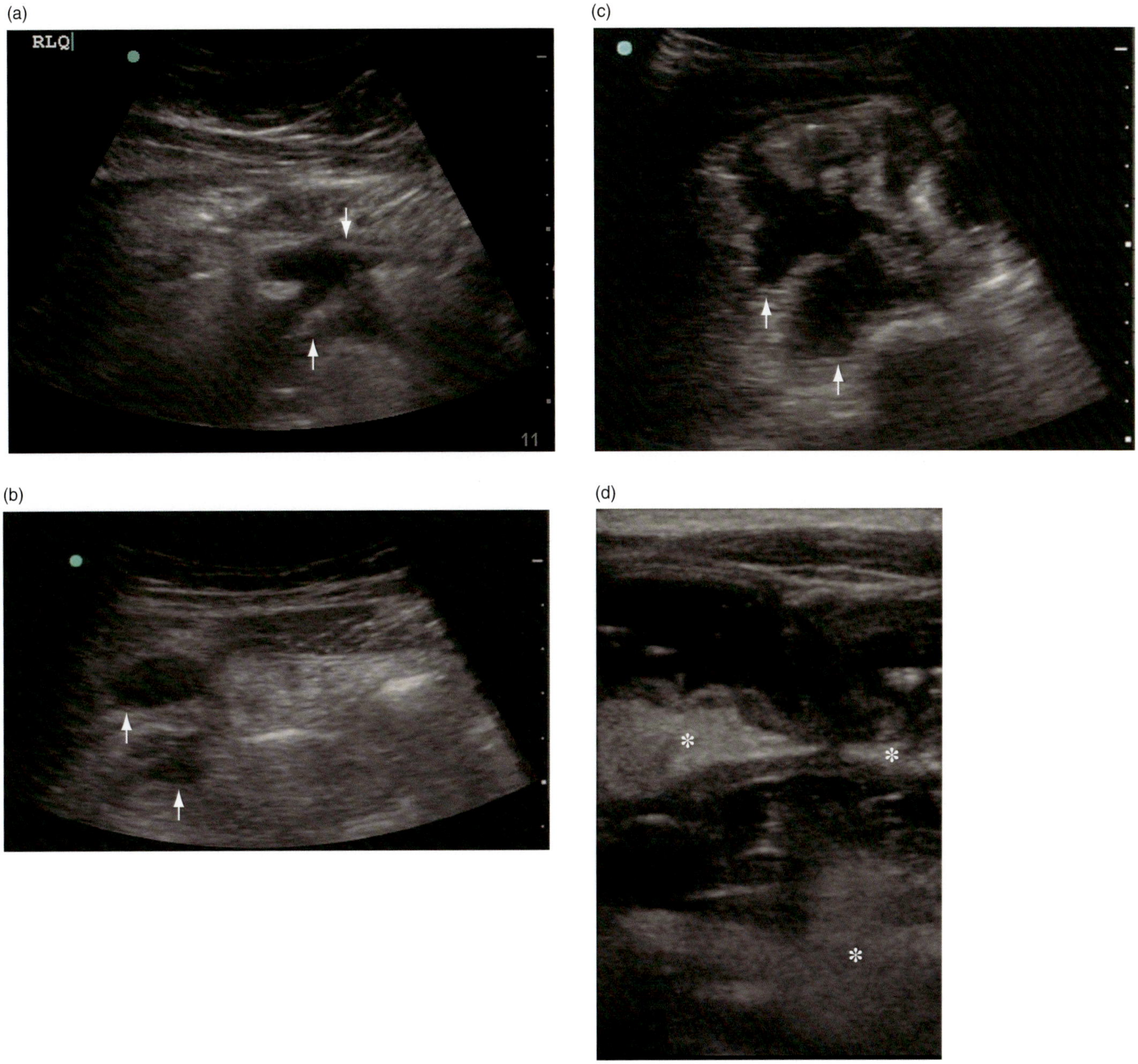

Figure 10.14 Ruptured appendicitis. (a–c) Signs of ruptured appendicitis without direct visualization of an appendix. Transverse views are obtained with the low-frequency transducer, in order to obtain a greater field of view. All with noted fluid collections (arrows) suggesting perforations. (d) Small intestinal ileus with wall thickening and hyperechoic mesenteric inflammation (*).

PYLORIC STENOSIS

Background

Hypertrophic pyloric stenosis (HPS) is the most common cause of intestinal obstruction in infants. An overgrowth of the muscle around the pyloric channel causes a progressive gastric outlet obstruction. It is seen in 3 / 1000 live births, and males, particularly first born, are affected five times more often than females. Patients typically present during the initial two to six weeks of life, with a progressively worsening non-bilious emesis that occurs after each feeding, which eventually becomes "projectile." The presence of a palpable "olive" (the hypertrophied pylorus) is diagnostic for the condition, but it is often difficult to palpate without first decompressing the stomach with a nasogastric tube. Additionally, a peristaltic wave may be seen on examination in advanced cases (Figure 10.16). Laboratory abnormalities of a hypochloremic, hypokalemic metabolic alkalosis, are pathognomonic for the disorder. To date, there is no absolute etiology for the development of pyloric stenosis, though many have been postulated. In 1912, Ramstedt performed the first successful pyloromyotomy, which, a century later, continues as the standard surgical treatment. Surgical techniques have advanced though, from open to laparoscopic approaches, both involving minimal morbidity with curative results.

Radiologists have been using ultrasound to diagnosis HPS since 1977, when it replaced the upper gastrointestinal (UGI) barium study as the gold-standard diagnostic test. While the typical history has not changed, the physical examination findings have been discovered less frequently and the classic laboratory findings rarely, with the availability of early ultrasound investigation. Ultrasound has been shown to have a sensitivity and specificity near 100%, making it the ideal screening test. The ultrasound examination is straightforward, and recent literature has described both the emergency physician and resident surgeon's ability to accurately diagnose HPS by point-of-care ultrasonography. Most recently, Sivitz *et al.* investigated pediatric emergency physician-performed sonography for pyloric stenosis, and found a sensitivity and specificity both of 100%. There were also no differences found between emergency physician-performed and radiologist-performed measurements of the pylorus in these patients. Further research needs to be performed in order to evaluate the accuracy of emergency physicians' ability to detect pyloric stenosis at the bedside.

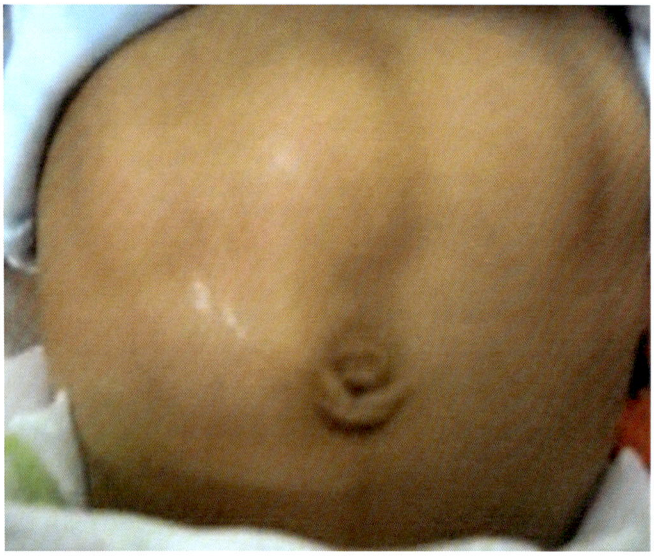

Figure 10.15 Peristaltic wave seen with pyloric stenosis.

Anatomy

When evaluating for pyloric stenosis, it is important to recognize the structures of the stomach. In particular, these are the antrum, the greater and lesser curvature of the stomach, and the pylorus. The pyloric muscle is in continuity with the gastric wall and arises to the right of midline (Figure 10.16).

Technique

Point-of-care questions

1. Can the pylorus be identified?
2. Does the pylorus measure **greater than 11 mm × 3 mm × 14 mm**?
3. Is pyloric stenosis present?

Transducer selection and orientation

In general, sonography of the abdomen for pyloric stenosis, intussusception, and appendicitis are all best performed using a high-frequency (5–10 MHz), linear transducer. The investigation should start with an anterior approach, starting just below the xiphoid process in a transverse view. The indicator should initially be oriented towards the patient's right side (Figure 10.17a).

Patient position and preparation

The patient should be in a supine position. It is common for infants to be irritable and crying. It may be helpful to place the infant in their parents' lap for comfort, or to use sucrose water

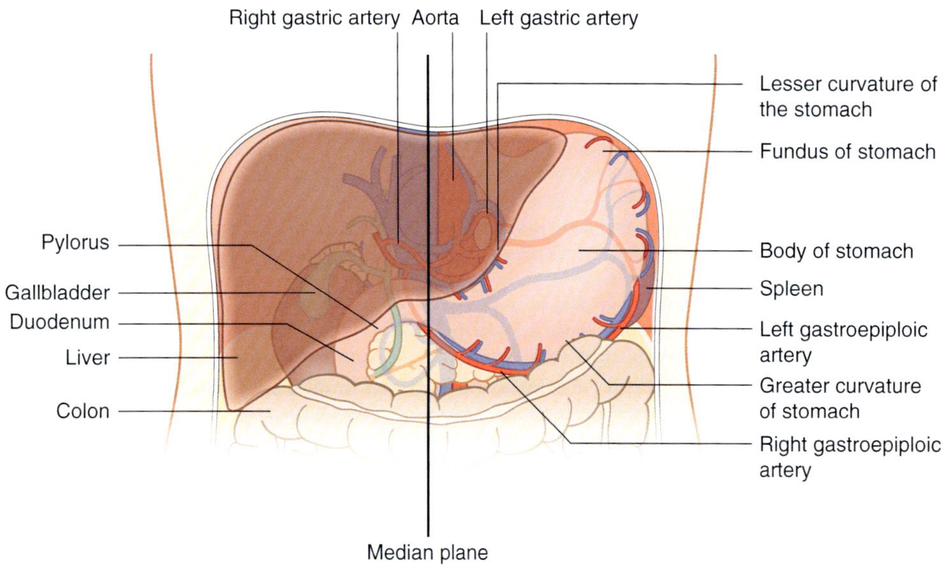

Figure 10.16 Anatomy of the stomach. Important structures are the body of the stomach, the pylorus, and the duodenum. *Artwork created by Emily Evans © Cambridge University Press.*

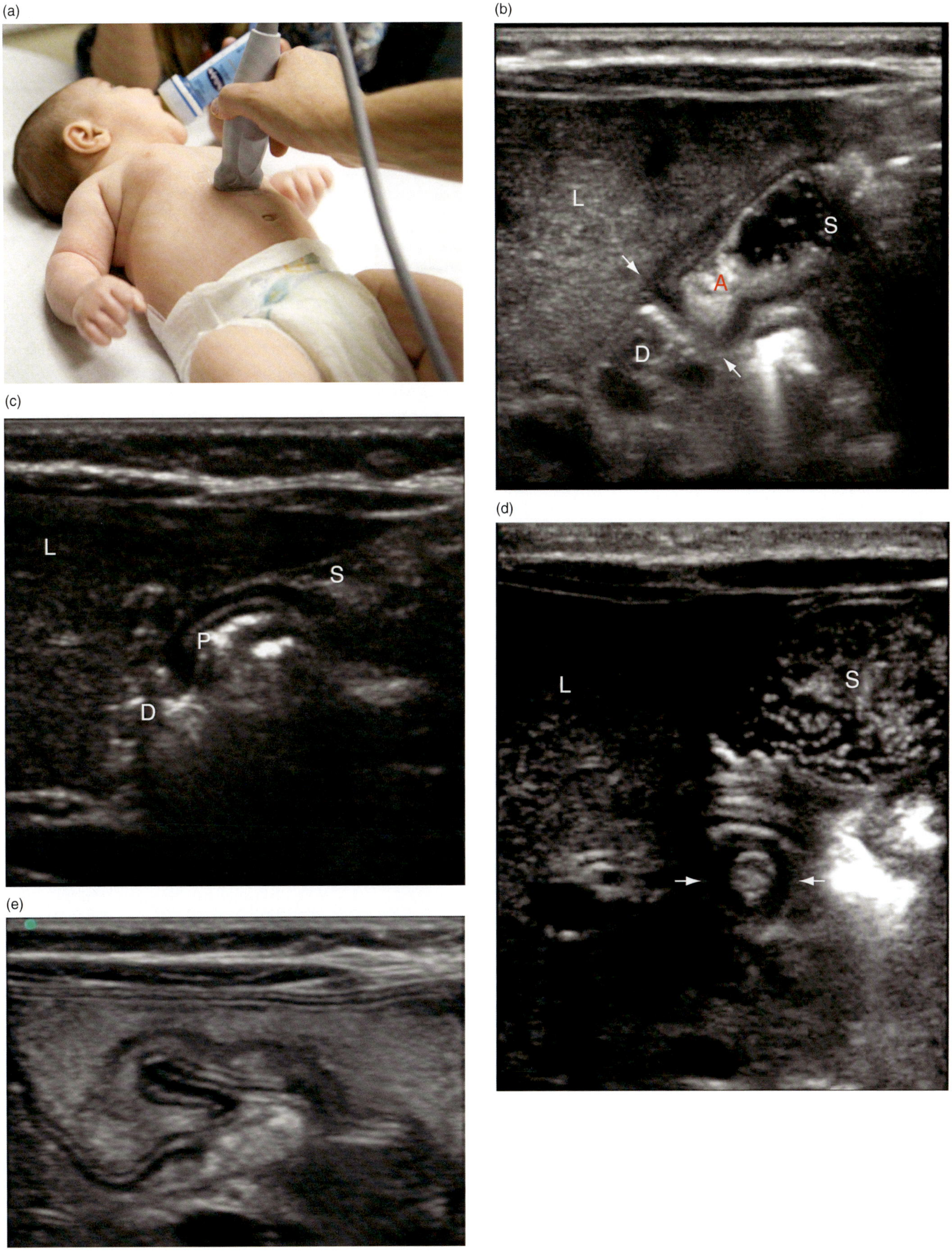

Figure 10.17 The evaluation for pyloric stenosis. (a) Transducer placement at the subxiphoid location, with the indicator towards the patient's right side. It is often helpful to give the baby Pedialyte® and to roll the baby slightly towards a right lateral decubitus position, in order to preferentially fill the pyloric antrum with gastric fluid. (b) Ultrasound image, the long-axis view of the gastric outlet. The stomach (S) and pyloric antrum (A) run beneath the edge of the liver (L). The pyloric muscle terminates at the pyloric sphincter (white arrows) before the beginning of the duodenum (D). (c) Long-axis view of pyloric canal (P). When air passes through, only the anterior wall is visible as secondary to gas shadowing. (d) Transverse view of the pylorus (arrows). Adjacent structures are the liver (L) and stomach (S). (e) Posteriorly pointing pylorus.

solution on a pacifier (i.e. Sweet-Ease™). In addition, administering a clear fluid such as Pedialyte® may be used to fill the stomach, and serve as an acoustic window to better visualize the pylorus.

Ultrasound imaging

The pyloric muscle is in continuity with the gastric wall and arises to the right of midline. Using the liver as a sonographic window, the gastric wall is identified overlying the gas- or fluid-filled stomach. The echogenicity of the gastric contents is variable, or even mixed, depending on the type of liquid the infant has recently ingested. Once the gastric wall has been identified, it is then traced caudally to the right of midline, along the lesser curvature of the stomach, until it meets the antrum (Figure 10.17b). The pylorus is classically shown arising off the stomach in a horizontal plane, but, in cases of over distention, it may be directed in a more posterior position (Figure 10.17e). In cross-section, the muscle appears as a "target" shape with the pylorus muscle uniformly surrounding the hyperechoic, directly opposed layers of mucosa (Figure 10.17d).

A normal pylorus may be observed passing gastric contents through the pyloric canal with gastric peristalsis, or changing in size and thickness with pylorospasm (Figure 10.18a). These observations may require viewing the pylorus for an extended period of time to visualize gastric peristalsis or relaxation from pylorospasm (Figure 10.18b). Neither of these findings is seen with pyloric stenosis. Pyloric stenosis has a markedly thickened muscular wall, and an elongated pyloric channel (Figure 10.19). In addition to thickened walls and elongated channel, the "antral nipple sign" (Figure 10.20) may be visualized, which represents prolapsed, hypertrophied pyloric mucosa protruding into the gastric antrum. Finally, the failure of gastric contents to pass through the pyloric channel can be visualized on real-time ultrasound imaging.

Ultrasound imaging: measurements

The diagnostic measurements for hypertrophic pyloric stenosis include the hypoechoic pyloric muscle diameter and pyloric channel length. The pyloric muscle diameter should be measured in both the transverse and longitudinal views, with careful attention to making sure the view is midline or perpendicular to the respective plane of view (Figure 10.21). A pyloric muscle diameter measurement of greater than **3 mm** is considered to be abnormal (Figure 10.22). In a normal patient, the channel length may be more difficult to measure and a less reliable measurement than the more easily appreciated pyloric muscle diameter. A channel length of greater than **14 mm** is considered to be abnormal (Table 10.1). It is important to note that premature or small infants may have smaller measurements, and that a falsely thickened and elongated pylorus may be seen with pylorospasm. Generally, however, pylorospasm does not cause diameters to be larger than 2–3 mm.

(a) (b)

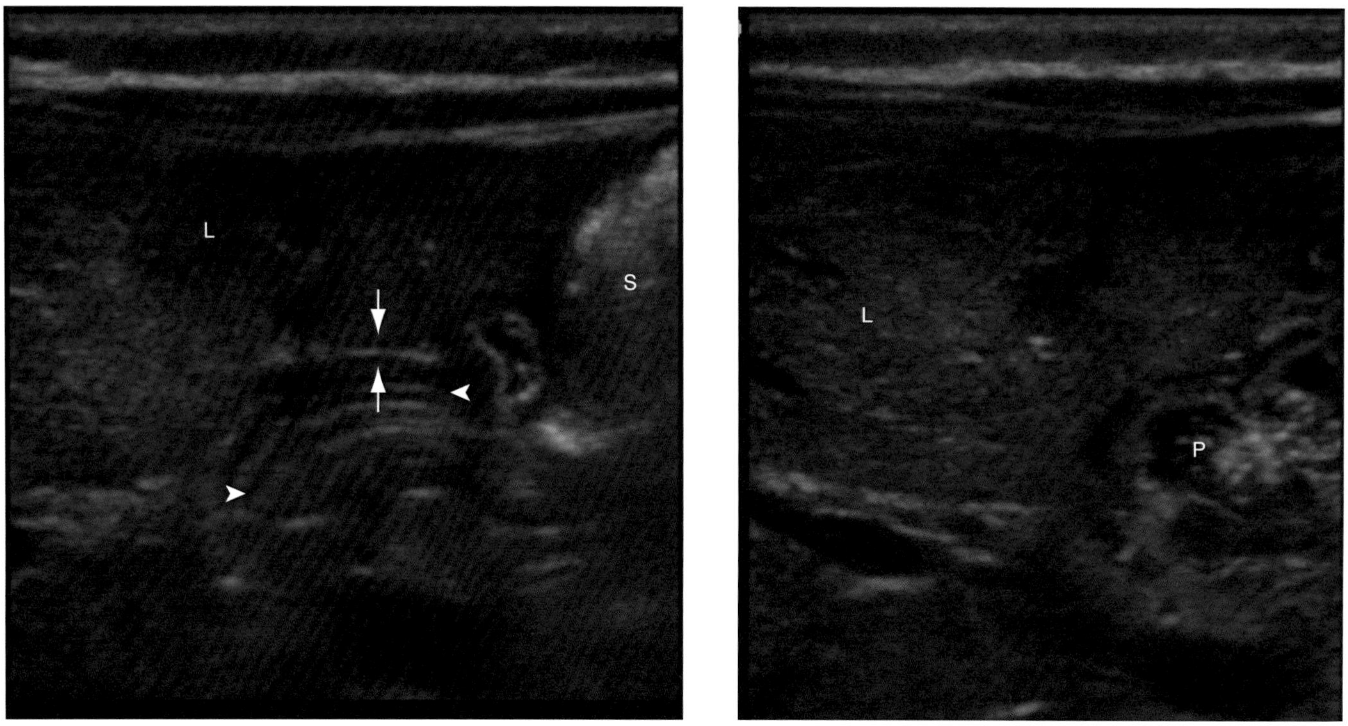

Figure 10.18 Pylorospasm. (a) Pyloric muscle measuring 25 mm (arrow heads) during pylorospasm. Note that the channel appears long, but the muscle wall (arrows) is not thickened. Surrounding structures are the liver (L) and stomach (S). (b) View of the same patient 30 seconds later with decreased pyloric wall thickness and fluid and air passing through the open pyloric channel. Note the pylorus (P) is adjacent to the liver (L).

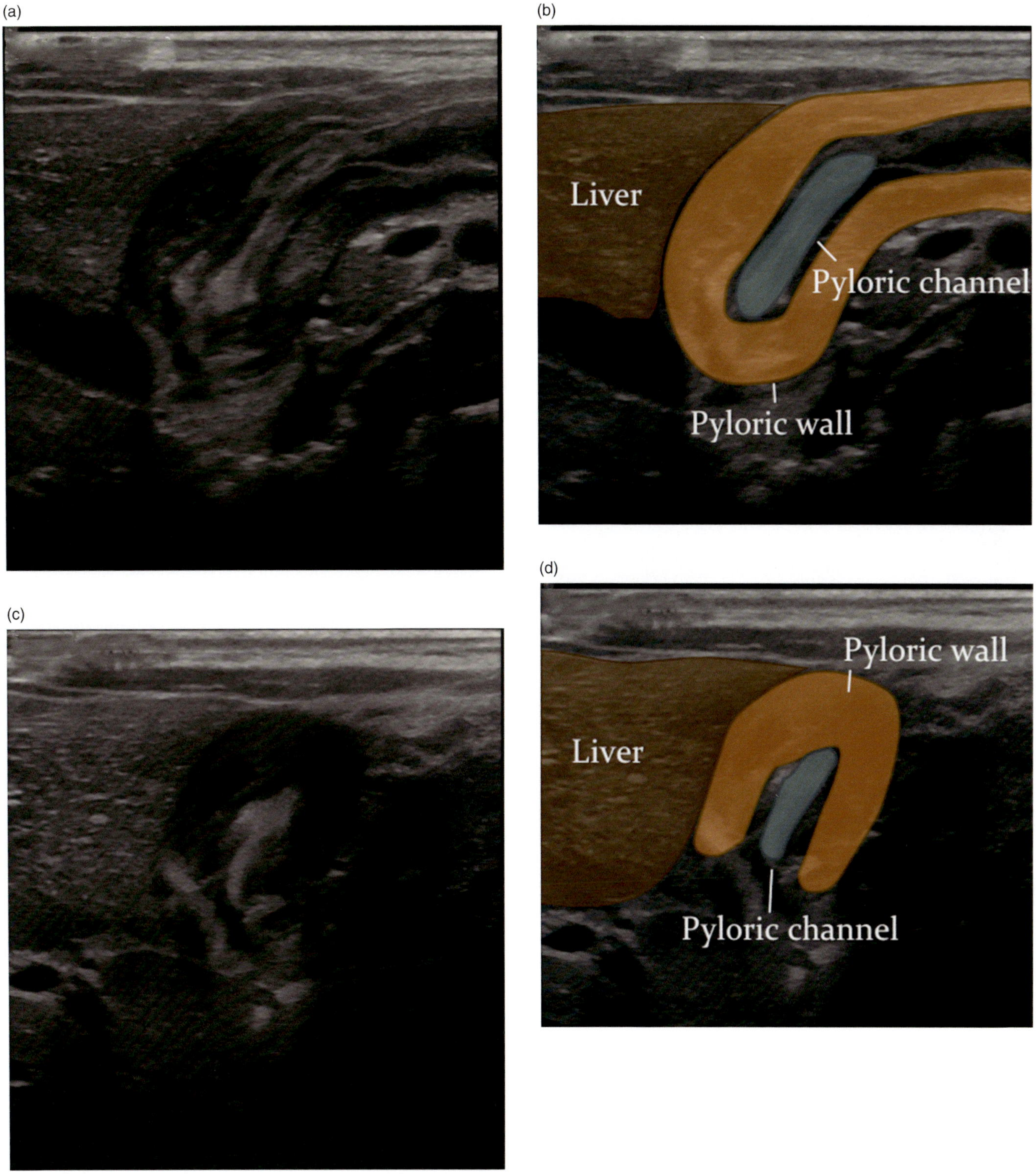

Figure 10.19 **Pyloric stenosis**. (a) In the longitudinal view, the pyloric channel is elongated and the muscle wall is hypertrophied. (b) Illustration depicting the pyloric channel and muscle wall. This is most commonly located adjacent to the liver. (c) Transverse view of the hypertrophied pylorus. (d) The transverse view is referred to as the "target" sign. *Illustrations by Laura Berg, MD.*

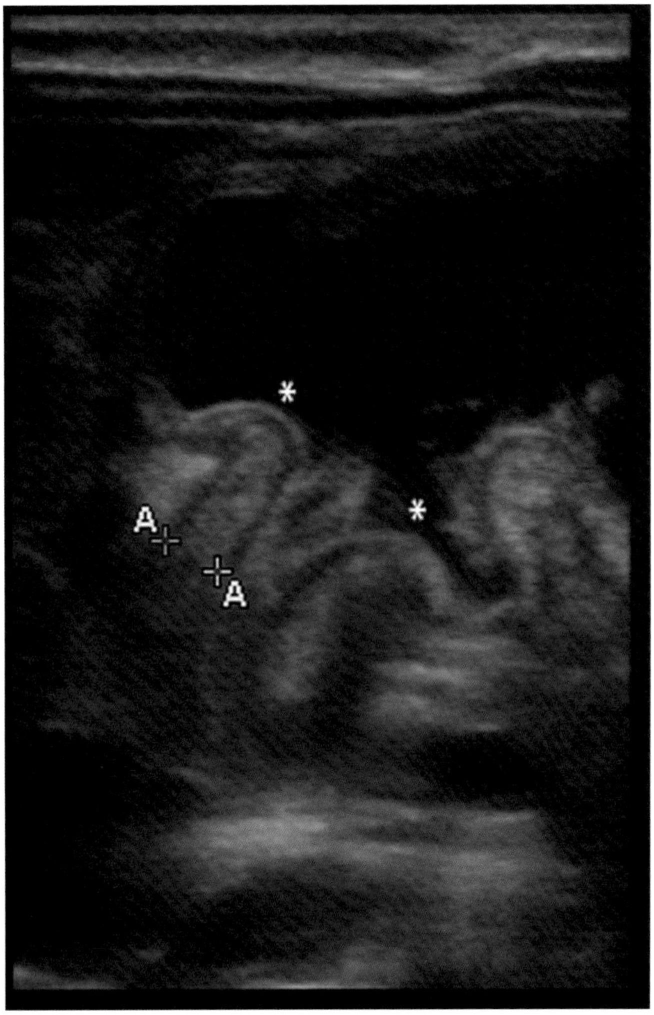

Figure 10.20 Pyloric stenosis: "antral nipple" sign. The "antral nipple" sign (*) represents prolapsed, hypertrophied pyloric mucosa protruding into the gastric antrum.

Scanning tips

Pitfalls

- False-positive findings may occur with views that produce erroneously enlarged muscle widths.
- Not waiting long enough during pylorospasm may also lead to a false-positive examination. However, pylorospasm should still not produce measurements greater than 3 mm (Figure 10.18).
- False-negative findings may arise from misidentifying the small bowel or an inflamed gastric wall instead of the pyloric channel. This may occur with gastritis or other inflammatory processes, or from an over-distended stomach or a posteriorly displaced pylorus.
- The muscle surrounding the pyloric channel may appear hyperechoic as opposed to hypoechoic when viewed perpendicularly, due to anisotropy. This effect is seen at the 12 and 6 o'clock positions on cross-sectional imaging,

Table 10.1 Sonographic pylorus measurements required for the diagnosis of pyloric stenosis.

Pylorus	Measurement (mm)
Diameter	>11
Muscle thickness	>3
Canal length	>14

sparing the 3 and 9 o'clock views (Figure 10.23). On longitudinal views, this effect may make identification and differentiation of the anterior and posterior wall borders difficult, though with modern equipment this should not preclude accurate measurements.

Tips to improve scanning

- ✓ Taking time to enhance patient comfort is crucial to obtaining an adequate scan. This can be attained through proper positioning in the parents' lap, warmed gel, sucrose solution on a pacifier, and patience.
- ✓ In the case of gaseous distention, the administration of a clear fluid such as Pedialyte® can help to fill up the stomach with a sonographic medium to create a better acoustic window.
- ✓ To improve visualization, the infant can be turned to a right anterior oblique position to preferentially fill the antrum with gastric contents.
- ✓ In the case of stomach over-distention with fluid, visualization can be obtained by preferentially positioning the patient in a left posterior oblique position.
- ✓ While a diameter measurement of less than 3 mm rules out HPS at that moment, it is an evolving process and should warrant re-examination at a later date if typical symptoms persist.

Cases

1. A one-year-old, previously healthy child presents with bouts of screaming and drawing up his legs that last 5–10 minutes, followed by periods of somnolence. He has also had two episodes of non-bloody, non-bilious emesis. Upon arrival to the emergency department, the child appears comfortable, but refuses to drink. On physical examination, the vital signs are normal for age, and, while the abdomen feels soft, there is a palpable mass in the right upper quadrant. His stool guaiac is positive. A plain radiograph with upright and decubitus views shows no signs of obstruction or free air. It is unclear whether air completely fills the ascending colon. On point-of-care ultrasonography, a layered, target-shaped mass is visualized, extending from the cecum to the hepatic flexure (Figure 10.24). A confirmatory radiologist-performed ultrasound finds trapped fluid, outer wall thickening, and decreased blood flow to the bowel wall. An air contrast enema study is attempted, but cannot completely reduce the

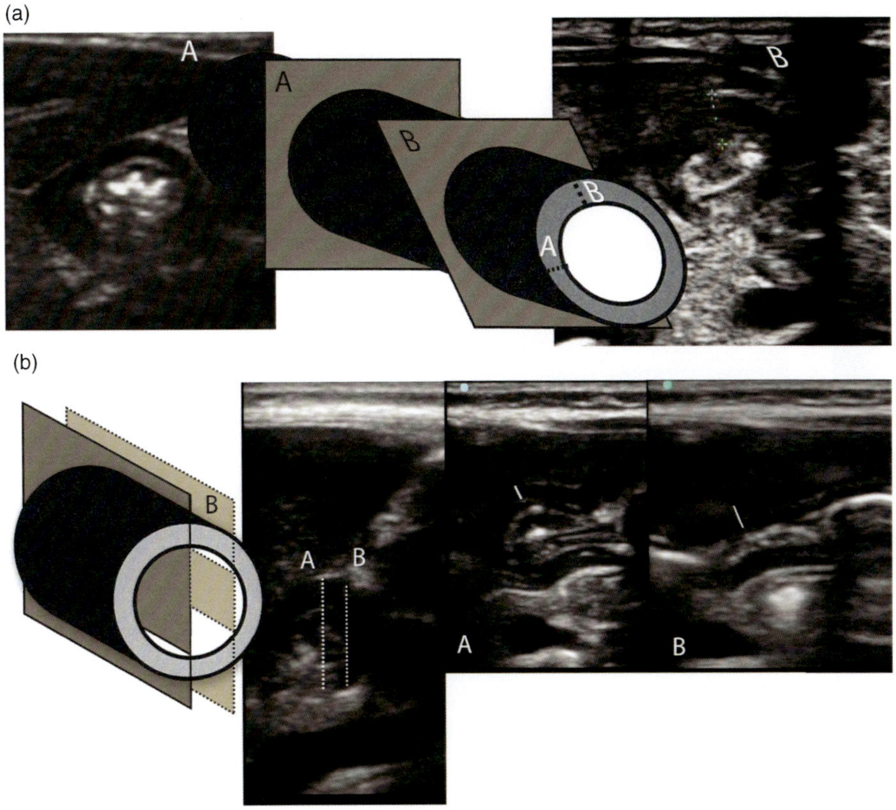

Figure 10.21 Measurements in pyloric stenosis. (a) Two different transverse viewing angles are compared. The view in A is perfectly perpendicular with bowel wall (gray circle) diameters equal on all sides. In B, this tangential view produces an apparent wall diameter at the 12 and 6 o'clock positions that is falsely wider than at the 3 and 9 o'clock positions. The bowel diameter measured through line B would also be falsely enlarged compared to the diameter drawn through line A. (b) This is shown in the longitudinal view. Through plane A, a true wall and bowel diameter are measured. Through plane B the bowel diameter would appear falsely narrower, while the wall diameters would appear wider. *Illustrations by Adam Sivitz, MD.*

intussusception. The child's vital signs are stable and the patient remains in the emergency department waiting for admission. After four hours, a second attempt is made at enema reduction with similarly unsuccessful results. The pediatric surgeons take the child to the operating room, where an ileocolic intussusception is manually reduced without requiring any bowel resection.

This case describes the classic, though uncommon, triad of vomiting, colicky abdominal pain, and a palpable mass in the right upper quadrant seen with ileocolic intussusception. In this case, the child had sonographic characteristics that have been suggested to predict non-operative failure, with surrounding fluid and decreased blood flow to the bowel wall. If the patient is clinically stable, a repeat air or contrast enema reduction can still be attempted, even with these findings. In a clinically unstable patient, or in the presence of free air, enema reduction is contraindicated. It is also important to remember that 10% of patients will have recurrence of intussusception, with 50% having the event after hospital discharge. A return of any characteristic sign or symptom should make the treating clinician highly suspicious for a re-intussusception.

2. A four-year-old girl presents with a three-day history of vomiting and diarrhea, with recent worsening of the abdominal pain. Her pediatrician saw her two days ago and diagnosed her with a "stomach virus." On presentation, she appears uncomfortable and has abdominal distention on examination. She cries during the entire examination, and there is no identifiable point of maximal tenderness. While in the emergency department, she develops a fever and vomits during attempts at oral hydration. Therefore, intravenous fluids are started and laboratory studies are drawn. After a dose of morphine is given, a focused point-of-care ultrasound of the right lower quadrant is performed. Free fluid and diffusely dilated bowel loops are noted on graded compression examination, but the appendix cannot be visualized. Compression of overlying bowel to locate the psoas muscle and iliac vessels is performed, but is notably difficult. A formal radiology ultrasound study is performed, noting free fluid. The appendix is identified, measuring 5.6 mm in diameter, but the appendix tip cannot be identified (Figure 10.25). Therefore, acute appendicitis cannot be ruled out. At the request of the surgical consultant, a CT with oral and intravenous contrast is performed. The child has a ruptured appendicitis and is taken to the operating room.

This case highlights both the difficulty of definitive visualization by ultrasound, and the high frequency of perforation in young children with acute appendicitis. The complete visualization of the appendix necessitates localizing the blind end of the appendix, which may be the only site of inflammation. The failure to visualize the entire appendix results in an equivocal study. With an equivocal ultrasound and if clinical suspicion remains high, further imaging and surgical consultation should be considered. Non-visualization of the appendix on ultrasound should only be considered a definitively negative study when done by an experienced radiologist, in a patient

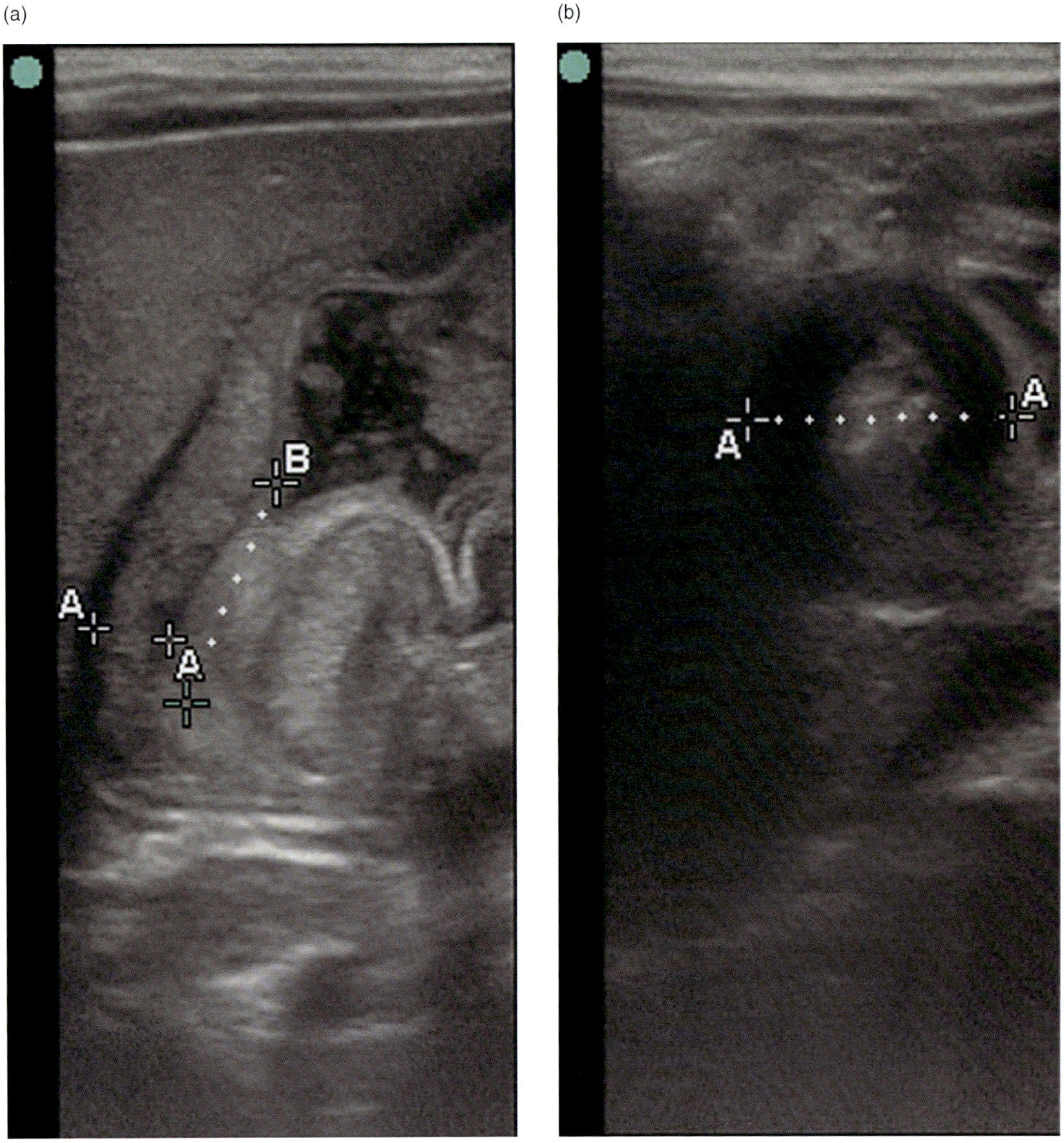

Figure 10.22 Measurements in pyloric stenosis. (a) In the long-axis the pyloric channel length and the muscle layer should be measured. (b) Pylorus visualized in the transverse view, with the diameter being measured.

with a low probability of disease. In these select cases, the patient may be discharged home with instructions to return for an abdominal CT if clinical conditions worsen. Alternatively, the patient may be admitted for observation. In the case above, the patient is at high risk for complications of peritonitis and delay is not indicated.

3. An obese 16-year-old boy presents with constant abdominal pain for one day. He has experienced anorexia, and has vomited twice. He reports periumbilical pain, but on examination he has distinct right lower quadrant tenderness to palpation. After requesting a pediatric surgery consultation, an intravenous line is started, laboratory studies are drawn, and morphine is given. A point-of-care ultrasound reveals the appendix as an aperistaltic, non-compressible, tubular structure originating from the cecum. The appendix measures 1 cm in diameter, and there is diffuse periappendiceal inflammation (Figure 10.26). The surgeon reviews the history, examines the patient, and reviews the point-of-care ultrasound. A decision is made to take the boy to the operating room. An acutely inflamed, non-perforated appendix is removed and the patient is discharged the day after surgery.

This case highlights the classic history associated with acute appendicitis. In unequivocal cases, formal imaging studies should be obtained only if requested by the surgical consultant. Waiting hours for a CT with oral contrast may only add unnecessary delay. It may also expose the patient to unnecessary ionizing radiation. The decisions for imaging should be arranged in consultation with both radiology and surgery. While this patient was obese and may not be considered an optimal candidate for ultrasonography, a point-of-care examination can quickly determine whether the appendix

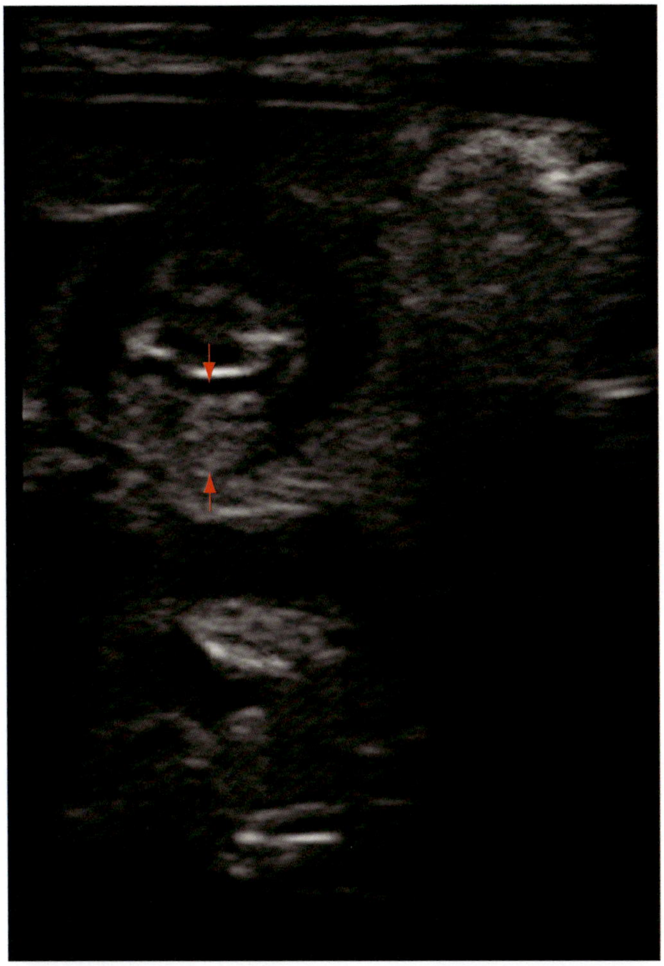

Figure 10.23 Anisotropic effect. A patient with pyloric stenosis that is posteriorly directed. In the transverse view, the thickened muscle wall (arrows) appears hyperechoic due to anisotropic effect from perpendicular orientation to the ultrasound beam, and this is most prominent at the 6 o'clock positions.

can be readily visualized, and whether additional imaging is warranted.

4. A 40-day-old female infant presents with a one-week history of non-bilious, non-bloody vomiting only after formula feeding. The mother is both breast and bottle-feeding since the child always seems hungry. There was no history of reflux prior to the introduction of cow-milk-based formula two weeks earlier. The patient was seen five days before at another emergency department, and diagnosed with "reflux." Since that time, she has lost 300 g in weight. On examination the vitals are normal for age, and the abdomen is non-tender but scaphoid in appearance. Stool guaiac is negative. A point-of-care ultrasound is performed, which shows a 4 mm pyloric muscle diameter and channel length of 2 cm, without the passage of gastric contents through the pyloric canal throughout the examination (Figure 10.27). The pediatric surgery service is consulted and the patient undergoes an uneventful pyloromyotomy.

   This case reflects the index of suspicion that is required for making the diagnosis of HPS. Children with reflux rarely have acute weight loss. Ultrasonography is a quick, non-invasive, and accurate test for pyloric stenosis. A prompt diagnosis of HPS will prevent worsening morbidity associated with the inevitable dehydration from a gastric outlet obstruction. While this child will need intravenous fluids, there is no indication to wait for laboratory results, or use them as a screening tool to rule out HPS.

Summary/key points

1. Exercise patience during the ultrasound examination of the abdomen, and wait until the child is quiet and comfortable. Change patient positioning as needed to improve visualization.

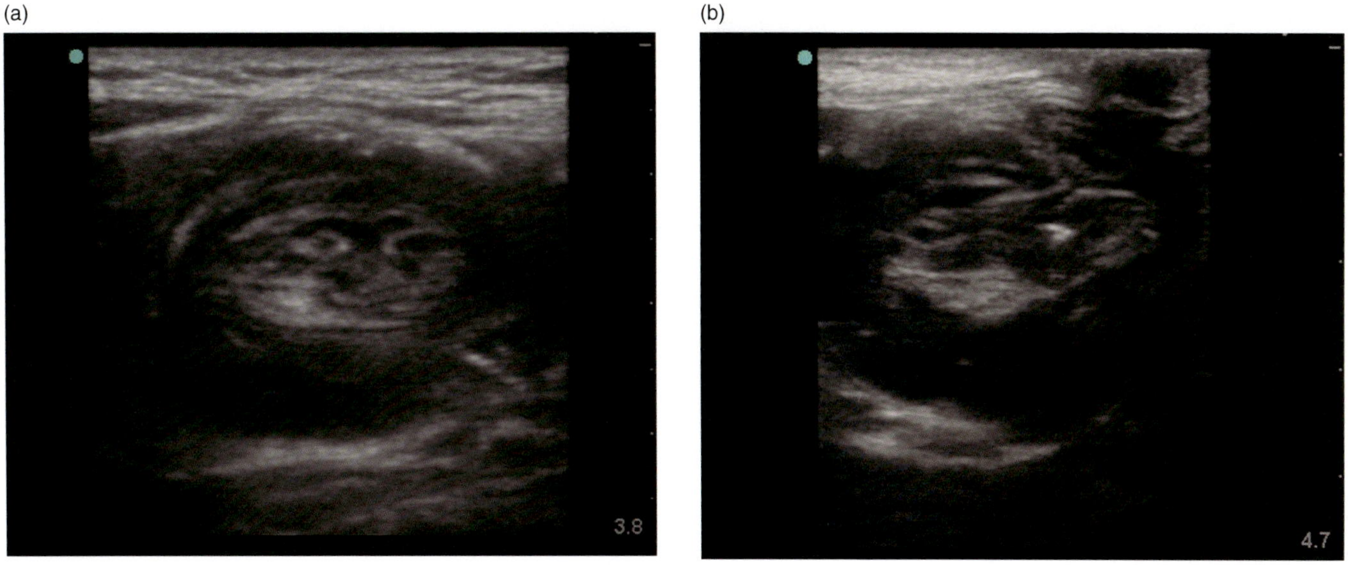

Figure 10.24 Case 1: intussusception. (a) Transverse view at the right upper quadrant reveals a "target" or "doughnut" sign: an intussusception. (b) Longitudinal view reveals the "hayfork" or "pseudokidney" sign.

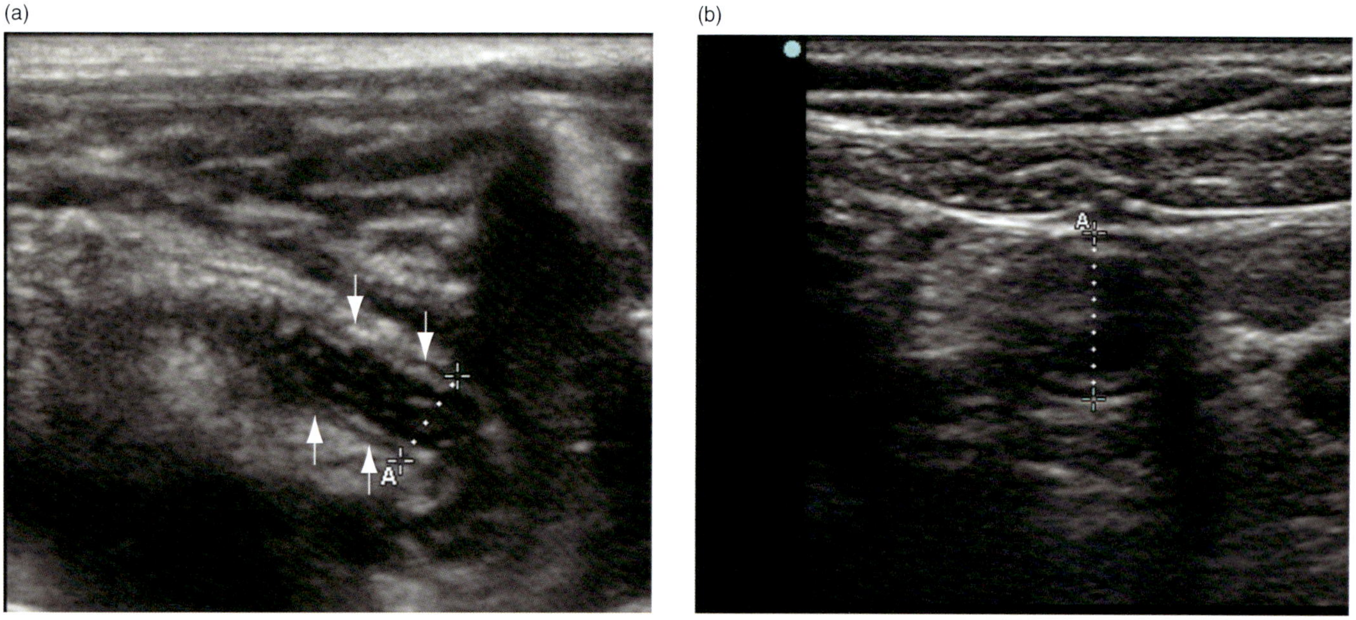

Figure 10.25 **Case 2: enlarged appendix**. An enlarged appendix without secondary signs of inflammation. (a) Longitudinal view of the appendix without visualization of the appendix tip. (b) Transverse view of the appendix measuring greater than 0.6 cm but without secondary signs of inflammation.

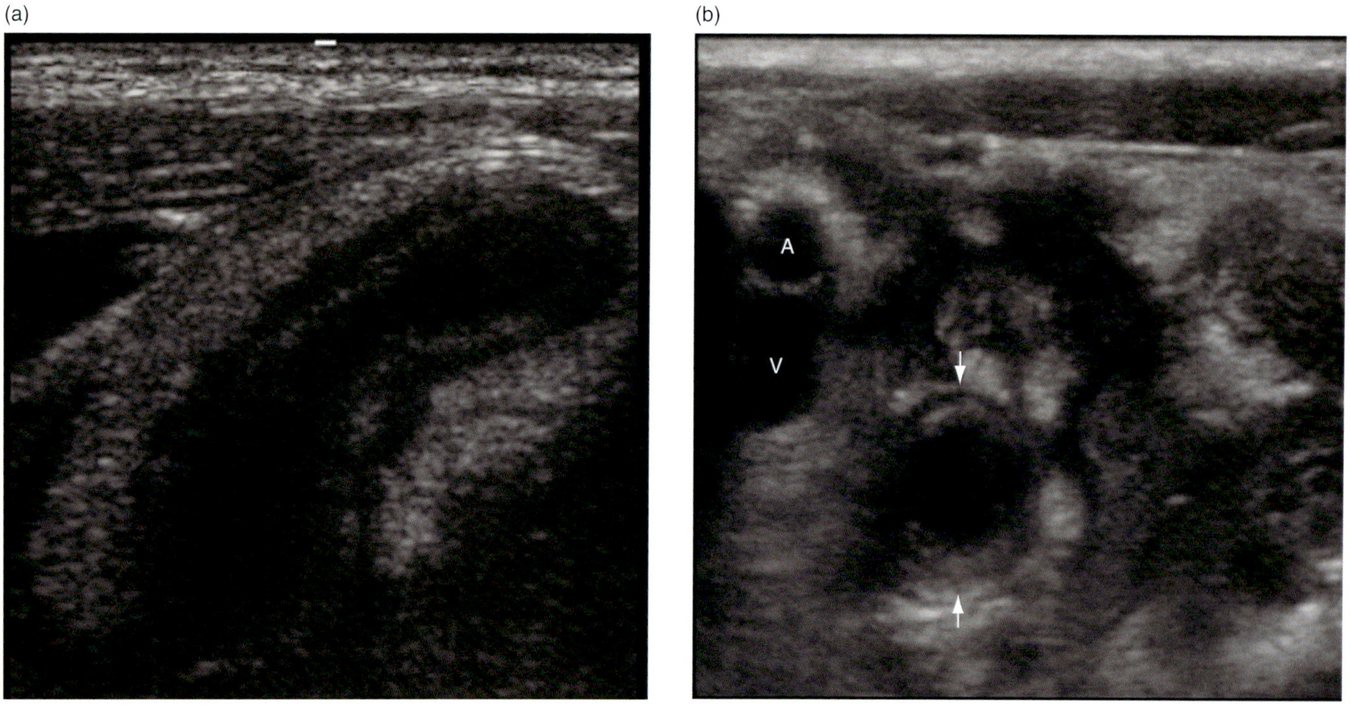

Figure 10.26 **Case 3: appendicitis**. (a) The longitudinal view of the appendix, which measures under 6 mm but the tip is not identified. (b) Transverse view of the appendix tip (arrows), 1.2 cm with loss of distinct hyper–hypoechoic pattern and hazy submucosal layer. Surrounding structures are the iliac artery (A) and iliac vein (V).

2. It is important to recognize the typical appearance of a large, layered mass consistent with intussusception, which is usually located at the hepatic flexure. It is important to differentiate small bowel from ileocolic intussusception by tracing down to the ileocecal valve. In transverse view the intussusception appears as a "target" or "doughnut"; while in longitudinal view it appears as a "hayfork" or "pseudokidney."

3. The adequate visualization of the appendix requires utilizing the graded compression technique. A positive study for appendicitis includes the identification of a blind-ending, tubular, non-compressible structure that arises from the cecum and measures **greater than 6 mm** in diameter. Additional evidence of periappendiceal inflammation and free fluid are helpful in making the diagnosis.

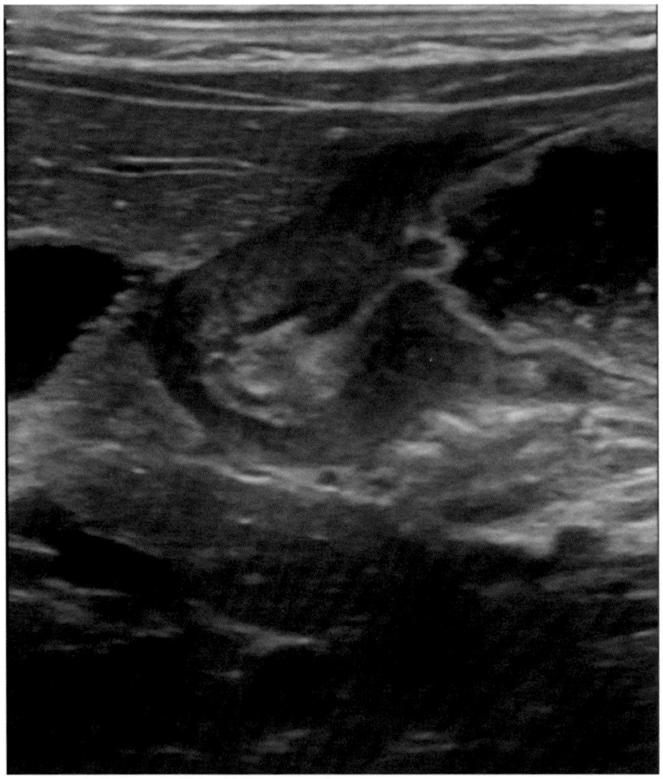

Figure 10.27 Case 4: pyloric stenosis. The pyloric channel is elongated, and the muscle hypertrophied. Also, on real-time visualization, there is failure of passage of gastric contents through the channel into the duodenum.

4. The non-visualization, or visualization, of the appendix in a patient with a high index of suspicion for acute appendicitis should not exclude the diagnosis and should warrant further workup. The appendicitis ultrasound should not be used as a rule out, but rather as a rule in study.
5. A pyloric muscle diameter of **3 mm** or greater and channel length of **14 mm** or greater is the sonographic diagnostic criterion for HPS. Take multiple measurements in order to ensure that the most perpendicular plane is measured. If muscle thickening is noted, observe the pylorus for an extended period of time to ensure it is not thickened due to pylorospasm. There should be no fluid passing through the channel, or muscle relaxation during prolonged observation.

Selected references

Eshed, I., Gorenstein, A., Serour, F., *et al.* (2004) Intussusception in children: can we rely on screening sonography performed by junior residents? *Pediatr Radiol* **34**: 134–7.

Fox, J. C., Hunt., M. J., Zlidenny, A. M., *et al.* (2007) Retrospective analysis of emergency department ultrasound for acute appendicitis. *W J Emerg Med* **8**(2): 41–5.

Fox, J. C., Solley, M., Anderson, C. L., *et al.* (2008) Prospective evaluation of emergency physician performed bedside ultrasound to detect acute appendicitis. *Eur J Emerg Med* **15**(2): 80–5.

Justice, F. A., de Campo, M., Liem, N. T., *et al.* (2007) Accuracy of ultrasonography for the diagnosis of intussusception in infants in Vietnam. *Pediatr Radiol* **37**(2): 195–9.

Krishnamoorthi, R., Ramarajan, N., Wang, N. E., *et al.* (2011) Effectiveness of a staged US and CT protocol for the diagnosis of pediatric appendicitis: reducing radiation exposure in the age of ALARA. *Radiology* **259**(1): 231–9.

Malcom, G. E., Raio, C., Del Rios, M., *et al.* (2009) Feasibility of emergency physician diagnosis of hypertrophic pyloric stenosis using point-of-care ultrasound: a multi-center case series. *J Emerg Med* **37**: 283–6.

Mittal, M. K., Dayan, P. S., Macias, C. G., *et al.* (2013) Performance of ultrasound in the diagnosis of appendicitis in children in a multicenter cohort. *Acad Emerg Med* **20**(7): 697–702.

Riera, A., Hsiao, A. L., Langhan, M. L., *el al.* (2012) Diagnosis of intussusception by physician novice sonographers in the emergency department. *Ann Emerg Med* **60**(3): 264–8.

Shuh, S., Man, C., Cheng, A., *et al.* (2011) Predictors of non-diagnostic ultrasound scanning in children with suspected appendicitis. *J Pediatr* **158**: 112–18.

Sivitz, A. B., Tejani, C., Cohen, S. G. (2013) Evaluation of hypertrophic pyloric stenosis by pediatric emergency physician sonography. *Acad Emerg Med* **20**(7): 646–51.

Chapter

11

Hepatobiliary

Alexander C. Arroyo

Objectives/indications

Abdominal pain is one of the most common complaints encountered in the pediatric emergency department. Unlike in adult patients, with the exception of certain conditions, hepatobiliary disease is infrequent in pediatric patients. There are only 1.3 cases of pediatric cholecystitis for every 1000 adult cases. However, with the increasing prevalence of childhood obesity, diseases of the biliary tract are increasingly becoming more prevalent in children. The approximate incidence of gallstones in children is 1.5%, with 85% of these children having an underlying disease predisposition to gallstone formation. Older children and adolescents may present classically with right upper quadrant (RUQ) pain and vomiting. In contrast, infants and young children may present with more nonspecific symptoms, such as jaundice and irritability.

The most common reasons to order an ultrasound of the biliary tract are jaundice or right upper quadrant pain. In neonates, a few causes of cholelithiasis include: total parenteral nutrition (TPN) administration (40% of infants receiving TPN develop cholelithiasis), anomalies of the biliary tract, and short gut syndrome. In younger children, diseases that have a predilection for pigment gallstone formation include the hemolytic anemias, sickle cell anemia, and hereditary spherocytosis. Other conditions such as cystic fibrosis or Crohn's disease can cause gallstones as well in this age group. Cholesterol stones are more often seen, and lead to cholecystitis, in adolescent girls than in their male counterparts. Enteric bacterial infections and vasculitis syndromes can lead to cholecystitis without the presence of any gallstones. Gallbladder hydrops, or the abnormal distention of the gallbladder, is one of the lesser known findings seen in children with Kawasaki disease. While applications for right upper quadrant ultrasound are evolving for pediatric patients, other potential indications for gallbladder and liver ultrasonography include: congenital abnormalities such as biliary atresia or choledochal cysts, and hepatic tumors. While these applications may require a comprehensive examination, they may be encountered in a clinician's point-of-care evaluation and should prompt further evaluation.

Ultrasonography of the right upper quadrant can be very challenging. At times, all of the pertinent structures are easily identified, but it may be difficult to isolate one or more key structures. Structures like the common bile duct (CBD) and the neck of the gallbladder may be especially difficult to locate and/or differentiate from other surrounding structures. The objectives of this chapter are to review the basic normal sonographic anatomy of the liver, gallbladder, and surrounding structures. This chapter also reviews the sonographic appearance of gallstones (cholelithiasis), an acutely inflamed, diseased gallbladder (cholecystitis), and biliary ductal dilatation.

Background

Traditionally, formal ultrasonography has been the study of choice for the evaluation of the right upper quadrant. However, with the advent of portable ultrasonography, gallbladder, or right upper quadrant ultrasound has been one of the most important applications in point-of-care ultrasound in rapidly diagnosing gallbladder pathology at the bedside. In the radiology literature, the diagnostic accuracy of ultrasound is based upon individual sonographic signs. Shea *et al.* performed a review which found formal ultrasonography to be 97% sensitive and 95% specific for gallstones. With the introduction of focused emergency department right upper quadrant sonography, the diagnostic accuracy of biliary disease increased from 28% to 70%, with decreased return visits secondary to pain, and decreased complications from stones. Further, a focused right upper quadrant ultrasound can shorten emergency department stays in patients like these by guiding further testing and eliminating other potential diagnoses. Blaivas *et al.* performed a large retrospective study, which showed a decreased length of stay of 7% in those patients who received an ultrasound performed by the emergency physician. Moreover, multiple studies have proven that adult emergency physicians can correctly diagnose the absence or presence of biliary disease. Kendall *et al.* showed that an average right upper quadrant ultrasound can be performed by emergency physicians in less than 10 minutes, with a sensitivity of 96% and a specificity of 88%. The ultrasound performed by the emergency physicians had a higher sensitivity for detecting a sonographic Murphy's sign (75%), when compared with formal ultrasonography (sensitivity 45%). When compared with clinically important outcomes such as pathology reports and clinical follow-up, point-of-care ultrasonography is comparable to formal radiographic studies.

Early studies of point-of-care ultrasound for pediatric patients with suspected biliary disease seem promising, but further studies are needed to assess its accuracy. Thus far, the literature is limited

Pediatric Emergency and Critical Care Ultrasound, ed. Stephanie J. Doniger. Published by Cambridge University Press.

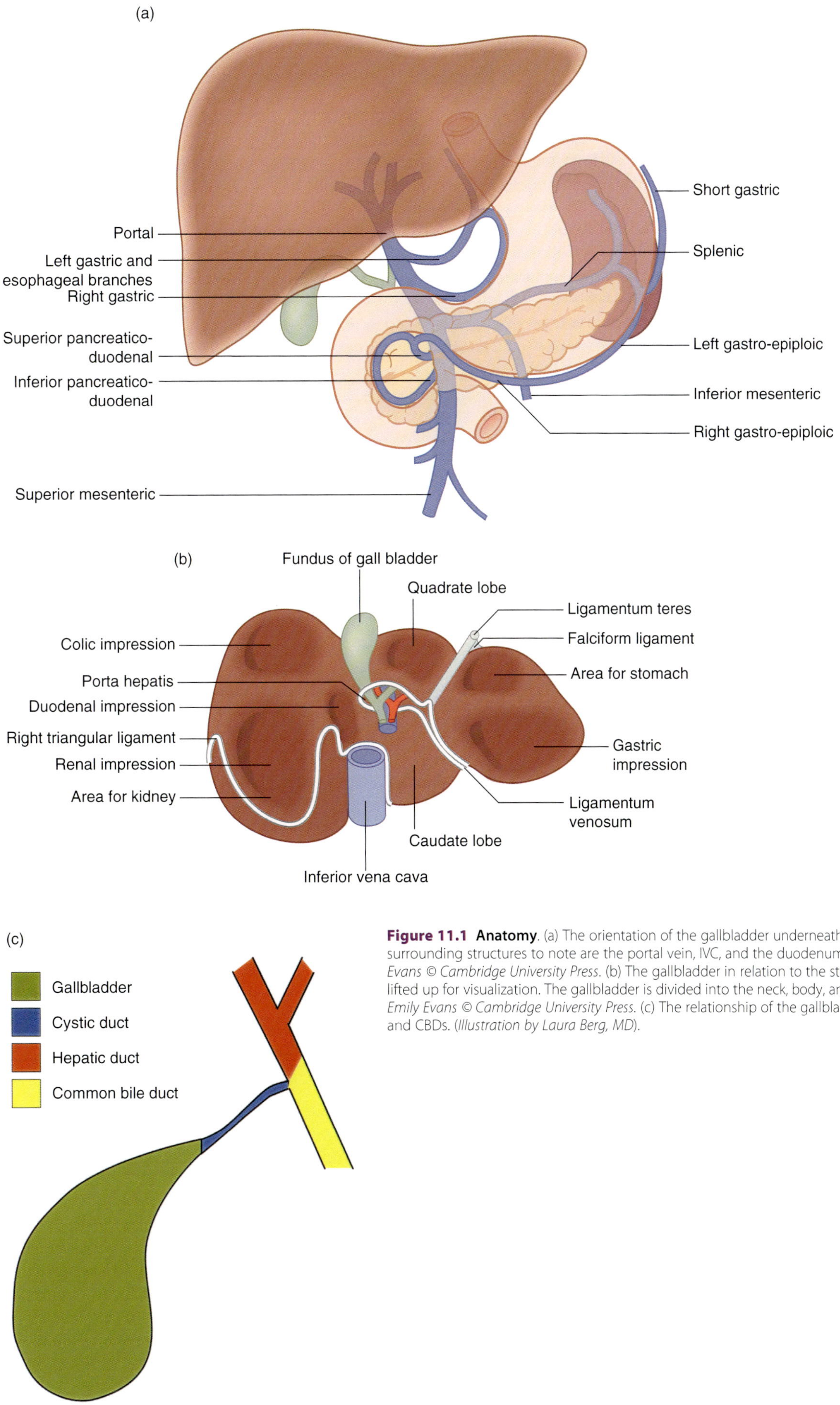

Figure 11.1 Anatomy. (a) The orientation of the gallbladder underneath the liver. Important surrounding structures to note are the portal vein, IVC, and the duodenum. *Artwork created by Emily Evans © Cambridge University Press.* (b) The gallbladder in relation to the stomach and liver; the liver is lifted up for visualization. The gallbladder is divided into the neck, body, and fundus. *Artwork created by Emily Evans © Cambridge University Press.* (c) The relationship of the gallbladder, and the cystic, hepatic, and CBDs. (*Illustration by Laura Berg, MD*).

to case series, and data to support sonographic diagnostic criteria in children are limited. Until further studies are performed, the measurements and sonographic diagnostic criteria have been extrapolated from adult data.

Anatomy

The gallbladder is usually found on the lower border of the liver, in between the right and left lobes. Other pertinent structures in the vicinity are the liver, IVC, duodenum, and the components of the portal triad: the hepatic artery, portal vein, and CBD (Figure 11.1a). The gallbladder has three components: the fundus, the body, and the neck (Figure 11.1b). The neck of the gallbladder is continuous with the cystic duct. The cystic duct merges with the hepatic ducts coming from the liver, to form the CBD (Figure 11.1c). Since the gallbladder is not a fixed organ, it may have various orientations and locations within the right upper quadrant.

Technique

Point-of-care questions

1. Are gallstones present? Is pericholecystic fluid present?
2. Does the patient have a sonographic Murphy's sign?
3. Is there thickening of the anterior gallbladder wall greater than **3 mm**? Is the CBD dilated more than **6 mm**?
4. Is an abnormal mass or echotexture present in the liver?

Transducer selection and orientation

For most children, using the low-frequency (2–5 MHz), curvilinear transducer or the high-frequency (5–10 MHz), linear transducer is adequate. At times, it may be helpful to use the phased-array transducer in order to view the gallbladder in between the ribs if there is difficulty in obtaining images.

Transducer placement can be at the subcostal region, right flank, or the "X-7" approach. In the subcostal region, the indicator is oriented towards the patient's right shoulder. Begin scanning at the subxiphoid region, and slide subcostally towards the patient's right side (Figure 11.2a). At the right flank, orient the transducer with the indicator towards the patient's head (Figure 11.2b). In the "X-7" approach, the transducer is placed at the right anterior chest, 7 cm to the patient's right. This is generally in the midclavicular line, using the intercostal space to scan. Initially the indicator is oriented in the transverse plane, towards the patient's right side (Figure 11.2c). Regardless of the approach to scanning, the gallbladder must be visualized in two views: its long-axis and its short-axis. Once the gallbladder is identified in its short axis the transducer can be rotated clockwise in order to visualize the gallbladder in its long-axis.

Patient position and preparation

The initial position can be supine, but, frequently, to visualize the gallbladder and liver properly the patient may need to be placed in the left lateral decubitus position where gravity brings the gallbladder anterior (Figure 11.2d). If it is still difficult to locate the pertinent structures, having the patient lie nearly prone on the transducer may help. A deep inspiration pushes the liver and gallbladder inferiorly and may make them easier to locate.

(a)

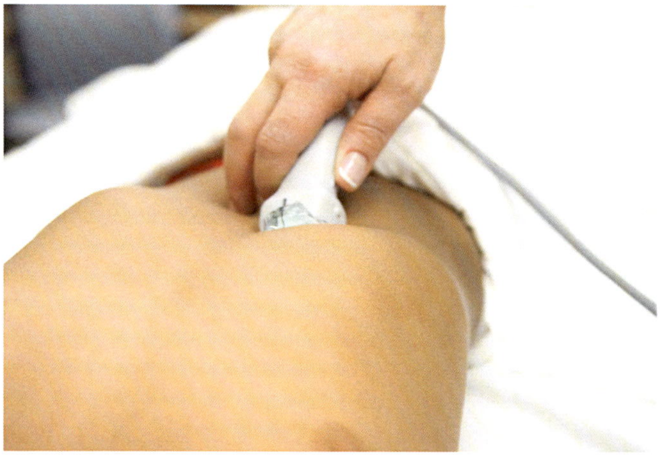

(b)

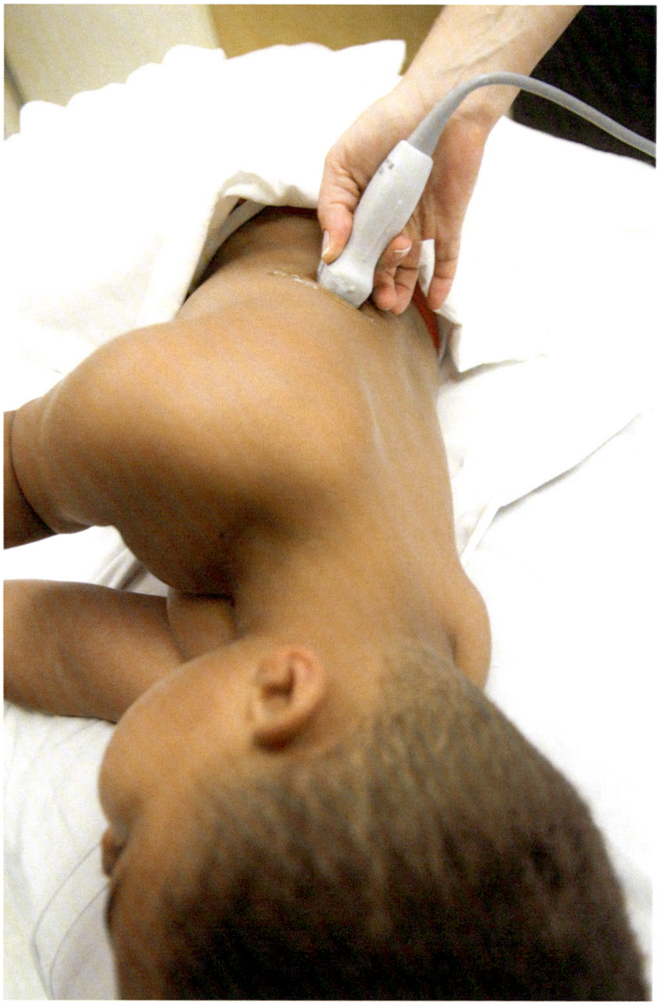

Figure 11.2 Ultrasound examination of the gallbladder. (a) The subcostal approach, with the indicator oriented towards the patient's right shoulder. (b) The right flank. The patient may be supine or in the left lateral decubitus position, with the indicator pointing cephalad. (c) "X-7" approach, with the transducer in the transverse plane, with the indicator towards the patient's right side. (d) Rotating the patient in the left lateral decubitus position may improve visualization of the gallbladder.

(c)

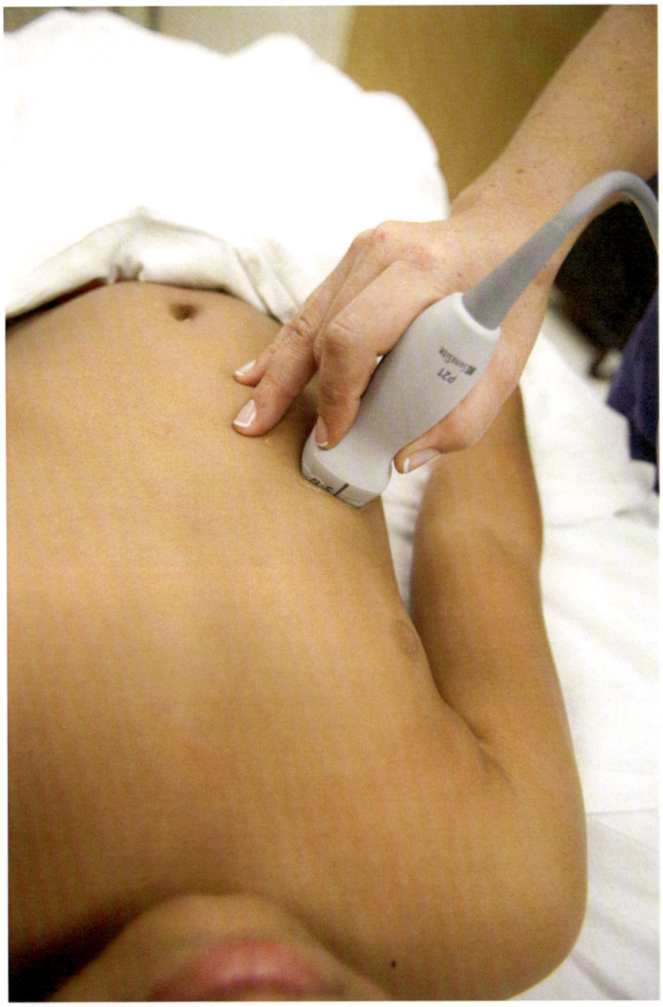

(d)

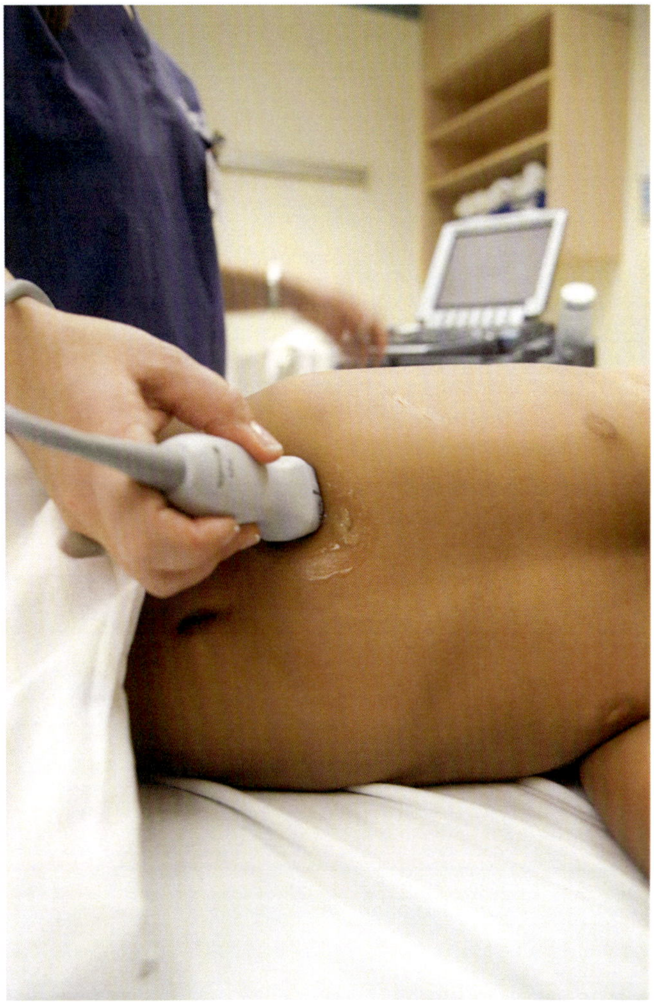

Figure 11.2 (cont.)

Rolling the patients also helps distinguish a polyp from a stone and also whether a stone is simply sitting near the neck of the gallbladder or is impacted in the neck.

Traditionally, it was taught that it was best to visualize the gallbladder after a fast of four to six hours; at this point it will be filled with bile and easily seen. If the patient has just eaten, the gallbladder may be difficult to visualize since contraction may have occurred. This has recently come into question, with a study showing that no significant difference in gallbladder size is seen after ingestion of a fatty meal. Plus, fasting in the emergency department setting would make the examination prohibitive.

Ultrasound imaging

By applying gentle pressure and fanning the through the liver, the gallbladder should be visualized. If it is not visualized readily, slide the transducer down along the costal margin scanning through the dome of the liver. Sweep through the entire gallbladder in the transverse view (Figure 11.3a,d). When completed, rotate the transducer 90° to obtain the longitudinal view of the gallbladder. In the longitudinal view the gallbladder neck, body, and fundus can be visualized (Figure 11.3c,d). The major lobar fissure leads to the gallbladder, and can serve as a landmark in identifying the gallbladder (Figure 11.3e) and right portal vein should appear as an exclamation point (Figure 11.3d,e). Because it is filled with bile, a normal gallbladder has several of the sonographic qualities of a cyst: smooth, thin, well-defined walls, an anechoic internal lumen, bright echogenic posterior walls, and posterior acoustic enhancement (Figure 11.4). Frequently, the tear-drop shaped gallbladder may contain one of a few variant folds. A junctional fold can be seen as an echogenic line in the middle of the gallbladder (Figure 11.5a). A Hartmann's pouch is a fold near the neck of the gallbladder, where gallstones can collect (Figure 11.5b). A Phrygian cap is a small fold near the distal end of the fundus (Figure 11.5c).

The liver is straightforward to visualize with sonography. Its dense structure serves as a good sonographic window, allowing the other portions of the right upper quadrant to be visualized. It appears dense on ultrasound with multiple small and large anechoic "holes" distributed throughout the organ. These are the many ducts and vessels that comprise the liver and give it a homogeneous "salt and pepper" appearance (Figure 11.6a). When this appearance is disrupted, an abnormality probably exists in the liver, such as cancer or hepatitis (Figure 11.6b). The IVC is

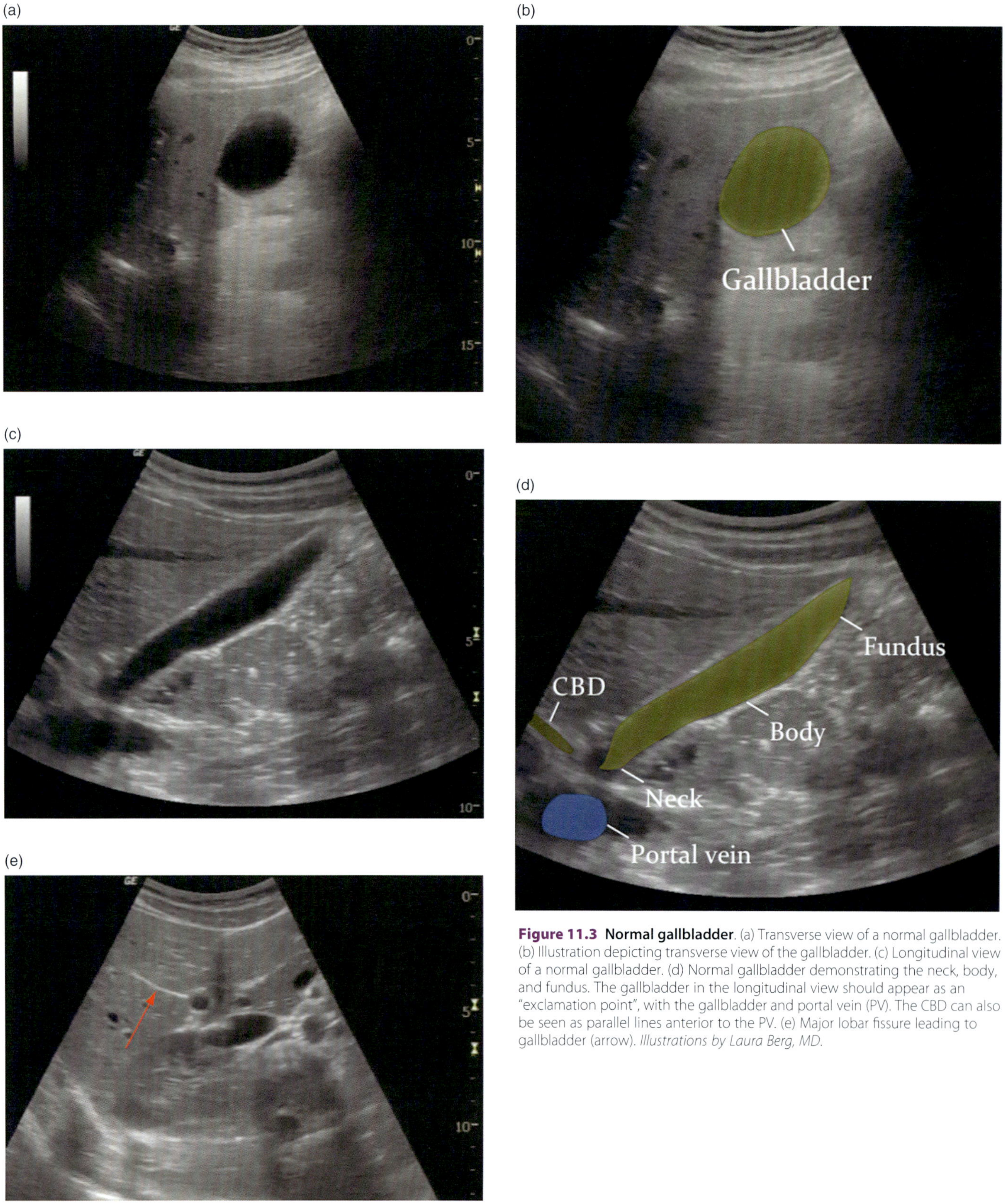

Figure 11.3 Normal gallbladder. (a) Transverse view of a normal gallbladder. (b) Illustration depicting transverse view of the gallbladder. (c) Longitudinal view of a normal gallbladder. (d) Normal gallbladder demonstrating the neck, body, and fundus. The gallbladder in the longitudinal view should appear as an "exclamation point", with the gallbladder and portal vein (PV). The CBD can also be seen as parallel lines anterior to the PV. (e) Major lobar fissure leading to gallbladder (arrow). *Illustrations by Laura Berg, MD.*

the largest vessel seen in this area; its course can be traced from the lower abdomen, posterior to the liver, where it enters the right atria (Figure 11.7). The right, middle, and left hepatic veins branch off the IVC as it enters the abdomen; this branching has been nicknamed the "Playboy bunny" sign because it takes the appearance of rabbit ears (Figure 11.8). Like the gallbladder, the duodenum lies on the lower left border of the liver. Frequently it is mistaken for the gallbladder, but observing it for a time should

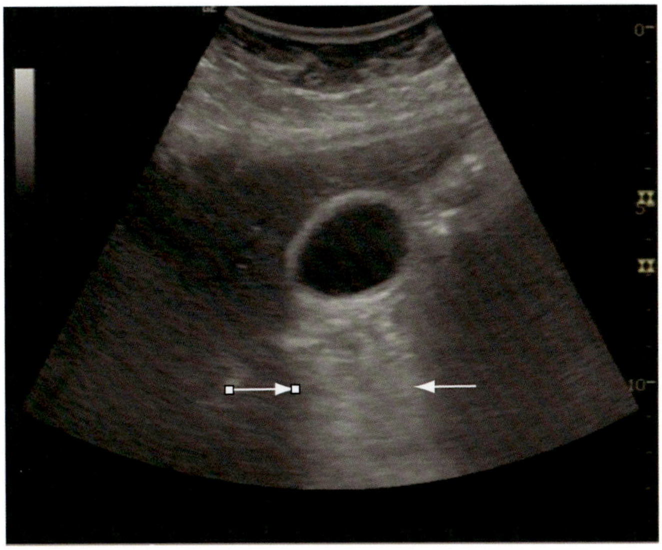

Figure 11.4 Gallbladder demonstrating posterior acoustic enhancement (arrows).

demonstrate peristalsis (Figure 11.9). The portal vein is the largest component of the portal triad, with hyperechoic walls that make it easy to locate in the liver. If traced out further into the liver, the portal vein branches off into the right and left portal veins. The second structure in the portal triad, the hepatic artery, has a limited role in emergency sonography. The neck of the gallbladder is continuous with the cystic duct, which merges with the hepatic ducts coming from the liver to form the CBD (Figure 11.10). Sonographically, the CBD usually lies between the gallbladder and the portal vein. It can be seen as two hyperechoic lines running on top of and parallel to the portal vein (Figure 11.11a). Often it is difficult to distinguish the CBD from the hepatic artery or other vessels in the area. Magnifying the area with your machine's zoom capability can help enhance the smaller portions of the examination. Another helpful way to recognize the duct is to use color Doppler, since the CBD will not demonstrate any color flow (Figure 11.11c). In transverse view, the portal triad takes on the appearance of three circles, affectionately called the "Mickey Mouse" sign (Figure 11.12).

Once the gallbladder and its surrounding structures are located, it should be determined whether there is the presence or absence of certain sonographic features to assess for acute cholecystitis:

1. **Stones**: noting location and mobility (Figure 11.13). By rolling the patient, stones should move to a more dependent portion of the gallbladder.
2. **Gallbladder wall edema** or wall thickening.
3. **Pericholecystic fluid** – in a diseased gallbladder, fluid often accumulates as a hypoechoic halo around the gallbladder, which may be a subtle finding. This represents subserosa and hepatic edema and cellular infiltration (Figure 11.14).
4. **Sludge** – thick viscous bile that layers out in the dependent portion of the gallbladder. When compared to stones, sludge appears less hyperechoic and does not exhibit posterior shadowing. Sludge may appear grayish white and

(a)

(b)

(c)

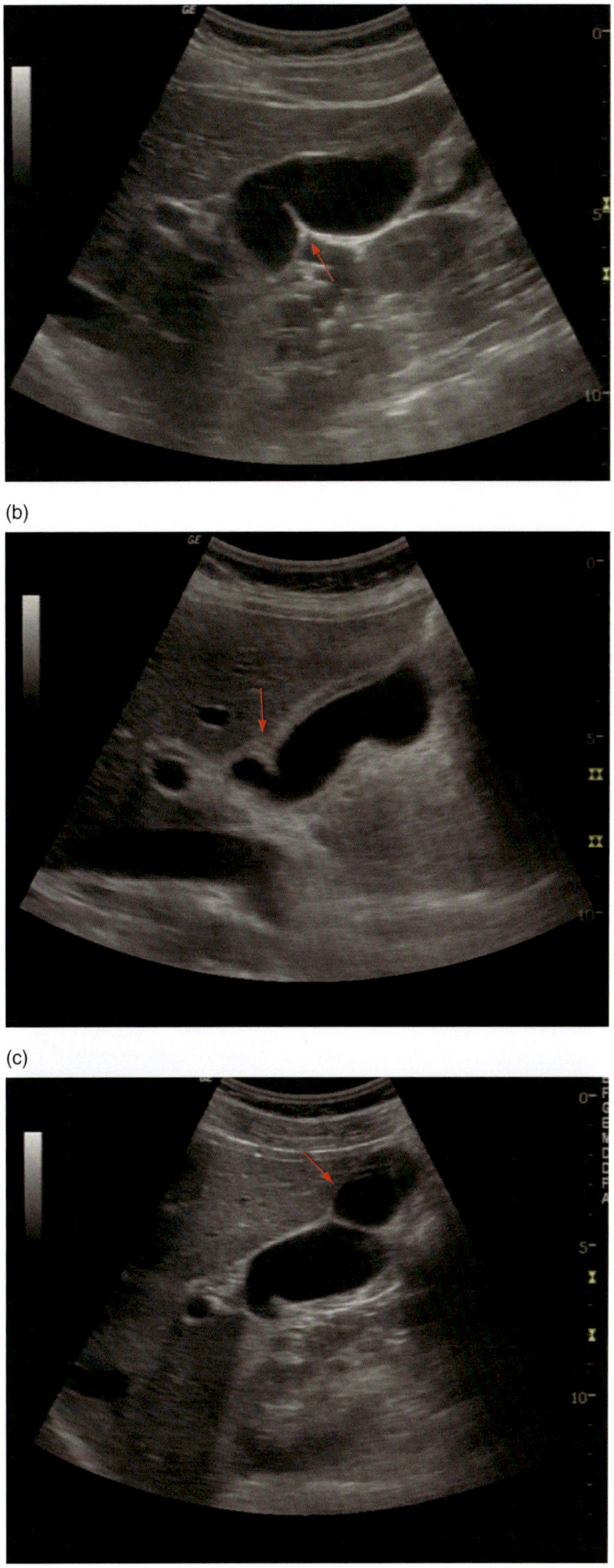

Figure 11.5 Normal variants of the gallbladder. (a) A junctional fold in the middle of the gallbladder (arrow). (b) A Hartmann's pouch near the neck of the gallbladder (arrow). (c) A Phrygian cap seen at the fundus of the gallbladder (arrow).

(a) (b)

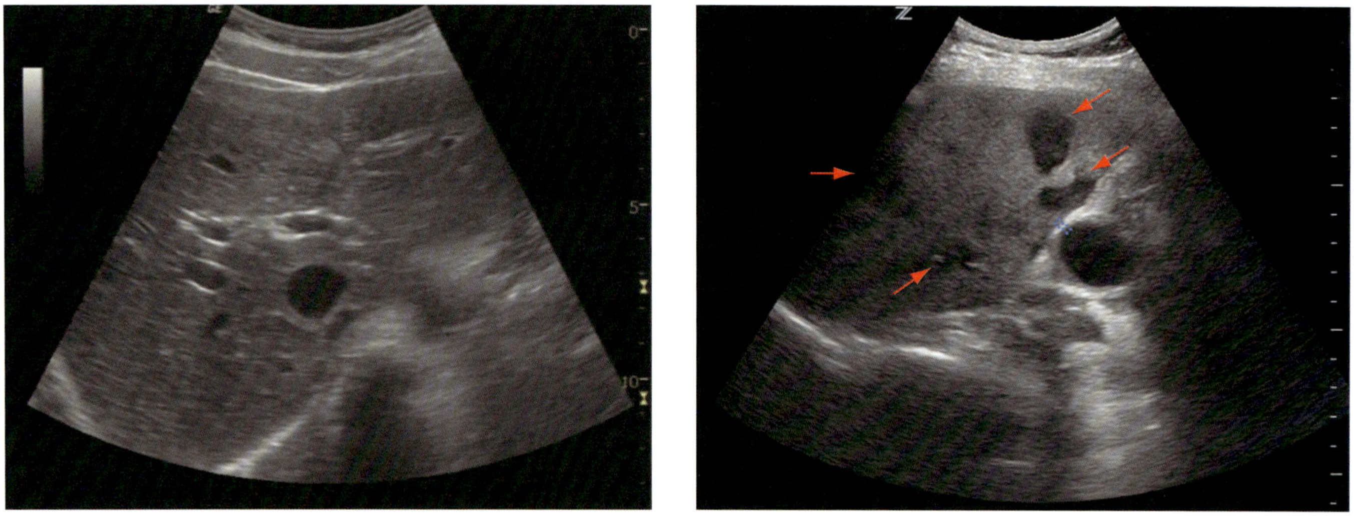

Figure 11.6 Normal liver. (a) Normal liver with homogeneous appearance. (b) Liver demonstrating cancer metastases (arrows). Notice the very heterogeneous appearance of this diseased liver.

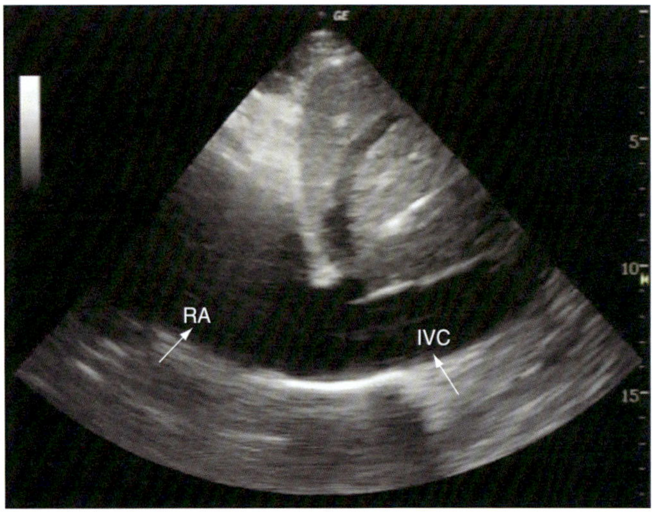

Figure 11.7 Inferior vena cava (IVC). Inferior vena cava emptying into the right atria (RA). The liver and diaphragm are seen in the upper portion of this image.

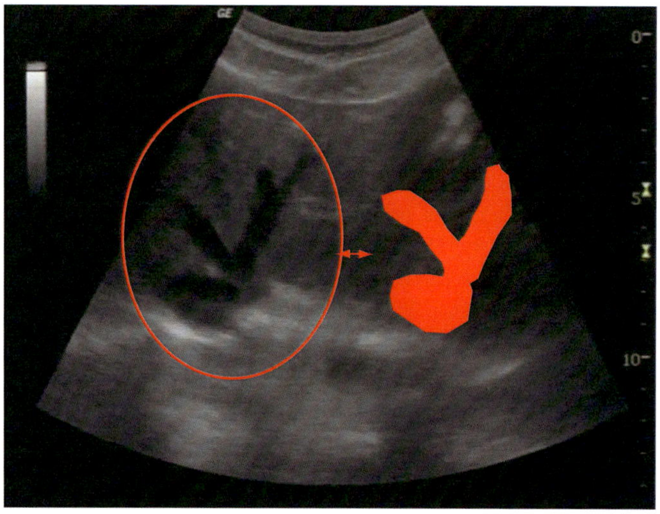

Figure 11.8 Hepatic veins. The branching hepatic veins give the appearance of a bunny with ears, referred to as the "Playboy bunny" sign.

have a "dirty" shadow posteriorly when mixed with small stones (Figure 11.15). Sludge is not a normal finding and usually signifies a diseased gallbladder.

5. **Sonographic Murphy's sign** – a variation of the physical examination finding, when pain is elicited and respiration is halted when pressing on the gallbladder with the transducer. Some consider this the most specific sign for cholecystitis.
6. **Gallbladder distention** – using size to asses for biliary disease in children is of little use because of the variations of normal measurements (Figure 11.16).
7. **Biliary ductal (CBD) dilatation** – secondary to a stone obstructing bile flow. Sometimes the stone in question can be visualized, but more often only the dilatation is observed. On sagittal view, with a dilated CBD, the portal triad has been described as an "olive sandwich," in which the CBD is the top slice of bread, the hepatic artery is the olive in the middle, and the portal vein is the bottom slice of bread (Figure 11.17c,d).

Ultrasound imaging: measurements

In order to perform a thorough right upper quadrant ultrasound examination, and appropriately determine whether there is the presence of gallbladder pathology, measurements of the anterior gallbladder wall and the CBD must be performed. This measurement is performed at the anterior wall, in the near field where the liver meets the gallbladder. Posterior acoustic enhancement will falsely thicken the posterior wall of the gallbladder and should not be measured (Figure 11.4). The CBD should be measured from the inner wall to the inner wall. The upper limit of normal size for the CBD is **3 mm** in children and **4 mm** in adults (Figure 11.18).

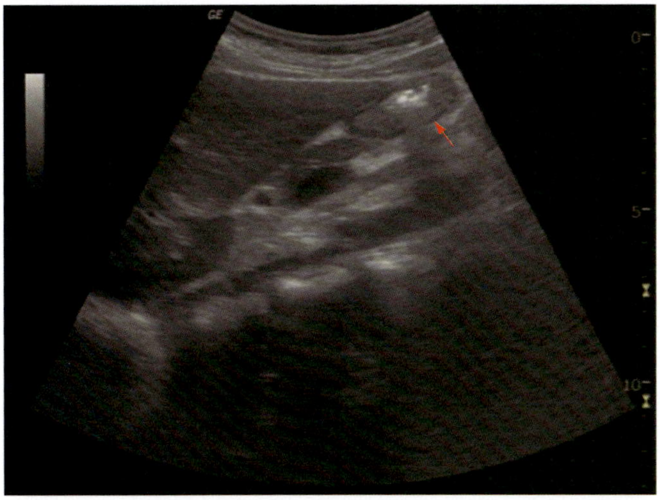

Figure 11.9 Duodenum. The duodenum (arrow) is frequently mistaken for the gallbladder because of its appearance and location.

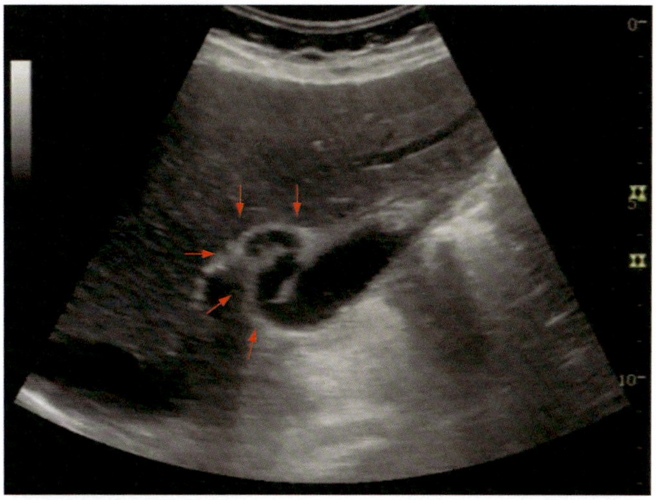

Figure 11.10 Biliary ducts. The cystic duct (arrows) is seen at the neck of the gallbladder.

(a) (b)

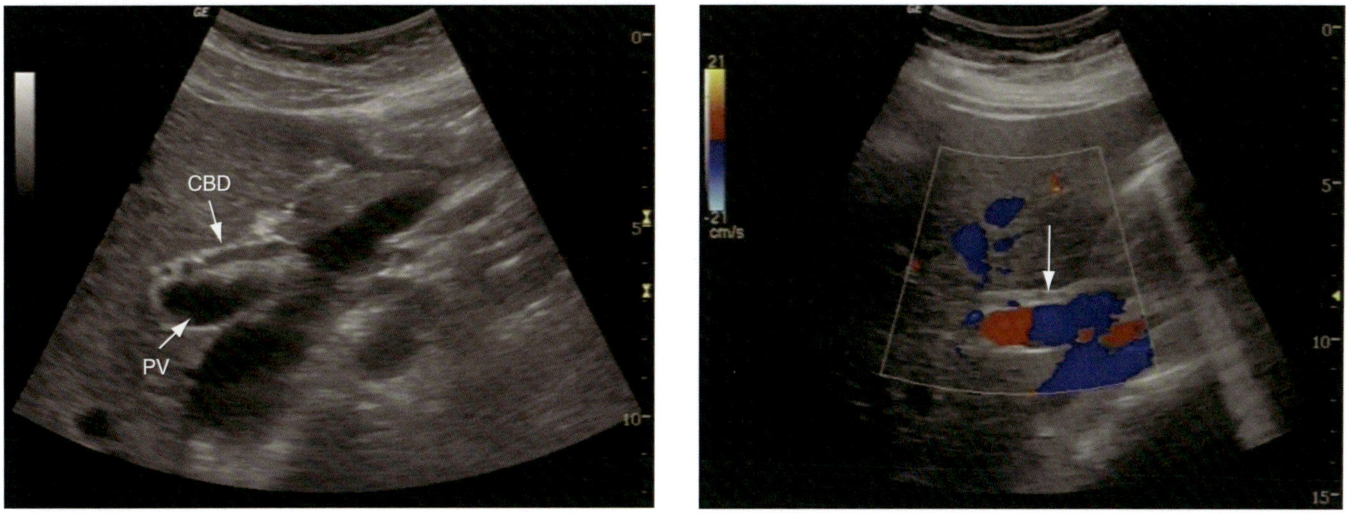

Figure 11.11 Common bile duct (CBD). (a) A sagittal view of the CBD is seen superior to the portal vein (PV). (b) Color Doppler can be utilized to locate the CBD. Note how the CBD does not demonstrate color flow (arrow).

Additionally, the gallbladder length may be helpful in this assessment. In a neonate/young infant the gallbladder can be 1.3–3.4 cm in length (mean 2.5 cm) and 0.5–1.2 cm in width (mean 0.9 cm). In children 2–16 years old, the gallbladder can be 2.9–8 cm in length (mean 5 cm) and 1–3.2 cm in width (mean 1.8 cm) (Figure 11.18c).

Training and education

It has been shown that emergency physicians can accurately perform right upper quadrant ultrasounds with some training and experience, in as little as 25 ultrasounds. This recommendation is largely a result of consensus opinion. A recent study by Jang *et al.* investigated right upper quadrant point-of-care ultrasound test characteristics in order to determine how many examinations should be performed by residents in order to attain competence. They showed that the learning curve starts to flatten out after performing 50 examinations, resulting in an accuracy of approximately 90% in detecting cholelithiasis. Therefore, it is suggested that more than 25 scans may be necessary, and a significant proportion of those scans should be "true-positives." Another method other than an arbitrary number of scans might be needed in order to assess for competency. This needs to be investigated further especially in pediatric patients.

Scanning tips

Pitfalls

- Duodenal gas often obscures structures of interest. Gentle pressure with the transducer may displace bowel gas, and turning the patient to the left decubitus position, or time, can help alleviate this problem.
- The duodenum or the IVC may be mistaken for the gallbladder. The duodenum will demonstrate peristalsis.

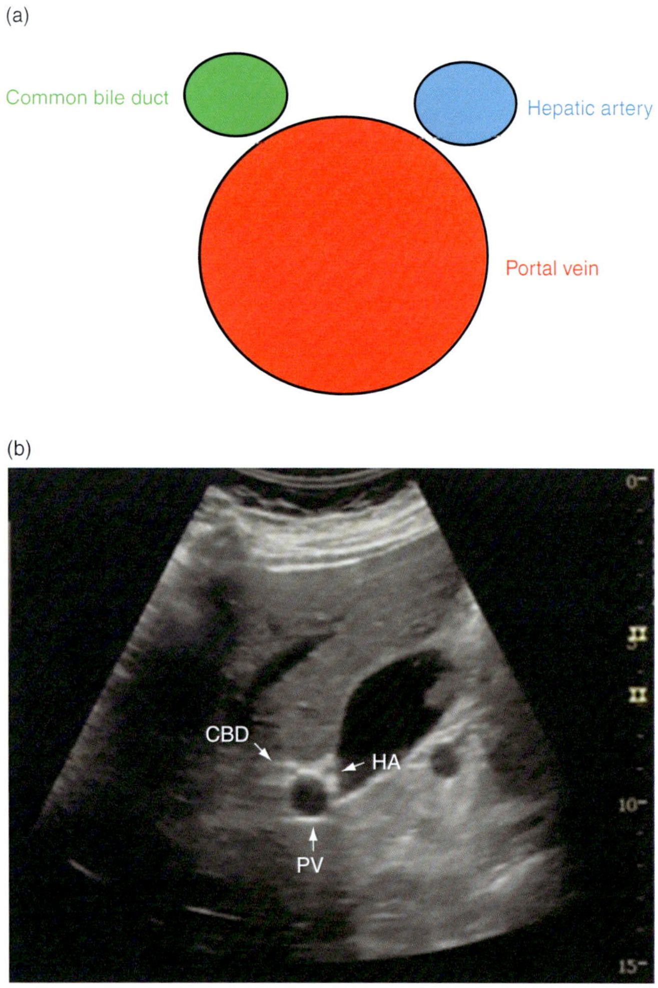

Figure 11.12 **Portal triad**. (a) Drawing demonstrating the "Mickey Mouse" sign of the portal triad. (b) Portal triad on transverse image demonstrating the "Mickey Mouse" sign: portal vein (PV), common bile duct (CBD), hepatic artery (HA).

The IVC will demonstrate color flow and can be seen emptying into the right atrium.

- Assessing a contracted gallbladder: the contracted gallbladder will be difficult to locate and appear to have thickened walls.
- The posterior wall may appear falsely thickened due to posterior acoustic enhancement. Therefore, it is recommended to only perform measurements at the anterior gallbladder wall.
- Beware of acalculous cholecystitis. In the absence of gallstones, patients can still have gallbladder disease; about 50% of acute cholecystitis cases in children lack gallstones. Conditions leading to this are burns, sepsis, recent surgery, or debilitation.
- Many things can be missed when incomplete scans are performed. Subtle pericholecystic fluid or a stone impacted in the neck of the gallbladder are notables.
- Mistaking a polyp or fold for a gallstone; polyps will usually not shadow and will remain stationary.
- Mistaking artifact for sludge or stones: a round, cyst-like structure such as the gallbladder often has "side lobe artifact," which will leave a dark shadow on the sides of the cyst. This shadowing is commonly mistaken for gallstone shadowing.

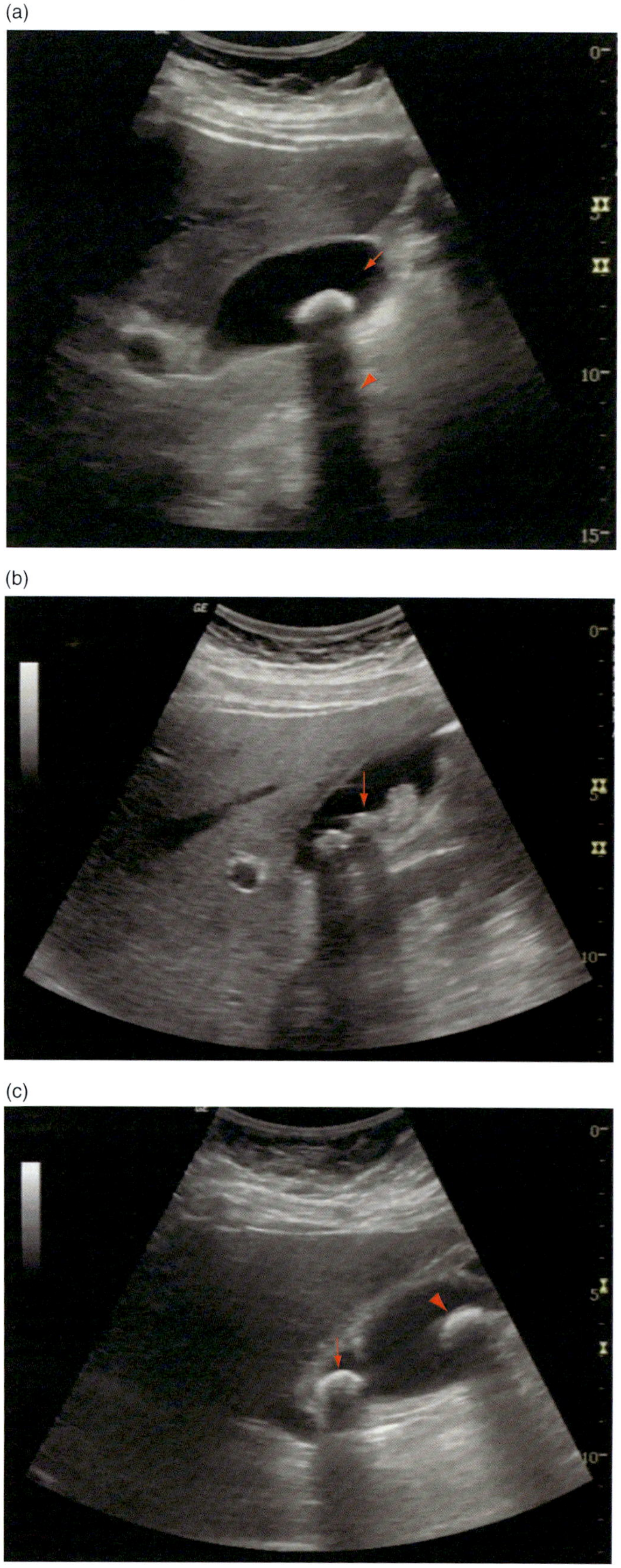

Figure 11.13 **Gallstones**. (a) Stone in the gallbladder (arrow) with "clean shadowing" (arrowhead); notice how hyperechoic the stone is. (b) Multiple stones are seen in this gallbladder (arrow); notice the shadow cast down by the gallstones. (c) Stone impacted in the neck of the gallbladder (arrowhead). When this patient was asked to roll, the stone in the body of the gallbladder (arrowhead) moved, but the stone in the neck (arrow) did not.

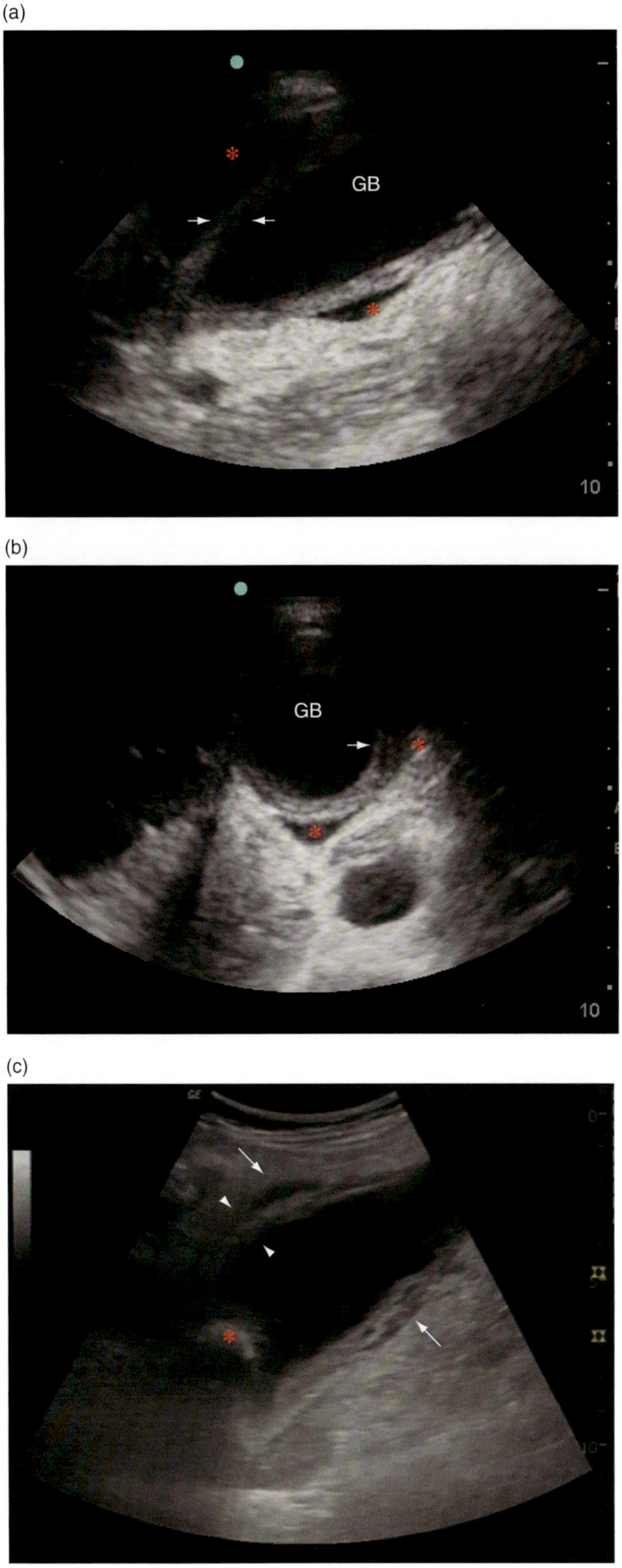

Figure 11.14 Pericholecystic fluid. (a) Pericholecystic fluid (*) collects around a diseased gallbladder (GB); notice the thickened wall (arrows). (b) Transverse view of the same gallbladder with thickened wall (arrows) and pericholecystic fluid (*). (c) A large gallstone (arrowhead) is seen in the neck of the gallbladder. Pericholecystic fluid (*) and a thickened anterior gallbladder wall (arrows) are noted.

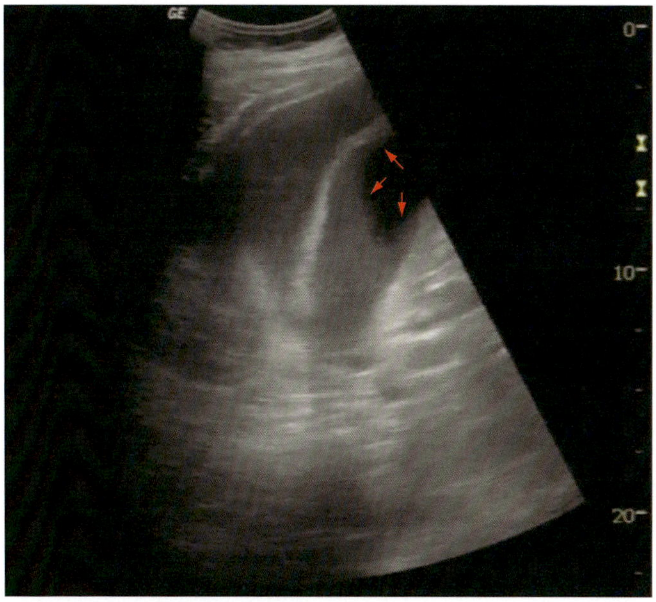

Figure 11.15 Gallbladder sludge. A large amount of viscous sludge is seen filling this otherwise normal gallbladder (arrows).

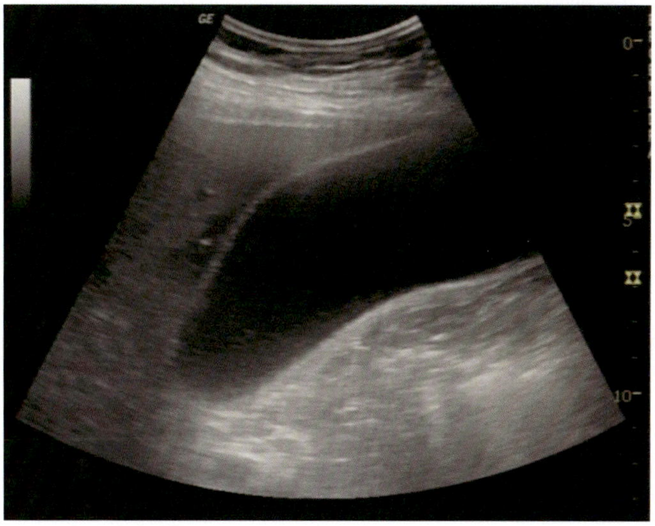

Figure 11.16 Gallbladder distension. This gallbladder is so distended it cannot be fully visualized on screen. In children the size of the gallbladder varies by age; the upper limits of size are listed in the text.

Tips to improve scanning

✓ Angle the transducer between the ribs. If it is difficult to see the gallbladder at the inferior costal margin, placing the transducer between the patient's ribs can be helpful. A switch from the curvilinear transducer (2–5 MHz) to the smaller-footprint phased-array transducer (2–8 MHz) can aid in this, especially in small children.

✓ Know when to roll. If image acquisition is inadequate with the patient supine, place him/her in the left decubitus position. This will greatly help in locating the portal triad.

✓ Scan on deep inspiration. Asking the patient to take a deep breath and hold it, will expand the lungs, pushing

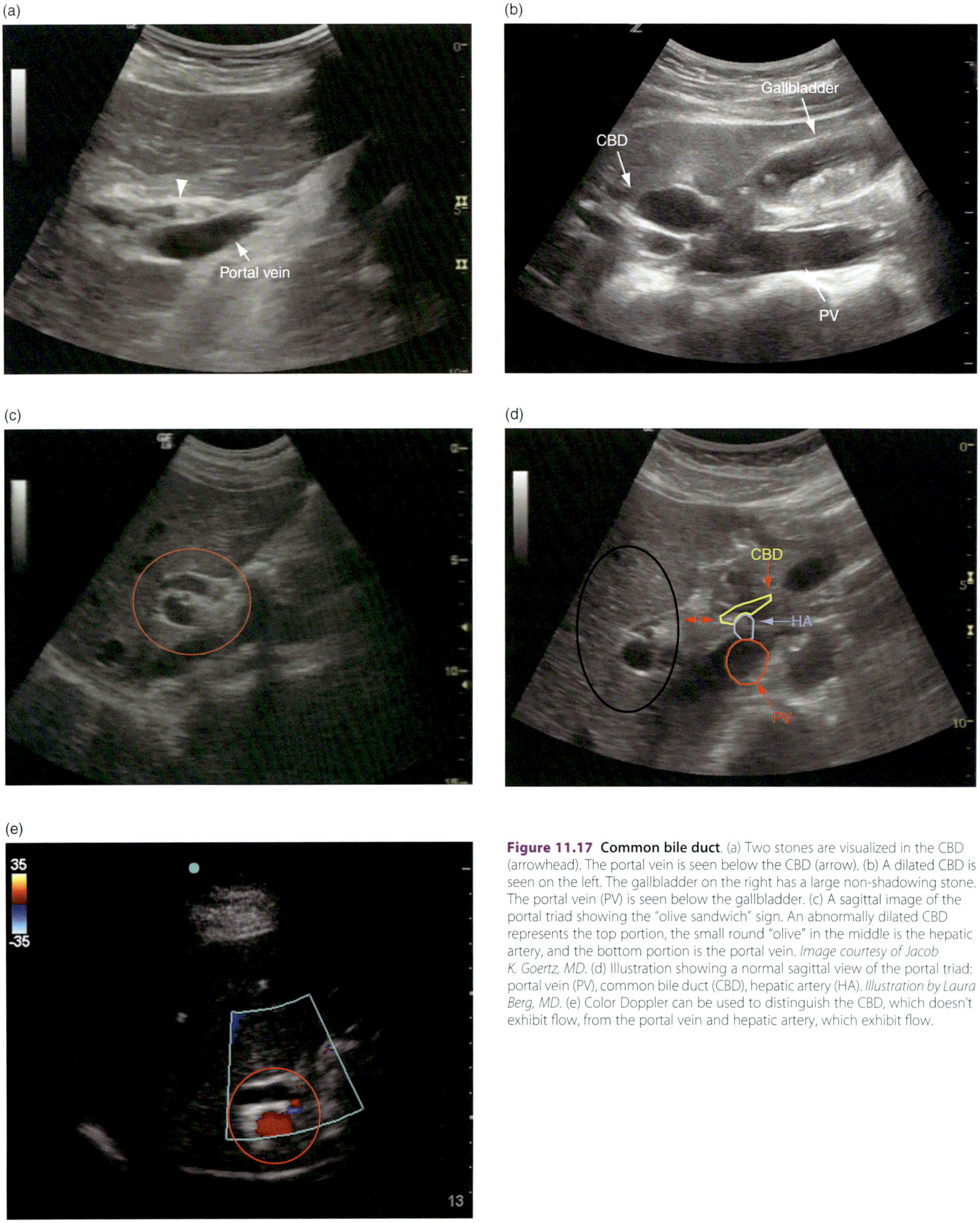

Figure 11.17 Common bile duct. (a) Two stones are visualized in the CBD (arrowhead). The portal vein is seen below the CBD (arrow). (b) A dilated CBD is seen on the left. The gallbladder on the right has a large non-shadowing stone. The portal vein (PV) is seen below the gallbladder. (c) A sagittal image of the portal triad showing the "olive sandwich" sign. An abnormally dilated CBD represents the top portion, the small round "olive" in the middle is the hepatic artery, and the bottom portion is the portal vein. *Image courtesy of Jacob K. Goertz, MD*. (d) Illustration showing a normal sagittal view of the portal triad: portal vein (PV), common bile duct (CBD), hepatic artery (HA). *Illustration by Laura Berg, MD*. (e) Color Doppler can be used to distinguish the CBD, which doesn't exhibit flow, from the portal vein and hepatic artery, which exhibit flow.

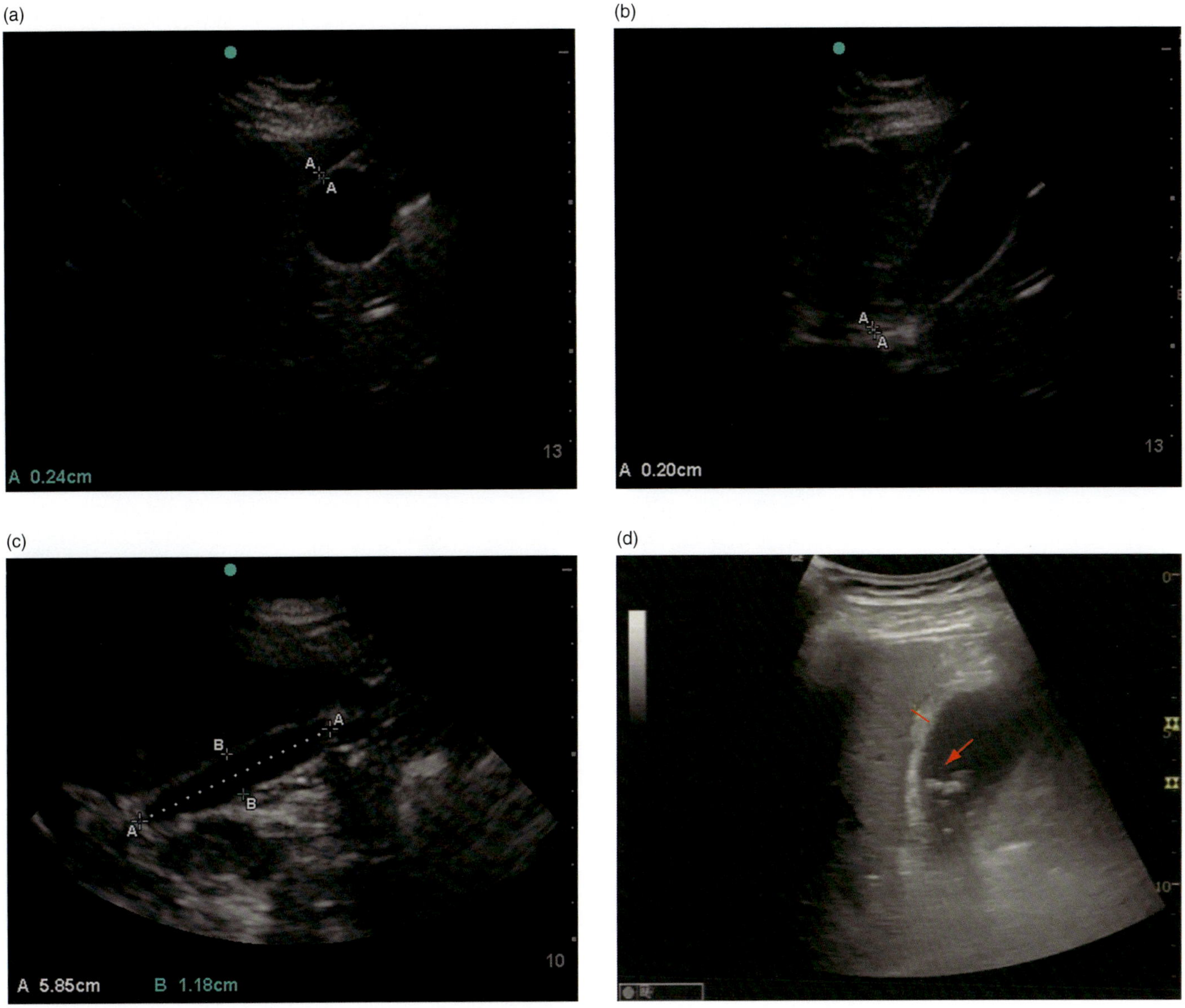

Figure 11.18 **Measurements.** (a) Measurement of the anterior gallbladder wall. (b) Measurement of the CBD. (c) Measurement of the gallbladder dimensions. (d) Gallstones (arrow) in a gallbladder demonstrating a thickened wall (solid line).

down the diaphragm and subsequently the liver and gallbladder, making them easier to locate.

✓ Distinguishing the CBD. Color Doppler can be helpful in differentiating the CBD from the surrounding vessels. The absence of flow through a structure in the portal triad makes it the CBD (Figure 11.17e).

✓ Magnify the small areas. Magnification can significantly improve localization and measurement of the portal triad.

Pathology

Cholelithiasis, choledocholithiasis

Cholelithiasis is the presence of gallstones within the gallbladder. Choledocholithiasis involves the presence of at least one stone in the CBD. This occurs in up to 20% of patients with cholelithiasis. Choledocholithiasis often causes obstruction of the biliary tree, resulting in an ascending cholangitis.

It is important to distinguish cholelithiasis from cholecystitis, which involves inflammation of the gallbladder often with the additional finding of gallstones. Sonographically, the majority of stones appear hyperechoic with dense posterior shadowing, and are mobile. In small stones less than 4 mm in diameter, this shadowing may be absent. Another finding is the "WES" sign, or "wall-echo-shadowing." The "WES" sign is seen in a contracted gallbladder that is filled with stones, producing a large amount of shadowing that prevents a thorough evaluation of the gallbladder. The anterior gallbladder wall is "the wall," the hyperechoic gallstones are "the echo," and the shadow produced from the gallstones is "the shadow" (Figure 11.19).

Cholecystitis

Cholecystitis involves the inflammation of the gallbladder, with or without the presence of stones. This inflammation may be caused by obstructing stones, polyps, sludge, or tumors.

Sonographic signs of acute cholecystitis include wall thickening, pericholecystic fluid, and, commonly, stones (Figure 11.20a). Gallbladder sludge (Figure 11.20b) may also be seen, which consists of cholesterol crystals, calcium bilirubinate pigment, and other calcium salts. Gallbladder sludge may eventually develop into stones, or disappear, depending on the causative etiology. Acute acalculous cholecystitis involves the presence of an inflamed gallbladder without stones. Certain conditions predispose patients to developing acalculous cholecystitis, including TPN. Sonographic findings of acalculous cholecystitis are the same as with cholecystitis, but without the presence of stones and shadowing. With acalculous cholecystitis, sludge may be visualized, which layers out in dependent portions of the gallbladder (Figure 11.21). Acalculous cholecystitis is the cause of gallbladder disease in up to 50% of pediatric patients.

Polyps

Polyps may commonly be visualized in an otherwise normal gallbladder (Figure 11.22). However, upon initially encountering a mass within the lumen of the gallbladder, it may be difficult to distinguish it from a gallstone. The majority of polyps do appear hyperechoic, but there is no posterior shadowing. A polyp will also be non-mobile with changes in patient positioning. A free-floating stone in the gallbladder will move around as the patient is rolled, whereas a polyp will stay stationary regardless of patient position (Figure 11.13c).

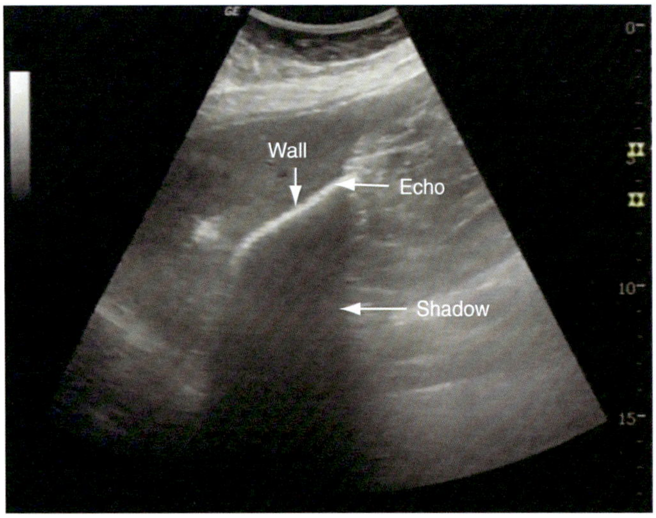

Figure 11.19 Wall-echo-shadow sign (WES). This gallbladder is filled with multiple stones, obscuring the rest of the gallbladder.

(a)

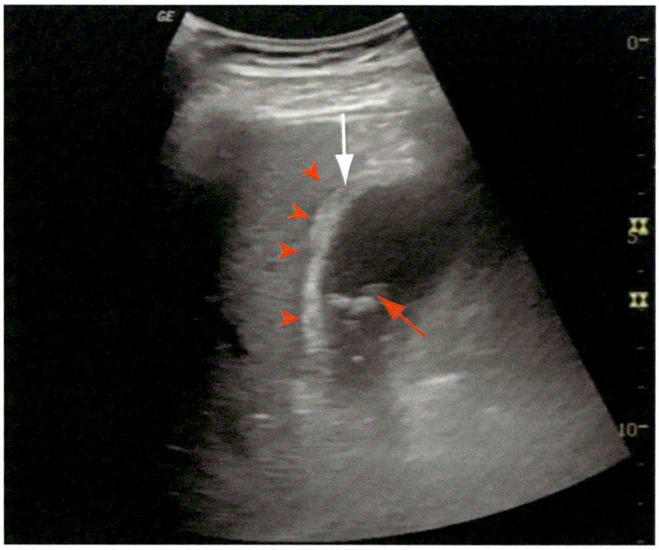

Figure 11.20 Cholecystitis. (a) Classic findings of acute cholecystitis: shadowing gallstones (red arrow), thickened anterior gallbladder wall (white arrow), and pericholecystic fluid (arrowheads).

(b)

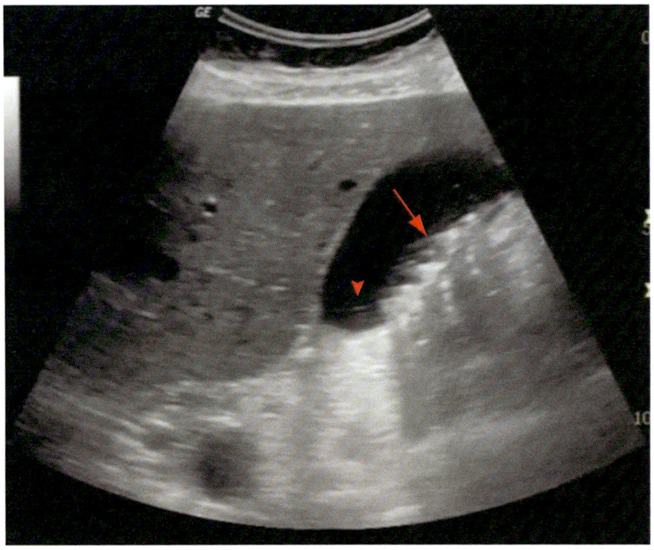

Figure 11.20 (cont.) **Cholecystitis.** (b) Gallbladder sludge (arrowhead), which appears hyperechoic without posterior shadowing. This patient also has tiny gallstones (arrow), which exhibit posterior shadowing.

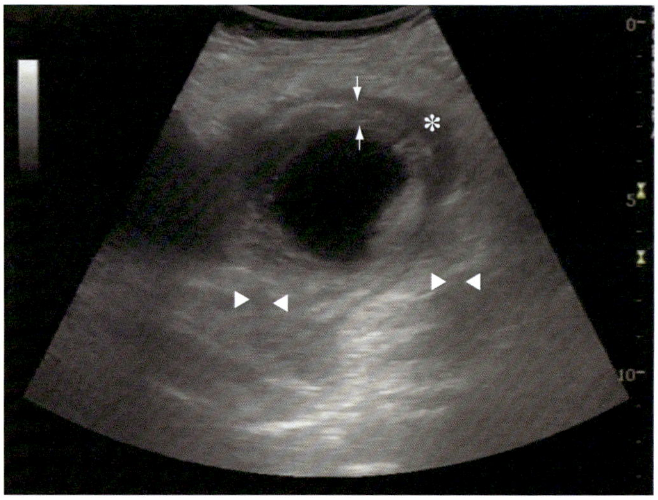

Figure 11.21 Acalculous cholecystitis. Transverse image of the gallbladder shows a thickened gallbladder wall (arrows) with surrounding pericholecystic fluid (*). The side-lobe artifact (arrowheads) can also be seen. This patient did not have any visible gallstones on thorough examination.

Gallbladder polyps are extremely rare in pediatric patients; sometimes they can be inflammatory or consist of cholesterol and triglycerides. If one encounters a patient with polyps, the patient should be followed with serial right upper quadrant ultrasounds to assess for enlargement of the polyp or the development of gallbladder disease.

Congenital disorders of the biliary tree

While it is beyond the scope of the emergency physician to diagnose congenital abnormalities of the biliary system, they may occasionally encounter a child who presents with these conditions. The most important concept is that the clinician become familiar with what is a "normal" right upper quadrant ultrasound, and what is "abnormal." When abnormalities are encountered, it is important to refer the patient for more comprehensive and definitive imaging studies. Such congenital abnormalities include biliary atresia, and Alagille syndrome (intrahepatic biliary hypoplasia), which cause obstructive jaundice in the neonate. Infants and children may also present with choledochal cysts. This involves cystic dilatations of the extrahepatic biliary system (Figure 11.23), with approximately 25%

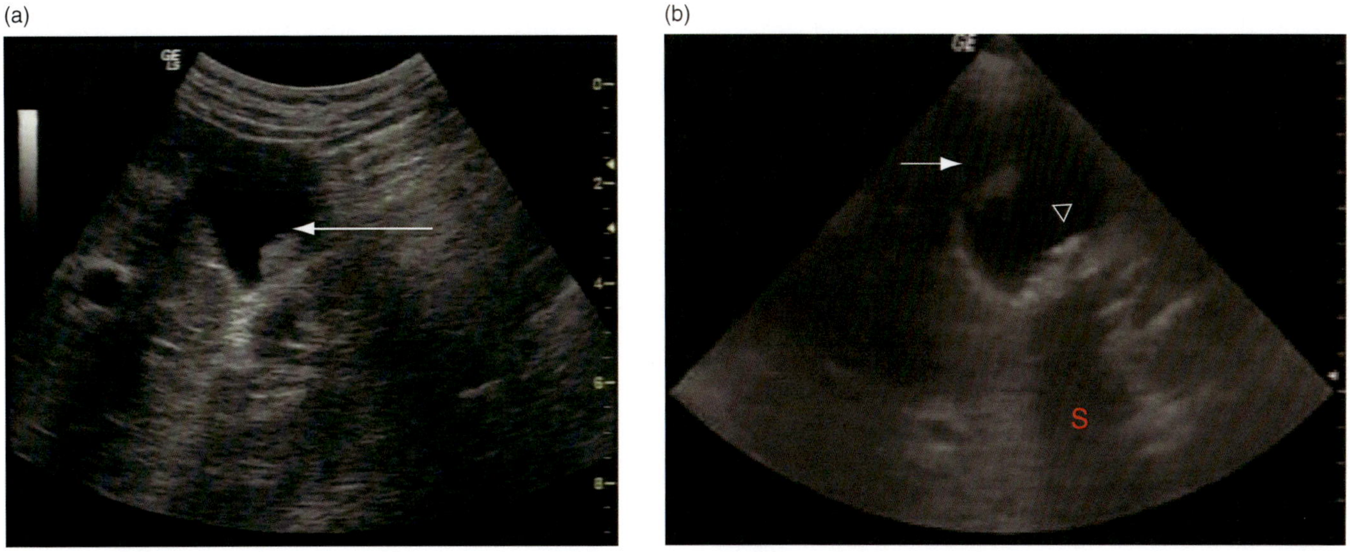

Figure 11.22 Polyp. (a) A polyp (arrow) in an otherwise normal gallbladder; note that there is no shadowing and will be no changes in position. *Image courtesy of Jacob K. Goertz, MD.* (b) A polyp arrow noted in the superior aspect of the gallbladder, with stones (arrowhead) in the posterior gallbladder, with posterior shadowing (S). *Image courtesy of St. Luke's Roosevelt Hospital Emergency Ultrasound Division.*

(a)

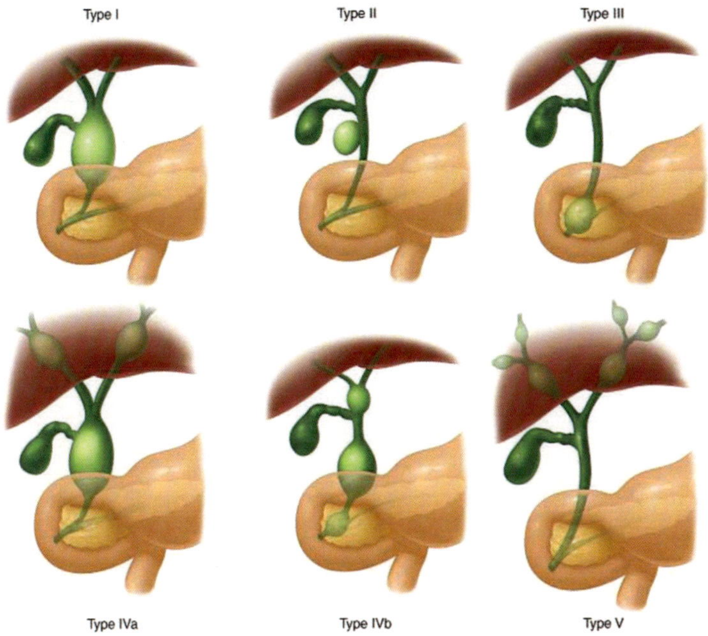

Figure 11.23 Choledochal cysts. (a) Illustration of the different classifications of choledochal cysts. © *Schwartz's Principles of Surgery* McGraw Hill 2009. (b) Ultrasound image: transverse view of the gallbladder (GB) and ductal dilatation. This is a type IV choledochal cyst. (c) Ultrasound image: longitudinal view of the gallbladder and ductal dilatation.

(b) (c)

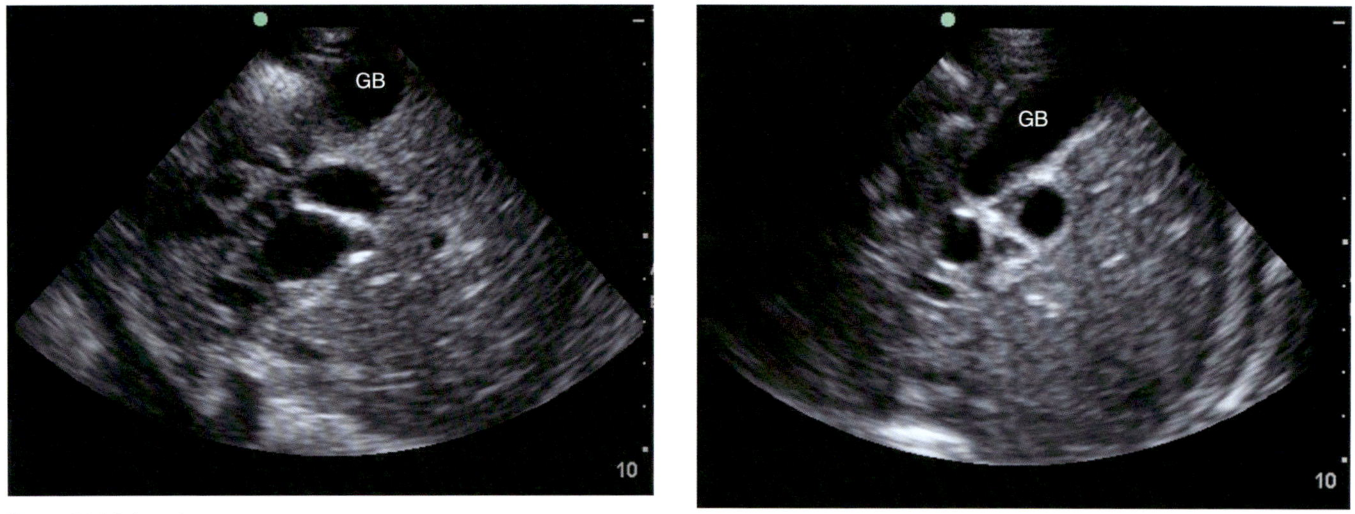

Figure 11.23 (cont.)

(a) (b)

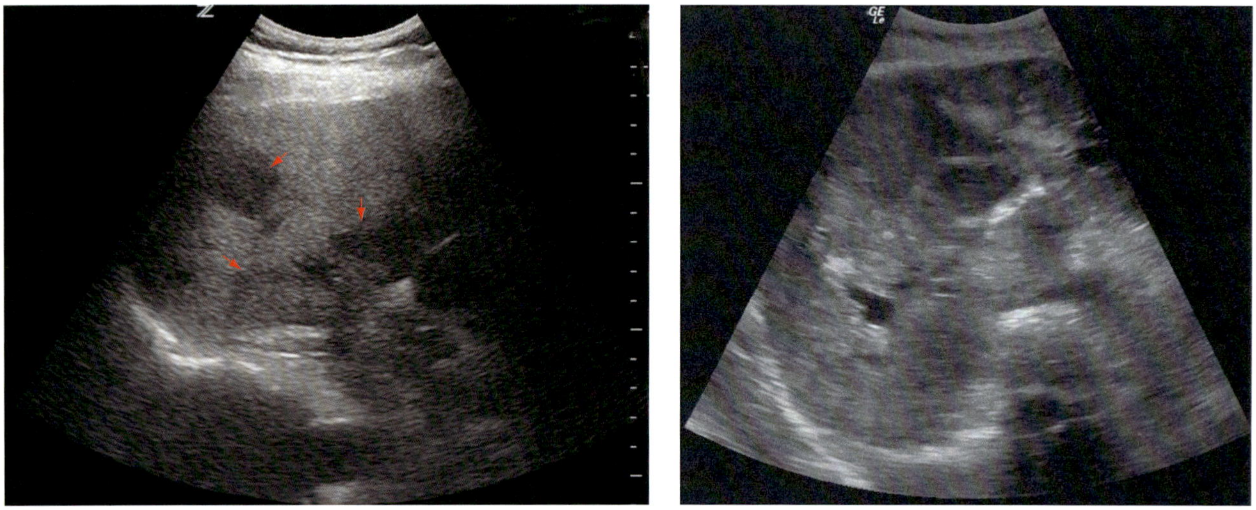

Figure 11.24 Liver infiltration. (a) The normal homogeneous appearance of the liver is interrupted by hypoechoic metastases from the patient's prior condition (arrows). (b) Multiple diffuse, hyperechoic lesions can be seen throughout the liver parenchyma in a patient with metastatic cancer.

of patients presenting in the neonatal period with cholestasis. Children may present with fever, vomiting, jaundice, and abdominal pain, which may be due to secondary pancreatitis or cholangitis (an ascending infection of the bile ducts).

Hepatic masses: tumors, abscesses, cysts

While the goal of point-of-care ultrasound is not necessarily to be comprehensive and identify malignancies, occasionally abnormalities such as these are encountered. As a result, it is crucial to refer the patient for further, formal radiographic studies. A clinician may occasionally encounter a focal abnormality within the liver. Examples of common pediatric tumors include hemangiomas, hepatoblastomas, neuroblastomas, and hepatocellular carcinomas. A hemangioma is a benign hepatic mass, primarily seen within the first six months of life. Sonograpically, there is a wide spectrum of features, which includes single or multiple hyperechoic nodules, with calcification seen in 15%. In contrast, hepatoblastomas are malignant tumors. Sonographically, they appear as solid, well-defined lesions with increased vascularity. Neuroblastomas may be found in infants. Sonographically, the liver appears enlarged, with a heterogeneous appearance. Similarly, metastatic tumors disrupt the normal homogeneous appearance of the liver (Figure 11.24). It is important always to look closely at the liver and ensure it appears uniform.

Other benign conditions such as cysts and abscesses can disrupt the normal appearance of the liver. Cysts are rare in children, but may appear as single or multiple lesions. Sonographically, they appear as well-defined anechoic structures. Abscesses may be present, and are often difficult to distinguish from hemangiomas. Sonographically, there may be single or multiple abscess cavities, with thickened walls and

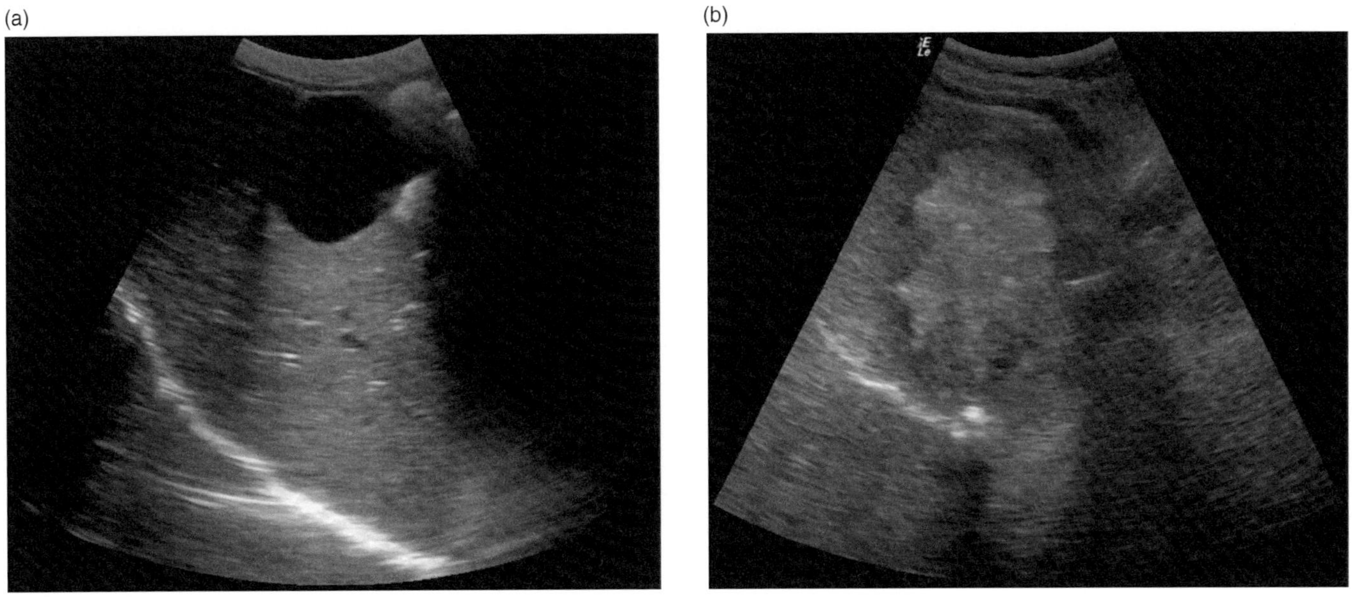

Figure 11.25

internal echoes and debris (Figure 11.25b). Particular types of lesions worldwide include hydatid cysts and amebic abscesses.

Diffuse infiltrative processes

Several conditions in childhood and adulthood may cause diffuse infiltrative diseases of the liver. Appearances of the liver may be nonspecific. Etiologies of diffuse infiltration of the liver include, but are not limited to: hepatitis, cirrhosis, fatty infiltration, portal hypertension, and veno-occlusive disease. Sonographically, an increased echogenicity of the liver may be seen with fatty infiltration and cirrhosis, while hepatitis generally causes an enlarged liver with a hypoechoic appearance.

Hydrops of the gallbladder

Hydrops of the gallbladder is an extremely rare condition, but is associated with Kawasaki disease, scarlet fever, typhoid, leptospirosis, burns, sepsis, and prolonged TPN administration. Hydrops involves the massive dilatation of the gallbladder, without associated gallbladder wall thickening, stones, or ductal dilatation (Figure 11.16). Sludge may occasionally be present (Figure 11.15). Surgery is not indicated for hydrops of the gallbladder, and it usually resolves within one to two weeks of treatment of the underlying cause.

Cases

1. A 17-year-old, obese female presents to the emergency department with four days of epigastric and right upper quadrant pain after eating large meals. She has acute intense pain that lasts for one to two hours, which is not alleviated by changes in position. She has also had a low-grade fever, nausea, and vomiting for the last two days. On examination, she does not appear jaundiced, and her abdominal examination is significant for epigastric and right upper quadrant tenderness to palpation. You are able to elicit a positive Murphy's sign. The remainder of the physical examination is normal. Laboratory studies reveal a leukocytosis (WBC: 22,000), with a normal bilirubin level. A point-of-care ultrasound is performed by the treating physician (Figure 11.26). This ultrasound image of the right upper quadrant demonstrates some classic findings of acute cholecystitis: gallstones, a thickened anterior gallbladder wall, and pericholecystic fluid.

   While gallbladder disease is uncommon in children, it must be considered in the appropriate clinical scenario. It is important to assess for the presence of stones, and for acute cholecystitis. These findings warrant surgical consultation, and inpatient admission for intravenous antibiotics.
2. A five-year-old, previously healthy female is referred from an outside hospital, with right upper quadrant pain, vomiting, and fever. They had performed a formal ultrasound that was read by the referring hospital as "acute cholecystitis with cholelithiasis," but images are unavailable for review. Shortly after arrival, the clinician performs a point-of-care ultrasound that shows multiple cystic structures with hyperechoic stones within the lumen (Figure 11.27). On further evaluation, there appears a markedly dilated biliary system with a CBD measuring 12 mm. Additional laboratory studies are obtained, which show a total bilirubin of 3.3 and a lipase of 16,340. Formal ultrasonography is obtained, followed by magnetic resonance cholangiopancreatography (MRCP). The child is diagnosed with a choledochal cyst, with cholelithiasis. The patient's pancreatitis is due to an obstructing lesion at the extrahepatic pancreatic duct.

   This case highlights the importance of recognizing "normal" from "abnormal." While it is beyond the scope of the clinician to identify specific lesions of the biliary

(a) (b)

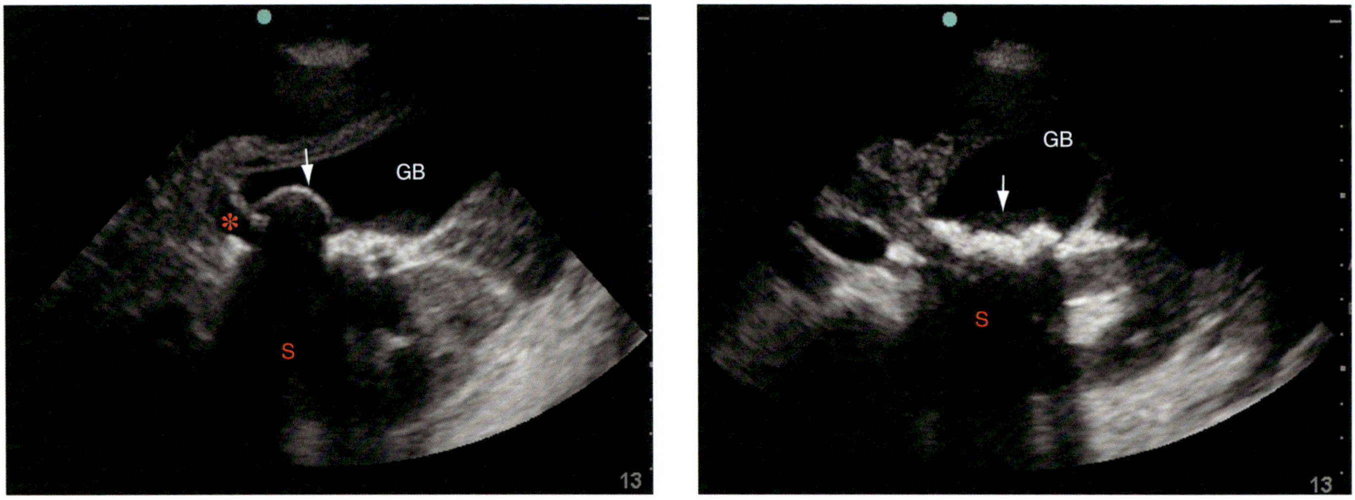

Figure 11.26 **Case 1: acute cholecystitis with cholelithiasis.** (a) Longitudinal view of the gallbladder (GB) showing hyperechoic gallstones (arrow) with posterior shadowing (S), thickened gallbladder wall, and pericholecystic fluid (*). (b) Transverse view of the gallbladder in the same patient.

(a) (b)

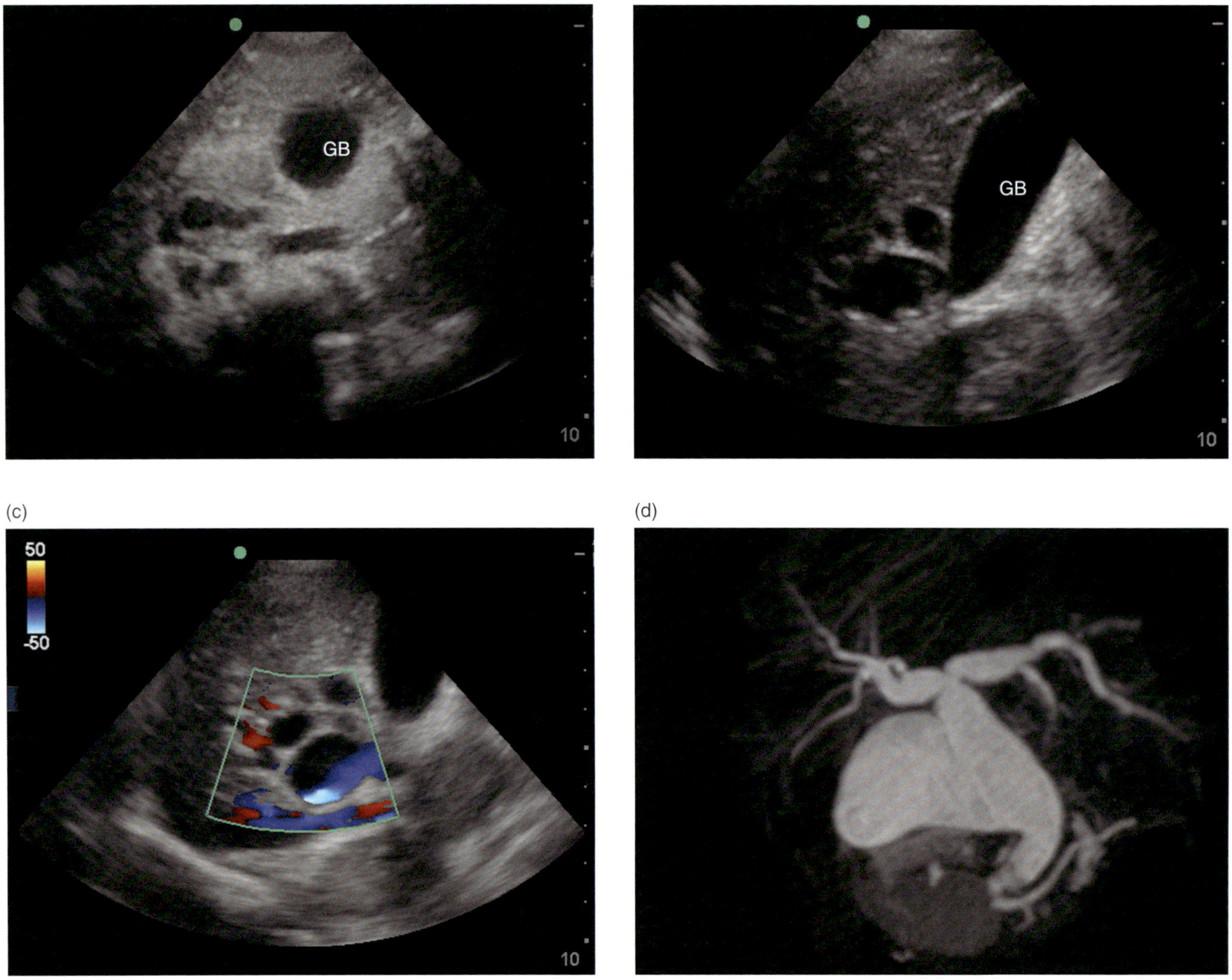

Figure 11.27 **Case 2: choledochal cyst, stones.** (a) Transverse view of the gallbladder (GB) with ductal dilatation. (b) Longitudinal view of the gallbladder (GB) and adjacent ductal dilatation. (c) Color Doppler flow helps to distinguish blood vessels from the dilated biliary ductal system. (d) An MRI three-dimensional reconstruction of the choledochal cyst. *Image courtesy of Ken Martin, MD.*

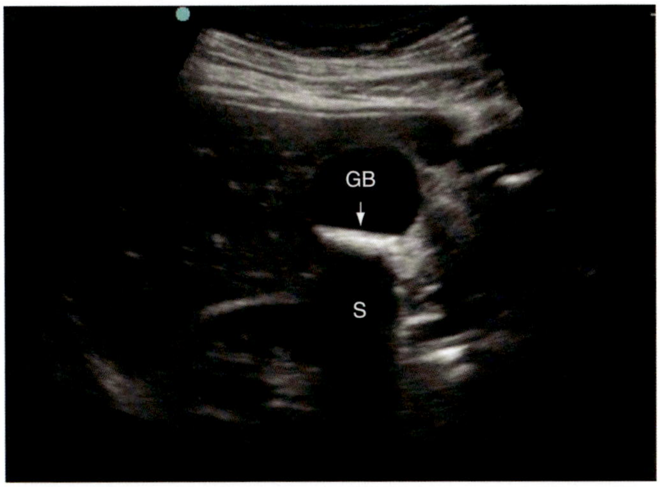

Figure 11.28 **Case 3: unexpected gallstone.** In this patient with colicky abdominal pain, given the child's age, there was concern for intussusception. Though the ultrasound scan was negative for an intussusception, the gallbladder (GB) was visualized with this gallstone (arrow), with posterior shadowing (S), when scanning at the liver edge.

tree, it is important to be aware of certain abnormalities, in order to obtain the appropriate definitive study. Though the anatomy was initially difficult to identify, the patient also had superimposed cholelithiasis and acute cholecystitis in addition to the choledochal cyst.

3. A nine-month-old male, with history of prematurity, presents with intermittent abdominal pain, vomiting, and "drawing his legs up." He has not had any fevers or grossly bloody stools. Given the clinical history, the clinician is concerned about intussusception. During an ultrasound evaluation for intussusception, a hyperechoic lesion is incidentally found within the gallbladder, which exhibits posterior shadowing (Figure 11.28). The remainder of the ultrasound evaluation is negative for intussusception.

While exceedingly rare in this age group, it is important to keep gallbladder disease on the differential diagnosis for abdominal pain. It is especially important to recognize that certain medical conditions such as sickle cell disease and cystic fibrosis predispose children to developing gallbladder disease. In this case, the child had been on prolonged TPN while in the neonatal ICU, which predisposed him to developing gallstones.

Summary/key points

1. Ultrasonography of the right upper quadrant can be challenging, but it has been proven that emergency physicians can diagnose cholecystitis and cholelithiasis accurately after focused training and practice.
2. Properly locate the gallbladder and scan completely through it in both sagittal and transverse orientations. Ensure you are not confusing it with the IVC or duodenum.
3. Ensure that you have evaluated the gallbladder for all possible signs of cholecystitis: stones, anterior wall edema, pericholecystic fluid, sludge, a sonographic Murphy's sign, and hydrops. Also, visualize the CBD for any signs of dilation. Be sure to perform measurements of the anterior gallbladder wall and the CBD.
4. Utilize all the tools at your disposal: roll the patient on the left side or nearly prone, scan on inspiration, use the phased-array transducer in between the ribs, magnify the small areas, and use color Doppler to distinguish the CBD from the surrounding vessels.
5. Acalculous cholecystitis is the cause of gallbladder disease in up to 50% of pediatric patients, and should be considered in patients with right upper quadrant pain. While gallbladder disease is rare in children, its incidence is increasing, and should be considered in the appropriate clinical scenario.

Selected references

Blaivas, M., Harwood, R. A., Lambert, M. J. (1999) Decreasing length of stay with emergency ultrasound examination of the gallbladder. *Acad Emerg Med* **6**: 1020–3.

Breyer, M. J., Giordano, M., Tinjum, B., *et al.* (2010) Emergency medicine resident performed bedside ultrasonography of the gallbladder in non-fasted healthy volunteers. *J Emerg Med* **39**(1): 65–9.

Durston, W., Carl, M. L., Guerra, W., *et al.* (2001) Comparison of quality and cost-effectiveness in the evaluation of symptomatic cholelithiasis with different approaches to ultrasound availability in the ED. *Am J Emerg Med* **19**: 260–9.

Jang, T. B., Ruggeri, W., Dyne, P., *et al.* (2010) The learning curve of resident physicians using emergency ultrasonography for cholelithiasis and cholecystitis. *Acad Emerg Med* **17**: 1247–52.

Kendall, J. L., Shrimp, R. J. (2001) Performance and interpretation of focused right upper quadrant ultrasound by emergency physicians. *J Emerg Med* **21**: 7–13.

McGahan, J. P., Phillips, H. E., Cox, K. L. (1982) Sonography of the normal pediatric gallbladder and biliary tree. *Radiology* **144**: 873–5.

Poffenberger, C. M., Gausche-Hill, M., Ngai, S., *et al.* (2012) Cholelithiasis and its complications in children and adolescents. *Pediatr Emerg Care* **28**(1): 68–76.

Rosen, C. L., Brown, D. F, Chang, Y., *et al.* (2001) Ultrasonography by emergency physicians in patients with suspected cholecystitis. *Am J Emerg Med* **19**: 32–6.

Summers, S. M., Scruggs, W., Menchine, M. D., *et al.* (2010) A prospective evaluation of emergency department bedside ultrasonography for detection of acute cholecystitis. *Ann Emerg Med* **56**(2): 114–22.

Tsung, J. W., Raio, C. C., Ramirez-Schrempp, D., *et al.* (2010) Point-of-care ultrasound diagnosis of pediatric cholecystitis in the ED. *Am J Emerg Med* **28**(3): 338–42.

Chapter 12

Male genitourinary: scrotal pain, swelling

Joshua Rempell and Andrew S. Liteplo

Objectives/indications

Acute scrotal pain makes up approximately 0.5% of all complaints presenting to the emergency department. Patients with acute scrotal pain often present a diagnostic dilemma, as the history and physical examination alone are often not enough to confidently make a timely diagnosis. Historical features of such disease processes as testicular torsion, orchitis, and epididymitis, for example, often overlap in the duration of symptoms, type of onset, clinical features, and physical examination findings.

The use of ultrasound plays an integral role in differentiating between many of these disease processes, and determining the appropriate treatment. The many benefits of ultrasound include excellent resolution of the scrotum, the lack of ionizing radiation, and it is inexpensive in comparison to other imaging modalities. Moreover, ultrasound is reliably able to distinguish testicular torsion from epididymitis. Testicular torsion is the most time-sensitive and emergent diagnosis, and prompt diagnoses may reduce the risk of testicular loss and infertility. It is also important to identify certain benign intratesticular lesions and thus spare patients from exploratory invasive surgical procedures, which were common before the current advances in scrotal ultrasound. However, it is important to note that the majority of these indications involve formal ultrasonography examinations performed in the radiology suite. As emergency physicians and intensivists become more familiar with point-of-care ultrasound, its use in making timely diagnoses in scrotal pain and swelling is a logical advance in practice, especially in those departments lacking 24-hour imaging services. Scrotal ultrasound performed by clinicians has the potential of allowing clinicians to accurately diagnose organ-threatening conditions in a timely fashion, when faced with the diagnostic dilemma of scrotal pain and swelling.

This chapter reviews the scrotal anatomy and the ultrasonographic technique in a variety of pathologic entities. Scrotal ultrasound with the use of pulsed and color Doppler modes plays an integral role in the evaluation of many disease processes that present clinically with scrotal pain and/or swelling. In addition to the anatomy and technique, this chapter focuses on the use of scrotal ultrasound in the diagnosis of testicular torsion, torsion of the appendix testes, epididymitis, hernias, hydroceles, varicoceles, tumors, and testicular trauma.

Background

Ultrasound is the imaging modality of choice in the evaluation of scrotal pain and swelling. The radiology-based literature has made it clear that ultrasound with pulsed color, and pulsed wave Doppler, is the modality of choice for the evaluation of acute scrotal pain and swelling, and is highly accurate when compared with surgical exploration. Yagil *et al.* performed a retrospective review of 620 patients who presented to the emergency department with acute scrotal erythema, swelling, or pain. All of the patients received a scrotal ultrasound with Doppler performed at the ultrasound unit in the radiology department. The authors found that the most common diagnoses were epididymitis, hydrocele, varicocele, and orchitis. Doppler ultrasound was found to be 94% sensitive and 96% specific for the diagnosis of testicular torsion. Confirming both arterial and venous blood flow is even more challenging in prepubertal patients, as the detection of testicular blood flow is inconsistent and shows variability. The sensitivities of color Doppler ultrasonography for the diagnosis of testicular torsion in prepubertal patients have been reported to be between 84% and 91%. For the diagnosis of testicular malignancy, Doppler ultrasound was 92% sensitive and 95% specific. While it is unclear how this applies to point-of-care ultrasound performed by the clinician, it does show the important role of scrotal ultrasound in the emergent evaluation of patients with testicular complaints.

There remain instances when ultrasound alone is not adequate in the evaluation of scrotal pain and swelling, and additional studies may be indicated. Testicular radionuclide scintigraphy and MRI are other imaging modalities that have been used. While more research is needed, past studies have shown a higher sensitivity and specificity of nuclear studies when compared to ultrasound. Scinitigraphy has been shown to have a sensitivity and specificity of 100% and 97% respectively. Additionally, unless a definitive diagnosis of epididymitis or orchitis can be made in boys and young men with acute scrotal pain, immediate surgical exploration may be necessary.

There is limited evidence to determine what role point-of-care ultrasound will play in the bedside evaluation of these pathologies. It is suggested that the clinician utilize point-of-care ultrasound with caution, as a screening tool. Studies on emergency physicians' use of scrotal ultrasound are limited in number, and primarily

Pediatric Emergency and Critical Care Ultrasound, ed. Stephanie J. Doniger. Published by Cambridge University Press.

consist of case reports and retrospective studies comparing its accuracy to surgical findings and radiology-performed ultrasound. A retrospective chart review of 194 patients presenting with a complaint of scrotal pain evaluated point-of-care ultrasound performed on 36 patients. Results revealed a sensitivity of 95% and specificity of 94% when compared with confirmatory studies. While the majority of studies are small and retrospective, the limited data support the notion that emergency physicians with appropriate training are able to use point-of-care ultrasonography to accurately evaluate patients presenting with acute scrotal pain.

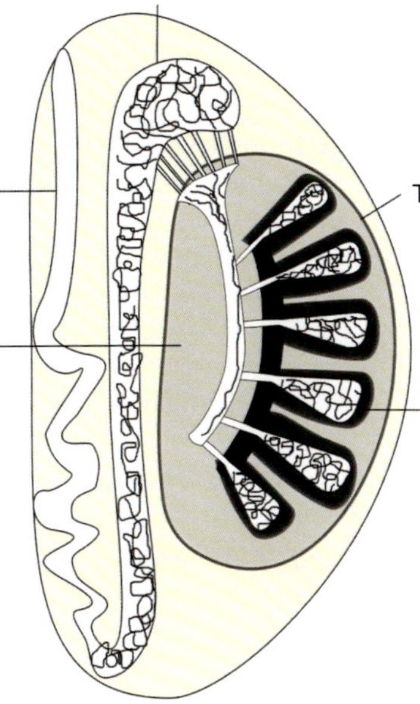

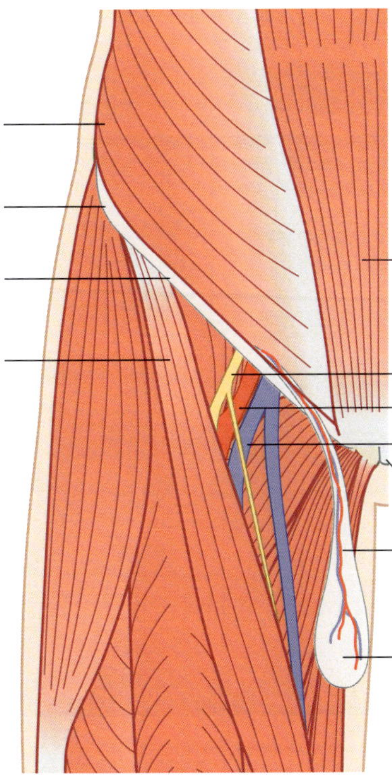

Anatomy

A normal scrotum is relatively symmetrical and oval in shape. It is important to become familiar with the contents of the scrotum: the testes, epididymis, vas deferens, spermatic cord, and appendix testes (Figure 12.1a). The scrotum is separated by a midline septum, with each half of the scrotum containing a testis and associated structures. The two testicles are usually of equal mass and volume, and are found in the vertical axis with a slight forward tilt. The left testicle is often higher than the right, since its blood flow empties into the low-pressure vena cava, rather than the high-pressure renal vein. Testicular size depends on age and state of sexual development. At birth, the testis measures approximately 1.5 cm × 1 cm × 1 cm. The adult testis measures approximately 3–5 cm × 2–4 cm × 3 cm. Normal scrotal wall thickness ranges from 2 to 8 mm. The testes are surrounded by the tunica albuginea, a dense, white, fibrous capsule. Multiple septations arise from the tunica albuginea and run through the testis to converge posteriorly to form the mediastinum testis. The mediastinum testis comprises the support for the entering and exiting testicular vessels and ducts.

Additional structures in the scrotum should be recognized. The epididymis is an extratesticular curved structure, that measures 6–7 cm in length and lies posterolateral to the testis. The tail of the epididymis turns into the vas deferens as it moves superiorly out of the scrotum. The spermatic cord consists of the vas deferens, the arteries supplying the testes, a plexus of veins, the lymphatics, and the nerves of the testes. The normal spermatic cord lies just beneath the skin and is difficult to distinguish from the adjacent soft tissues of the inguinal canal on examination or with ultrasound. Finally, the appendix testis

Figure 12.1 **Anatomy of the scrotum with blood supply.** (a) Diagram of the normal scrotal anatomy showing tunica albuginea surrounding the testis and the extratesticular epididymis. *Illustration by Laura Berg, MD.* (b) Testicular blood supply. *Artwork created by Emily Evans © Cambridge University Press* is a small ovoid structure located most commonly on the superior pole of the testis or in the groove between the testis and the head of the epididymis.

The blood supply of the testis is important to understand, in order to accurately interpret ultrasound with Doppler (Figure 12.1b). The supply of blood comes from the testicular, deferential, and cremasteric arteries. The majority of the blood flow to the testis is supplied by the testicular artery, which enters the spermatic cord at the deep inguinal ring and continues along the posterior surface of the testis. A transmediastinal arterial branch of the testicular artery is present in approximately one-half of normal testes; it courses through the mediastinum to supply the periphery of the gland. The deferential and cremasteric arteries primarily supply the epididymis and extratesticular tissues of the structures of the scrotum, but they also supply a small portion of the arterial supply to the testicle through anastomoses with the testicular artery. Venous drainage of the testes is via the pampiniform plexus of draining veins, formed around the upper half of the epididymis, and continues as the testicular vein through the deep inguinal ring. The right testicular vein empties into the IVC, while the left testicular vein empties into the renal vein.

Technique

Point-of-care questions

1. Is normal flow to the testicle present? Increased/absent?
2. Is there an abscess, tumor, or hernia present?
3. Is there a urologic emergency, as a cause of scrotal pain/ swelling?

Transducer selection and orientation

Optimal results are obtained using a linear, high-frequency (5–10 MHz) transducer with the capabilities of performing power, color, and pulsed-wave Doppler ultrasonography. If greater penetration is needed because of scrotal swelling, a lower-frequency transducer may be helpful. Power Doppler is helpful in scrotal ultrasound as, unlike color Doppler, it is insensitive to direction of flow, and more likely to register low-pressure blood flow, as that found in testicles.

The scan is begun in the longitudinal axis to the testicle, with the indicator oriented towards the patient's head. This will reveal the epididymis on the left side of the ultrasound screen (Figure 12.2a.) The testicle is then scanned through in its entirety, paying careful attention to any changes in the normally homogeneous organ. The scan is then repeated with the transducer turned 90° towards the patient's right, giving a short-axis view of the testicle (Figure 12.3a).

Patient position and preparation

Scrotal ultrasound is performed with the patient in the supine position, traditionally with the scrotum supported by a towel placed between the thighs. If a young child is anxious or difficult to control, having a parent hold him may be advantageous.

Ultrasound imaging

Scrotal ultrasound is highly dependent on the skill of the operator. The detection of blood flow, which is integral in the assessment of testicular torsion, depends on the patient's age, testicular volume, and the sensitivity of the equipment and type of Doppler used. Scanning is performed with the transducer in direct contact with the skin. The testes are examined in at least two planes, along the longitudinal (Figure 12.2b) and transverse (Figure 12.3b) axes. It is important to scan through the entire testicle so that any small areas of pathology are not missed. It is preferable to scan the unaffected scrotum first. Not only does this provide an important comparison of anatomy and blood flow, but also it helps to ease any patient anxiety regarding the ultrasound. When scanning the asymptomatic side first, the

(a) (b)

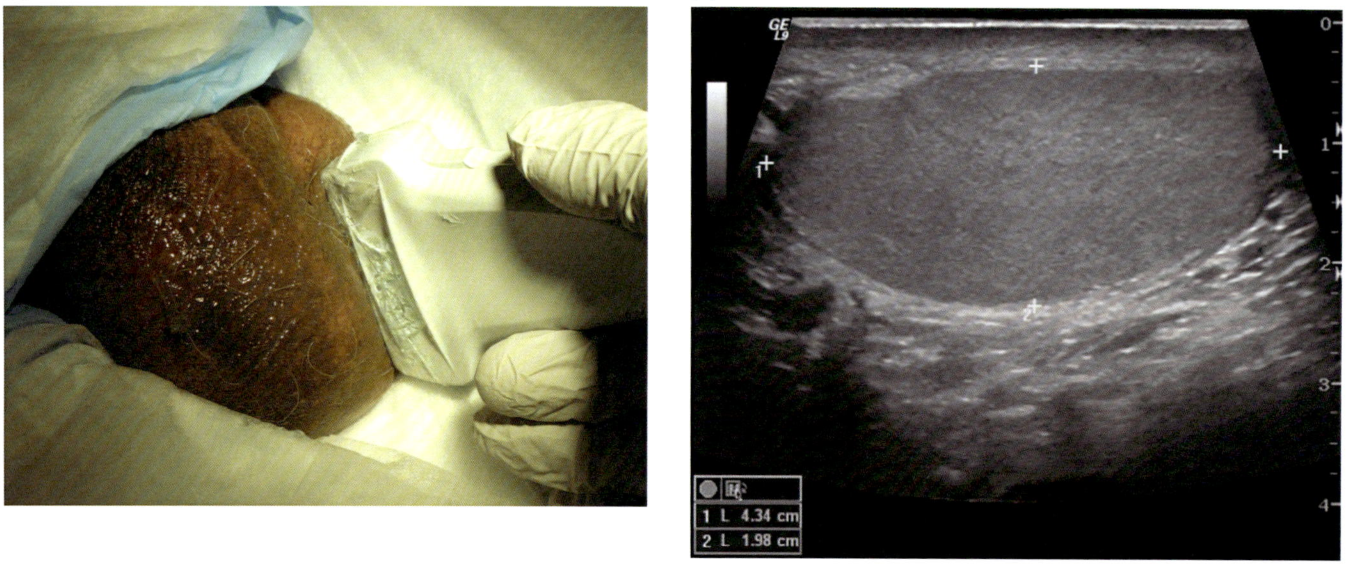

Figure 12.2 Scrotal imaging, sagittal view. (a) Transducer placement for the sagittal view with indicator towards the patient's head. (b) Normal right testis in the sagittal view. Note the homogeneity of the testicular tissue.

(a)

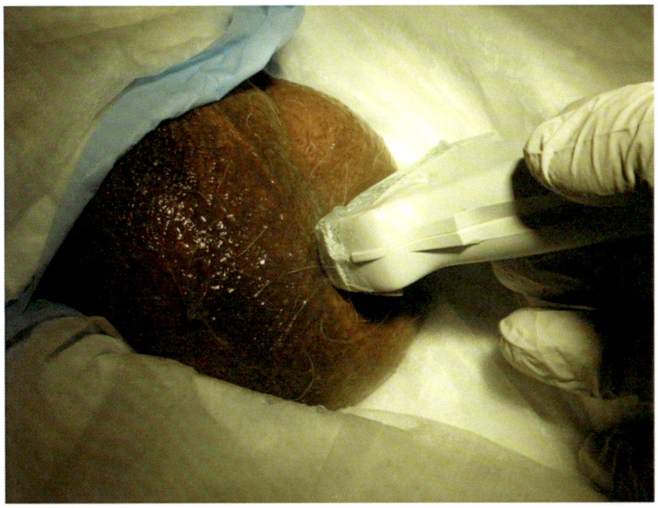

(b)

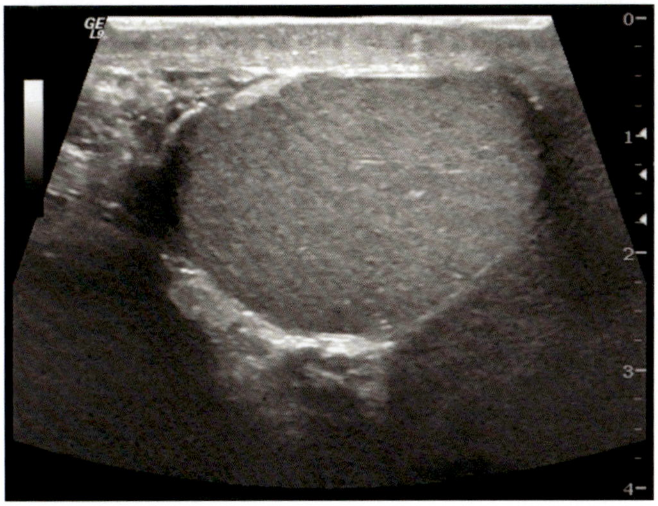

(c)

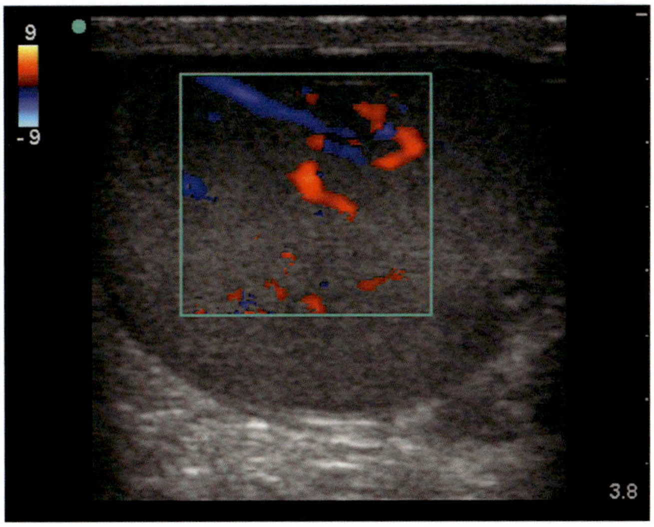

Figure 12.3 Scrotal imaging, transverse view. (a) Transducer placement for the transverse view, with the indicator towards the patient's right side. (b) Normal testis in the transverse view. (c) Color Doppler flow to the testis in the transverse view.

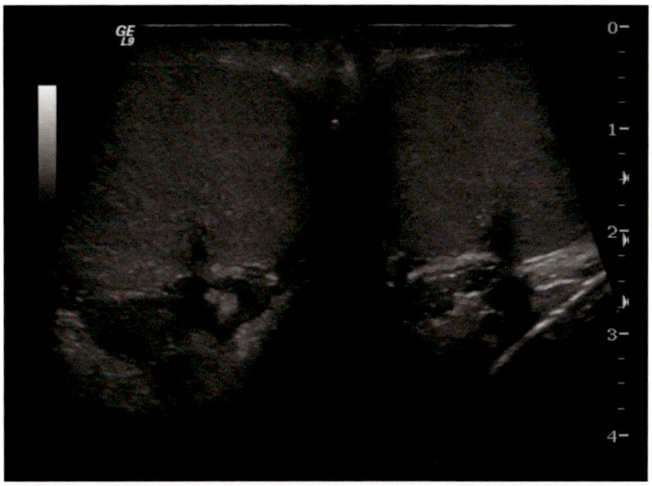

Figure 12.4 Scrotal imaging, "buddy" view. Transverse view showing both testes side-by-side in a single image, allowing for direct comparison.

operator should set the grayscale and Doppler gain settings, in order to allow the highest sensitivity to detect blood flow with the least amount of artifact (Figure 12.3c). It is also helpful to obtain one image that contains both testicles side by side in the transverse or short-axis, also referred to as the "buddy" view (Figure 12.4). This allows for a more direct comparison of the size and echogenicity between the two testes and epididymis. The structures within the scrotal sac are also examined to detect extratesticular masses or other abnormalities. In patients presenting with palpable masses or nodules, the scan should include the region of concern. A finger may be placed beneath the nodule and the transducer placed directly over the nodule for scanning.

The normal testis on ultrasound has a homogeneous appearance, and is composed of uniformly distributed medium-level echoes (Figure 12.2b, 12.3b). Its echogenicity is often compared with that of the liver or the thyroid gland. However, prepubertal testes typically have lower echogenicity than that of adults. The mediastinum testis is sometimes seen as a linear echogenic band extending through the center of the testicle in a caudo-cranial direction (Figure 12.5a). The epididymis is normally isoechoic or slightly hyperechoic to the testis. The epididymal head can often be distinguished from the rest of the testis as it often appears slightly brighter and is located atop the superior pole of the testis. The body of the epididymis is usually isoechoic and indistinguishable from the surrounding tissue (Figure 12.5b,c). The appendix testis is normally hidden by the epididymal head and often not seen by ultrasound, unless surrounded by anechoic fluid in such cases as a hydrocele (Figure 12.5d). The layers covering the scrotum are normally indistinguishable by ultrasonography, and are seen as a single echogenic stripe. In some cases of testicular torsion, a rotated spermatic cord may be visualized.

Ultrasound imaging: Doppler

An integral part of scrotal ultrasound is the use of power and spectral Doppler. Testicular perfusion can be evaluated with

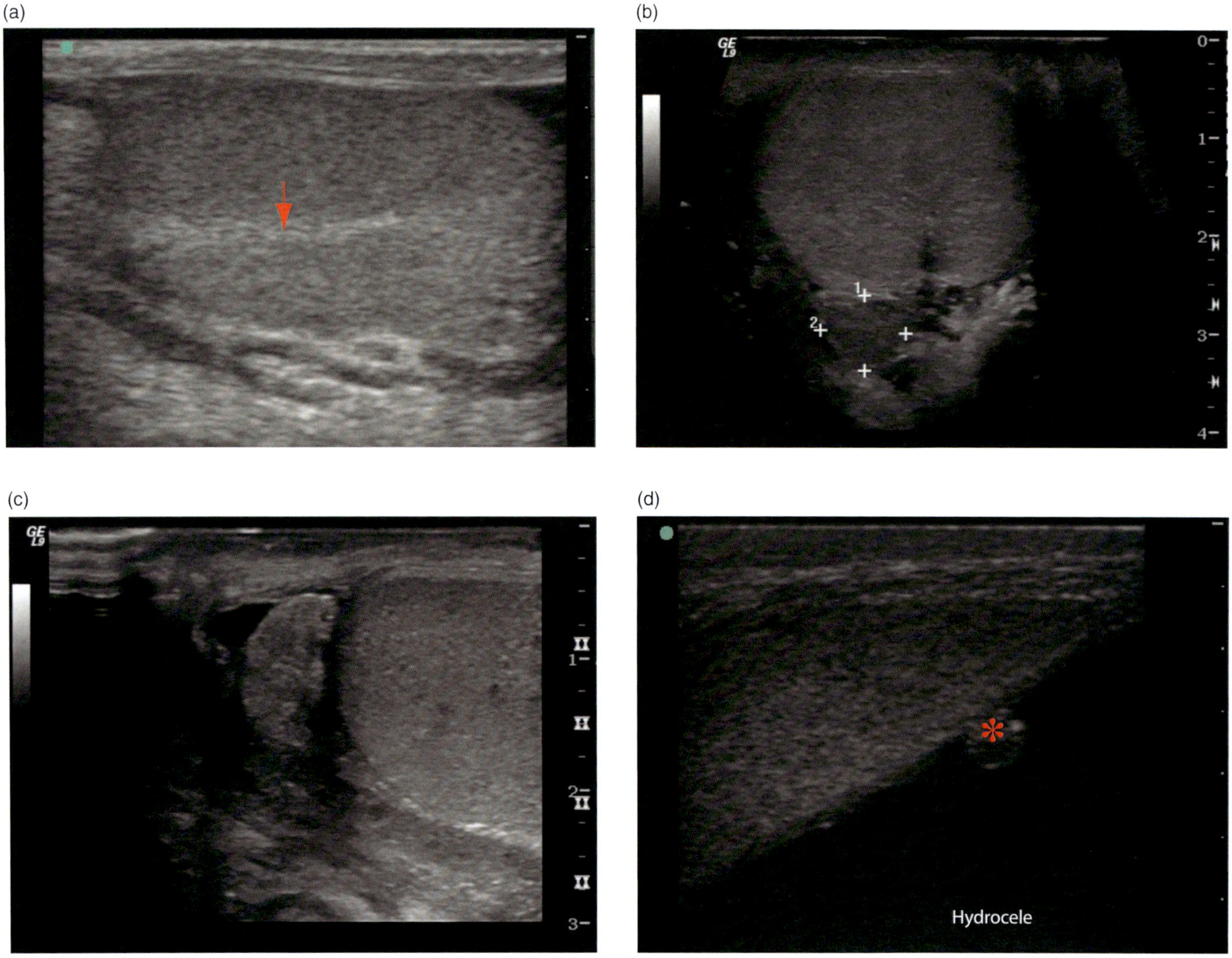

Figure 12.5 Normal structures within the scrotum. (a) The hyperechoic line extending horizontally is the mediastinum testis (arrow). (b) A view of a normal testicle showing the epididymis body and tail (calipers), in the transverse view. (c) The epididymis in sagittal orientation. (d) A normal appendix testis (*), seen in the presence of a hydrocele.

power, color, or pulsed-wave Doppler and is easily detected in both normal and pathologic testes. One of the most challenging aspects of scrotal ultrasound is confirming both arterial and venous blood flow. The failure to confirm the presence of both arterial and venous blood flow can lead to false-negative ultrasound examinations, when assessing for testicular torsion (Figure 12.6a,b). It is also important to recognize that flow is much more difficult to detect in prepubertal children and infants. Prepubertal boys have smaller testicular vessels and lower blood-flow velocities. The use of higher-frequency transducers and more careful examination may be necessary to detect blood flow. In the pediatric patient, it may be difficult to detect blood flow even in the normal testis.

The evaluation of blood flow is a key aspect in the diagnosis of testicular torsion, as well as in diagnosing epididymitis, and orchitis. Higher power gains are more likely attained with power Doppler, yielding a higher sensitivity in detecting blood flow than with color Doppler (Figure 12.7). While power Doppler is helpful in detecting blood flow and comparing the two testes, spectral or pulsed-wave Doppler is becoming the modality of choice. Pulsed-wave Doppler is able to distinguish between venous and arterial flow, which is essential in assessing for testicular torsion. The assessment of blood flow, in general, must be interpreted with caution. In situations of ongoing torsion and detorsion or with spontaneous detorsion, as the testicle regains its blood supply an increased blood flow may be seen and interpreted as a false-negative finding for testicular torsion. This increased blood flow must be differentiated from the hyperemia seen in inflammatory and infectious etiologies. In these cases, serial clinical and ultrasound examinations are essential, and the patient should still be evaluated for potential surgical management.

Scanning tips

Pitfalls

- Hyperemia may be seen with spontaneous detorsion and even in a necrotic testis. This may be mistaken for the hyperemia seen with epididymitis.

(a) (b)

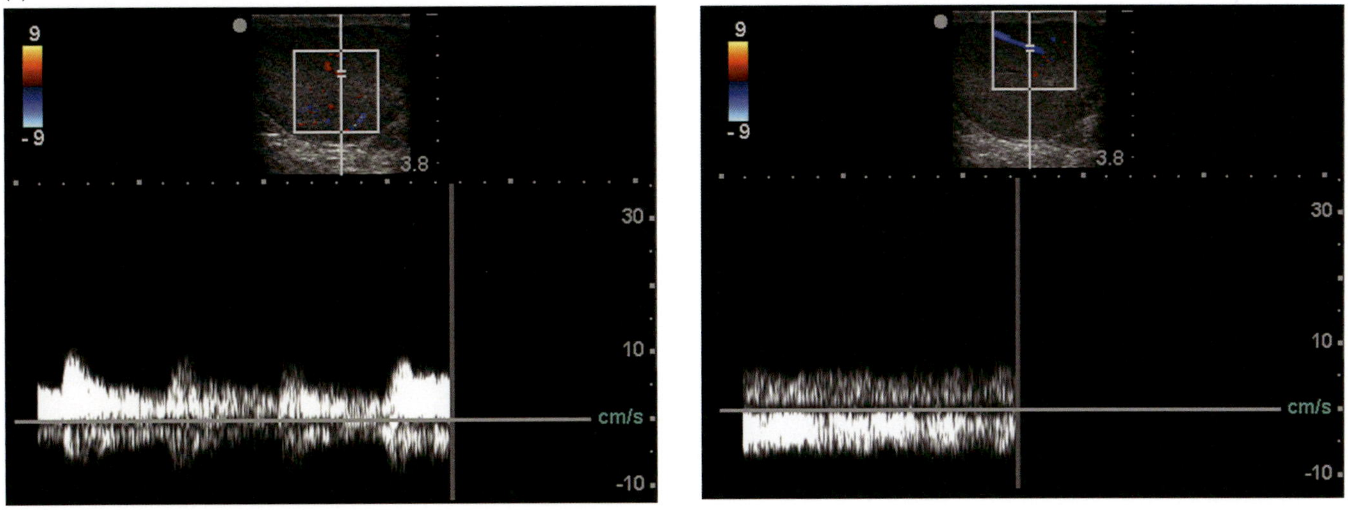

Figure 12.6 Doppler with arterial and venous waveforms. (a) Spectral Doppler showing the arterial waveform, which is more pulsatile than the (b) venous waveform, showing low continuous flow.

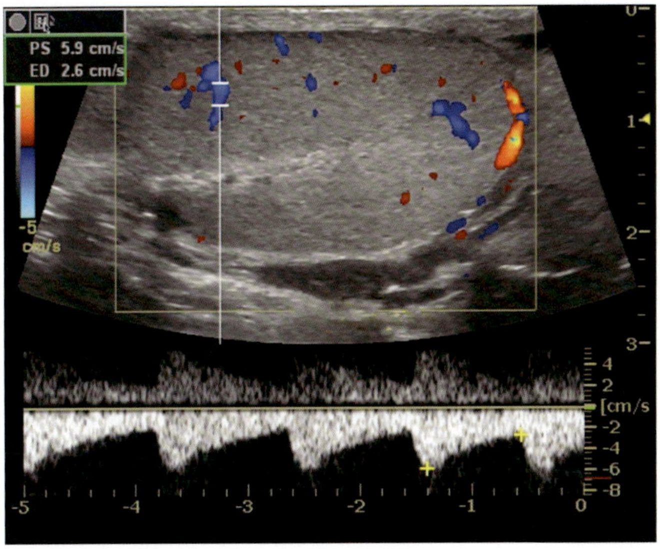

Figure 12.7 Doppler scanning of a normal testis. Sagittal view of a homogeneous right testicle showing both color and pulsed wave Doppler.

- There are reports of false-negative studies for torsion in cases of decreased blood flow in both testes, and in cases of incomplete or intermittent torsion where there is preserved blood flow.
- Failure to confirm the presence of both arterial and venous blood flow can lead to false-negative ultrasound examinations when assessing for testicular torsion in the patient presenting with a painful scrotum.
- Relying solely on a point-of-care ultrasound to rule in or rule out testicular torsion: the majority of portable ultrasound machines do not have high enough power to adequately assess for venous and arterial blood flow.

Tips to improve scanning

✓ It is important to become familiar with the anatomy of the testis, the surrounding structures, and the blood flow to the testicles.

✓ Start by scanning the unaffected side. Evaluate the testes in both longitudinal and transverse views and be sure to fan through the entire testicle.

✓ When a mass or nodule is suspected, place a finger underneath the mass and scan directly over the suspicious region.

✓ One of the most challenging aspects of diagnosing testicular torsion is detecting both venous and arterial blood flow. It is important to calibrate the Doppler settings in order to maximize the sensitivity to detect blood flow, without creating artifact.

✓ Use power Doppler and pulsed-wave Doppler whenever available, in order to evaluate for the presence of both arterial and venous blood flow to the testicle.

Pathology

Testicular torsion

Testicular torsion is the twisting of the testicle around the spermatic cord, leading to the blockage of vascular flow, and is the most important diagnosis that must be excluded emergently, since any delay in treatment is associated with increased risk of testicular loss and infertility. This can even occur in neonates. Of the cases of testicular torsion that occur in the neonatal population, 70% occur prenatally and 30% occur post-natally. The physical examination will often reveal a loss of the cremasteric reflex. However, it is important to check the cremasteric reflex on the unaffected side, since some patients do not have a cremasteric reflex on either side at baseline. Patients may also present with a tender, firm testicle that may be higher riding than the asymptomatic testicle. The twisting around the spermatic cord can leave the testicle in the transverse position. Following the twisting of the spermatic cord, initially, the venous return is blocked; with ongoing torsion, arterial obstruction develops, ultimately leading to ischemia and necrosis of the testicle. The duration of vascular

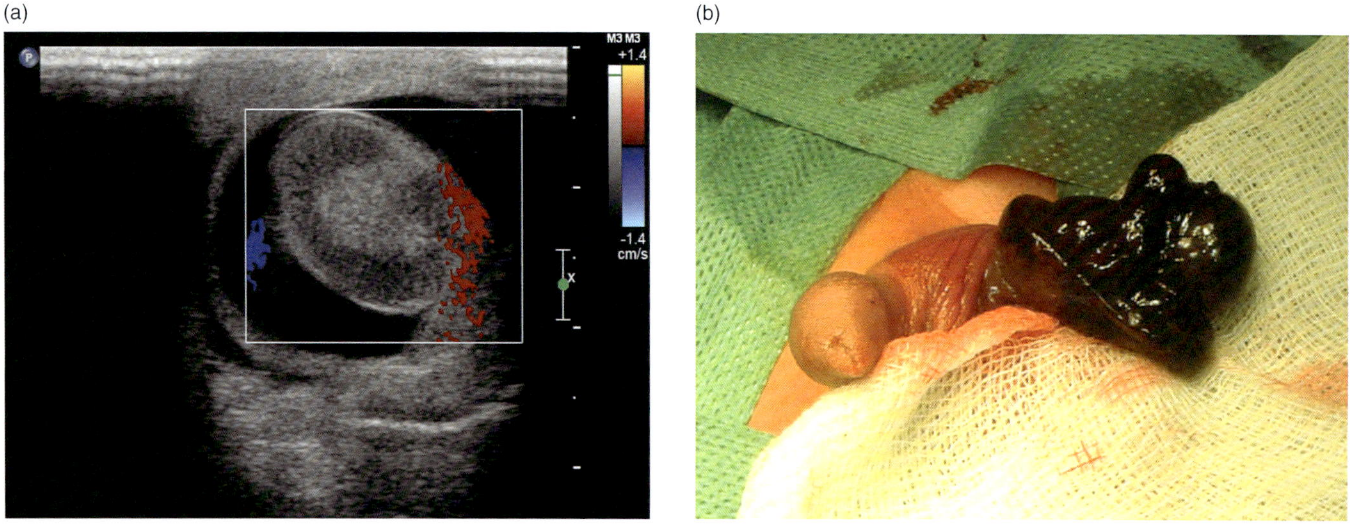

Figure 12.8 Neonatal testicular torsion. (a) The Doppler flow of the left testicle of a newborn, with absent blood flow in the intratesticular arteries and severely decreased venous blood flow. (b) Finding of testicular infarction at surgery with a black testicle and infarcted epididymis. *Images courtesy of Mahmoud Elbarbary, MD MSc PhD.*

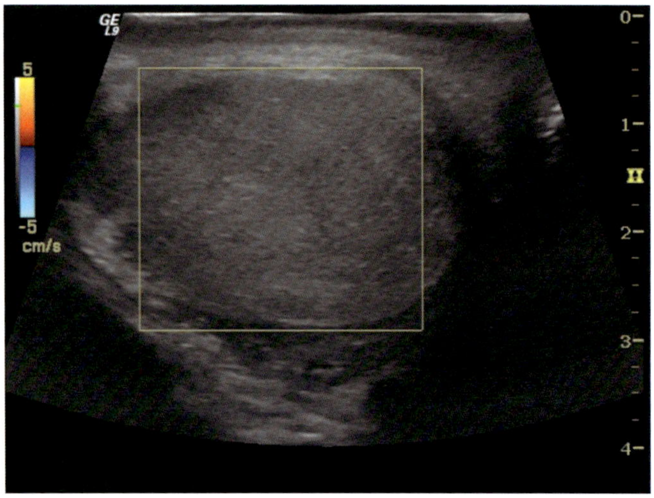

Figure 12.9 Testicular torsion. Heterogeneous-appearing testis, without blood flow, using color Doppler.

obstruction is associated with the salvage rate of the testicle. Typical testicular salvage rates are quoted at between 80 and 100% if surgery is performed within 5–6 hours of the onset of pain, 70% if surgery is performed within 6–12 hours, and only 20% if performed within 12–24 hours. There is a nearly universal loss of the testicle if torsion is left untreated for 24 hours or longer.

Ultrasound remains the gold standard in the evaluation for a possible testicular torsion. The sensitivity of ultrasound diagnosis is 90–100%, with specificity approaching 90%. Ultrasound findings will depend on the stage of the torsed testicle. In the early stages of torsion, the more compliant veins are obstructed before arterial blood flow. This leads to early vascular engorgement and edema of the testicle. Within the first six hours of torsion, there are several changes seen. Initially the testis becomes enlarged with a normal echogenicity and later becomes heterogeneous and hypoechoic. Once it has become hypoechoic, the testis may no longer be salvageable. Over time, the testicle will become even more hypoechoic and the overall size of the testicle will increase due to edematous changes. Thus, comparing the echogenicity and size of the two testicles side to side is of utmost importance.

In torsion, the use of color or pulsed-wave Doppler is essential. In the early stages when only venous return is obstructed, it is possible to see flow on power Doppler and assume there is no torsion. However, careful examination with pulsed-wave Doppler will reveal that venous waveforms are absent while arterial waveforms are present. This is a critical distinction to identify, and one that can be easily missed. Thus, in early or partial torsion, pulsed-wave Doppler may reveal arterial but no venous waveforms. Partial torsion or cases of torsion/detorsion pose additional challenges. For complete arterial occlusion to occur, there must be torsion of at least 540°. With an incomplete torsion, of 360° or less, it is possible to see dampened arterial waveforms, which may be mistaken for venous waveforms. Therefore it is not sufficient to see only what appear to be venous waveforms, as these may represent dampened arterial pressures as in the case of partial torsion. In cases of subacute or chronic torsion, color flow Doppler shows no flow in the testicle, but an increased flow in the paratesticular tissues, including the epididymis (Figure 12.8). There is also enlargement of the testis, and it takes on a heterogeneous echogenicity due to vascular congestion, hemorrhage, and infarction. Other indicators of subacute or chronic torsion include the presence of scrotal wall thickening and a reactive hydrocele (Figure 12.9).

Torsion of the appendix testes

The normal scrotum has several vestigial appendages that can also twist and become ischemic, resulting in acute scrotal pain. The most common is torsion of the appendix testis, which occurs between 7 and 14 years of age. The appendix testis is a small structure that is a remnant of the paramesonephric duct. It is located on the superior aspect of the testicle, between the testis and the epididymis. With torsion of the appendix testes, there is ischemia and eventually necrosis. However, torsion of the appendix testes has not been shown to affect fertility. It may however, lead to inflammation of the overlying epididymis head, leading to epididymitis in prepubertal boys. On physical examination, torsion of the appendix testes often leads to a hard, tender, 2–3 mm nodule at the superior aspect of the testicle. The cremasteric reflex is often intact. One may occasionally appreciate the "blue dot" sign, which refers to the blue appearance of the ischemic or black appendix with transillumination of the scrotum. This, however, is not a reliable indicator of a torsed appendix testis.

Ultrasound examination may reveal an avascular hypoechoic mass next to a normally perfused testis and surrounded by an area of increased color flow. However, depending on the location of the appendix testis, it may not be visualized on ultrasound unless it is outlined by fluid from a hydrocele.

Epididymitis

Epididymitis is the inflammation or infection of the epididymis. It is a common cause of acute scrotal pain in adolescent boys and adults, and the most common intrascrotal inflammatory disease. Nearly one-half of cases of epididymitis arise in men between the ages of 20 and 29 years, though it affects children and men of all ages. The epididymis becomes infected when organisms travel retrograde from the bladder or prostate via the vas deferens. The organism involved in the infection depends largely on the age and sexual activity of the patient. In sexually active men, many cases are due to sexually transmitted organisms such as *Chlamydia trachomatis* and *Neisseria gonorrhoeae*. In prepubertal boys, the majority of cases are due to viruses or urinary tract pathogens. If left untreated, epididymitis can lead to orchitis, or infection of the testicle itself. Epididymitis can also lead to a testicular abscess and, rarely, systemic infections. Epididymitis often presents with scrotal pain that is of more gradual onset compared to torsion, though this is an unreliable indicator of epididymitis. In patients with sexually transmitted diseases (STDs), urinary symptoms and urethral discharge are found in approximately one-third of cases. On physical examination, the epididymis may be palpated as an enlarged, tender structure separate from the testis coursing along the posterior aspect of the testis. Later in the disease process, the pain and tenderness spreads to the adjacent testis. The scrotum may become edematous, erythematous, and tender. The diagnosis of epididymitis and orchitis based on history and physical examination alone is unreliable.

Scrotal ultrasound plays a prominent role in distinguishing epididymitis from testicular torsion. The affected and unaffected sides should be compared to each other, to evaluate for differences in echogenicity and blood flow. In epididymitis, ultrasonography shows enlargement of the epididymis with decreased echogenicity, due to associated edema. Other findings may include a reactive hydrocele, though this is not specific

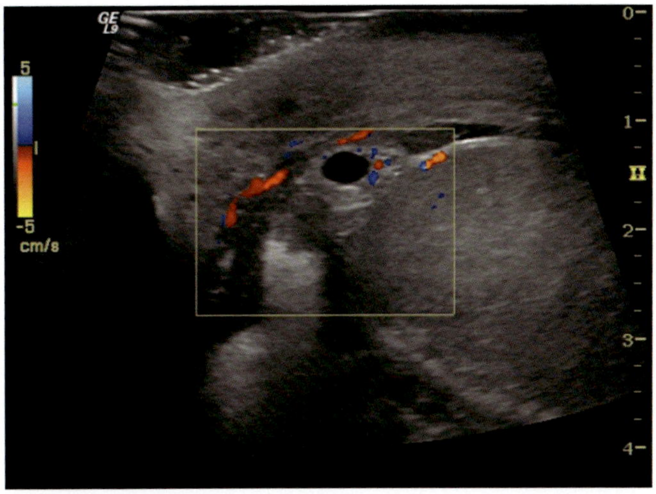

Figure 12.10 Epididymitis. The sagittal view, showing an enlarged and heterogeneous-appearing epididymis with increased blood flow.

to epididymitis. When the infection has spread to the testis, ultrasonography may show testicular enlargement, heterogeneous testicular echogenicity, and increased testicular blood flow. These grayscale ultrasound findings, however, are not specific to epididymitis or orchitis (Figure 12.10). Most importantly, the use of Doppler may distinguish epididymitis from testicular torsion. Increased blood flow to the epididymis using Doppler is a well-established criterion for the diagnosis of epididymitis. Grayscale images may be normal or nonspecific, and hyperemia is the key diagnostic finding on ultrasound using color or power Doppler. Analysis of the spectral waveform is also helpful, since inflammation of the epididymis leads to decreased vascular resistance compared with the healthy scrotum. However, it is important to remember that using Doppler to distinguish testicular torsion from epididymitis or orchitis can be misleading. While increased blood flow is usually associated with infection, as with epididymitis or orchitis, hyperemia may transiently be seen in testicular torsion immediately following spontaneous detorsion. If there is doubt, serial examinations and correlation with symptoms will decrease the likelihood of misinterpreting hyperemia following detorsion, and allow the two entities to be differentiated.

Scrotal infection

Infection of the scrotum itself is fairly uncommon and usually associated with diabetes mellitus. The major concern where ultrasonography may play a role is in the diagnosis of a scrotal abscess or Fournier's gangrene. Scrotal abscesses are focal infections involving the skin, typically originating from an infected hair follicle, but they may also originate from the internal contents of the scrotum such as the testis or epididymis. Fournier's gangrene is a polybacterial infection of the scrotum that typically originates from the skin, rectum, or urethra/prostate. It is a rapidly progressing infectious process that leads to necrosis and is a surgical emergency. In cases of scrotal abscesses, ultrasonography will show a focal fluid collection. It is important to determine if such sites are associated with internal scrotal pathology such as an abscess inside the scrotum (Figure 12.11). Sonographic findings of a Fournier's gangrene consist of skin edema throughout the affected area. Gas appears as areas of "dirty" shadowing that can be seen even in small amounts.

Testicular trauma

Trauma to the scrotum can result in damage to the testis or the peritesticular structures. Trauma is a common cause of acute scrotal pain, and can result from assault, athletic injury, or motor vehicle collisions. Trauma can cause contusions, lacerations, hemorrhage, testicular fracture, or even testicular rupture. The goal of scrotal ultrasound in trauma is to evaluate for damage to the testis. When rupture of the testis occurs, fertility is potentially compromised and early exploration can result in improved outcomes. Point-of-care ultrasound will typically show irregular borders when testicular rupture has occurred. Any abnormalities seen within the testis in the context of trauma should be considered rupture until proven otherwise. Surrounding the testicle, there will often be an associated hydrocele, a hypoechoic area or areas in the testicle, and scrotal thickening. An actual fracture line may be seen in only a minority of cases (Figure 12.12). Trauma can also lead to testicular torsion. Therefore, blood flow must be carefully evaluated through the use of Doppler ultrasound in all cases of testicular trauma.

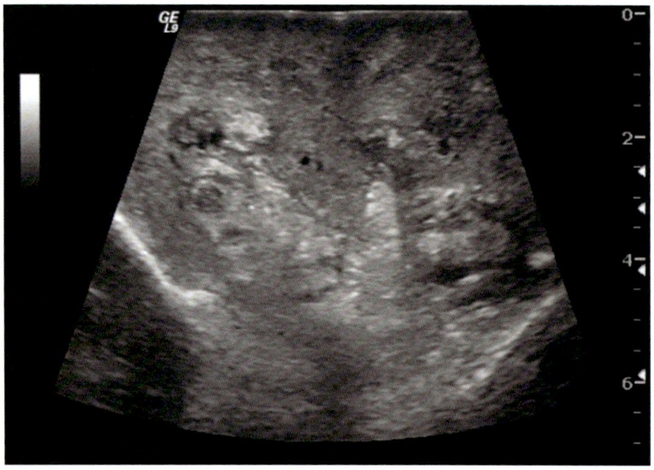

Figure 12.11 Scrotal abscess. Areas of anechoic texture superior to the testis are visualized within the scrotum of a patient with diabetes mellitus. Scanning is performed superior to the testes.

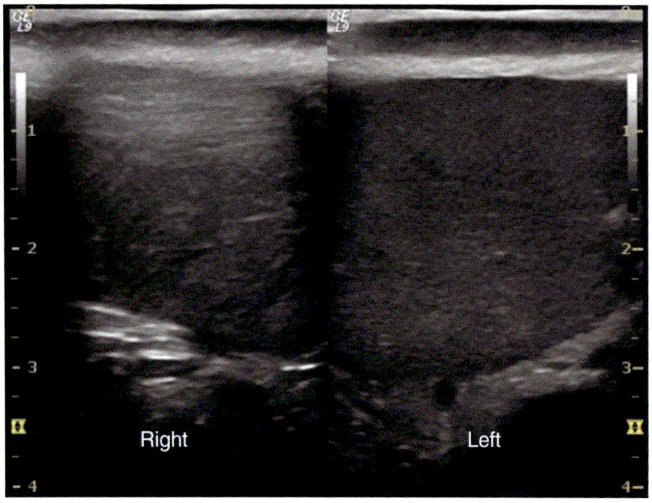

Figure 12.12 Testicular fracture. In comparison to the unaffected left testis, the right testis appears heterogeneous, with a small hydrocele, in the context of trauma. This image shows the importance of direct comparison between the two testicles, in the transverse views.

Scrotal masses: hernias, varicoceles, and tumors

Scrotal masses may be accompanied by testicular pain, but a painless mass is more common. The initial determination of a scrotal mass as intratesticular or extratesticular is important, since the majority of malignant tumors are intratesticular. Testicular cancer is the primary cancer affecting young men, and scrotal ultrasound is extremely sensitive in its diagnosis.

Hernias

The most common extratesticular scrotal masses are inguinal hernias, cysts of the epididymis, and varicoceles. Herniation of bowel can develop suddenly and present with significant pain. Most commonly, herniation into the scrotum involves bowel, though it can also commonly include omentum. Ultrasonography can be of critical help when the onset of pain and swelling is acute. Hernias have a variable appearance depending on luminal contents. Bowel hernias containing air or solid stool may appear hyperechoic with posterior shadowing

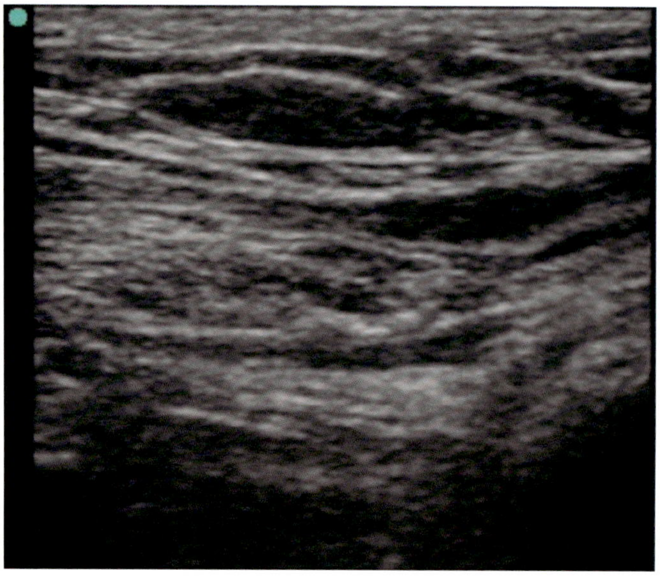

Figure 12.13 Hernia. Ultrasound image showing bowel contents within the inguinal canal, just superior to the upper portion of the scrotum. Bowel contents appear as a finger-like projection, and appear hypoechoic. Bowel extends from the left side of the image to the right side, towards the testes. When viewed in real time, the bowel wall should be examined for peristalsis and movement with cough or Valsalva maneuver.

(Figure 12.13). Peristalsis is often visualized and confirms the diagnosis of bowel herniation. The use of color or power Doppler is helpful to identify flow in the bowel wall, supporting continued perfusion to the bowel. However, a significant increase in blood flow to the bowel wall may represent early strangulation. Studies have shown that identifying a dilated, akinetic loop of bowel on scrotal ultrasonography is associated with a strangulated hernia.

Varicoceles

Varicoceles refer to dilation of the veins of the pampiniform plexus located in the spermatic cord. They are seen in up to 15% of healthy adult men, and 40% of infertile men. The majority of cases are left sided, due to the longer left testicular vein, its angle of entry in the left renal vein, and because of its greater risk of compression by the left renal vein. Patients in their late teens or early 20s with a varicocele may present after discovering a scrotal mass during a testicular self-examination. On ultrasonography, varicoceles appear as multiple, dilated, serpiginous veins in the spermatic cord and around the epididymis, with diameters larger than 2 mm (Figure 12.14). Using color or power Doppler, flow in these veins is slow, and low-flow settings must be used to detect the flow using Doppler. They will often enlarge during the Valsalva maneuver and will show reversal of blood flow.

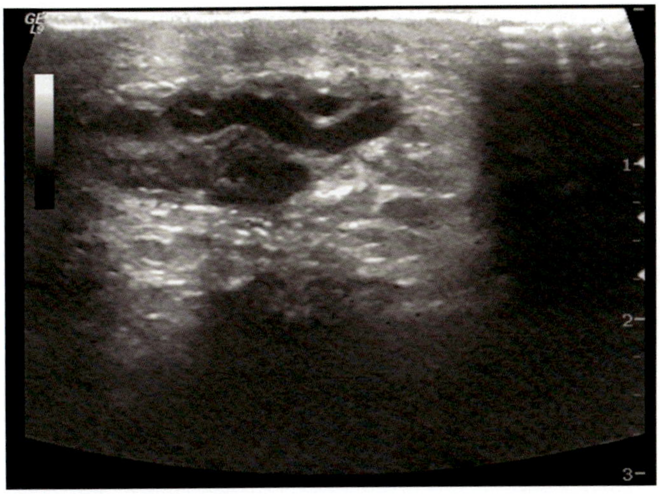

Figure 12.14 Varicocele. Ultrasound image of the lower portion of the scrotum. Multiple dilated veins in the spermatic cord.

Hydroceles

Normally, a small amount of fluid may be seen within the sac of the tunica vaginalis. This small amount of fluid can be visualized in over 80% of normal male patients. However, larger amounts of fluid are known as hydroceles. A hydrocele is the most common cause of scrotal swelling and may be unilateral or bilateral. Hydroceles may be idiopathic or seen in neonates due to a persistent communication between the scrotum and peritoneal cavity. They may also be the result of trauma, infection, neoplasms, radiation therapy, undiagnosed torsion, or congenital anatomic variations. Most hydroceles are anechoic in nature and therefore appear as black fluid surrounding the testicle (Figure 12.15). Hydroceles are most commonly seen in the anterolateral aspect of the scrotum. Since the testis is posteriorly attached to the epididymis and scrotal wall, a hydrocele does not develop posteriorly. Simple hydroceles appear anechoic or may contain low-level echos from fibrin bodies or cholesterol crystals. Complex hydroceles may contain a greater amount of internal echos with septations and loculation and, when chronic, may have calcifications present.

Tumors

Tumors of the testes are the most common malignancy in young men, but account for only 1% of all cancers in men. Testicular neoplasms are the fifth leading cause of death in men aged 15–34 years. Approximately 65–94% of patients with testicular neoplasms present with painless unilateral testicular

(a)

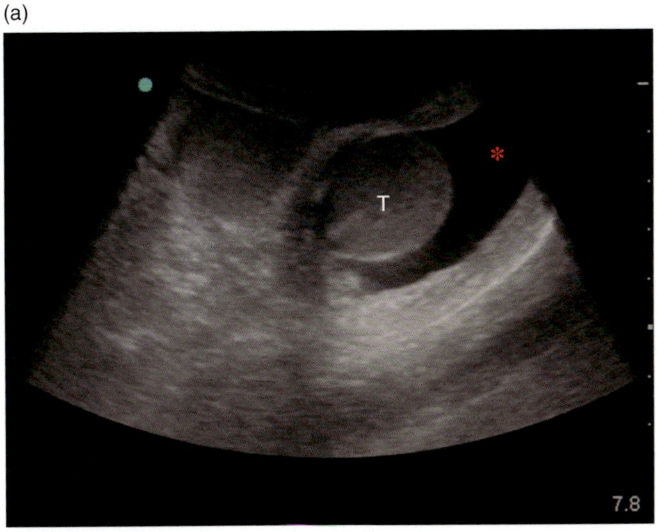

(b)

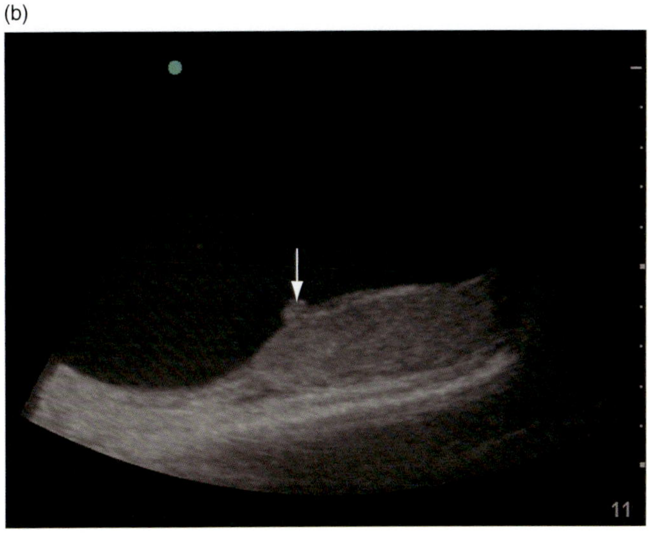

Figure 12.15 Hydrocele. (a) Simple anechoic hydrocele (*) surrounding a testis (T). Note, in this side-by-side comparison view, the right scrotum is seen without a hydrocele. (b) An extremely large hydrocele in a patient who presented with rapidly enlarging hemiscrotum. The appendix testis (arrow) can be seen adjacent to the testicle.

masses or diffuse testicular enlargement, and 4–14% present with symptoms of metastatic disease. Approximately 95% of tumors are germ cell tumors, with half of these being seminomas and the other half being mixed types. The remaining 5% of testicular tumors are sex cord stromal tumors. With ultrasonography, masses can be detected with a sensitivity of nearly 100%. The most important distinction is between intratesticular and extratesticular masses. All intratesticular lesions should be considered malignant until proven otherwise. Most malignant testicular neoplasms appear more hypoechoic than normal testicular parenchyma. However, hemorrhage, necrosis, calcification, or fatty changes can produce regions of increased echogenicity within tumors (Figure 12.16). The key finding to look for is any heterogeneity in testicular echogenicity – the absence of this does not rule out cancer, but the presence should prompt further evaluation.

Case

1. A 15-year-old male presents to the emergency department with four days of right testicular pain and swelling. He denies any trauma or recent sexual activity. On examination, the patient is well appearing, but uncomfortable with examination of his left testicle. The testicle appears enlarged, red, and is moderately tender to palpation. No cremasteric reflex can be appreciated on either the right or left sides. A point-of-care ultrasound is performed, which reveals a thickened scrotal layer. The architecture

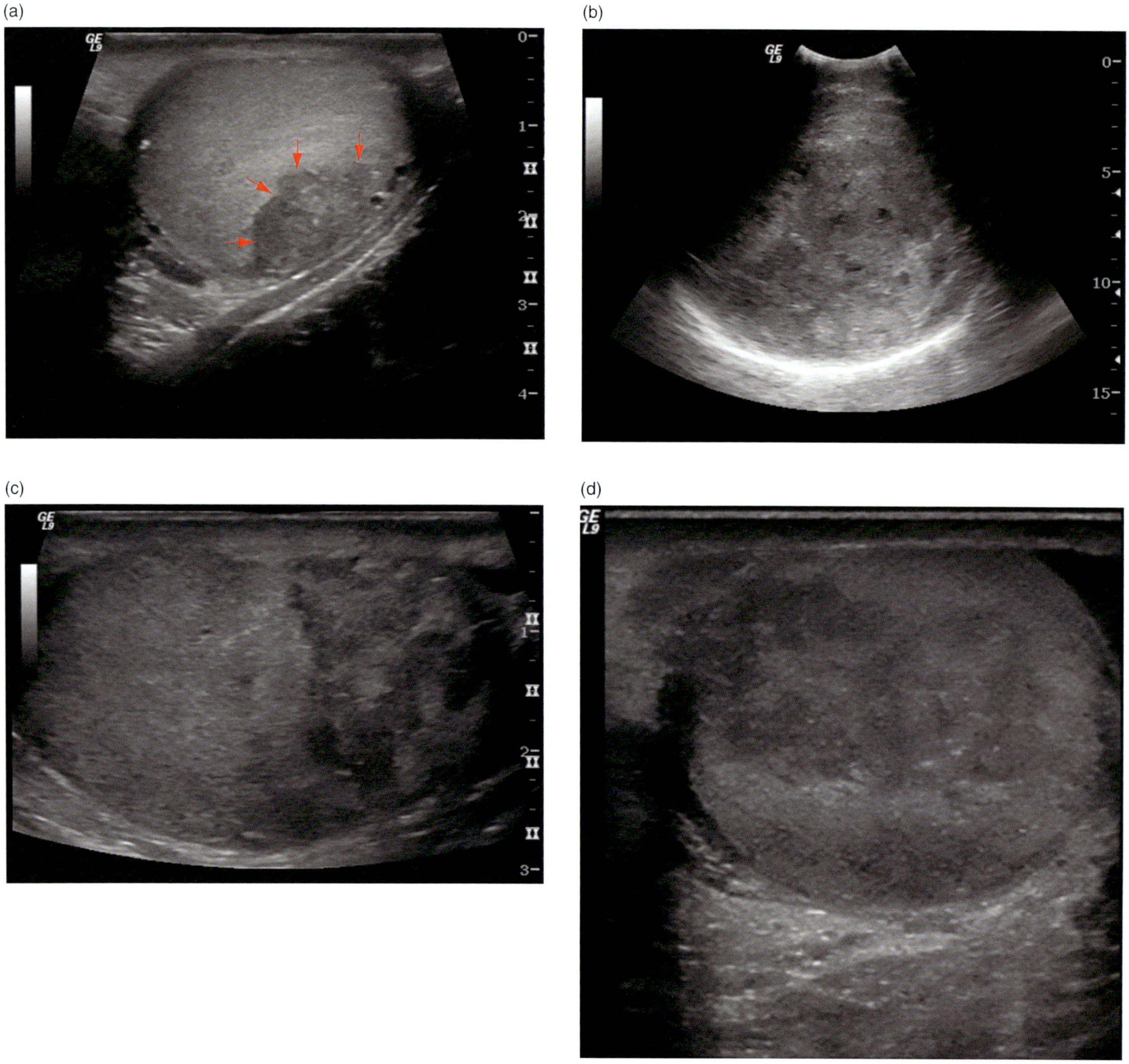

Figure 12.16 Tumors. (a) Transverse view of a large intratesticular hypoechoic mass (arrows) in a patient who presented after feeling a testicular mass and pain. (b) Diffusely heterogeneous-appearing mass found to be a metastatic testicular neoplasm. (c) Multiple hypoechoic masses found to be a seminoma. (d) Heterogeneous-appearing mass representing a mixed type of germ cell tumor.

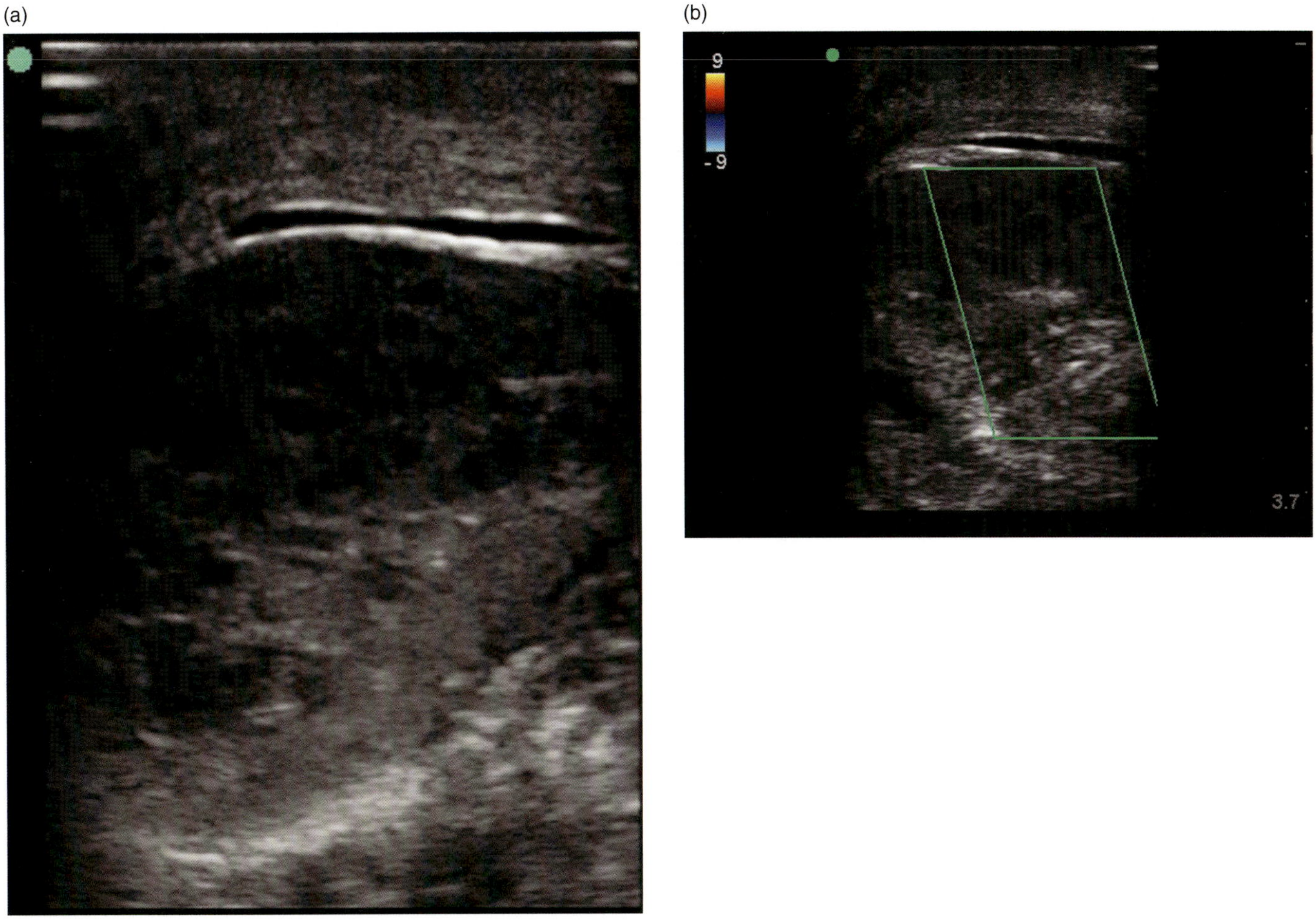

Figure 12.17 Case 1: torsion. (a) An initial ultrasound image was obtained of the painful, swollen right testicle. The architecture is disrupted and heterogeneous. (b) Color Doppler was used, which failed to show any blood flow. These findings were confirmed with formal ultrasonography.

of the testicle itself is disrupted and markedly different from the unaffected right side (Figure 12.17a). Doppler evaluation is performed, on which it is difficult to appreciate blood flow in the left side (Figure 12.17b). The urology service is immediately contacted, for concern of testicular torsion, given the appearance on point-of-care ultrasonography. Since formal ultrasonography is not immediately available, the technician needs to be called in emergently, in order to perform the scan. One hour later, a formal radiology ultrasound study confirms the findings of testicular torsion. Unfortunately, given the prolonged delay in seeking medical care, the testicle is not salvageable.

This case highlights the utility of point-of-care ultrasound in the immediate evaluation of a patient presenting with scrotal pain. While it does not replace formal radiographic studies, it provides the clinician with the ability to mobilize resources more efficiently and rapidly. It is also important to emphasize that the majority of smaller, portable machines do not have the capabilities of having high enough power that is needed to adequately assess for both venous and arterial testicular flow. Therefore, point-of-care ultrasound should not be relied upon to rule-in or rule-out testicular torsion.

Summary/key points

1. Scrotal ultrasound with color, power, and pulsed-wave Doppler is the test of choice for the assessment of scrotal pain and swelling. While the history and physical examination will always remain critical, it is clear that many disease processes overlap in their presentations in the emergency department.
2. Scrotal ultrasound is paramount to the diagnosis of organ-threatening disease states, and the radiology literature supports ultrasound as the fundamental imaging modality in the assessment of scrotal pain and swelling.
3. Evaluation of blood flow to the testes using pulsed-wave Doppler is essential to distinguish testicular torsion from other entities.
4. While point-of-care ultrasound may be limited, it may serve as a triage tool in rapidly identifying pathologic processes, allowing for mobilization of resources and facilitating patient care.
5. As the use of point-of-care ultrasound continues to expand in the emergency department, more research and training is needed to make scrotal ultrasound a part of the bedside evaluation of the patient presenting with scrotal pain or swelling.

Selected references

Blaivas, M., Sierzenski, P. (2001) Emergency ultrasonography in the evaluation of the acute scrotum. *Acad Emerg Med* **8**(1): 85–93.

Edelsberg, J. S., Surh, Y. S. (1988) The acute scrotum. *Emerg Med Clin North Am* **6**(3): 521–46.

Fisher, R., Walker, J. (1994) The acute paediatric scrotum. *British J Hosp Med* **51**(6): 290–2.

Gislason, T., Noronha, R. F., Gregory, J. G. (1980) Acute epididymitis in boys: a 5-year retrospective study. *Journal Urol* **124**(4): 533–4.

Kadish, H. A., Bolte, R. G. (1998) A retrospective review of pediatric patients with epididymitis, testicular torsion, and torsion of testicular appendages. *Pediatrics* **102**(1 Pt 1): 73–6.

Lewis, A. G., Bukowski, T. P., Jarvis, P. D., *et al.* (1995) Evaluation of acute scrotum in the emergency department. *J Pediatr Surgery* **30**(2): 277–82.

Likitnukul, S., McCracken, G. H. Jr, Nelson, J. D., *et al.* (1987) Epididymitis in children and adolescents. A 20-year retrospective study. *Am J Dis Child* **141**(1): 41–4.

Nussbaum Blask, A. R., Bulas, D., Shalaby-Rana, E., *et al.* (2002) Color Doppler sonography and scintigraphy of the testis: a prospective, comparative analysis in children with acute scrotal pain. *Pediatr Emerg Care* **18**(2): 67–71.

Petrack, E. M., Hafeez, W. (1992) Testicular torsion versus epididymitis: a diagnostic challenge. *Pediatr Emerg Care* **8**(6): 347–50.

Yagil, Y., Naroditsky, I., Milhem, J., *et al.* (2010) Role of Doppler ultrasonography in the triage of acute scrotum in the emergency department. *J Ultrasound Med* **29**(1): 11–21.

Chapter 13

Pelvic obstetrics

Heidi Ladner and Tony Berger

Objectives/indications

In the female adolescent patient presenting with acute, non-traumatic abdominal pain, the ultrasound examination can be of great utility. While lower abdominal pain in this patient population may be caused by appendicitis, bowel obstruction, constipation, peritonitis, inflammatory bowel disease, or a mass, it is essential to determine whether the patient is pregnant. A careful medical history and a urine pregnancy test are important first steps to be taken with any adolescent female presenting with abdominal pain. Pelvic sonography is an essential tool, in conjunction with the physical examination and laboratory testing, in the workup of these patients. The most common reason to perform a pelvic ultrasound in the pregnant adolescent patient is to evaluate first trimester bleeding (<12 weeks) and/or abdominal pain. Patients may present with vaginal bleeding alone, which is quite common in early pregnancy, occurring in up to 40% of women. In such patients, ultrasound is useful for assessing whether a patient has an intrauterine pregnancy (IUP). Overall, the clinical goal of evaluating a symptomatic pregnant patient during the first trimester is to determine whether she is having a spontaneous abortion, threatened abortion, ectopic pregnancy, or a ruptured ectopic pregnancy, since all four diagnoses may present with vaginal bleeding and/or abdominal pain.

The primary immediate goal of point-of-care pelvic ultrasonography is to evaluate for the presence of an ectopic pregnancy, which carries a high maternal morbidity and mortality. The prevalence of ectopic pregnancy is approximately 2% of all pregnancies, but is as high 3–13% in symptomatic first-trimester emergency department patients. The goal of the examination is not necessarily to identify an ectopic pregnancy but, rather, to confirm the presence of an IUP, since an ectopic implantation is often not directly identified. When an IUP is identified, it nearly completely excludes the presence of an ectopic (extrauterine) pregnancy, and is the cornerstone in the evaluation of patients with presentations concerning for ectopic pregnancy. It is important to understand that the presence of an IUP does not entirely eliminate the possibility that a patient has a simultaneous extrauterine pregnancy, a rare entity known as a *"heterotopic pregnancy."* This is more common in patients who have undergone fertility treatments, with an incidence as high as 1 / 900. In patients who have not undergone fertility treatments, the incidence is extremely rare, and is estimated to be 1 / 30000. Once an IUP is identified, secondary objectives of pelvic ultrasonography include determining the gestational age and evaluating for the presence of a fetal heartbeat. When no IUP has been identified, the secondary objective is to identify a tubal ring, complex adnexal mass, pelvic free fluid, or, in some instances, a live extrauterine pregnancy, all of which are highly suggestive of an ectopic pregnancy. Most importantly, the absence of these findings does not exclude the possibility of ectopic pregnancy, and pregnant patients with vaginal bleeding and no identifiable IUP are considered to have an ectopic pregnancy until proven otherwise, irrespective of the beta human gonadotrophin (β-hCG) level. If an ectopic pregnancy or a fetal demise is suspected, one should obtain an obstetrics consultation.

If a woman is bleeding but has evidence of fetal cardiac activity on ultrasound and a cervical os that is closed on bimanual examination, then she is considered to have a "threatened abortion." Ultimately, 77–90% of these patients will go on to have normal term pregnancies. If the cervical os is found to be open, then the pregnancy is known as an "inevitable abortion," regardless of whether an IUP has been identified by ultrasound. Conversely, one may discover by ultrasound, or by decreasing serum β-hCG levels, that a fetus is no longer viable despite a lack of miscarriage symptoms. These cases are referred to as "missed abortions." This diagnosis is more commonly made in the emergency department if the patient has had a live IUP seen on a prior ultrasound. The greatest diagnostic challenge in a pregnant patient with vaginal bleeding occurs in early pregnancy, since sonographic evaluation may not reveal an IUP, even in the case of a normal pregnancy. This can represent one of the following scenarios:

1. The pregnancy is too early to be identified by ultrasound;
2. The patient has completed a spontaneous abortion and passed all of the products of conception; or
3. The patient has an ectopic pregnancy.

Quantitative serum β-hCG levels are a fundamental part of the workup of vaginal bleeding/abdominal pain in the first-trimester pregnant patient. Although there is some correlation between β-hCG levels and ultrasound findings, a single β-hCG level is never enough to exclude ectopic pregnancy in a patient without evidence of IUP on ultrasound. The serum level of β-hCG at which one should definitively be able to identify an

Pediatric Emergency and Critical Care Ultrasound, ed. Stephanie J. Doniger. Published by Cambridge University Press.

Table 13.1 Embryologic structures seen by ultrasound. Embryologic structures appear earlier with transvaginal ultrasonography than transabdominal ultrasonography. Generally, their appearance may be correlated with expected gestational ages and β-hCG levels, otherwise known as the "discriminatory zone."

		Expected gestational age at appearance (wks)		β-hCG level (mIU/mL)
		Transabdominal	Endovaginal	
IUP ↓	Gestational sac	5.5–6	4.5–5	>2,000
	Yolk sac	6–6.5	5–5.5	7,000
	Fetal pole	7	5.5–6	11,000
	Cardiac activity	7	6	
	Fetal parts	>8	8	

IUP on ultrasound is known as the β-hCG discriminatory zone (Table 13.1). It is the level at which, in the absence of an IUP on sonographic examination, one's index of suspicion for ectopic pregnancy should be extremely high. Mistakenly, some clinicians misinterpret the discriminatory zone as the β-hCG level below which one should not be able to identify an IUP. This is incorrect and it must be understood that there is no "safe" β-hCG level below which one can rule out an ectopic pregnancy. If a patient is found to have a low β-hCG with no IUP and is hemodynamically stable with assured appropriate follow-up, discharge from the emergency department for a repeat β-hCG level in two days is a reasonable strategy, since this is the amount of time it takes for the β-hCG level to double in a normal IUP. At follow-up, if the β-hCG level is decreasing, then the patient is presumed to have had a miscarriage. If the level is doubling, then she likely has an IUP that will be followed until identified on ultrasound. If, however, the β-hCG is increasing more slowly, then an ectopic pregnancy is the presumed diagnosis and can be managed by obstetricians as an outpatient.

In addition to the assessment of vaginal bleeding and abdominal pain in early pregnancy, the emergency physician may occasionally be called upon to perform sonographic evaluations of patients in their second or third trimester. The differential diagnosis for vaginal bleeding and abdominal pain changes during this crucial period and largely consists of placenta previa and placental abruption. It is highly recommended that an obstetrician perform the evaluation of symptomatic pregnant patients of greater than 20 weeks gestational age, since the fetus may be viable. Understandably, many practitioners work in remote or austere environments where an immediate obstetrics consultation is not available. In addition, many children's hospitals do not have an obstetrics service immediately available. Therefore, learning to identify these clinical entities is an important skill for emergency physicians, depending on their region or scope of practice.

This chapter reviews the indications for pelvic ultrasonography in the pregnant patient. The techniques for the evaluation, including the transvaginal and transabdominal approaches, are reviewed. It is important to recognize the limitations of ultrasonography in evaluating the pregnant adolescent patient and in diagnosing an IUP. Readers are encouraged to explore the topic further to enhance their knowledge and comfort level with the use of ultrasound in the evaluation of the complicated pregnant patient.

Background

Point-of-care pelvic ultrasonography has become part of the standard workup for a pregnant patient presenting to the emergency department. Emergency physicians have been shown to reliably and accurately be able to identify an intrauterine pregnancy. A 1997 study was the first to prospectively evaluate all first-trimester pregnancy patients for ectopic pregnancy using point-of-care ultrasound when presenting to the emergency department with complications. Durham *et al.* showed that point-of-care ultrasonography correlated with formal ultrasonography in 97% of patients, thereby showing that emergency physicians can perform and interpret pelvic ultrasonography with reliable and accurate results. Shortly thereafter, Dart *et al.* found that the presence of echogenic material seen within the endometrial cavity on point-of-care ultrasound could reliably exclude the diagnosis of a normal IUP. However, this finding did not exclude the possibility of an ectopic pregnancy. The vast majority of the patients (93%) had abnormal IUPs and 5% had ectopic pregnancies. Tayal *et al.* investigated the outcomes of patients with first-trimester pregnancy complications and "indeterminate" emergency department ultrasounds, when an IUP was not identified. They found that there was a substantial proportion of embryonic demise (53%) and ectopic pregnancy (15%), with a low proportion of IUP as the final diagnosis. Therefore, an indeterminate pelvic ultrasound yields poor outcomes, with high rates of fetal demise and ectopic pregnancy. Recently, Wang *et al.* investigated indeterminate ultrasounds in conjunction with a "discriminatory zone" for β-hCG. Using a discriminatory zone of 3,000 mIU/mL yielded a sensitivity of only 35% and specificity of 58% for ectopic pregnancy. The overall sensitivity and specificity for detection of an IUP was 71% and 99%, respectively. Therefore, when point-of-care ultrasonography does not demonstrate an IUP, β-hCG levels are not reliable in differentiating an IUP from an ectopic pregnancy. Overall, Stein *et al.* performed a meta-analysis showing that point-of-care ultrasonography has a pooled sensitivity of 99.3% and negative predictive value of 99.96%. As a result, point-of-care pelvic ultrasonography is a reliable screening tool, with the visualization of an IUP being sufficient to rule out an ectopic pregnancy. To date, there have been no lawsuits against emergency physicians resulting directly from performance of or incorrect interpretation of point-of-care pelvic ultrasounds. The only identified lawsuit was for failure to perform a pelvic point-of-care sonogram in a patient who had a ruptured ectopic pregnancy a few days later.

Additional components of pelvic ultrasonography in the emergency department include the evaluation of the fetal heart rate and gestational age in order to determine fetal viability and the possibility of miscarriage or spontaneous abortion. In 2000, Choi *et al.* sought to determine the outcome of pregnancies that had documented fetal heartbeats on first-trimester transvaginal ultrasonography. Previously, the obstetrics literature reported a 90% delivery of normal, full term infants among patients with first-trimester complications who had an ultrasound finding of a fetal heartbeat documented at their presentation. In contrast, in the higher-risk emergency department population, they ultimately found that 23% of the pregnancies were non-viable and only 77% were viable and carried to full-term delivery. Recently, Saul *et al.* showed that emergency physicians can accurately perform a gestational age measurement. When compared with formal ultrasound studies (by radiologists), the median discrepancy was only two days, with a correlation coefficient of 0.978. In 2012, Mallin *et al.* performed the first prospective evaluation of emergency department patients with a documented IUP and fetal heart tones. The spontaneous abortion rate of 14.8% is consistent with previously reported rates. This information may help to guide the clinician and give some prognostic information to patients.

Thus far, there is no specific research to be found on the use of point-of-care ultrasound examination in pregnant adolescent patients. A recent study showed that pelvic ultrasonography performed by emergency medicine or pediatric emergency medicine physicians reduced lengths of stay. However, the burgeoning art of point-of-care ultrasound has yielded peer-reviewed research on the use of ultrasound for pregnant patients in the emergency department in general, and the results of these studies may be carefully applied to the adolescent population.

Embryology and anatomy

It is important to recognize the normal anatomy of the uterus and ovaries, and their relationship to the iliac vessels and bladder (Figure 13.1).

The common convention when referring to pregnancy age is to count from the first day of the last menstrual period (LMP). Ovulation occurs approximately 14 days after the LMP (two weeks of gestational age), and fertilization of the oocyte must occur within 24 hours of this event. Once the spermatocyte and oocyte fuse, they become a zygote. During the week following fertilization, the early zygote transforms into a ball of 16 cells, known as the morula, as it travels down the fallopian tube (Figure 13.2). The morula proceeds to develop into the blastocyst, a structure containing an outer ring of trophoblast cells and an inner cell mass, which are destined to become the placenta and embryonic stem cells, respectively. The blastocyst implants into the maternal endometrium approximately seven days after fertilization (three weeks of gestational age). After implantation, the embryo begins to produce β-hCG. By four weeks of gestational age, many home urine pregnancy tests, which measure β-hCG, may be positive. The embryo continues to develop and differentiate the major organs until the end of the 11th gestational week, at which time the pregnancy becomes known as a fetus.

The structure to develop first includes the **gestational sac**, which appears at approximately four weeks of gestational age. The endometrium changes as a result of the influence of progesterone and creates a "double decidual sign," which is the apposition of the decidualized endometrium layer against the outer layer of the gestational sac. It is important to recognize that the decidual sign may be present in ectopic pregnancies, in which case it represents a pseudo-gestational sac. The first embryologic structure to appear within the gestational sac is the **yolk sac**. This is the first reliable indicator of an IUP. The next structure to appear is the **fetal pole**. Initially it is juxtaposed next to the yolk sac but, as the pregnancy progresses, it can appear connected to the yolk sac by a linear structure known as the vitelline duct. The amniotic sac may be seen as a separate membrane around the embryonic structure at approximately six weeks of gestation. By 14 to16 weeks of gestational age, the amniotic sac has grown to fill the entire chorionic cavity and no

(a)

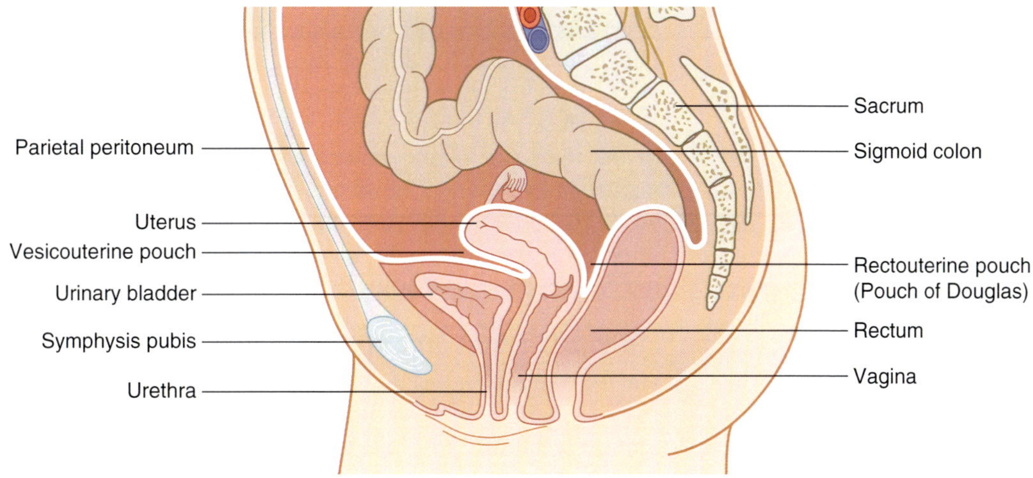

Figure 13.1 Anatomy of the female pelvis. Note the uterus and ovaries and their relationship to the iliac vessels. (a) Median section of the pelvic contents. Note the relationship between the uterus, bladder, and rectum. (b) Transverse section of the pelvic contents. Note the orientation of the uterus, ovaries, bladder, and rectum. *Artwork created by Emily Evans © Cambridge University Press.*

(b)

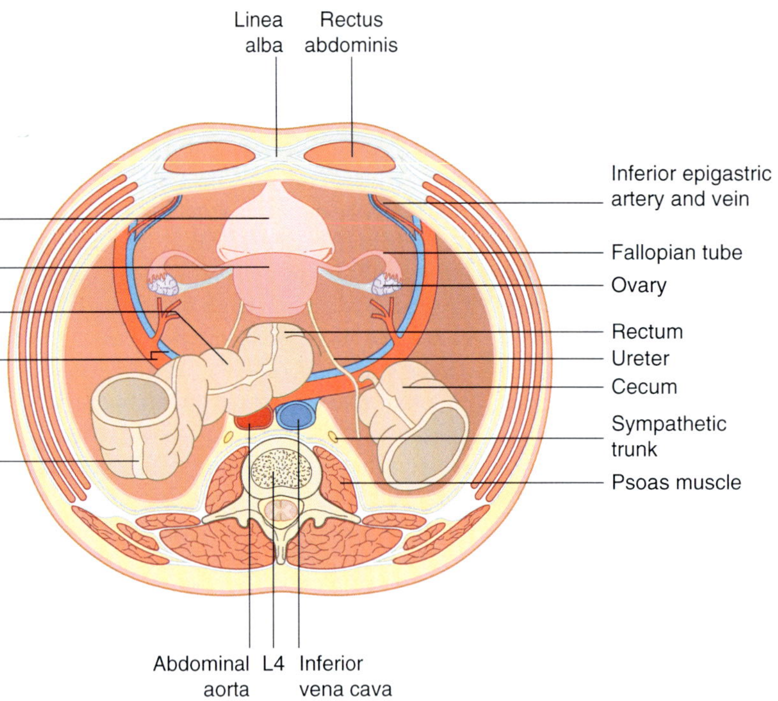

Figure 13.1 (cont.)

longer appears as a separate membrane. It is helpful to recognize at what gestational age one can expect certain embryonic structures to appear, and when they can be visualized by both transabdominal and transvaginal ultrasonography (Table 13.1).

Technique

The first sonographic approach to a patient should always be transabdominal. If the transabdominal examination yields the required information, then the more invasive transvaginal examination is not necessary. However, if the transabdominal approach does not unequivocally reveal an IUP, then the practitioner should perform a transvaginal examination. A particularly useful sequence for the performance of obstetric ultrasound in the emergency setting is to first perform the transabdominal examination while the patient is supine with a filled bladder. Next, the patient is asked to void her bladder, as the examination table and the ultrasound machine are prepared for the transvaginal examination. The practitioner then performs a speculum and bimanual examination, followed by the transvaginal sonographic examination, if required.

Imaging in the late second and third trimesters is almost exclusively performed via the transabdominal approach. Many emergency departments will triage pregnant patients with an estimated gestational age greater than 20 weeks and apparent obstetric complaints such as vaginal bleeding, cramping, or decreased fetal movement, directly to the labor and delivery ward. However, some small or remote community settings may not have immediate obstetric consultation available, in which case the emergency physician may be called upon to evaluate second- and third-trimester patients. As such, there are several conditions that present later in pregnancy that emergency clinicians should be aware of and trained to evaluate if necessary.

Point-of-care questions

1. Is an intrauterine pregnancy (IUP) present? Is a yolk sac/fetal pole/fetal heart rate present?
2. Is an ectopic pregnancy present? Is free fluid present?

Transabdominal

Transducer selection and orientation: transabdominal

For the transabdominal examination, a low-frequency (2–5 MHz) curvilinear or phased-array transducer is best used, since it provides the necessary penetration to evaluate abdominal structures (Figure 13.3). As in most abdominal ultrasound examinations, it is important to visualize the structures of interest in two planes in order to get a three-dimensional understanding of structures in space. The initial placement of the transducer is in the suprapubic region of the abdomen. In the transverse view, the indicator will be oriented to the right side of the patient (Figure 13.4a), while in the sagittal abdominal view it will be oriented towards the patient's head (Figure 13.5a). For scanning in later pregnancy, the transducer is swept across the abdomen until the structures of interest (placenta, fetal heart, etc.) are visualized and identified.

Patient position and preparation: transabdominal

For the transabdominal examination, a full bladder can aid in the visualization of the uterus and ovaries by providing an acoustic window. The patient should be in a supine position or with slight reverse Trendelenburg position for better visualization of free fluid in the pelvis for the transabdominal portion of the examination.

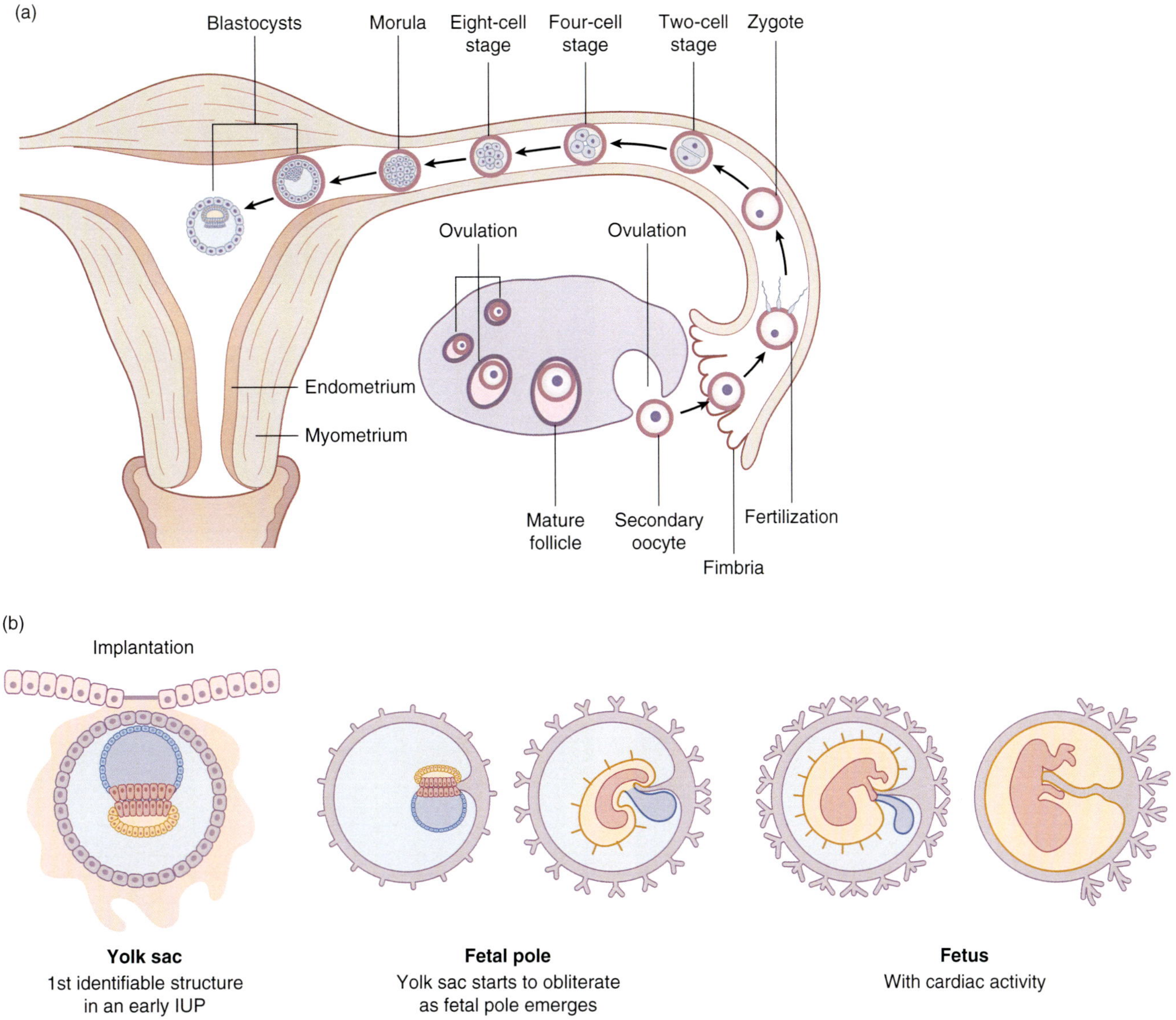

Figure 13.2 Embryologic structures. (a) Illustration depicting path of an egg from fertilization to implantation. (b) The development of embryologic structures: a yolk sac is the first identifiable form of an intrauterine pregnancy, followed by the fetal pole, and finally the fetus with cardiac activity. *Artwork created by Emily Evans © Cambridge University Press.*

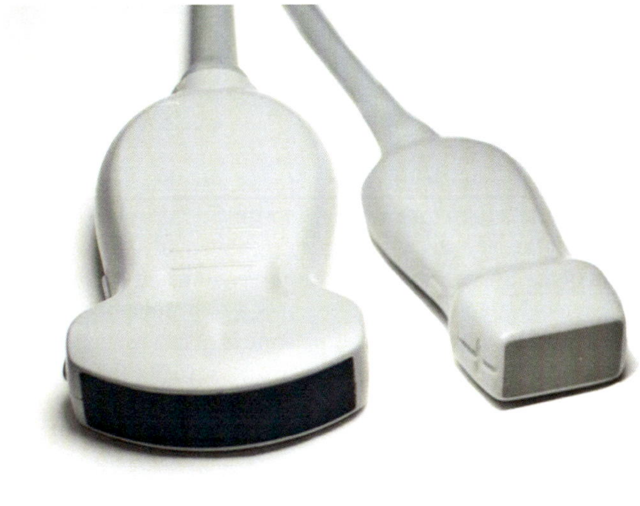

Figure 13.3 Low-frequency transducers utilized for the transabdominal pelvic ultrasound examination.

Ultrasound imaging: transabdominal

It is important to recognize key structures on the normal transabdominal pelvic ultrasound. In the transverse view, the bladder appears as an anechoic rectangular or trapezoidal structure. The uterus and ovaries are located posterior, or deep to the bladder (Figure 13.4b). On the sagittal view, the bladder appears as a wedge. The uterus is to the left of the bladder (Figure 13.5b). It is important to have the patient with a full bladder, since it will act as an acoustic window to better visualize the uterus and ovaries.

Transvaginal

Transducer selection and orientation: transvaginal

The endovaginal probe (Figure 13.6) is a high-frequency (5–9 MHz) transducer that provides higher-resolution images for superficial structures. The transvaginal approach allows for

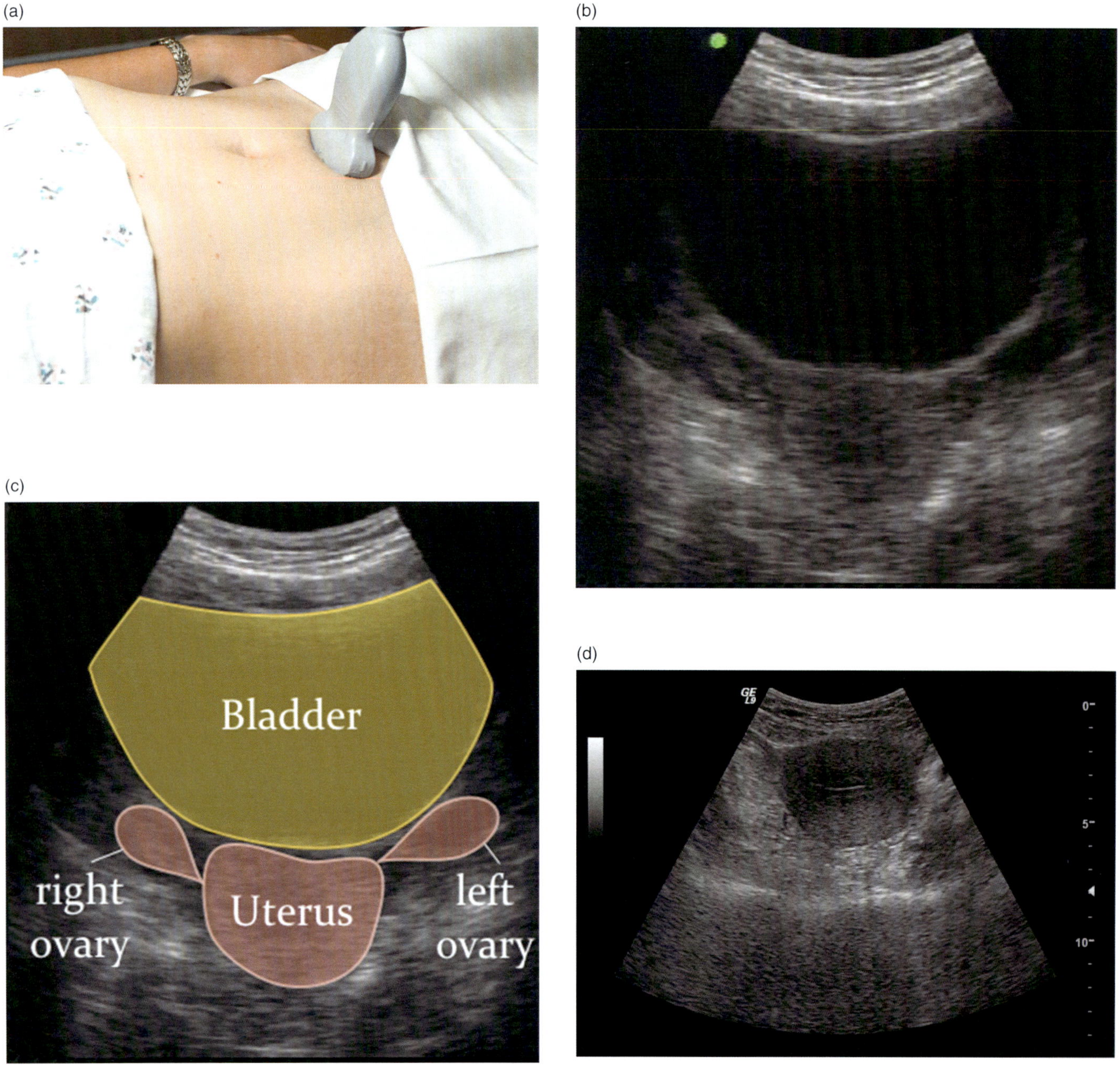

Figure 13.4 Transabdominal pelvis imaging, transverse view. (a) Transducer placement, with the indicator towards the patient's right side. (b) Ultrasound image of the transverse pelvic view. (c) Illustration of the structures visualized in the ultrasound image: uterus, bladder, and ovaries. *Illustration by Laura Berg, MD.* (d) Ultrasound image of the transverse view or cross-section of the uterus itself.

near immediate approximation of the transducer against the uterus, so the depth of essential anatomic structures is rarely an issue in the first trimester. In addition to providing a more detailed view of the uterus, it allows for clearer imaging of the ovaries as there is no intervening bowel gas and the transducer is in closer proximity to the ovaries.

The endovaginal transducer requires special preparation given its use within the vagina. A moisture impermeable cover must be placed over the transducer. A layer of gel is needed within the probe cover: a layer of sterile gel is also needed on the outside of the probe cover (Figure 13.7). It is crucial to eliminate as many bubbles as possible between the transducer and the cover in order to obtain adequate images. Otherwise, the air will cause bright ring-down artifacts through sectors of the image. Additionally, the cleaning and disinfecting of the endovaginal transducer requires a well-thought-out and institutionally approved infection control plan, as the transducer can come into contact with many sexually transmitted microbes. Once the probe cover is removed and discarded, the transducer is washed with water and/or soap and then soaked in or wiped with a disinfecting agent e.g. Cidex®, according to machine-specific manufacturer recommendations.

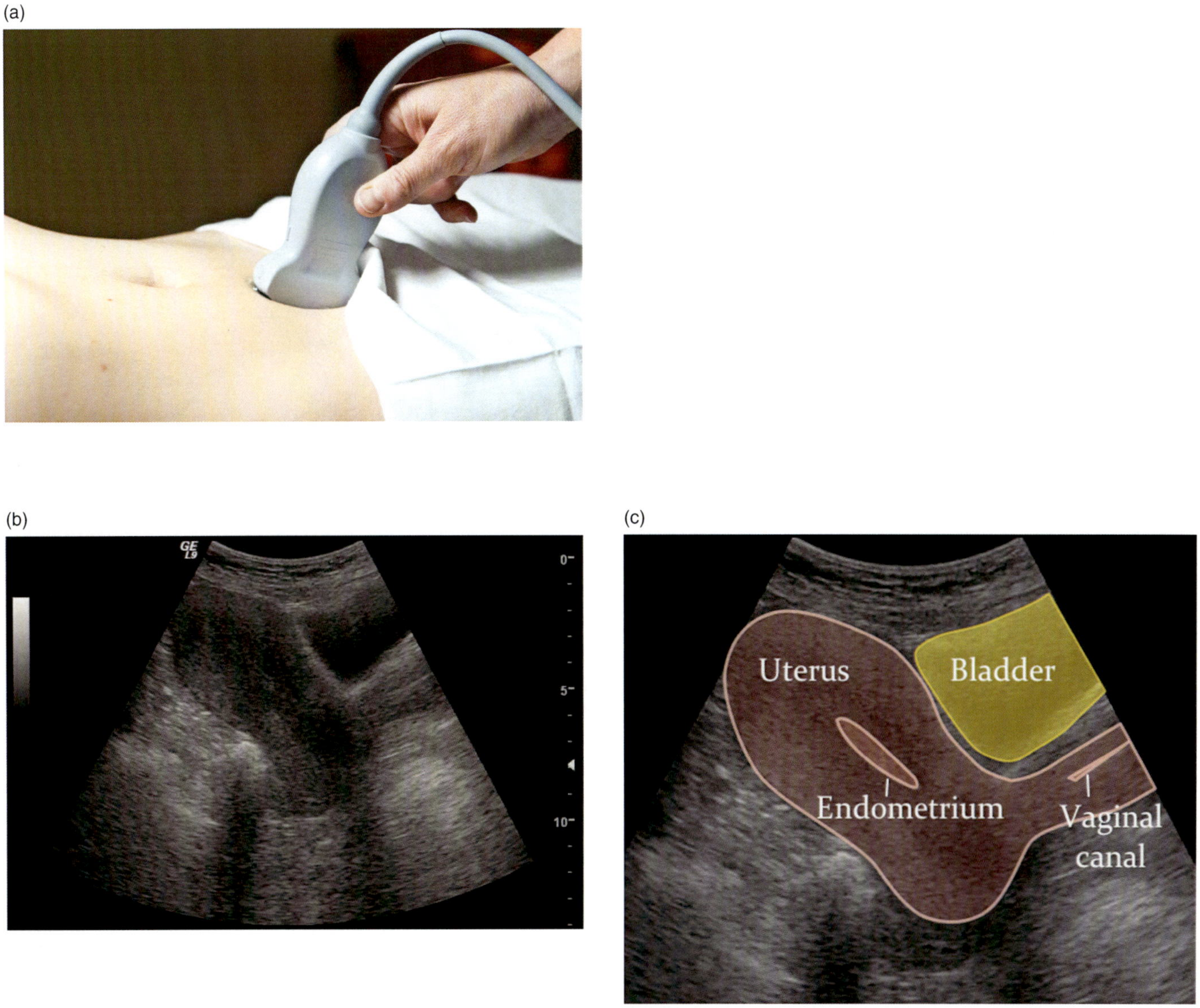

Figure 13.5 Transabdominal pelvis imaging, sagittal view. (a) Transducer placement, with the indicator towards the patient's head. (b) Ultrasound image of the sagittal pelvic view. (c) Illustration of the structures visualized in the ultrasound image: uterus and bladder. *Illustration by Laura Berg, MD.*

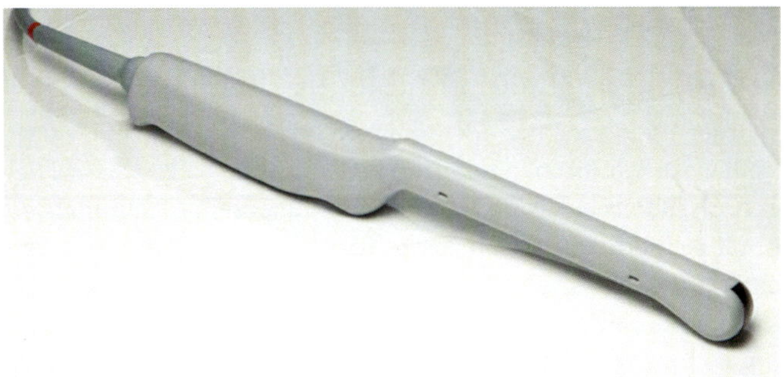

Figure 13.6 Endovaginal, or endocavitary, probe, 5–9 MHz is used to perform the transvaginal ultrasound examination. The higher frequency allows for high resolution of structures in near proximity to the transducer, such as the ovaries and uterus. Note the indicator on the transducer handle.

The orientation of the endocavitary probe may at first seem complex to the novice sonographer. As the transducer is introduced into the vaginal orifice, the indicator should be pointing "up" towards the ceiling to produce a sagittal view through the uterus (Figure 13.8a). At the same time, the index finger "trigger" grip is in the 6 o'clock position. The transducer is then fanned from right to left in order to locate the uterus, which is not always a midline structure. This transducer orientation allows for easier localization of the uterus within the pelvis and is performed first. Next the transducer is rotated 90° counterclockwise, such that the indicator is now oriented towards the patient's right side (Figure 13.9a); the index finger "trigger" is oriented towards the patient's left side. This transducer position is commonly referred to as the transverse position but, anatomically speaking, is actually a coronal view of the pelvis.

(a) (b)

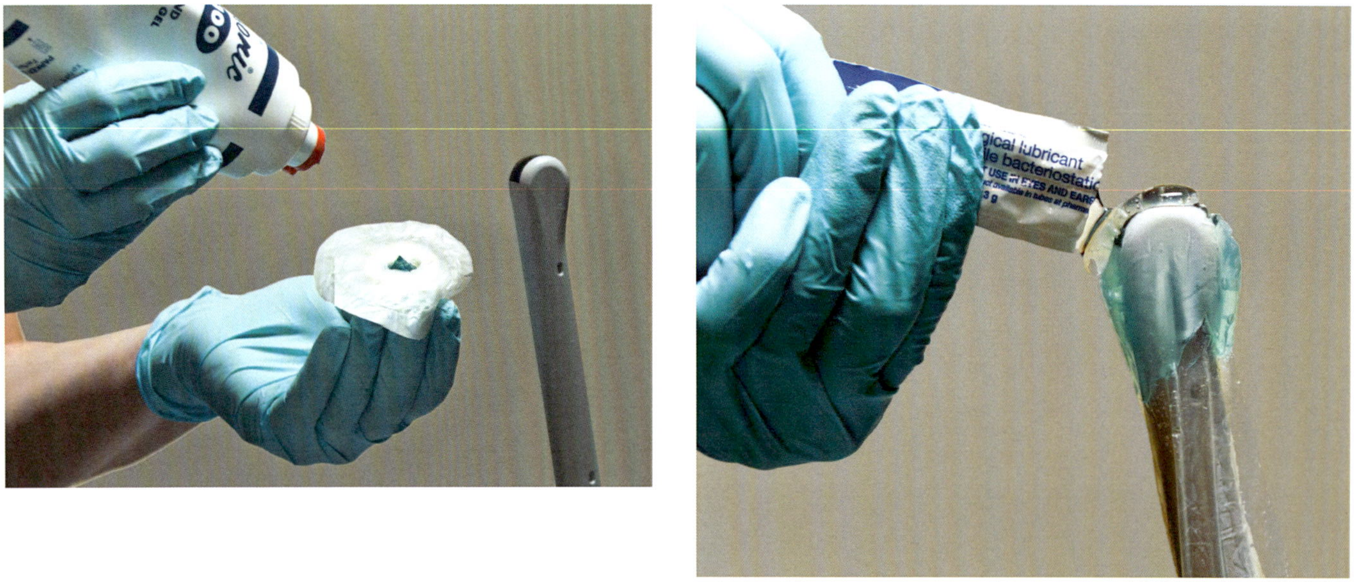

Figure 13.7 Endocavitary probe preparation. Proper preparation of the endocavitary probe is required in order to perform the transvaginal ultrasound examination. Note that the gel is placed (a) inside and (b) sterile lubricant on the outside of the probe cover, in order to allow for conduction of the sound waves.

Patient position and preparation: transvaginal

For the transvaginal examination, the patient should be comfortably positioned in the lithotomy position. The patient should void their bladder prior to the examination, as it is more comfortable for the patient and prevents the bladder from dominating the image in the pelvis. As the examination may feel awkward for a teenaged patient, it is appropriate to ask whether she would like to introduce the endovaginal probe herself. A female chaperone or a person designated by the patient should be present to provide security and comfort during the examination.

Ultrasound imaging: transvaginal

Begin scanning the uterus in the sagittal view. Once localized, a detailed examination through each section of the uterus is performed in the sagittal view, in order to detect a gestational sac (Figure 13.8). The transducer is then rotated in order to obtain the coronal view (Figure 13.9). The transducer is fanned in an up-and-down, sweeping motion through the uterus in an attempt to localize the gestational sac. If no such structure is identified, one must again obtain an image with a clear outline of the endometrial stripe free of any evidence of an IUP. Finally, when imaging the uterus in any view or orientation, it is important to adjust the depth appropriately, in order to visualize the rectouterine space, or the pouch of Douglas, which lies posterior or deep to the uterus. If this is not accomplished, one might miss the presence of free fluid in the pelvis (Figure 13.8).

In order to visualize the ovaries, the transducer is maintained in the coronal orientation, and is fanned towards the patient's right in an attempt to localize the right ovary. The internal iliac artery serves as a landmark for finding the ovary. The right ovary is located anterior and medial to the artery (Figure 13.10). Once the ovary is identified, it is possible to obtain images in both planes by keeping the ovary in the center of the screen and rotating the transducer clockwise such that the indicator is again pointing up towards the ceiling. To view the left ovary, the transducer is fanned towards the left of the uterus (the patient's left side), and the above procedure of scanning the ovary in two planes is repeated. Diameter measurements of the ovary are taken along its long and short-axis in both views. Any cystic structures are measured from just interior to hyperechoic rim. In the first-trimester female, it is common to see a corpus luteum cyst (Figure 13.11), which is usually a simple, thin-walled anechoic structure. This is the remnant of the follicle from which the oocyte was derived and is at its maximum size at approximately 7 weeks of gestational age and resolves by the middle of the second trimester (18 weeks).

Ultrasound imaging: intrauterine pregnancy

In order to confidently document the presence of an IUP, one should, at a minimum, visualize a yolk sac. If no yolk sac is visible on transabdominal examination, then transvaginal examination should be performed. In order to identify a true IUP, one must identify the first structure to appear within the gestational sac, which is the yolk sac. The yolk sac appears as a brightly echogenic ring within the anechoic gestational sac (Figure 13.12). After the yolk sac appears, the fetal pole emerges as a moderately echogenic structure within the gestational sac (Figure 13.13).

In order to correctly identify an IUP, one must demonstrate certain structures in each sonographic view. In the event that no IUP is identified after a complete examination, which

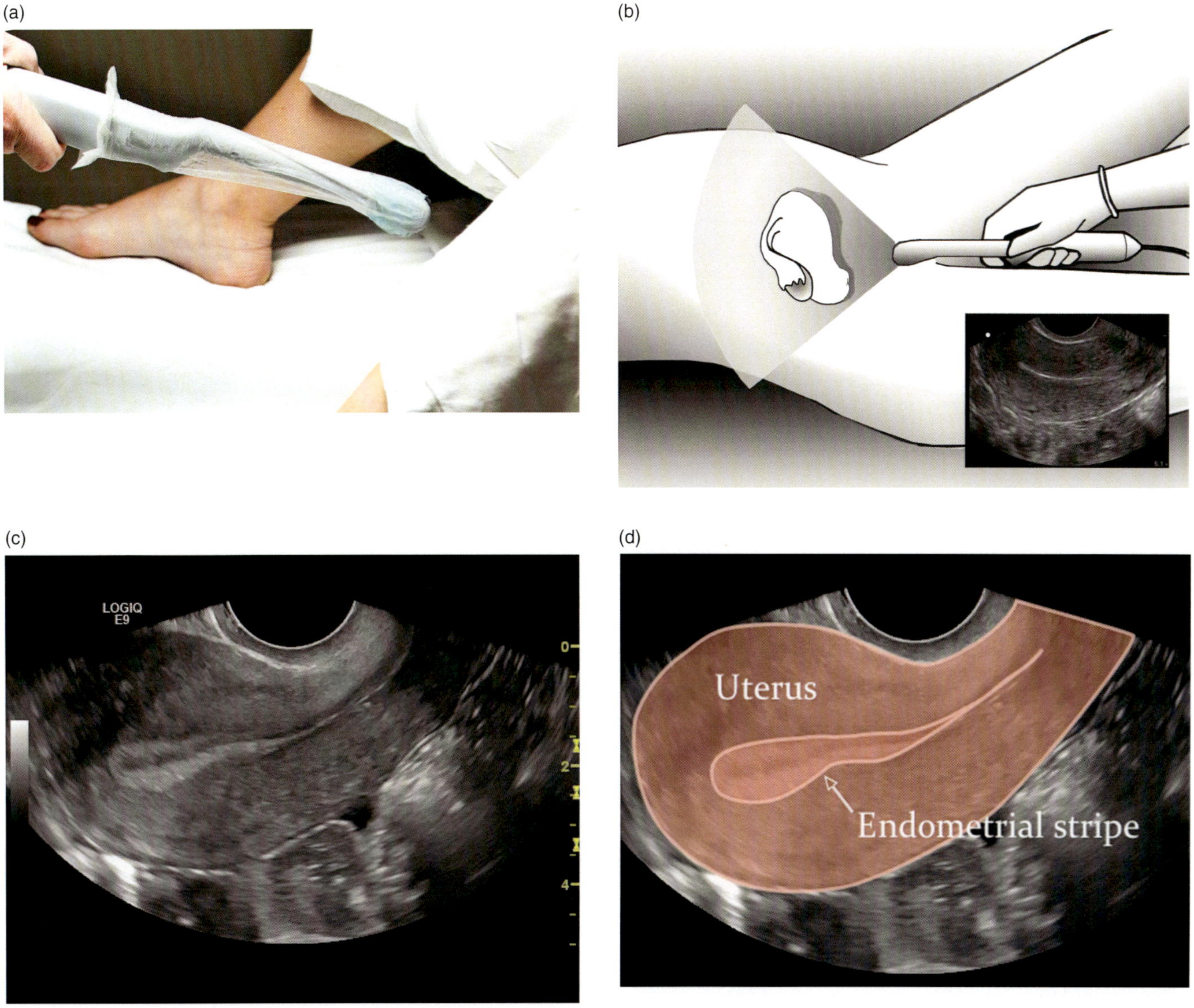

Figure 13.8 Transvaginal pelvis imaging, sagittal view. (a) Transducer placement, with the indicator towards the ceiling in a 12 o'clock orientation. (b) Illustration depicting how the sagittal orientation of the endovaginal probe in the pelvis results in the anterior aspect of the patient on the left of the monitor screen and the more caudal structures being located near the bottom of the image. Note the hyperechoic endometrial stripe within the myometrium. Additionally, trace free fluid is noted in the rectouterine space. *Illustration by Tony Berger, MD.* (c) Sagittal transvaginal view of the uterus. (d) Illustration depicting the transvaginal sagittal image of the uterus. *Illustration by Laura Berg, MD.*

includes fanning the transducer through the entire uterus in both the transverse and sagittal orientations, still images of both orientations of the uterus should be obtained in order to document the absence of an IUP. It is important that the endometrial stripe be fully visualized. Additionally, it is important to obtain an image of the cervix while performing the endovaginal examination in the sagittal orientation, to be sure there is no cervical ectopic pregnancy (Figure 13.14). A cervical ectopic pregnancy is identified by the presence of a fetal heart rate and in this way is differentiated from expelled products of conception in the cervical zone during a spontaneous abortion.

It is important to recognize certain embryonic structures and the timing of their expected appearance on transvaginal and transabdominal ultrasonography (Table 13.1). Initially, the gestational sac will appear, which is an anechoic structure within the body of the uterus. However, a gestational sac alone is insufficient in the diagnosis of an IUP, since ectopic pregnancies may have a similar-appearing "pseudo-gestational sac." Other, more subtle signs of early pregnancy include the "double decidual" sign (Figure 13.15), which is beyond the scope of this chapter. Therefore, a sonogram with a gestational sac alone should be considered indeterminate even when the timing of the LMP is consistent with a five-week pregnancy.

If no IUP is identified, it is considered an indeterminate scan. Since there is a high possibility of an ectopic pregnancy with an indeterminate scan, one should consult an obstetrician to discuss further management. If a simple, anechoic, sac-like

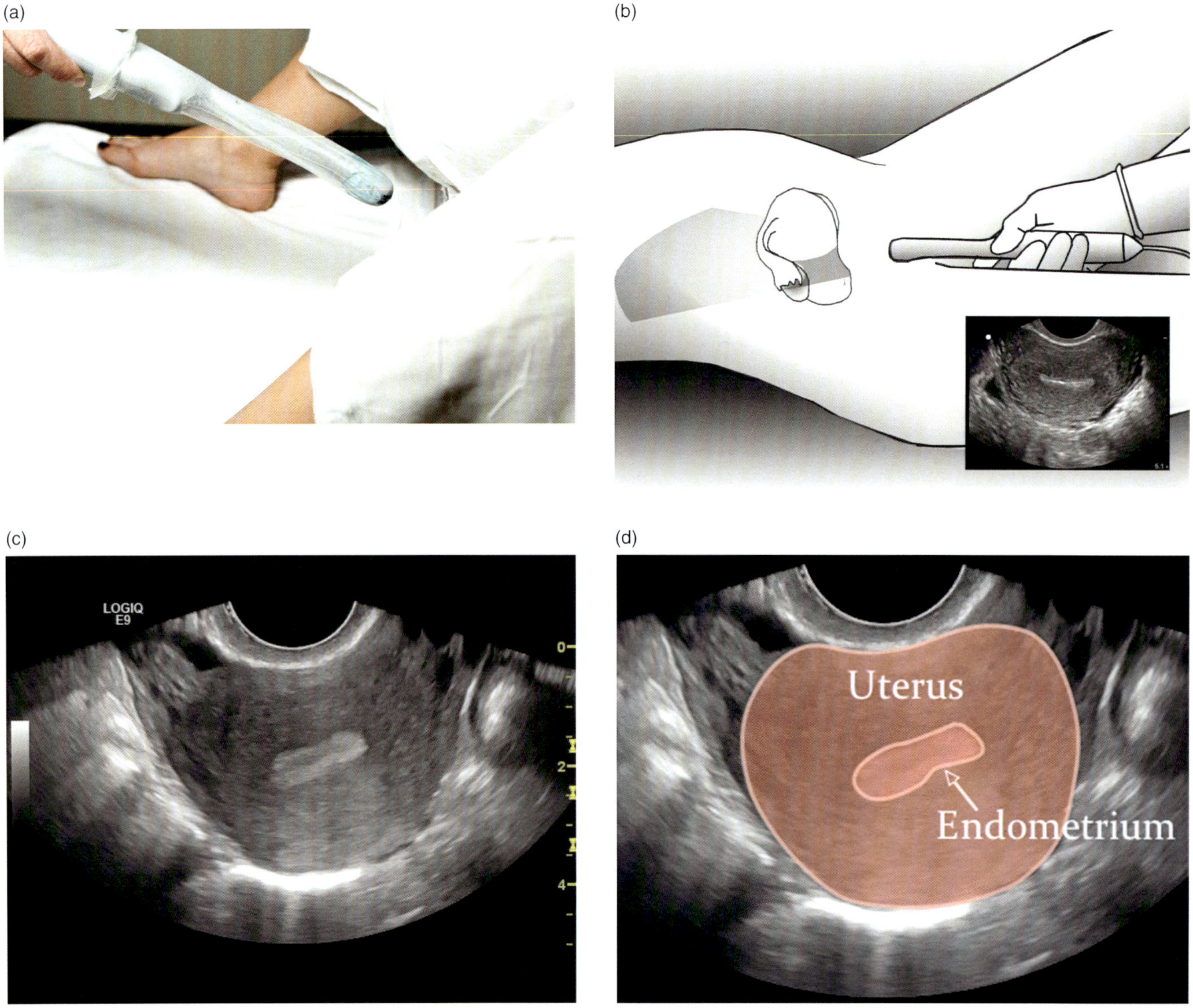

Figure 13.9 Transvaginal pelvis imaging, coronal view. (a) The indicator is rotated towards the patient's right side in order to obtain a coronal view of the pelvis. (b) Illustration depicting how the transverse orientation of the endovaginal probe results in the structures on the right side of the patient being located on the left side of the image. More caudal structures are located at the bottom of the image. *Illustration by Tony Berger, MD.* (c) Transvaginal coronal image of the uterus. A clear endometrial stripe is seen without any gestational sac or other evidence of IUP. (d) Illustration depicting the transvaginal coronal image of the uterus. *Illustration by Laura Berg, MD.*

structure is identified in the uterus without other signs of pregnancy, three possibilities exist:

1. Very early gestation.
2. A "blighted ovum," or an early pregnancy failure: the gestational sac measures greater than 20 mm on transabdominal ultrasonography and the patient is at approximately six weeks of gestational age (Figure 13.16).
3. Ectopic pregnancy, with a "pseudo-gestational sac," which is present in up to 20% of ectopic pregnancies. It is for this reason that it is strongly discouraged to confirm an intrauterine pregnancy solely based on the presence of an anechoic sac in the uterus.

Ultrasound imaging: measurements

Fetal heart rate

Embryonic cardiac activity can be identified between seven and eight weeks of gestational age. The heart appears as a small flicker within the fetal pole and allows for measurement of the fetal heart rate. The preferred method for obtaining the fetal heart rate is to utilize M-mode in order to get a linear representation of the beating heart over time. The screen marker should be placed across the flickering heart, resulting in a cyclical pattern of heart wall motion over time. The function "zoom" may be utilized in order to make the heart larger and to facilitate centering the cursor over the flickering heart. Most machines have calculation software that allows the sonographer

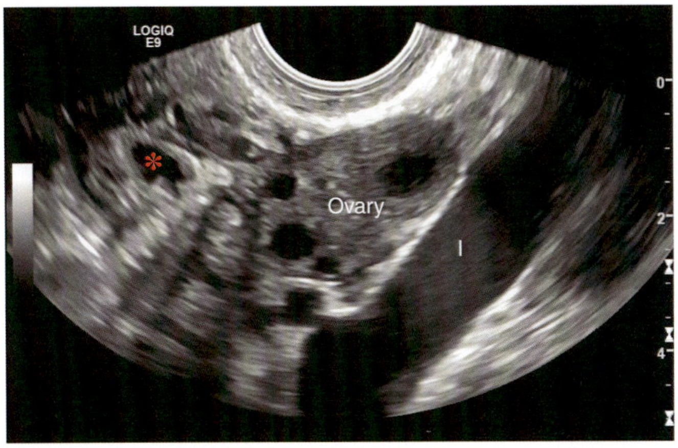

Figure 13.10 **Transvaginal image of the left ovary and adnexa**. Note the internal iliac artery (I) posterior to the ovary. Additionally, a tubal ring (*) is seen directly adjacent to the ovary in this patient who was found to have a ruptured ectopic pregnancy.

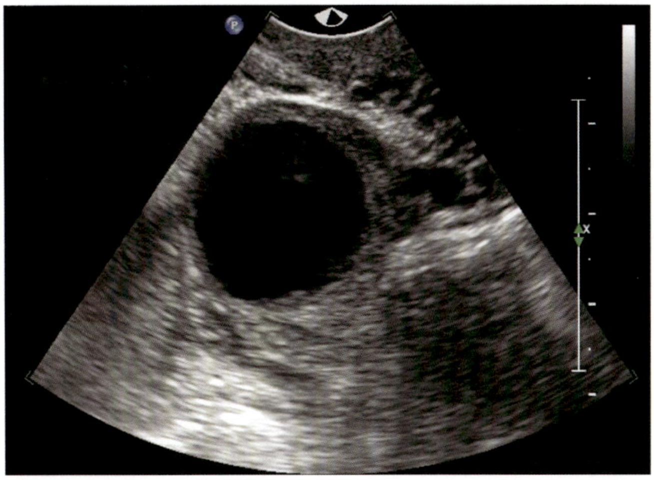

Figure 13.11 **Corpus luteum cyst**. A corpus luteum cyst is typically a thin-walled, simple anechoic cyst, but may contain internal echoes.

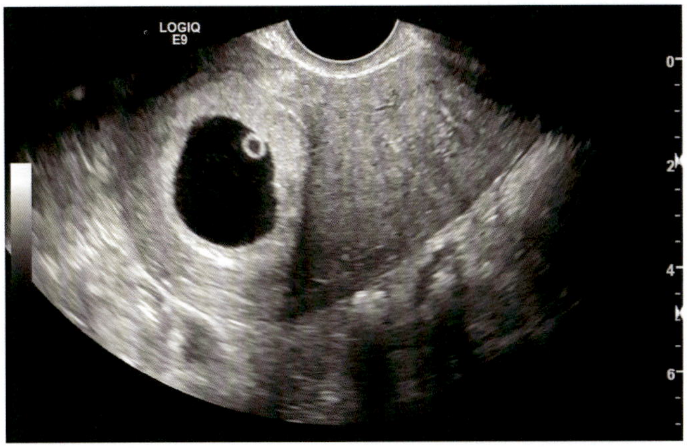

Figure 13.12 **Yolk sac**. A coronal transvaginal ultrasound demonstrating a yolk sac within the gestational sac. The yolk sac (arrow) appears as a hyperechoic ring within the anechoic gestational sac.

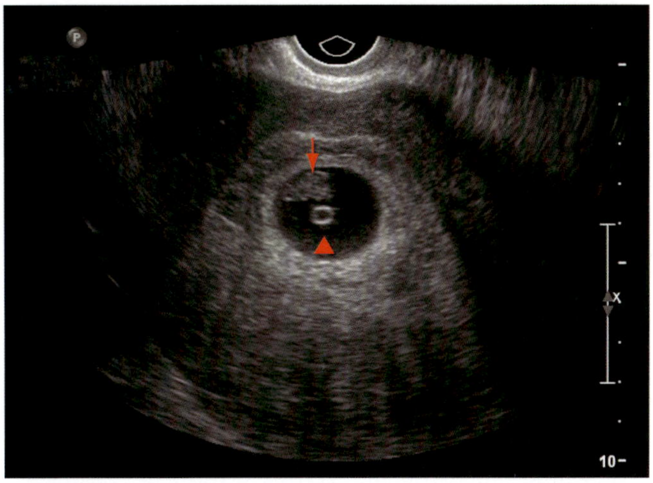

Figure 13.13 **Fetal pole and yolk sac**. A coronal transvaginal ultrasound demonstrating a fetal pole (arrow) adjacent to the yolk sac (arrowhead).

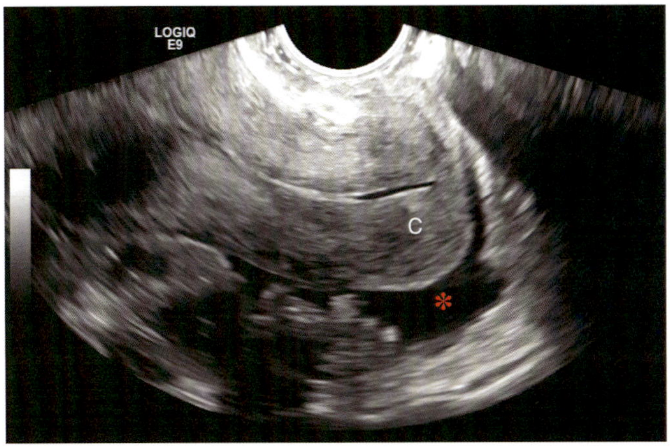

Figure 13.14 **Ruptured ectopic pregnancy**. This sagittal transvaginal image demonstrates the cervix (C) as well as free fluid (*) posterior to the cervix in a patient with a ruptured ectopic pregnancy.

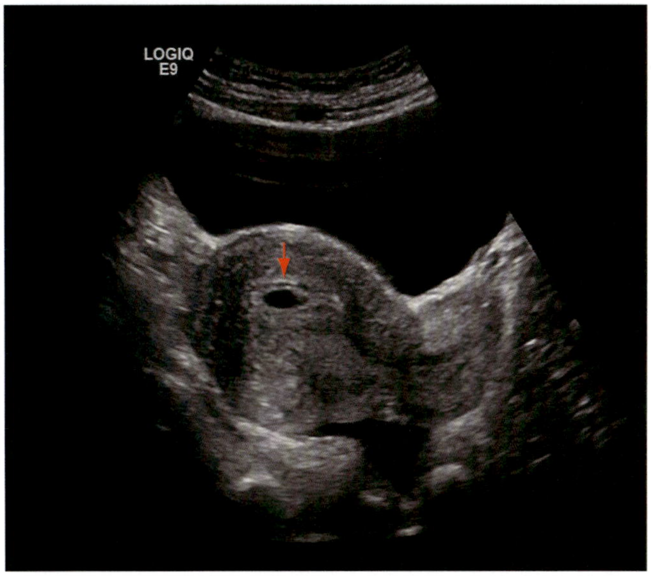

Figure 13.15 **Double decidual sign**. A sagittal transabdominal ultrasound view demonstrating a "double decidual sac" sign (arrow). Note that this is a subtle sign of early pregnancy, and should not be relied upon for the diagnosis of an IUP.

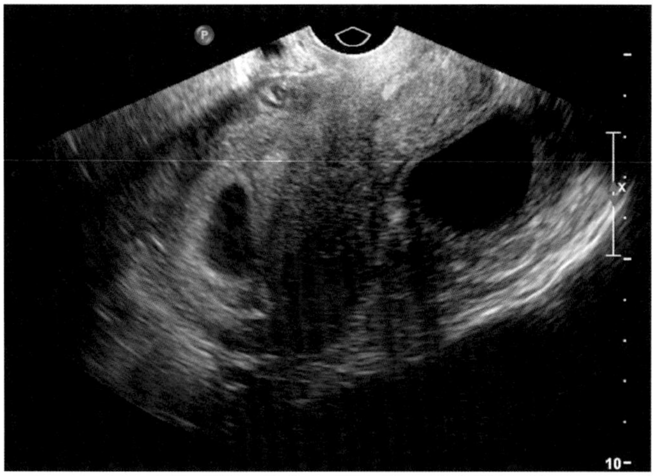

Figure 13.16 Blighted ovum. This gestational sac measures 22 mm on transabdominal ultrasonography, and is consistent with an early pregnancy failure, commonly known as a "blighted ovum."

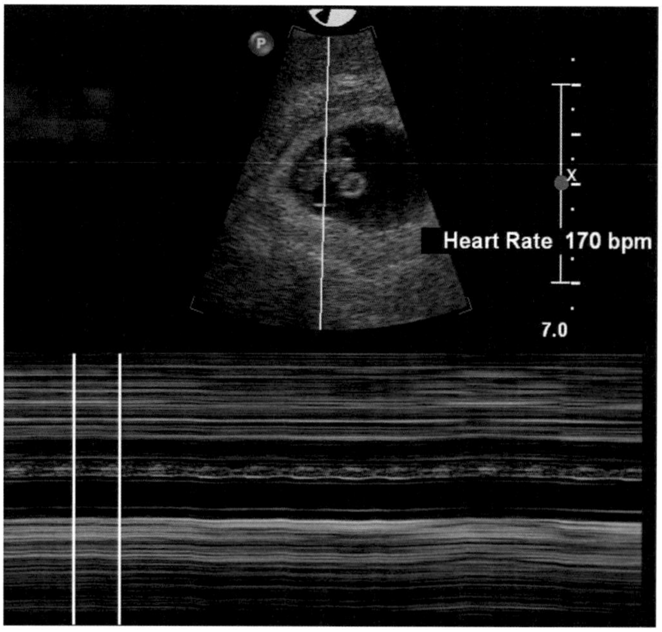

Figure 13.17 Fetal heart rate, M-mode. Note the cyclical pattern across the center of the M-mode screen. Using the machine's fetal heart rate calculator, one can obtain a still image demonstrating the fetal heart rate.

to freeze the M-mode screen and measure from the beginning of one cardiac cycle to the beginning of the next. Where one measures is not of particular importance as long as the placement of the calipers is consistent across the cardiac cycle. It is essential to include the entirety of a cycle and no more than a single cycle to calculate an accurate fetal heart rate (Figure 13.17).

M-mode is the preferred method, rather than pulsed-wave Doppler, since pulsed-wave Doppler concentrates the sound beam over a smaller area than M-mode. The acoustic energy is converted to heat within the tissue and, although no adverse effects have ever been demonstrated, there is a theoretical risk to the fetus of administering focused, high levels of energy. This is in keeping with the ALARA (as low as reasonably achievable) principle of reducing acoustic energy delivered to the fetus.

One should be cautious when diagnosing fetal demise by the absence of a fetal heart rate alone. If no heartbeat is identified on transabdominal ultrasound, a transvaginal examination should be performed next. If no heartbeat is identified during the transvaginal examination, obstetric consultation should be obtained.

Endomyometrial mantle

Another important criterion in the evaluation of an IUP is the measurement of the endomyometrial mantle (EMM), to exclude certain rare ectopic pregnancies such as an interstitial or cornual ectopic pregnancy. The EMM is the thinnest portion of uterus that surrounds the gestational sac. The measurement is taken from the edge of the gestational sac out to the outer edge of the myometrium. The measurement includes the endometrial and myometrial layers of the uterus on one side (Figure 13.18a,b). In a normal pregnancy, the width of the EMM should be greater than 5–7 mm. This measurement is used to evaluate for the possibility of an interstitial or cornual ectopic pregnancy.

Gestational age

Although the major objective for the emergency physician is to identify the presence an IUP, it is often useful to obtain an estimated gestational age by measuring the crown–rump length (CRL). In order to perform this measurement, obtain a sagittal view of the embryo, and measure from the crown of the head to the bottom of the torso or rump (Figure 13.19). This is the most accurate sonographic measurement of gestational age in the first trimester. By the time the CRL is 5 mm, one should generally be able to identify a fetal heartbeat on transvaginal examination, since the embryonic heart can be visualized by six weeks as a rapid flicker.

The mean gestational sac diameter can also be used to date a pregnancy, but it is less accurate and is not within the scope of emergency practice, since an empty gestational sac will require further consultation. It may be useful, however, to obtain this measurement for discussion with consultants. The gestational sac is measured from the inner aspect of the hyperechoic sac rim. Three measurements are obtained in three different planes, which are then averaged by the ultrasound machine.

Education and training

The cornerstone of education for most applications in ultrasonography includes a lecture component, competency examination, a total number of minimum scans performed, and supervised ultrasounds. MacVane *et al.* investigated one such training pathway for emergency residents in performing transvaginal ultrasonograpjy to detect an IUP. After residents performed 10 supervised transvaginal ultrasounds, had training, lectures, and a competency examination, residents were able to determine the presence or absence of an IUP that correlated with the emergency department ultrasound director's interpretation 93.3% of the time. In addition, the actual number of scans required comes into question. The

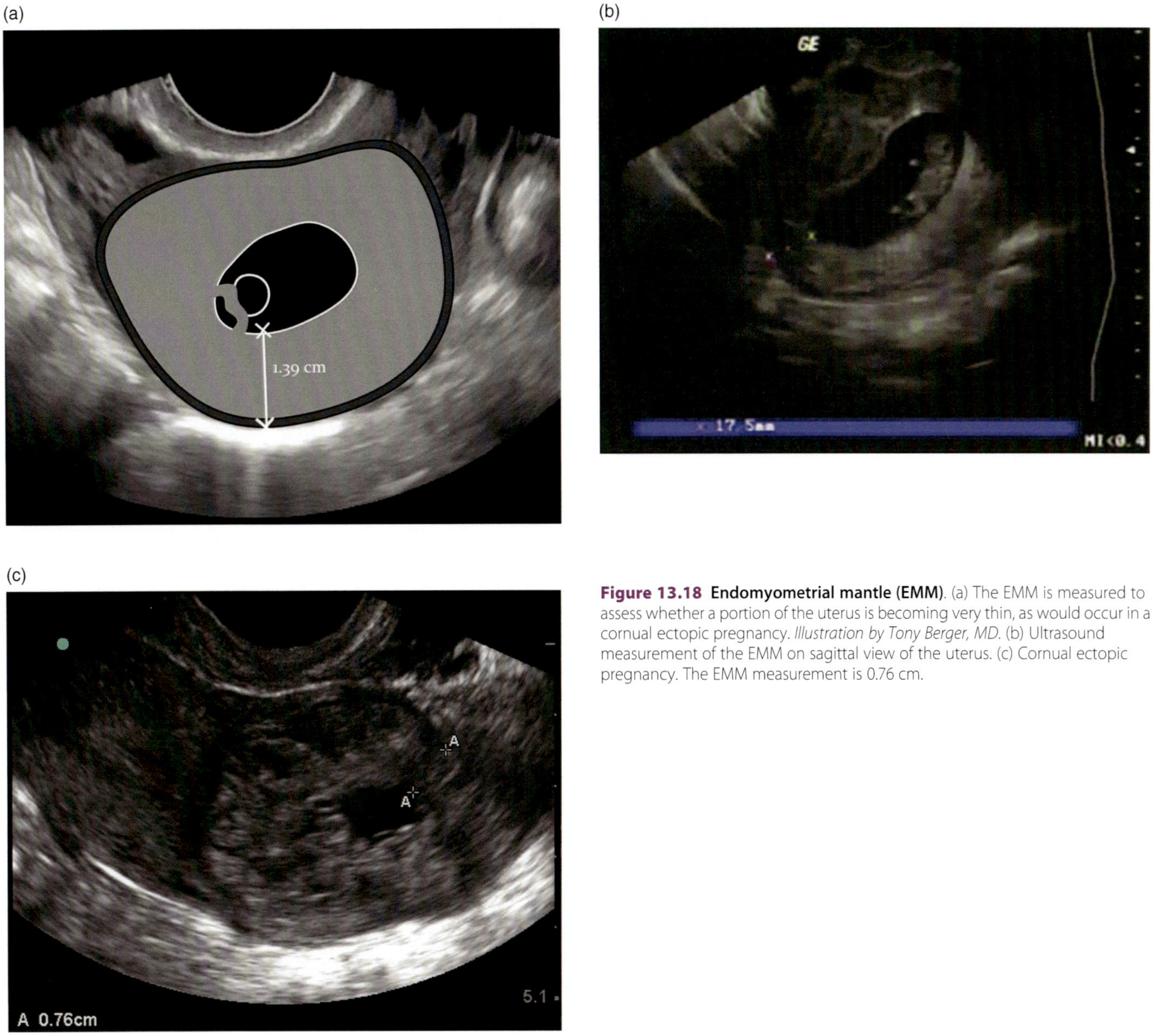

Figure 13.18 Endomyometrial mantle (EMM). (a) The EMM is measured to assess whether a portion of the uterus is becoming very thin, as would occur in a cornual ectopic pregnancy. *Illustration by Tony Berger, MD.* (b) Ultrasound measurement of the EMM on sagittal view of the uterus. (c) Cornual ectopic pregnancy. The EMM measurement is 0.76 cm.

American College of Emergency Physicians requires a minimum of scans for each basic application. However, with pelvic ultrasonography in particular, Jang *et al.* showed that, after an emergency physician's first 10 scans, their sensitivity for detecting an IUP was 80% and specificity 86%. After 40 scans, their sensitivity and specificity both increased to 100%. However, the detection of adnexal masses or ectopic pregnancy was 90% and remained unchanged with 40 examinations. Therefore, there is a significant learning curve that persists even past 40 performed examinations.

Scanning tips

Pitfalls

- A low β-hCG does not necessarily mean the absence of ectopic pregnancy.
- Avoid falsely identifying an IUP when just a gestational sac is visualized. The earliest that an IUP can be defined on sonogram is when a yolk sac is present.
- If a pregnancy is found in the uterus, one must confirm that it is not in the cornua or the cervix, by measuring the endomyometrial mantle. A measurement of less than 7 mm raises the possibility of a cornual, or interstitial ectopic pregnancy.
- The late second- and third-trimester pregnant patient with either vaginal bleeding or abdominal pain will require a transabdominal ultrasound for placental localization prior to speculum and digital examination. If the patient has placenta previa, cervical examination can lead to severe life- and fetus-threatening hemorrhage.
- Avoid "ruling out" placental abruption with ultrasound. Abruption is primarily a clinical diagnosis and, if suspected,

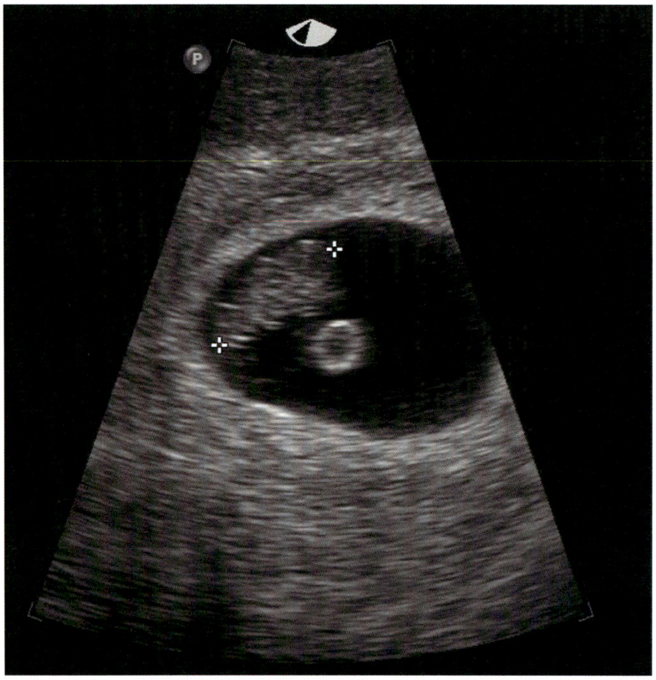

Figure 13.19 **Gestational age**. The crown–rump length is measured from head to bottom of the fetus (calipers). This measurement does not include extremities.

should be evaluated by fetal and maternal monitoring by the obstetric department.

- Do not utilize Doppler in the evaluation of the fetal heart. This offers potential risk to the fetus by delivering concentrated, high-energy sound waves to the fetus.

Tips to improve scanning

✓ In adolescent patients, a high index of suspicion for pregnancy must be maintained. All patients with a history of menarche should have a qualitative urine β-hCG test to determine whether they are pregnant, and a sexual history should be obtained without parents or other relatives present.

✓ A patient with an indeterminate ultrasound may be safely discharged from the emergency deprtment if she is clinically stable with normal vital signs, no noted hemoperitoneum on sonogram, a normal hemoglobin level or one that is stable over time, and no active hemorrhage on speculum examination. She must be reliable in following up, since she will need to have quantitative serum β-hCG repeated in two days, in order to make sure that it is doubling appropriately.

✓ Be sure to identify the yolk sac, in order to diagnose an IUP. The presence of a gestational sac alone is not sufficient to diagnose an IUP.

✓ Be sure to evaluate the uterus and both ovaries in two planes in order to evaluate for extrauterine pregnancies or other pathology.

✓ Additional measurements include the endomyometrial mantle, fetal heart rate by M-mode, and gestational age.

Pathology

Spontaneous or missed abortions

A **spontaneous abortion**, or miscarriage, is the spontaneous loss of an embryo or fetus prior to 20 weeks of gestational age. Prior to 20 weeks of gestational age, a fetus is unable to survive outside of the womb, as the respiratory and nervous systems are not sufficiently mature to sustain life. After 20 weeks but prior to 36 weeks of gestational age, the birth of a fetus is considered a preterm delivery. Spontaneous abortions can occur in up to 25% of pregnancies and are often thought to occur due to genetic abnormalities, although infections, trauma, toxins such as cocaine, and placental abnormalities may also be the cause. The great majority of spontaneous abortions occur during the first trimester while the pregnancy is in the embryonic stage. If the patient has passed all of the products of conception, the miscarriage is referred to as a **complete abortion**. When possible, in these cases, products of conception should be collected and sent to a pathology lab to be certain of their anatomic completeness.

Embryonic demise

Early pregnancy failure, commonly referred to as a **blighted ovum**, occurs when a fertilized egg implants and forms a gestational sac but forms no embryonic tissue. This is a common cause of miscarriage, and is usually due to multiple chromosomal abnormalities. It may be recognized on ultrasound by the presence of a large gestational sac without a yolk sac or fetal pole. A gestational sac greater than 20 mm on transabdominal scan without a yolk sac or fetal pole is consistent with the diagnosis (Figure 13.16). Further evidence suggestive of embryonic demise is the lack of cardiac activity. With transabdominal ultrasonography, cardiac activity should be seen in embryos greater than 5 mm by crown–rump length. With transvaginal ultrasonography, cardiac activity should be seen in embryos greater than 10 mm by crown–rump length. However, one should refrain from making the diagnosis of embryonic demise without further consultation from the obstetrics service.

Ectopic pregnancies

In the absence of an IUP, one must consider the possibility of an ectopic pregnancy. One may scan the adnexa and surrounding pelvis for specific signs of an ectopic pregnancy, which include a cyst, complex cyst, tubal ring, or an identified live ectopic pregnancy. A live ectopic pregnancy is characterized by the presence of either a yolk sac or a fetal pole with a fetal heart rate located in the extrauterine space. It must be emphasized, however, that the absence of these findings does not rule out an ectopic pregnancy. The most specific finding for an ectopic pregnancy is a live embryo in an extrauterine location (Figure 13.20a,b).

Another finding highly suggestive of ectopic pregnancy is a thick "tubal ring" within the adnexa (Figure 13.20c). This structure is formed by the fallopian tube and is found adjacent

(a)

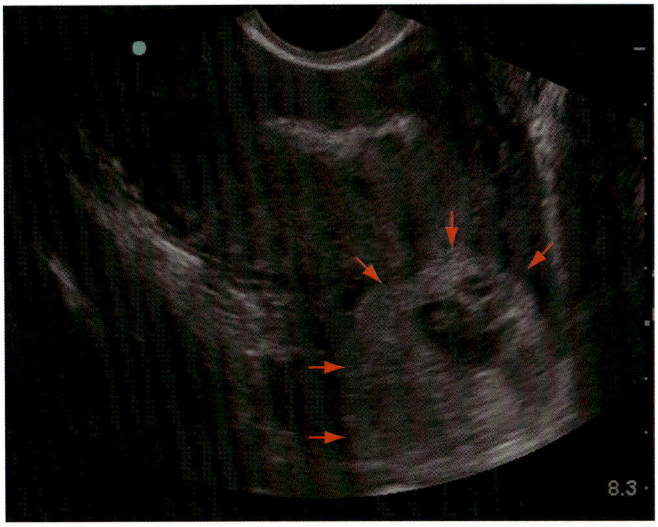

(b)

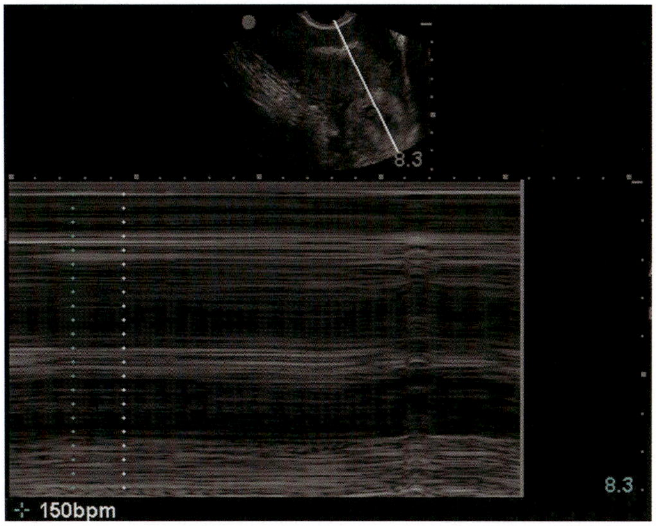

(c)

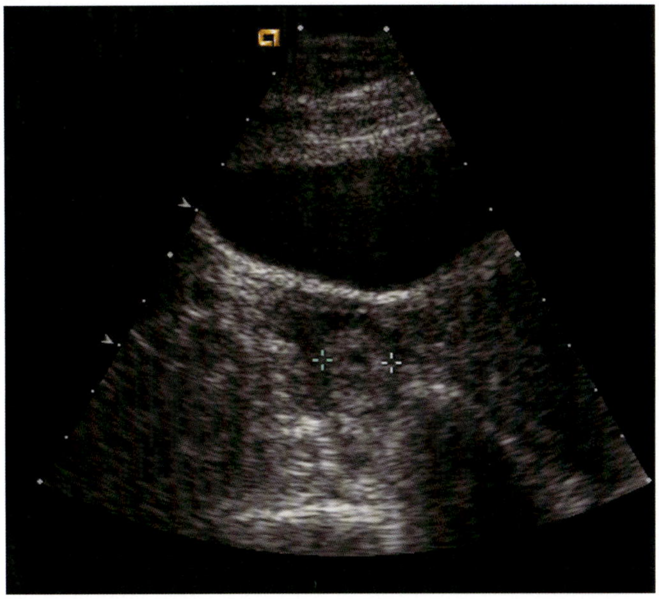

Figure 13.20 Ectopic pregnancies. (a) Extrauterine adnexal mass (arrows). An echogenic adnexal mass with internal debris is noted in the left adnexa. (b) Live ectopic pregnancy. M-mode demonstrates a heartbeat of 150 bpm, indicating a live ectopic pregnancy. (c) A 1.34 cm, adnexal tubal ring is identified; however, no fetal pole or cardiac activity is identified. A "tubal ring" (calipers) is a thick-walled, round structure within the adnexa, and is a specific finding for ectopic pregnancy.

to the ovary. The tubal ring often has increased perigestational blood flow, which can be seen with color or power Doppler and is called a "ring of fire". A tubal ring should not be mistaken for a corpus luteum cyst, which is typically thin-walled and anechoic, but may occasionally contain echogenic debris from hemorrhage within the cyst. Additionally, if one finds a large amount of peritoneal free fluid in a pregnant patient without an identifiable IUP, ectopic pregnancy is a very likely diagnosis. For this reason, it is worthwhile to perform an ultrasound scan of the right upper quadrant, Morison's pouch, looking for the presence of free fluid in the abdominal cavity.

A **cornual ectopic pregnancy** is a rare type of ectopic pregnancy in which the egg implants at the junction of the fallopian tube and the ovary. Although it may appear as though it is in the uterus, it is in fact an ectopic pregnancy that, if not properly identified, can have catastrophic consequences. These ectopic pregnancies tend to rupture later, are more vascular, and can result in severe hemorrhage. The mortality rate of cornual ectopic pregnancies is twice that of other ectopic pregnancies. As they grow, they invade the uterine wall and thin it out such that the endomyometrial mantle shrinks in size (Figure 13.18b). Additionally, the pregnancy will appear eccentrically located in the uterus. A pregnant women with an EMM of less than 7 mm should not leave the emergency department without a formal sonogram evaluated by a radiologist, or an obstetric consultation.

Although the quantitative serum β-hCG is helpful in the evaluation for an ectopic pregnancy, remember that a low value does not confirm the presence of an early IUP. The entire clinical picture must be evaluated, including such factors as

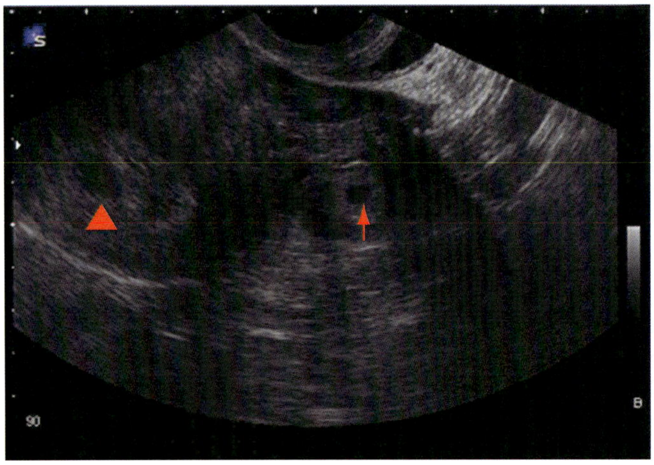

Figure 13.21 **Heterotopic pregnancy**. A heterotopic pregnancy is quite rare and involves an intrauterine (arrowhead) implantation in addition to an extrauterine (arrow), or ectopic, implantation. *Image courtesy of Alexis Langsfeld, MD.*

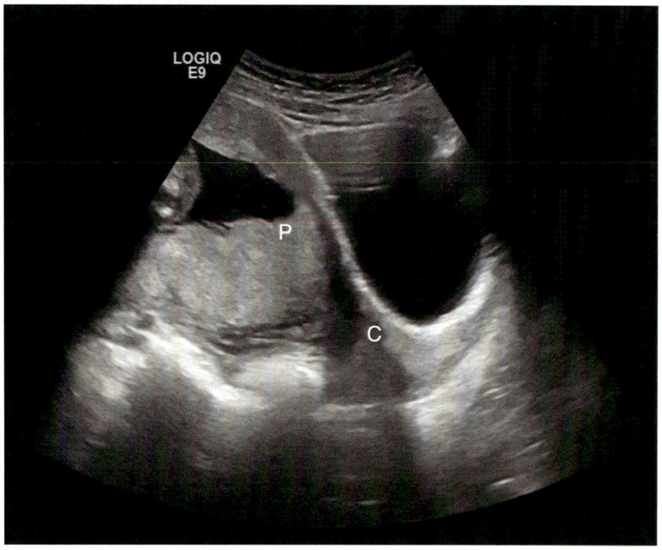

Figure 13.22 **Placenta previa**. Note the anterior placenta (P) and the tip overlying the cervical os (C).

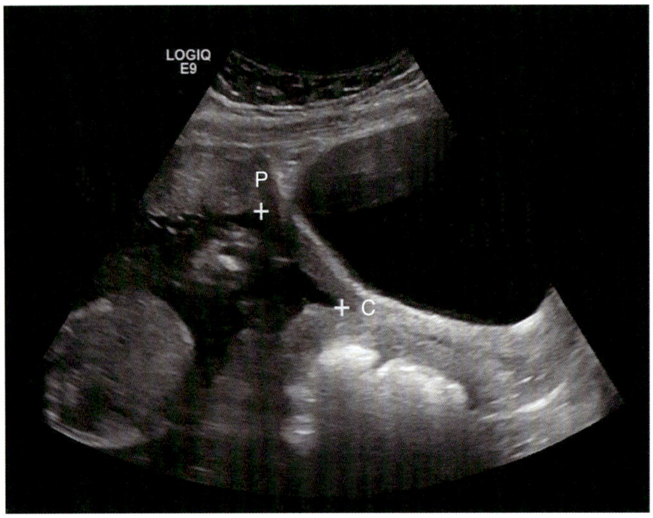

Figure 13.23 **Normal placenta**. The normal anterior placenta (P) is low lying but is located 4.5 cm from the cervical os (C).

hemodynamic stability, the presence of free fluid in the pelvis, the rate of blood loss noted on pelvic examination, and the reliability of the patient in obtaining follow-up. The case should be discussed with an obstetrician in order, at the very least, to arrange follow-up to obtain a repeat quantitative β-hCG in two days. It can't be emphasized enough that, there is no level of β-hCG at which a ruptured ectopic pregnancy is not possible. In fact, there is a case report of a β-hCG level of zero in a hypotensive critical patient with an ectopic pregnancy. However, if the β-hCG level is less than 700 mIU/mL, the patient has normal vital signs, there is minimal bleeding on physical examination, and the LMP is consistent with an early pregnancy, a reasonable strategy is to arrange follow-up in two days for a repeat β-hCG. It is important, in this circumstance, to communicate to the patient that the possibility of ectopic pregnancy remains and that any increase in bleeding, pain, or dizziness should prompt an immediate return to the emergency department.

Heterotopic pregnancy

One should consider the possibility of a heterotopic pregnancy in a patient with a confirmed IUP who has abdominal pain, hemodynamic instability, and free fluid present in the pelvis. In this situation, one should scan the adnexa and pelvis for other findings of ectopic pregnancy, such as a complex adnexal mass, pelvic free fluid, fetal heartbeat, and a tubal ring (Figure 13.21). Care should be taken not to confuse a tubal ring with bowel or a corpus luteum cyst. Although heterotopic pregnancy should theoretically be extremely rare in the pediatric population, given that this patient group rarely undergoes fertility treatment for conception, this possibility must be maintained in the astute clinician's differential diagnosis.

Placenta previa

Placenta previa is a condition in which the placenta is either very near or completely overlying the cervical os (Figure 13.22), when compared with the normal location of the placenta (Figure 13.23). It typically presents with painless vaginal bleeding in the late second, or early third, trimester but must be suspected in any pregnant patient who is beyond 20 weeks of gestational age. Often there is an initial self-limited episode of vaginal bleeding followed by a more severe episode of bleeding a few days later. Uterine cramping may be present; however, if the patient has significant pain, one must consider placental abruption (see below). An ultrasound examination must be performed prior to any pelvic examination – speculum or digital – as any manipulation of the placental tissue in a patient with placenta previa may induce severe hemorrhage.

To diagnose placenta previa, a transabdominal ultrasound examination should be performed. The preferred orientation is sagittal, as better visualization of the cervical os can be achieved. As stated above, this examination is generally beyond the scope of practice for the emergency physician/intensivist working in a

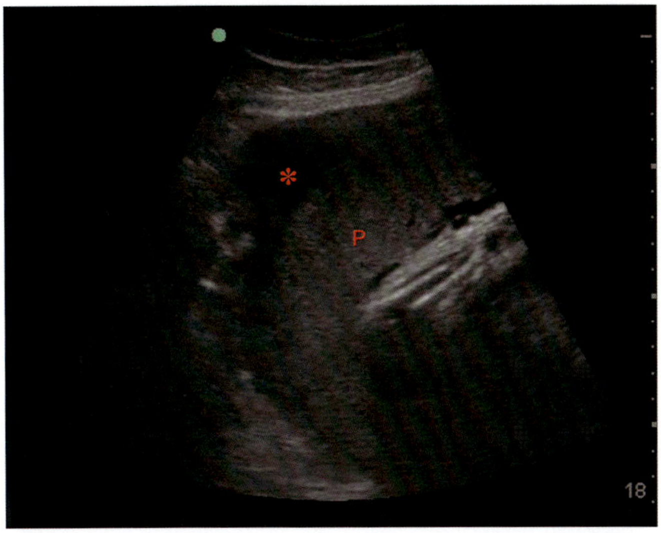

Figure 13.24 Placental abruption. Abruption is the separation of the placenta (P) from the uterine wall. In this image, hemorrhage (*) can be visualized. It is often unable to be seen by ultrasound. Therefore, ultrasound should not be relied upon to rule out an abruption. *Image courtesy of Rimon Bengiamin, MD RDMS.*

typical community or academic center where obstetric and radiologic consultations are readily available. The emergency physician's responsibility in most settings is to maintain hemodynamic stability by infusing crystalloid fluid and blood products as necessary, and to obtain immediate obstetric consultation.

Placental abruption

Another second- and third-trimester emergency is placental abruption, which occurs when the placenta separates from the uterine wall. Abruption may occur as a consequence of trauma, cocaine abuse, tobacco use, pre-eclampsia, or as a spontaneous occurrence. Placental abruption presents clinically as a range from mild cramping without bleeding to hemorrhagic shock, uterine tetany, and severe fetal distress. Ultrasound has only a limited role in the evaluation of placental abruption. This is due to the fact that, in mild cases, the separation may not even be visualized or the clotted blood between the placenta and the uterine wall may appear isoechoic to the placenta and invisible to the sonographer. In severe cases with hemodynamic instability and/or severe pain, the clinical picture, not the ultrasound, guides the diagnosis and treatment. When abruption is seen with ultrasound, it can appear as a variety of bright echogenic foci interposed between the placenta and the uterine wall (Figure 13.24). Again, the role of the emergency physician is to provide hemodynamic resuscitation and obtain emergent obstetric consultation.

Trauma

Patients presenting with abdominal pain after blunt abdominal trauma, such as after a motor vehicle collision, provide a particular diagnostic dilemma, since one must consider the possibility of intra-abdominal injury as well as placental abruption. In some instances, it may be necessary to obtain a CT scan to rule out splenic or liver injury, although the benefits of making the diagnosis must be weighed against the increased risk posed to the fetus by exposure to high levels of ionizing radiation. Conversely, patients may not have significant symptoms initially, but all pregnant patients greater than 20 weeks of gestation should be referred for fetal monitoring for a minimum of four hours in order to evaluate for fetal distress.

Cases

1. A 16-year-old female presents to the emergency department with left lower quadrant pain. The patient reports that her abdominal pain began 12 hours ago, and it has been increasing in severity since its onset. She is not quite sure when her last menstrual period was and reveals that she is sexually active. She and her boyfriend practice the "withdrawal method" of birth control. A urine β-hCG test is positive for pregnancy. She is unaware she is pregnant and as such has not had any prior ultrasounds. Her physical examination reveals normal vital signs, with mild general abdominal tenderness that is worse in the left lower quadrant. Her pelvic examination reveals a moderate amount of blood from the cervical os, which is closed on bimanual examination. Sonographic examination reveals an anechoic sac in the uterus, consistent with a gestational sac. There is no visible yolk sac or fetal pole within the gestational sac. There is moderate free fluid in the pelvis (Figure 13.25a). Right upper quadrant abdominal sonography also reveals free fluid in Morison's pouch (Figure 13.25b). Her serum β-hCG is 3000 mIU/mL. The obstetrics service is consulted for a patient with a ruptured ectopic pregnancy.

   This case highlights the importance of evaluating for an ectopic pregnancy. Since an intrauterine gestational sac may be present in ectopic pregnancies, it is crucial to identify a yolk sac and/or fetal pole within the gestational sac in order to diagnose an intrauterine pregnancy. It is often difficult to actually find the ectopic pregnancy, since it may be implanted in extrauterine locations other than in the adnexa. In cases of suspected ectopic pregnancies, it is also helpful to perform a FAST examination in order to evaluate for free fluid which would be suggestive of a ruptured ectopic pregnancy.
2. A 15-year-old female presents to the emergency department with a complaint of an irregular period and mild, cramping, suprapubic pain. She is not sure when her last period was, and believes that it might have been two months ago. A urine pregnancy test is performed and it is positive. Looking through the chart, you see that she was treated for a chlamydia infection four months ago. On physical examination, the patient is noted to have a small amount of blood from the cervix, and the os is closed. Transvaginal ultrasound examination reveals no IUP, no free fluid, and no adnexal masses present. Her β-hCG is 850 mIU/mL. The patient is informed that she is pregnant. The obstetrician is notified and recommends follow-up in clinic in two days to repeat the β-hCG and sonogram. She continues to have symptoms, and so in two days she returns and the β-hCG is 1100 mIU/mL. A repeat transvaginal ultrasound examination reveals a tubal ring located at the interstitium,

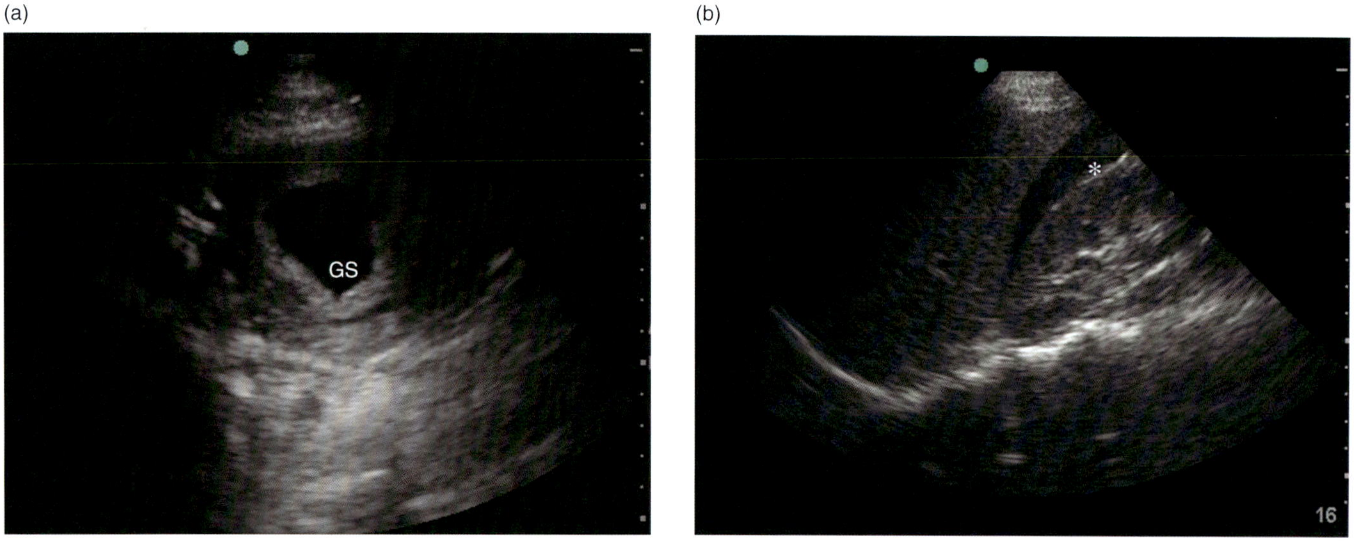

Figure 13.25 **Case 1: ruptured ectopic pregnancy**. (a) Anechoic sac seen within the uterus, consistent with a gestational sac (GS). However, no yolk sac or fetal pole may be visualized. (b) An additional view of Morison's pouch reveals free fluid (*), which is consistent with a ruptured ectopic pregnancy.

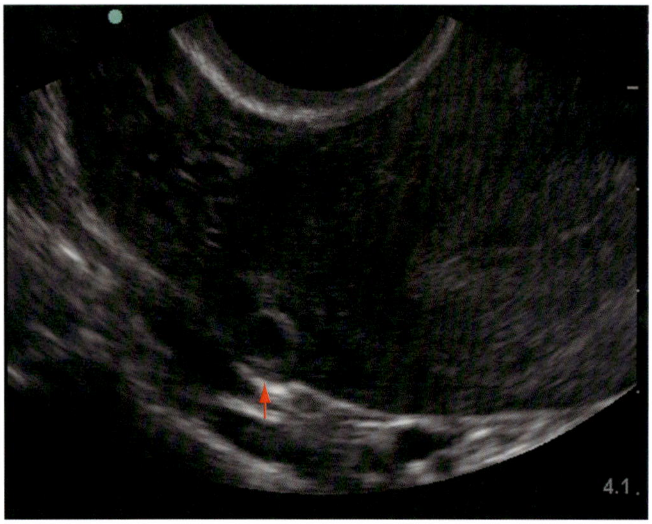

Figure 13.26 **Case 2: unruptured interstitial ectopic pregnancy**. A tubular ring (arrow) is located at the interstitium, the uterine portion of the fallopian tube.

the uterine portion of the fallopian tube. However, no fetal pole or cardiac activity is identified (Figure 13.26). No pelvic free fluid is identified. Her diagnosis is ectopic pregnancy (unruptured). She is treated with methotrexate and is counseled about birth control methods.

In stable patients who are reliable, they may be discharged home with close follow-up with an obstetrician. It is often difficult to differentiate an early IUP from an ectopic pregnancy. Therefore, it is crucial that patients follow-up with an obstetrician and have a repeat β-hCG, to make sure that it is increasing appropriately.

3. A 17-year-old female presents to the emergency department with intermittent vaginal bleeding. She states that she thinks she is pregnant because a home pregnancy test was positive; her period, which is very regular, is six weeks late. She also states that she has been feeling very nauseated and has had multiple bouts of emesis. Serum quantitative β-hCG is 1,314,414 mIU/mL. Transabdominal ultrasound reveals a uterus filled with an echogenic mass containing multiple small cystic structures or what is referred to as a "snowstorm pattern" (Figure 13.27).

   This pattern is consistent with a complete hydatiform mole. A hydatiform mole is a form of gestational trophoblastic disease, and is also referred to as a "molar pregnancy." Abnormal fertilization prevents the fetus from developing normally, and results in an abnormal placenta consisting of a mass of tissue with grape-like, swollen chorionic villi. Treatment of moles consists of ultrasound-guided suction evacuation by a trained obstetrician. The patient is scheduled for a dilatation and curettage (D&C), and serial quantitative serum β-hCG measurements are taken over the next six months to be sure that they do not increase or plateau, which is an indication of malignant transformation.

Summary/key points

1. Consider pregnancy in any adolescent female presenting with abdominal pain or abnormal vaginal bleeding. Identify early embryonic structures such as a yolk sac within the gestational sac prior to confirming the presence of an IUP.
2. Use quantitative serum β-hCG levels to increase your suspicion of an ectopic pregnancy, not to rule it out.
3. Recognize fetal demise by the lack of a fetal heartbeat at the appropriate gestational age, and arrange for proper obstetric consultation.
4. Recognize rare intrauterine-appearing ectopic pregnancies such as cornual or a cervical ectopic pregnancy by measuring the endomyometrial mantle and searching for a heartbeat if the gestational sac is located within the cervix.
5. In gestations older than 20 weeks with vaginal bleeding, perform transabdominal ultrasound to evaluate for placenta previa prior to physical examination. Perform fetal and maternal monitoring in suspected cases of placental abruption, which is a clinical diagnosis.

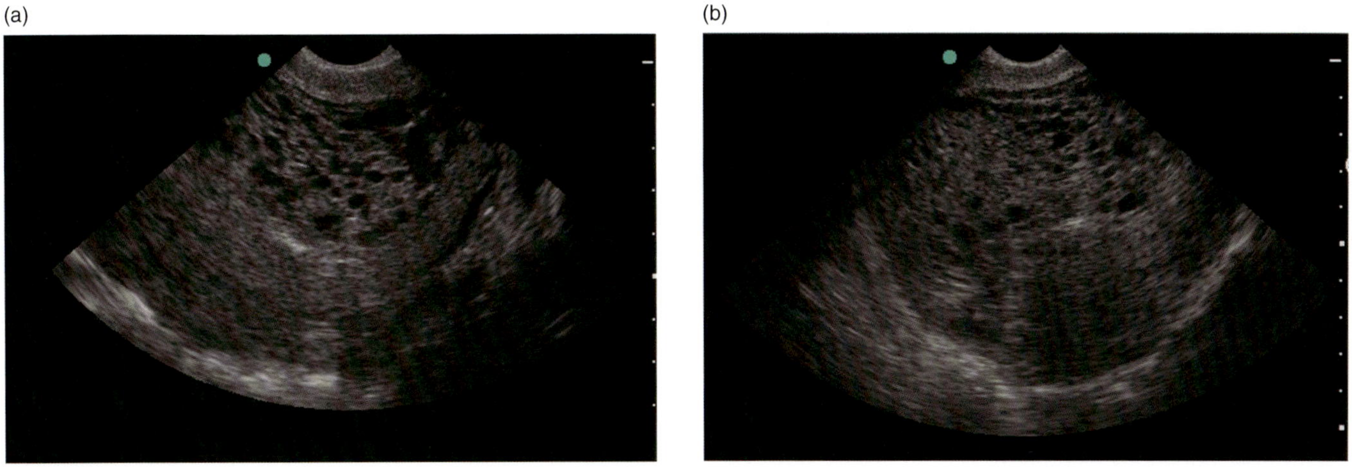

Figure 13.27 Case 3: hydatiform mole. (a) Sagittal transvaginal image of a molar pregnancy. (b) Coronal transvaginal image of a molar pregnancy. *Image courtesy of St. Luke's-Roosevelt Hospital, Emergency Ultrasound Division.*

Selected references

Choi, H., Blaivas, M., Lambert, M. (2000) Gestational outcome in patients with first-trimester pregnancy complications and ultrasound-confirmed live intrauterine pregnancy. *Acad Emerg Med* 7(2): 200–3.

Dart, R., Dart, L., Mitchell, P. (1999) Normal intrauterine pregnancy is unlikely in patients who have echogenic material identified within the endometrial cavity at transvaginal ultrasonography. *Acad Emerg Med* **6**: 116–20.

Durham, B., Lane, B., Burbridge, L., *et al.* (1997) Pelvic ultrasound performed by emergency physicians for the detection of ectopic pregnancy in complicated first-trimester pregnancies. *Ann Emerg Med* **29**: 338–47.

Hahn, S. A., Lavonas, E. J., Mace, S. E., *et al.* (2012) Clinical policy: critical issues in the initial evaluation and management of patients presenting to the emergency department in early pregnancy. *Ann Emerg Med* **60**(3): 381–90.

Mallin, M., Dawson, M., Schroeder, E., *et al.* (2012) Prospective outcomes of pregnant ED patients with documented fetal cardiac activity on ultrasound. *Am J Emerg Med* **30**: 472–5.

Saul, T., Lewiss, R. E., Rivera, M. D. (2012) Accuracy of emergency department bedside ultrasound in determining gestational age in first trimester pregnancy. *Crit Ultrasound J* **4**(1): 22. doi: 10.1186/2036-7902-4-22

Stein, J. C., Wang, R., Adler, N., *et al.* (2010) Emergency physician ultrasonography for evaluating patients at risk for ectopic pregnancy: a meta-analysis. *Ann Emerg Med* **56**: 674–83.

Tayal, V. S., Cohen, H., Norton, H. J. (2004) Outcome of patients with an indeterminate emergency department first-trimester pelvic ultrasound to rule out ectopic pregnancy. *Acad Emerg Med* **11**(9): 912–17.

Thamburaj, R., Sivitz, A. (2013) Does the use of bedside ultrasound decrease length of stay in the Emergency Department? *Pediatr Emerg Care* **29**(1): 67–70.

Wang, R., Reynolds, T. A., West, H. H. (2011) Use of a β-HCG discriminatory zone with bedside pelvic ultrasonography. *Ann Emerg Med* **58**: 12–20.

Chapter 14

Pelvic: gynecology

Katja Goldflam and Resa E. Lewiss

Objectives/indications

Adolescents and young women often present to the emergency department with abdominal complaints. Especially when they present with abdominal pain localized to the lower abdomen, this presents a particular challenge for the clinician. Pelvic pathology, including diseases of the uterus and adnexa, must be considered, along with the usual spectrum of gastrointestinal diseases, such as appendicitis and genitourinary diseases such as pyelonephritis. Pelvic pathology includes a vast possibility of differential diagnoses, ranging from ovarian cysts to infectious processes, such as pelvic inflammatory disease (PID) and tubo-ovarian abscesses (TOAs), to ovarian torsion. This differential should be expanded to include complications of pregnancy, such as ectopic or molar pregnancies, in patients with a positive pregnancy test (see Chapter 13).

Ultrasound has taken an increasingly important role in delineating many abdominopelvic disease entities. The benefits of ultrasound include a radiation-free evaluation, which is especially important in the pediatric and adolescent populations. It also involves an active scanning approach, unlike static CT or magnetic resonance imaging, and allows the sonographer to assess directly if pain or discomfort is reproducible in certain locations. Thus, for example, focal adnexal tenderness may be elicited, which can aid in making a diagnostic conclusion. In this instance, it is especially useful if the clinician, rather than an ultrasound technician, is able to perform the scan at the bedside, using it effectively as an integrated part of the physical examination. In conjunction with the history and physical examination, ultrasound can further aid in differentiating between multiple disease processes that often have similar clinical presentations. Useful adjuncts to the basic two-dimensional B-mode scanning include color Doppler or power Doppler. Color Doppler may be used to differentiate between different types of ovarian cysts and masses, as some will have a more vascular quality than others, as well as to evaluate vascular compromise to the adnexa when concern exists for ovarian torsion. Color power Doppler provides even greater sensitivity in low-flow states and may be used to confirm a diminished or an absent blood flow in some cases of ovarian torsion.

An evolving role for the emergency physician is in performing pelvic sonography in the non-pregnant patient. It is possible for the physician to correlate clinical presentations with sonographic findings, and to diagnose specific disease entities. However, it is important to recognize that gynecologic ultrasound requires skill and training beyond the basic emergency applications, specifically with Doppler ultrasound. However, even with limited expertise, point-of-care ultrasound may help direct the management of patients presenting with acute abdominal pain. In pre-pubetal pediatric patients, a sonographic evaluation may be limited to the transabdominal scanning approach, since the endovaginal approach requires insertion of an ultrasound transducer which may not be possible due to the patient's anatomical development, as well as undesired due to the potentially traumatic experience for the patient. In general, transvaginal scanning is reserved for the population of female patients who are physically mature, sexually active, and able to consent to the procedure. Transvaginal scanning allows for a higher-resolution image of the pelvic organs compared to the transabdominal approach, both due to physical proximity of the transducer to the uterus and ovaries, but also due to the higher-frequency transducer used during this approach. The method is therefore often especially valuable in obese patients, where trans-abdominal scanning may not provide adequate image quality.

This chapter reviews the indications for pelvic ultrasonography in non-pregnant females. Both the transabdominal and transvaginal approaches are discussed, with particular emphasis on gynecologic pathology commonly presenting to the emergency department.

Background

Pelvic ultrasonography has been utilized in the emergency department since the 1980s, to identify pathology in both pregnant and non-pregnant patients. In patients presenting with acute abdominal pain, ultrasound has been shown to be invaluable in detecting gynecologic disorders, and distinguishing them from other causes of acute abdominal pain that require surgical repair. Such disorders include ovarian torsion, pelvic inflammatory disease, tubo-ovarian abscesses, ovarian cysts, and ovarian masses. Ultrasound is a useful adjunct in the diagnosis of complicated pelvic inflammatory disease (PID). However, the sensitivity and specificity of ultrasound in the diagnosis of tubo-ovarian abscesses range widely from 56 to 93% and 86 to 98%, respectively. With this range of results, clinicians should be aware of the limitations of the technique. In addition, one of the most important indications for pelvic ultrasonography is in the evaluation for suspected ovarian torsion. However, there are significant limitations for

Pediatric Emergency and Critical Care Ultrasound, ed. Stephanie J. Doniger. Published by Cambridge University Press.

ultrasonography in diagnosing ovarian torsion. Typically, color Doppler is utilized to evaluate for the presence or absence of arterial and venous flow to the ovary. Additional findings suggestive of ovarian torsion include a lead point mass, an enlarged ovary, and a twisted vascular pedicle. Servaes *et al.* showed that color flow Doppler indicating either arterial or venous flow was obtained in 62% of torsed ovaries. Vascular flow was only absent in the remaining 38%, and a lead point mass (i.e. cyst or teratoma) was identified in only 55% of patients. Therefore, the physician's suspicion of the diagnosis should remain high even in the presence of venous and arterial flow and in the absence of a lead point mass.

Transvaginal pelvic ultrasonography, in particular, has become widely applied as an adjunct to transabdominal scanning of the pelvic organs. In addition to rapidly identifying life-threatening pathology, point-of-care ultrasound findings have been shown to significantly alter medical decision-making and patient management in an acute gynecology unit. In a prospective observational study of 1000 women, Haider *et al.* showed that a point-of-care transvaginal ultrasound changed the management plan in 38.1% of patients, thereby leading to a reduction in admission rates from 37.1 to 19.4%. As a result, the point-of-care ultrasound was shown to be both time saving and cost effective. Tayal *et al.* completed a similar prospective investigation in the emergency department, with patients over 17 years of age, presenting with right lower quadrant pain. Ovarian cysts and uterine fibroids were the most common pathologies identified; however, the majority of ultrasounds (70%) resulted in normal findings. Ultrasound findings overall only minimally changed management and consultation preferences. Overall, there was a mean reduction in 25% ($P < 0.001$) of gynecologic disease on the differential diagnosis, showing that transvaginal ultrasound had a significant impact on the diagnostic decision-making of the treating physician.

In the emergency department, Tayal *et al.* also showed that the transvaginal ultrasound examination provides improved confidence in key aspects of the pelvic examination. It performed better than traditional bimanual examination in assessing for cervical position, uterine size and position, uterine tenderness, ovarian size and tenderness, and the presence of an adnexal mass in patients with varying body mass indexes. In addition, several studies have illustrated the acceptance of this technique by patients in both the adult and adolescent population. Bellah *et al.* described their experience with non-pregnant patients, with ages ranging from 13 to 21 years. Patients were referred for evaluation for a variety of physician concerns, including possible PID, ovarian masses, irregular menses, and pelvic pain. Patients received a transabdominal scan, followed by a transvaginal scan. Image quality was improved on transvaginal scan compared to transabdominal scan in 86% of patients, and additional information was obtained in 58% of patients. Sixty percent of patients actually rated the comfort of transvaginal scanning higher than transabdominal scanning. Transabdominal scanning was limited primarily by overlying bowel gas or distorted pelvic anatomy, while transvaginal scanning had the advantage of using a higher-frequency transducer with better resolution as well as closer proximity to the pelvic anatomy. Ultimately, the authors' recommendation however was still to use transvaginal ultrasound as an adjunct and not in isolation. They also suggest considering transvaginal ultrasonography in the pediatric population on an individualized basis, taking into account the necessity of the examination and the emotional and physical maturity of the patient.

Anatomy

The pelvis may be divided into two regions: the true pelvis and the false pelvis (Figure 14.1). The true pelvis is bounded anteriorly by the pubic symphysis and the pubic rami, posteriorly by the sacrum and coccyx, and inferiorly by the perineal musculature. The false pelvis is located superior to the true pelvis. Within the true pelvis are the bladder, the uterus, and the ovaries. The uterus is a thick-walled muscular structure that varies in size according to cyclical menstrual changes. The ovaries are elliptical structures that are found in various positions, but are generally adjacent to the iliac vessels. The blood supply to the uterus is mainly provided by the uterine arteries. The ovaries have a dual supply, from the ovarian artery and a branch of the uterine artery (Figure 14.1b). The pouch of Douglas is the potential space in the posterior cul-de-sac of the pelvis. Since this is the most dependent portion of a supine female, fluid tends to collect in this region. A trace amount of free fluid is commonly seen here, and is normal, especially prior to menstruation.

Technique

The pelvic organs can be imaged in both a transabdominal and a transvaginal approach. The technique should be chosen based upon anticipated findings and organs of interest, as well as the age and sexual maturity of the patient. Transabdominal scanning may provide a broader field of view, as well as greater depth in imaging, and is useful in visualizing the ovaries, their vasculature, and the surrounding pelvic floor. Transvaginal scanning offers a greater resolution and more detailed imaging of the anatomy close to the transducer, including the cervix and endometrium. Each scanning technique and transducer type should be used to its full advantage and be allowed to complement one another, rather than limiting their utility by applying them in isolation. Also refer to Chapter 13 for the technique.

Begin with a transabdominal scan in order to gain a global impression of the positioning of the uterus. On occasion, the transabdominal view may also allow for better imaging of the adnexa and more lateral structures, as its range of motion is not as limited as with the transvaginal approach. Then, it is useful to perform the transvaginal examination when more detail of small structures, such as the ovaries, is necessary. It is important to image all pelvic structures in two planes, e.g. sagittal and transverse (transabdominal), or sagittal and coronal (transvaginal). This is the best means of gaining a view of three-dimensional objects such as the uterus and ovaries. The bladder plays an important role in both transabdominal and transvaginal scanning. A full bladder on transabdominal scan will act as

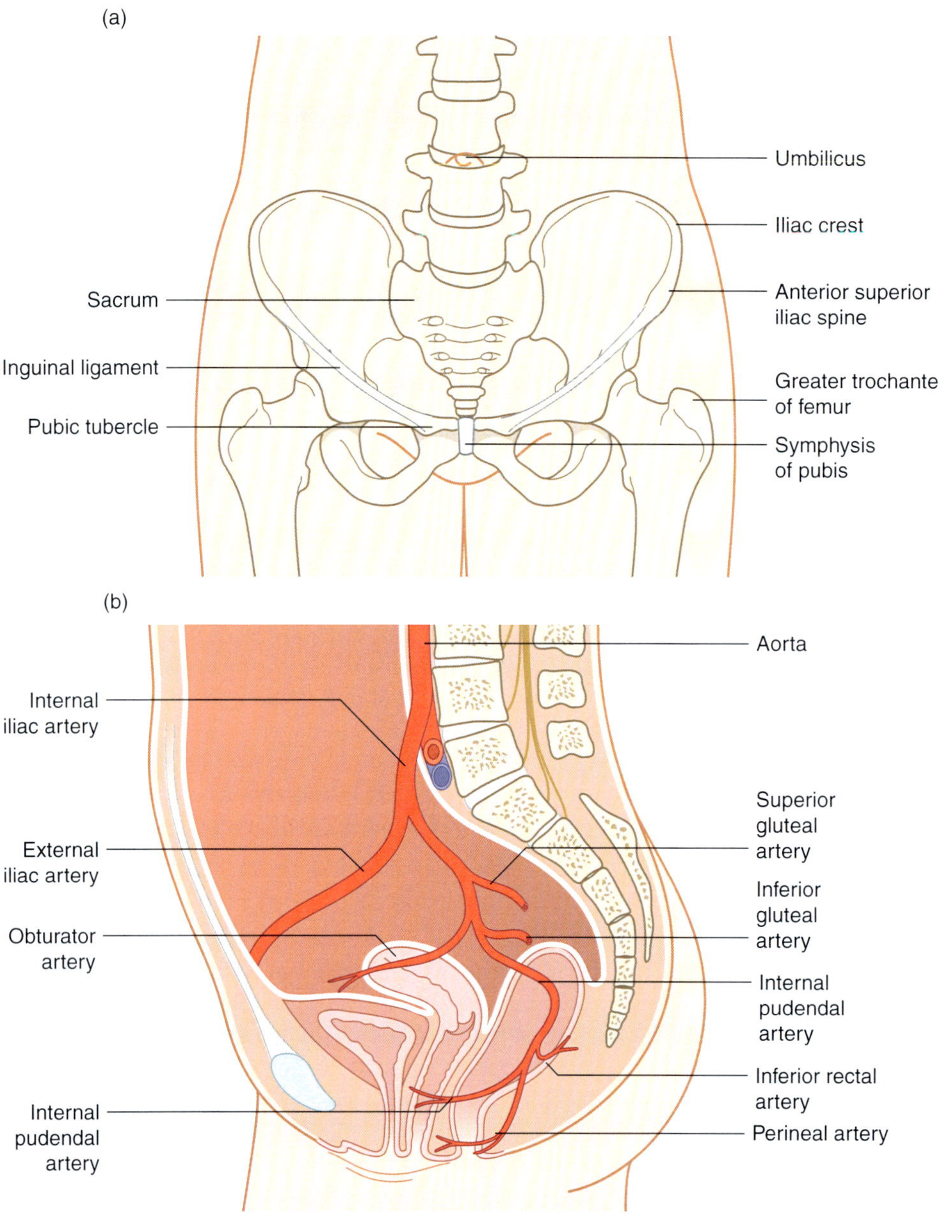

Figure 14.1 **Anatomy of the pelvis.** (a) The pelvis may be divided into the true pelvis and the false pelvis. The true pelvis is bounded anteriorly by the pubic symphysis and the pubic rami, posteriorly by the sacrum and coccyx, and inferiorly by the perineal musculature. Within the true pelvis are the bladder, the uterus, and the ovaries. (b) Blood supply to the uterus and ovaries. *Artwork created by Emily Evans © Cambridge University Press.*

an acoustic window, and allow for the improved visualization of structures such as the uterus and ovaries. An empty bladder on transabdominal scan may allow the uterus to fold up upon itself, distorting the anatomy and the relationship betweens structures. In contrast, a full bladder on endovaginal scanning may not only be uncomfortable for the patient, but may also obscure findings by retroverting the uterus and pushing it out of view or by taking up too much space to allow for the visualization of important structures.

Point-of-care questions

1. Are the ovaries enlarged? Are there cysts/masses present within the ovaries?
2. Does the uterus appear normal?
3. Is there abnormal pathology present that warrants an urgent/emergent referral to a gynecologist?

Transabdominal

Transducer selection and orientation: transabdominal

Transabdominal scanning allows for the visualization of organs further away from the transducer. A low-frequency (2–5 MHz) curvilinear transducer is utilized, which allows for deeper penetration of sonographic waves through the abdominal musculature and soft tissues.

Transabdominal images of the uterus and adnexa are obtained by placing the transducer immediately superior to the pubic symphysis, using the fluid-filled bladder as an acoustic window. A transverse image is obtained by placing the transducer with the indicator oriented towards the patient's right side (Figure 13.4a). A sagittal image is obtained by rotating the indicator cephalad directly towards the patient's head (Figure 13.5a).

Patient position and preparation: transabdominal

For transabdominal scanning, the patient is positioned comfortably in a supine position. This examination should, whenever possible, be performed on patients with a full bladder, since it provides an acoustic window through which to visualize the uterus and ovaries. For additional comfort, consider having the patient flex her legs at the hips and knees. This position also enhances the ability to utilize graded compression.

Ultrasound imaging: transabdominal

In the transverse view, the bladder appears as a dark, hypoechoic, oval or trapezoidal structure lying above the uterus (Figure 13.4b,c). In the sagittal view, the bladder appears as a wedge-shaped anechoic structure adjacent to the uterus. The bladder appears on the right and the uterus appears on the left when looking directly at the monitor (Figure 13.5b,c). The fluid-filled bladder is used as an acoustic window to scan the pelvic organs. As a fluid-filled structure, the bladder allows full through-transmission of the ultrasound beams to scan the deeper anatomy. A full bladder also aids indirectly by physically pushing bowel loops out of the way of the ultrasound window. When the bladder is empty, bowel loops may obscure the view by scattering of the echoes as they pass through the air-filled intestines, distorting the more distal image. It is important to remember that, due to the low attenuation of sound waves as they travel through the fluid-filled bladder, posterior acoustic enhancement may occur distal to the bladder. The image can be adjusted by decreasing the far-field gain (or time gain compensation), preventing the hyperechoic section behind the bladder from obscuring any important structures.

When scanning the pelvis for the presence of free fluid, such as in the case of a ruptured hemorrhagic cyst, the sonographer should be aware of the differing appearance that blood may have depending on the timing of the bleeding. While fresh blood will appear anechoic or hypoechoic (Figure 14.2), older pooled or clotted blood may appear more heterogeneous, with increasingly visible internal echoes as coagulation occurs. A collection of clotted blood may thus be confused with a loculated mass, bowel loops, or other anatomic structures.

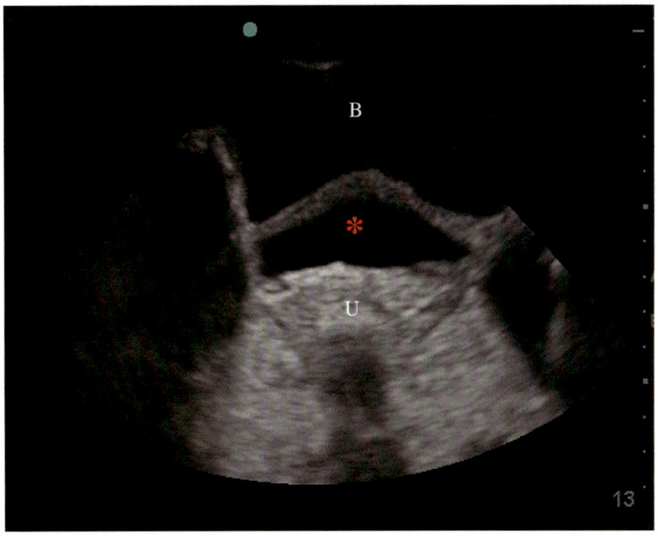

Figure 14.2 Free fluid. Transabdominal, transverse pelvic ultrasound showing anechoic blood (*) posterior to the bladder (B), and anterior to the uterus (U).

Transvaginal

Transducer selection and orientation: transvaginal

During transvaginal scanning, the pelvic anatomy of interest is much closer to the high-frequency transducer. The endovaginal or endocavitary probe therefore requires less depth penetration of the sound waves and employs a high frequency (5–9 MHz) which allows for higher image resolution. When using the endocavitary probe, identify the indicator prior to insertion. The sagittal view is obtained by pointing the indicator towards the ceiling (Figures 13.8, 14.3a). The coronal view is obtained by rotating the indicator counterclockwise, towards the patient's right side (Figures 13.9, 14.3b).

Patient position and preparation: transvaginal

Prior to the transvaginal scan, the patient should be asked to void and have an empty bladder. A full bladder on transvaginal scanning may not only be uncomfortable for the patient, but may also obscure findings by retroverting the uterus and pushing it out of view or by taking up too much space to allow visualization of important structures. The patient is placed in the lithotomy position to provide the sonographer with access to the vaginal introitus, as well as to allow for mobility of the transducer. Ideally, this portion of the ultrasound is performed in conjunction with the pelvic examination, in order to maximize the efficiency of the patient's evaluation.

Prior to insertion, an endocavitary probe should be covered with a clean, impermeable probe cover (i.e. glove, condom, or commercially available cover), in order to reduce contact and contamination with bodily fluids. There should be two layers of gel: one inside the probe cover, and a sterile lubricant gel on top of the covered transducer (Figure 13.7). In addition, it is crucial that the transducer be properly disinfected with chemical high-level disinfection immediately after each examination, in order to further minimize the risk of disease transmission. Such examples include immersion of the transducer in Cidex® or a sodium hypochlorite solution.

Ultrasound imaging: transvaginal

The transvaginal ultrasound examination can be useful in determining specific regions of patient discomfort, and the mobility of organs such as the ovaries. For example, adhesions from inflammation in the case of PID may reduce the mobility of the ovaries. Similarly, the ability of a mass to move with or separate from an adjacent ovary may aid in determining the etiology of this mass.

First, identify the longitudinal view of the uterus, in the sagittal view. The indicator is pointed towards the ceiling (Figure 13.8). Then, in order to obtain the coronal view, rotate the transducer counterclockwise, with the indicator towards the patient's right side (Figure 13.9). Find a plane of the uterus such that the uterine stripe is visible. Then, identify the ovaries by moving the transducer towards the lateral fornices. The ovaries will have a "chocolate chip cookie" appearance (Figure 14.4a).

(a)

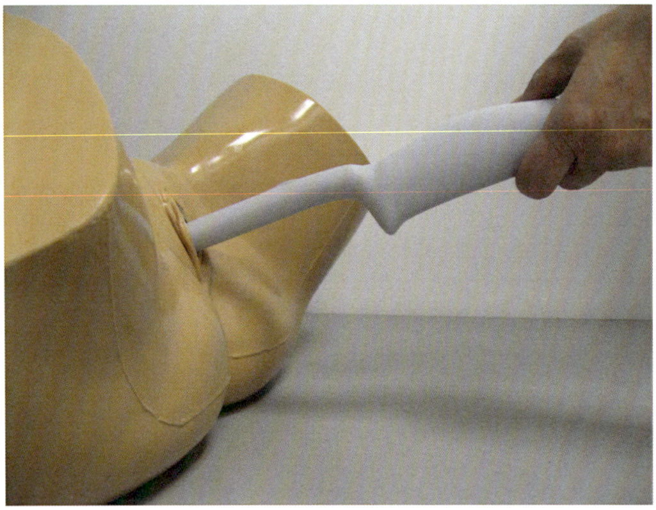

(b)

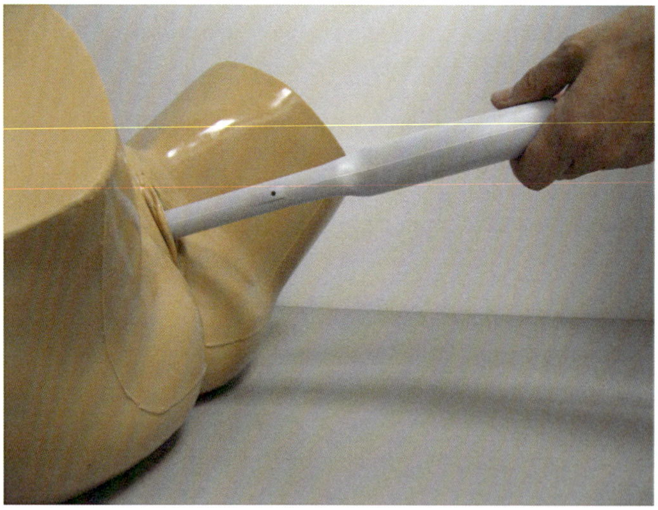

Figure 14.3 Phantom model, transvaginal scanning. (a) Sagittal view, with the indicator pointed towards the ceiling. (b) Coronal view, with the indicator oriented towards the patient's right side.

(a)

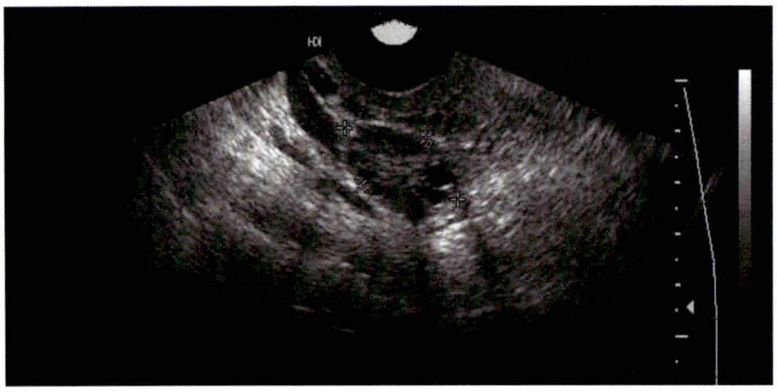

(b)

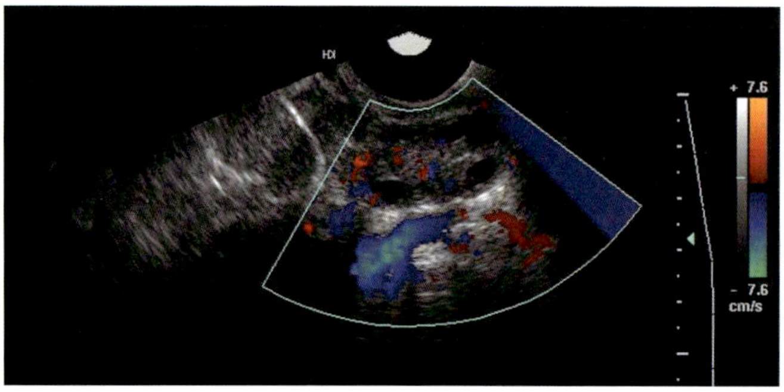

Figure 14.4 Normal ovaries. (a) Transvaginal scan of the ovaries demonstrating the "chocolate chip cookie" appearance. (b) Color Doppler showing normal flow to the ovary. *Images courtesy of Madhuri Kirpekar, MD.*

Color Doppler imaging may add significant information in pelvic pathology. While evaluating for ovarian torsion, color Doppler is utilized to assess for venous and arterial flow (Figure 14.4b). It is important to remember that the presence of venous and arterial flow does not "rule out" an ovarian torsion. In addition, color Doppler may be utilized in order to determine the etiology of masses, depending on their vascularity. Hyperemia may suggest inflammation and edema, such as in irritation of the endometrium and the adnexa in PID; while absence of vascularity may distinguish between a simple ovarian cyst and a more complex mass lesion.

Education and training

Training for transabdominal pelvic ultrasonography is easily performed with healthy volunteer models. However, it is often difficult to train clinicians in the use of transvaginal ultrasonography, and challenging to obtain live-patient model volunteers. Therefore, simulation has become increasingly important in the training of clinicians. Commercially available pelvic ultrasound trainers are available, which simulate pelvic anatomy and allow for transvaginal scanning (Figure 14.3). A recent study by Girzadas *et al.* introduced the combination of a high-fidelity scenario with a pelvic task trainer in order to train emergency medicine residents. Overall, both faculty and residents felt that this combination improved residents' skill in obtaining and interpreting transvaginal ultrasound images, and improved their overall education experience.

Scanning tips

Pitfalls

- An empty bladder on transabdominal scan may allow the uterus to fold up upon itself, distorting the anatomy and the relationship between structures.
- A full bladder on endovaginal scanning may not only be uncomfortable for the patient, but may also obscure findings.
- One of the main pitfalls for the novice sonographer is failing to verify findings in two planes. For example, a blood vessel seen in cross-section may be confused with a cyst if the longitudinal axis is not evaluated to allow the sonographer to see the tubular shape of the vessel.
- While fresh blood will appear hypoechoic, older pooled or clotted blood may appear more heterogeneous, with increasingly visible internal echoes as coagulation occurs.

A collection of clotted blood may thus be confused with a loculated mass, bowel loops, or other anatomic structures.

- A critical pitfall is relying on the visualization of venous or arterial flow on Doppler ultrasound to rule out ovarian torsion.

Tips to improve scanning

✓ Transabdominal scanning may provide a broader field of view, and greater depth in imaging. Transvaginal scanning offers a greater resolution and more detailed imaging of the anatomy close to the transducer, including the cervix and endometrium.

✓ With transabdominal scanning, the bladder should be full. In contrast, for transvaginal scanning the bladder should be emptied.

✓ The dynamic nature of pelvic ultrasonography can be used to assess for mobility of pelvic organs, and specific regions of discomfort.

✓ Any bowel loops that may be creating scattering of the ultrasound beam can usually be persuaded out of the way with gentle graded compression over the area of interest.

✓ The differential of pelvic pathology may include processes that result in bleeding or purulent drainage into the peritoneal cavity. In such situations, the sonographer should include a FAST examination as an adjunct to pelvic imaging.

✓ Doppler imaging may add significant information in pelvic pathology. The absence of venous and arterial flow to the ovary may suggest ovarian torsion; while hyperemia may suggest an inflammatory process.

Pathology

Ovarian torsion

Ovarian torsion is a surgical emergency constituting 3% of all gynecologic surgeries. The prompt identification of ovarian torsion may be critical to preserving future fertility in a woman of reproductive age. Torsion occurs either of the ovary alone, or of the fallopian tube/ovarian complex. Twisting occurs around the vascular pedicle containing the broad ligament of the uterus, the fallopian tube itself, the ovarian artery, and the adnexal branches of the uterine vein and artery. While most cases of torsion in adolescents and older women occur around the fulcrum of an ovarian mass or large cyst, the mechanism in younger children is thought to be as a result of increased laxity of the vascular pedicle. When related to a functional cyst, torsion is more common during the second half of the menstrual cycle. Torsion around the pedicle may be complete (i.e. a full 360°) or incomplete, and intermittent detorsing may occur, further complicating the presenting clinical picture.

On ultrasound, the affected ovary may appear enlarged and engorged, as obstruction of the lymphatic and venous drainage leads to edema of the adnexa (Figure 14.5a,b). When torsion occurs as a result of a cyst or mass acting as the fulcrum, these may be identified on ultrasound, along with multiple follicles along the periphery of the ovary, also typical for torsion. Occasionally the twisted pedicle itself can be visualized on ultrasound, giving a "whirlpool" appearance – one of the more definitive signs of torsion and 87% accurate for torsion. In later stages, infarction of the ovary may occur, leading to necrosis and free fluid that is visible in the pelvis. Occasionally, both ovaries can be imaged in a single sonographic plane, suggesting the significant displacement of one of the adnexa, which itself should raise suspicion for torsion.

Doppler ultrasound is a key adjunct in the sonographic evaluation for ovarian torsion (Figure 14.5c). Venous blockage is usually the initial insult, while arterial flow may only be affected later by mechanical obstruction from swelling and edema. Absence of both arterial and venous flow is quite specific to the disease process; however, since there is a dual blood supply of the ovary (by the ovarian artery and a branch of the uterine artery), the absence of arterial flow on Doppler imaging should not rule out torsion in a patient with a high clinical suspicion for torsion. Furthermore, arterial flow may be intermittently present in an ovary that is torsing and detorsing. Diminished arterial flow may be elicited by comparing Doppler imaging of both ovaries, increasing the sonographic sensitivity of the examination in patients with incomplete torsion. It is also important to recognize that smaller, portable ultrasound machines may not have sufficient power to detect the presence or absence of vascular flow to the ovary.

Ovarian cysts

Functional ovarian cysts are a frequent finding on pelvic ultrasound and are often incidental findings in an asymptomatic patient. Cystic structures of less than 2.5 cm should technically not be considered "cysts" but may be characterized as normal physiologic follicles in various stages of development as part of the woman's regular menstrual cycle. True cysts are larger than 2.5 cm and may reach up to 15 cm in size. Simple cysts are usually round and anechoic (Figure 14.6a). Complex cysts may appear septated (Figure 14.6b). In general, ovarian cysts are common and most often transient, resolving spontaneously over the course of the next one to two menstrual cycles. Discomfort occurs when there is rapid growth of the cyst, and from the resultant tension on the ovarian parenchyma. Follicular and corpus luteum cysts comprise the two most common functional varieties of cysts. Follicular cysts are the most frequent, resulting from the maturation of a follicle in the first half of the menstrual cycle in preparation for ovulation. When the follicle does not fully develop and fails to ovulate, a thin-walled, fluid-filled cyst remains. Corpus luteum cysts occur after ovulation, when the corpus luteum fails to completely involute during the second half of the menstrual cycle. These may also occur in neonates under the influence of maternal hormones. Corpus luteum cysts, in contrast to follicular cysts, have a thicker wall, and the periphery may appear more vascular on Doppler examination. In addition, patients may have multiple cysts throughout the ovary, as part of polycystic ovary syndrome (PCOS) (Figure 14.6c).

Occasionally cysts may hemorrhage within themselves or rupture, causing irritation of the peritoneum from blood and

(a)

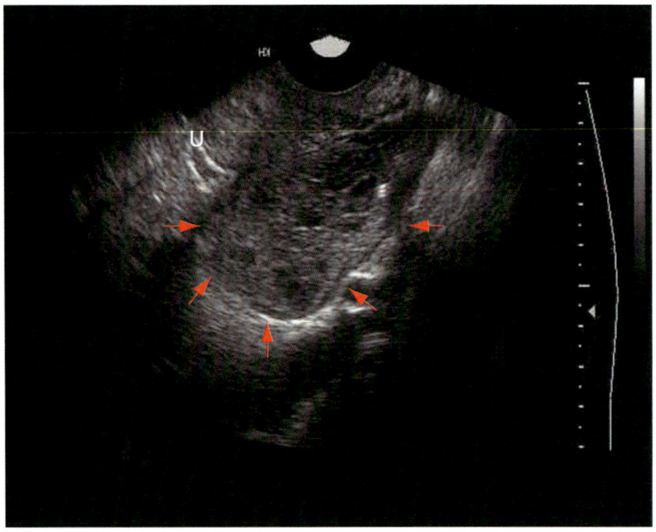

(b)

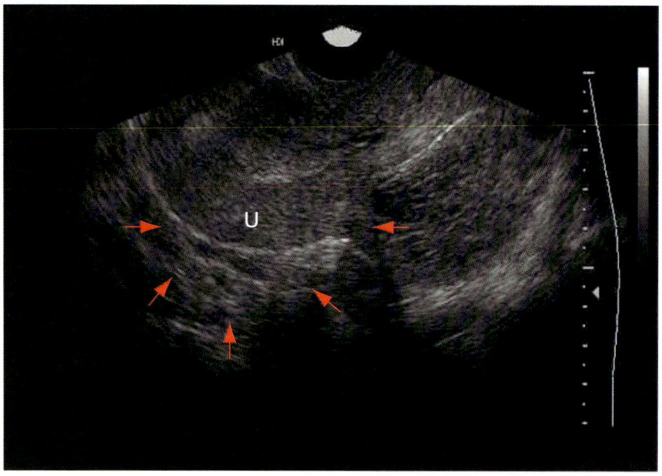

(c)

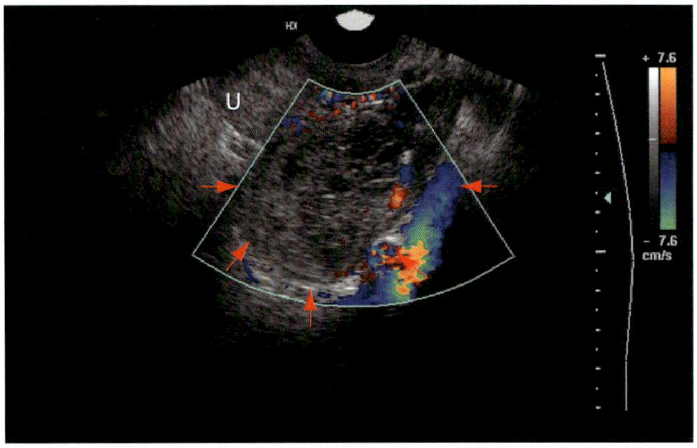

Figure 14.5 Ovarian torsion. (a,b) B-mode showing an enlarged ovary (arrows) and adjacent uterus (U). (c) Color Doppler. *Images courtesy of Madhuri Kirpekar, MD.*

inflammation. The patient may experience this as an abrupt worsening of the pain and discomfort. The clinical presentation may be similar to an ectopic pregnancy, so this possibility should always be excluded when the patient is not pregnant. On ultrasound, hemorrhagic cysts may have a varied appearance depending on the timing of the bleeding and depending on their age (Figure 14.6d). The content of the cyst may appear hypoechoic or anechoic immediately after the hemorrhagic event. However, as blood begins to clot the central area will develop more internal echoes in a reticular or "fishnet"-like pattern (Figure 14.6e). No central vascularity should be seen on Doppler, as this would suggest a more complex cyst or potentially a malignant mass. The sonographic evaluation should include a FAST examination to look for free fluid in the abdomen and pelvis. Such a finding of free fluid may help confirm the diagnosis of ruptured hemorrhagic cyst. Rarely, functional cysts may bleed enough to cause hemodynamic instability.

Pelvic inflammatory disease (PID)

Classically, patients presenting with PID will complain of acute pelvic discomfort, vaginal discharge, and fever. On bimanual and speculum examination, cervical motion tenderness and thick purulent vaginal discharge are present. Pelvic inflammatory disease presents as a spectrum of disease, ranging from simple cervicitis, to endometritis, salpingitis, and finally infection of the ovaries themselves.

Point-of-care ultrasound can provide information with regards to the various stages of the disease spectrum. Initially, the endometrium and endometrial stripe may appear thickened and heterogeneous, from edema and inflammation. Purulent material in the endometrial cavity may be seen as a hypoechoic, fluid- or debris-filled center within the uterus. Normal fallopian tubes may be difficult to image, especially with transabdominal scanning. As infection spreads to the fallopian tubes, fluid or purulent material causes enlargement of the tubular lumen, resulting in hydrosalpinx (Figure 14.7a,b) or pyosalpinx (Figure 14.7c,d), seen on ultrasound as a hypoechoic, debris-filled tubular structure adjacent to the adnexa. Inflammation further causes thickening of the tubular wall, making it much more easily identifiable and giving it a "cogwheeling" appearance, where the tubular folds appear prominently like small cogwheels contrasted against the fluid-filled center of the tube.

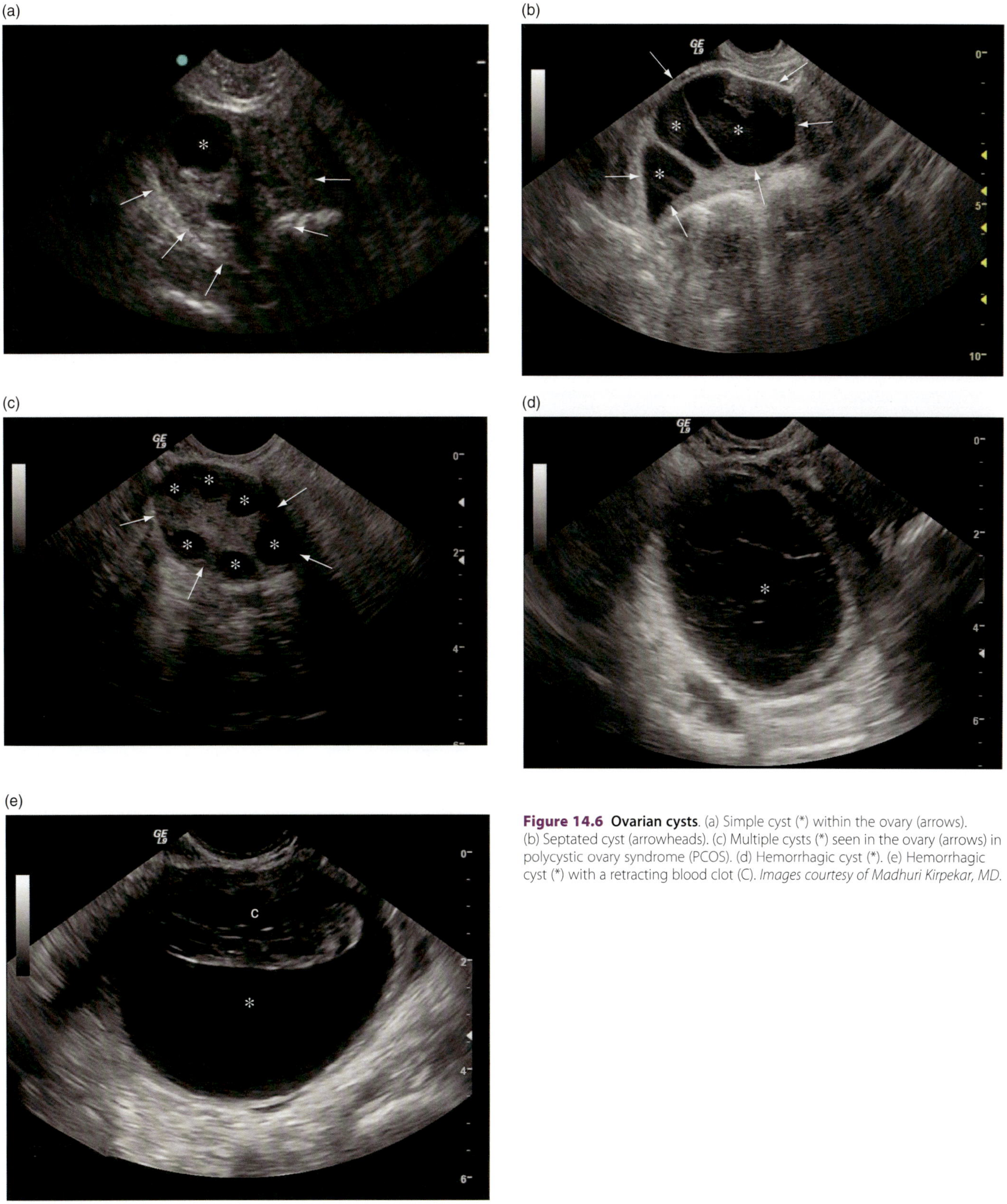

Figure 14.6 Ovarian cysts. (a) Simple cyst (*) within the ovary (arrows). (b) Septated cyst (arrowheads). (c) Multiple cysts (*) seen in the ovary (arrows) in polycystic ovary syndrome (PCOS). (d) Hemorrhagic cyst (*). (e) Hemorrhagic cyst (*) with a retracting blood clot (C). *Images courtesy of Madhuri Kirpekar, MD.*

Tubo-ovarian abscesses (TOAs)

The final stage in the spectrum of PID is the development of a tubo-ovarian abscess (TOA), which occurs in approximately 10–33% of patients. The clinical presentation may be similar to PID, making the distinction between simple PID and advanced PID complicated by an abscess difficult to achieve clinically. While some patients may have a palpable adnexal mass on physical examination, this is not sufficient to confirm or exclude TOAs. In the final stage of PID, the ovary and

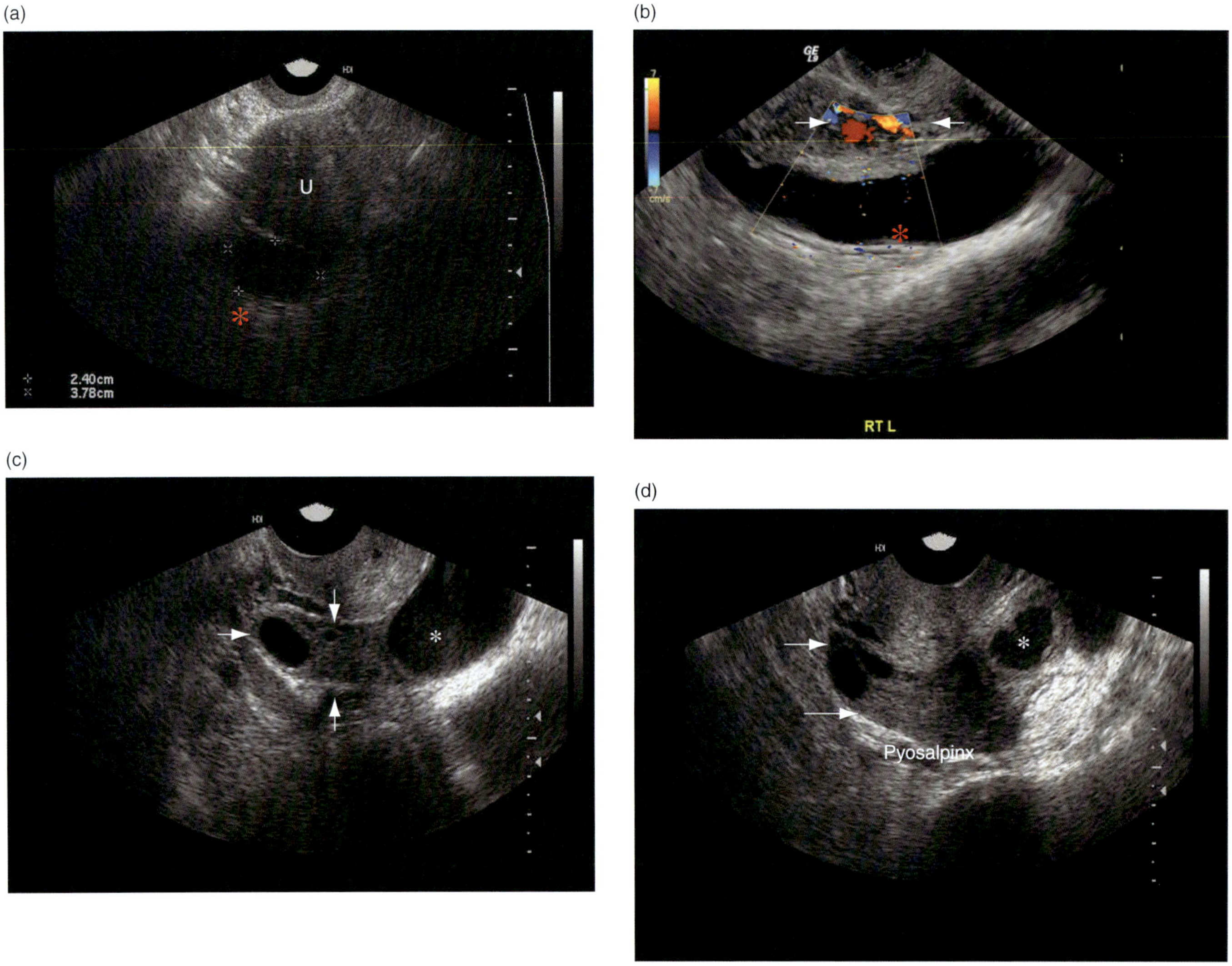

Figure 14.7 Pelvic inflammatory disease (PID). (a) Hydrosalpinx (*) with adjacent uterus (U) visualized. (b) Hydrosalpinx (*) adjacent to the ovary (arrows) with Doppler. (c) Pyosalpinx (*) adjacent to the ovary (arrows), sagittal view. (d) Pyosalpinx (*), coronal view adjacent to the ovary (arrows). *Images courtesy of Madhuri Kirpekar, MD.*

adjacent fallopian tube are infected and inflamed. The irritation and destruction of the surrounding tissue leads to adhesions, perforation, and ultimately to the formation of a tubo-ovarian complex. The diagnosis of the presence of an abscess is critical, since their management is significantly different from uncomplicated PID. Patients require admission for intravenous antibiotics and should also receive consultation in order to have surgical or interventional radiology-guided drainage of the abscess.

Sonographically, the tubo-ovarian complex is characterized by a loss of the normal distinct architecture of the individual structures of the ovaries and/or uterus. The abscess appears as a multiloculated cystic mass, usually closely adjacent to the uterus, and is partially fluid filled or with heterogeneous echoes from the purulent material contained within (Figure 14.8). While this is a bilateral disease process, a complex may be visualized at the site of either adnexa. The disease process is not always symmetric, and so one side usually has a more prominent mass visible on ultrasound. Using Doppler as an adjunct, the abscess displays prominent vascularity, as one would expect in an inflammatory process. Once perforation occurs, fluid may also be visualized in the posterior cul-de-sac, suggesting an advanced stage of the disease process.

Congenital abnormalities of the uterus

Approximately 0.5% of all females will have a congenital abnormality of the uterus, which frequently remains undiagnosed until the woman reaches reproductive age. Congenital abnormalities may range from anomalies in shape, to a complete absence of the uterus, where bilateral arrested development of the Müllerian duct results in uterine aplasia. Unilateral Müllerian ductal hypoplasia will produce a unicornuate uterus; while failure of the left and right Müllerian ducts to fuse results in a bicornuate uterus (Figure 14.9a). Failure of the median septum to resorb will cause a septated uterus (Figure 14.9b). A didelphys uterus can also be seen, in which a double uterus is present, with two separate cervices and often a double vagina (Figure 14.9c,d). An imperforate hymen or vaginal septa

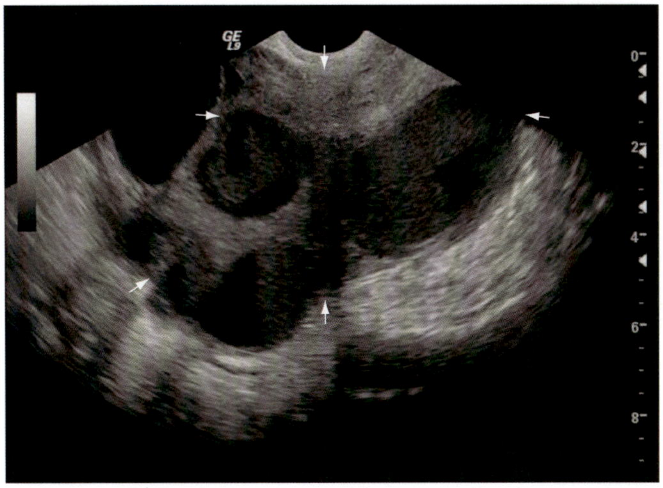

Figure 14.8 Tubo-ovarian abscess (TOA). A multiloculated, cystic mass (arrows) adjacent to the uterus, filled with the heterogeneous echoes of purulent material. *Image courtesy of Madhuri Kirpekar, MD.*

may cause fluid retention in pre-menarchal patients (hydrometrocolpos) and blood retention in post-menarchal patients (hematometrocolpos).

Ovarian masses

Infrequently, pediatric patients may present with ovarian masses. The majority of these consist of germ cell tumors, also known as teratomas (Figure 14.10). The mean age of diagnosis is around 10 years of age, with tumors developing slowly but occasionally growing as large as 30 cm in size. On imaging, these masses may be confused with benign cysts. However, certain anatomic features will help distinguish between the two. Cysts appear as anechoic and unilocular, fluid-filled structures with clearly defined margins, while malignant masses are more likely multilocular and septatated, with a thickened irregular wall. Teratomas may contain a cystic element of ectodermal tissue, such as dentin, hair, or skin, and hyperechoic calcifications may be identified within the mass.

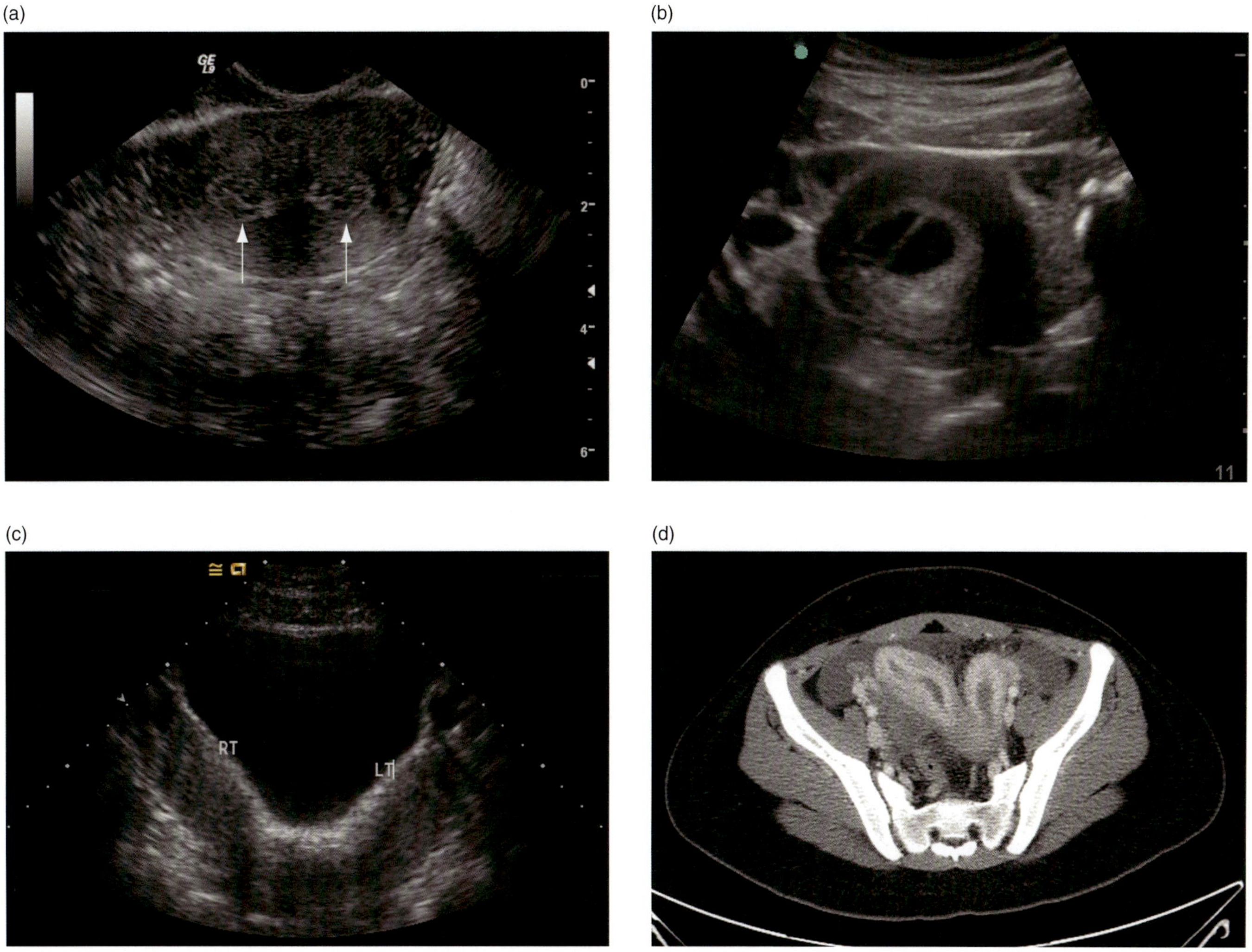

Figure 14.9 Congenital abnormalities. (a) Coronal view, showing the two "horns" (arrows) of a bicornuate uterus. *Image courtesy of Madhuri, Kirpekar, MD.* (b) Coronal view, showing septate (arrowhead) uterus (arrows). (c) Transverse view of the bladder (B) anteriorly, with a didelphys uterus: the right uterus (arrow) and the left (arrowhead). (d) Corresponding CT scan showing the didelphys uterus (arrows and arrowhead).

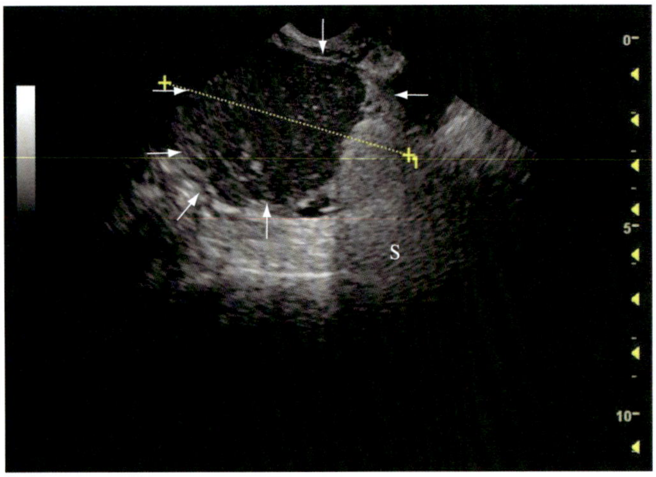

Figure 14.10 Ovarian masses. This large ovarian mass, a teratoma (arrows) exhibits different echogenicities and calcification with posterior shadowing (S).

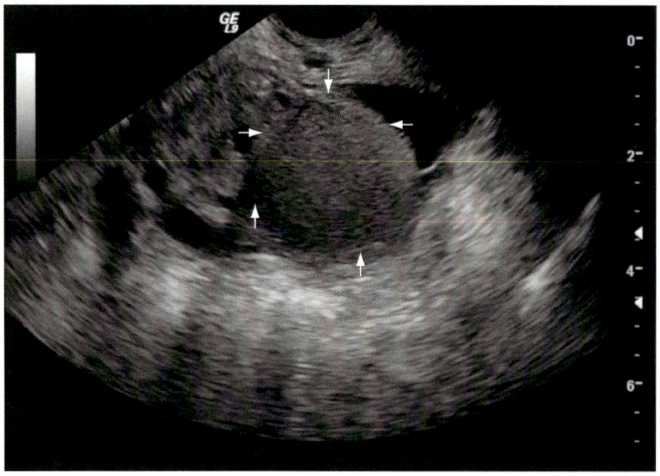

Figure 14.11 Endometrioma. Characteristic appearances of endometriomas are homogeneous, cystic masses that have a "ground glass" appearance.

(a) (b)

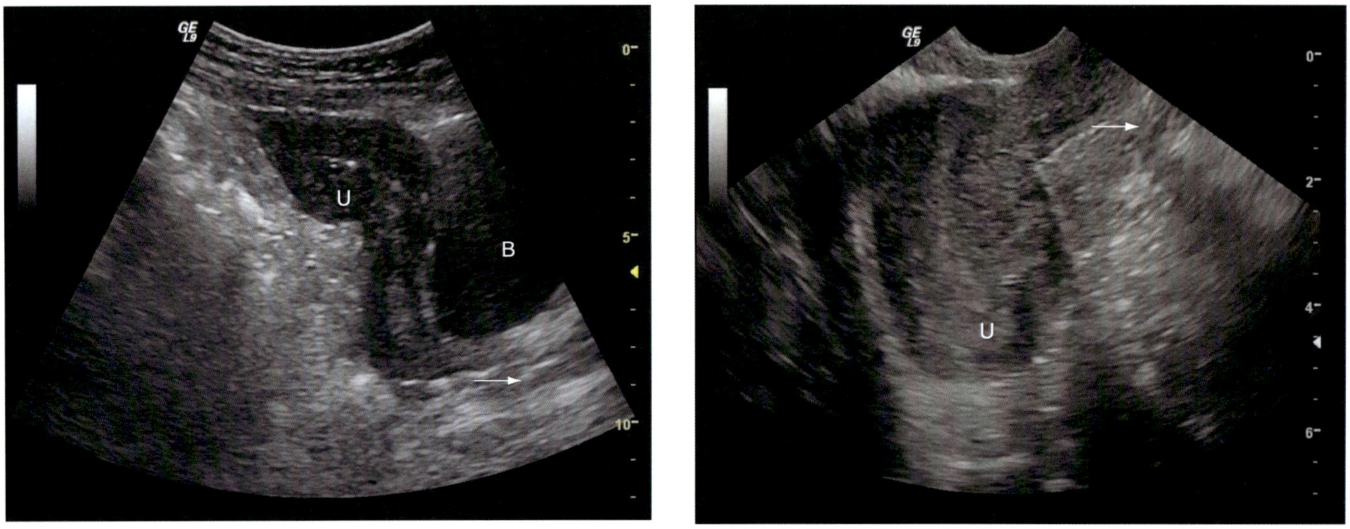

Figure 14.12 Retroverted uterus. (a) Transabdominal sagittal view with the uterus (U) bladder (B) and vaginal space (arrow) visualized. (b) Transvaginal sagittal view with the retroverted uterus (U) and vaginal space (arrow) visualized.

Endometriosis

Endometriomas, consisting of extrauterine endometrial tissue, are a frequent source of chronic pelvic pain in reproductively mature females. Patients present with discomfort or pain that is most prominent during menses, as endometriomas are hormonally stimulated similar to uterine endometrial tissue.

Ultrasound may not always reveal endometriomas, due to their small size and scattered locations. Eighty percent of the time these benign tumors are located on the ovaries. However, they may also be found on the ligaments and serosa of the uterus, on the fallopian tubes, in the peritoneal cavity or on the sigmoid colon. Sonographically, endometriomas appear classically as homogeneous cystic masses, with a hypoechoic center, and low-level internal echoes (Figure 14.11). Endometriomas are often described as having a "ground glass" appearance. This is in contrast to functional hemorrhagic cysts that contain more "lace"-like or "fishnet"-like internal echoes in a reticular pattern. Through transmission is increased in endometriomas, creating posterior acoustic enhancement distal to the mass. Punctate foci in the periphery that appear hyperechoic are an additional specific finding that helps confirm the diagnosis. Doppler imaging shows absent vascularity internally.

Normal findings

Many women have variations in the normal orientation of the uterus, the most common of which is a retroverted uterus (Figure 14.12). Many women have intrauterine devices (IUDs) for contraception. It is important to be familiar with their appearance, especially when there is suspicion that they may have become dislodged (Figure 14.13).

(a)

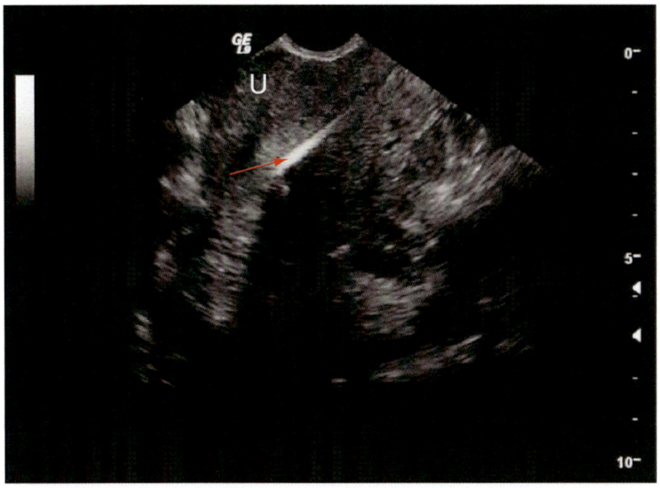

(b)

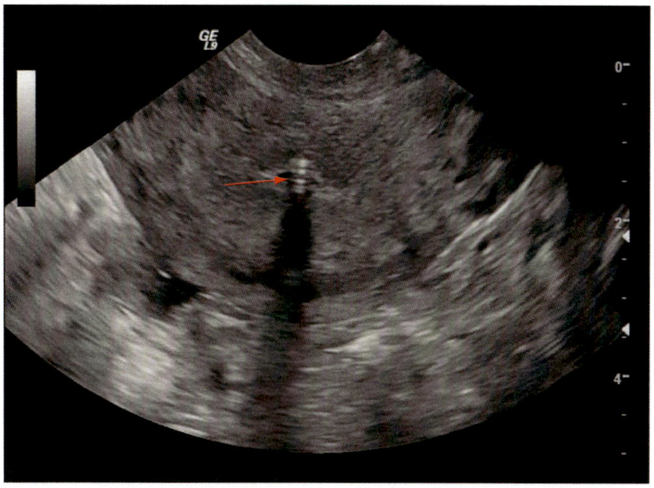

Figure 14.13 Intrauterine device (IUD). (a) Transvaginal, sagittal view of an IUD (arrow) within the uterus (U). Note the shadow artifact from the IUD itself. (b) Transvaginal, coronal view of an IUD (arrow).

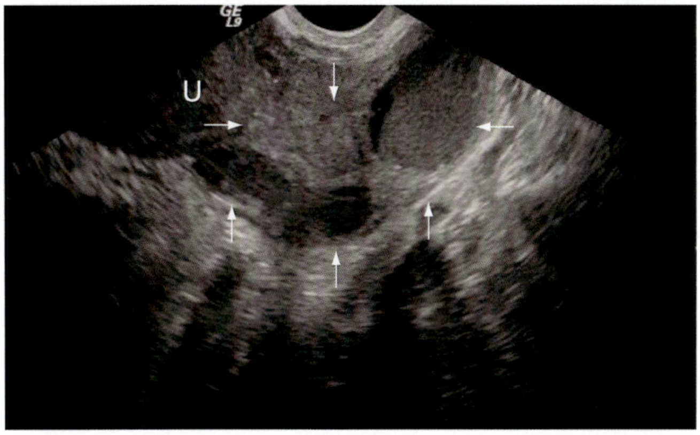

Figure 14.14 Case 1: tubo-ovarian abscess.

Cases

1. A 14-year-old female presents to the emergency department with two days of right lower quadrant abdominal pain. She also has had vaginal discharge and dysuria. She admits to having had unprotected intercourse on several occasions, and does not remember when her last menstrual period occurred. On examination, her vital signs are normal. She exhibits tenderness to palpation of the right lower quadrant and suprapubic regions, without palpable masses, rebound, or guarding. Her urine pregnancy test is negative. A bimanual and speculum examination is performed which reveals yellowish, foul-smelling discharge, marked discomfort, and a possible fullness at the left adnexa. A transabdominal pelvic ultrasound is performed at the bedside with a full bladder, which shows some trace fluid at the pouch of Douglas. An irregular mass is appreciated at the left ovary. The endovaginal probe is prepared with a probe cover and sterile gel. The left ovary has a multiloculated, cystic mass with heterogeneous echoes within the cystic cavities (Figure 14.14). The diagnosis is made of a tubo-ovarian abscess. The gynecology service is consulted, and the patient is admitted for intravenous antibiotics.

   This case highlights the wide range of diagnostic possibilities in a teenage female presenting with acute abdominal pain. Possibilities include appendicitis, urolithiasis, pyelonephritis, ovarian torsion, ovarian cysts, PID, and TOAs, just to name a few. Point-of-care ultrasonography can rapidly identify a TOA, which warrants gynecologic consultation and admission for intravenous antibiotics. It is helpful to first start with a transabdominal pelvic ultrasound to identify important structures, masses, and free fluid. Then, the transvaginal pelvic ultrasound further identifies details of suspected regions, as with this case a TOA.
2. A 12-year-old female presents with lower abdominal pain for the past week, worsening over the past few days. She describes the abdominal pain as intermittent and "crampy" at the suprapubic region, without radiation. She also endorses a history of small amounts of dark discharge on her underwear, and dysuria. She has not yet started her periods. She presents now, due to severe pain, and the inability to urinate. On examination, her vital signs are normal for age. She has moderate tenderness to palpation at the suprapubic region, with a palpable enlarged bladder. A Foley catheter is placed, which drains two liters of urine. A urine pregnancy test is negative. On external genitourinary examination, there is a protrusion from the vagina with no visible opening in the hymen (Figure 14.15a). A point-of-care ultrasound is then performed, which shows an irregular structure within the uterus (Figure 14.15b,c). These findings of hematocolpos secondary to an imperforate hymen are confirmed by formal ultrasonography. As there is no gynecology service available at your free-standing children's

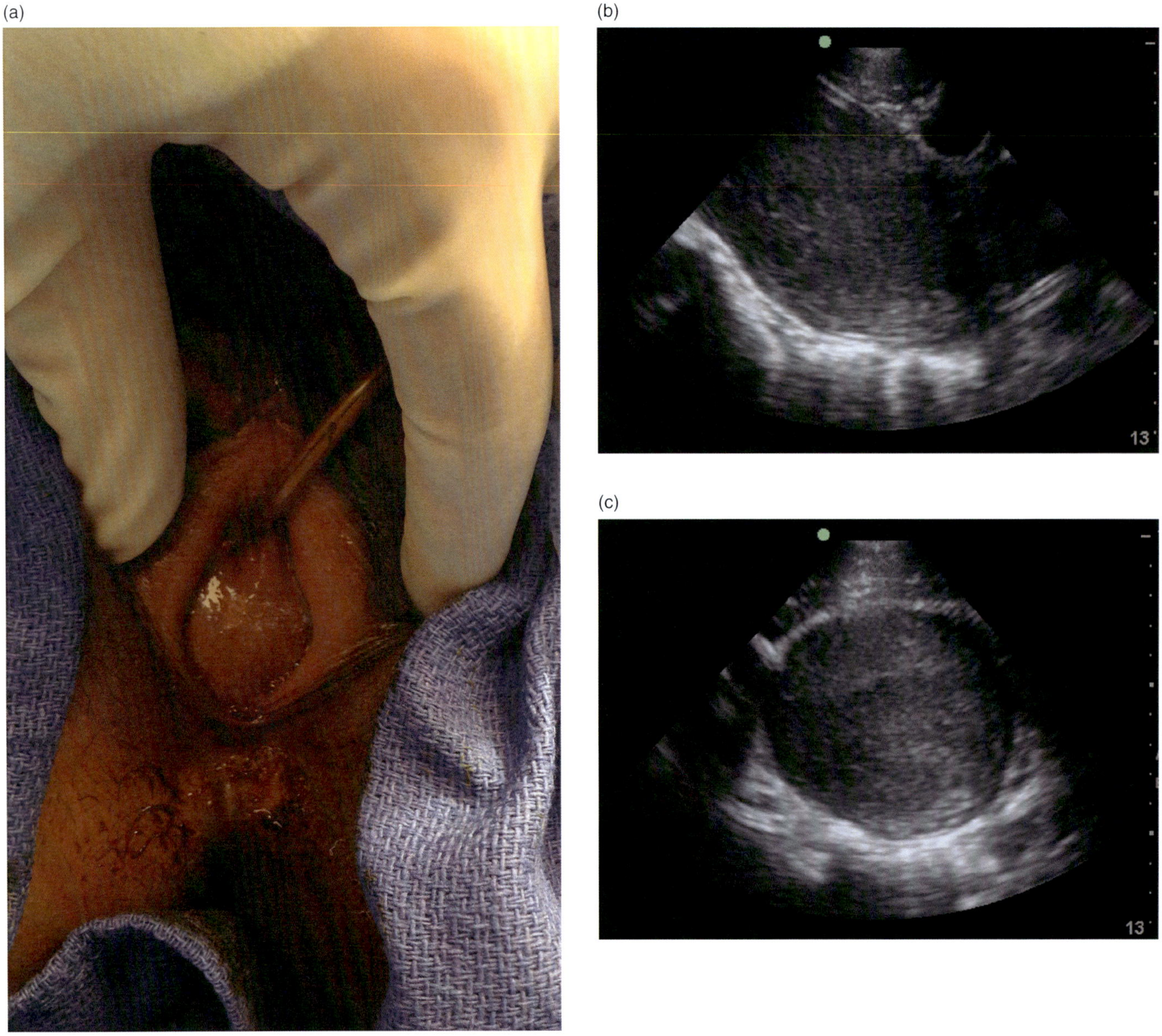

Figure 14.15 **Case 2: imperforate hymen and hematocolpos.** (a) Imperforate hymen, with Foley catheter in the urethra. *Image courtesy of Christopher Newton, MD.* (b) Transabdominal, sagittal view of the uterus with hematocolpos. (c) Transabdominal, transverse view of the uterus with hematocolpos.

hospital, the pediatric surgery service is consulted for operative intervention. The patient recovers uneventfully.

While the most common applications of pelvic ultrasonography are for ovarian torsion and tubo-ovarian abscesses, congenital abnormalities must be considered, especially in adolescent females. It is important to first obtain a urine pregnancy test, since the primary cause of amenorrhea is pregnancy. When the clinician encounters a rare or uncommon finding, it is important to confirm with formal ultrasonography whenever available.

3. A 15-year-old female presents with diffuse abdominal pain and weight gain over the past several months. Her family notices that she "looks pregnant." She has had irregular periods, the most recent of which was two months ago. On examination, she is thin with a protuberant abdomen. She has diffuse tenderness to palpation. A point-of-care transabdominal ultrasound examination is performed, which shows an extremely large, cystic mass extending from her suprapubic region down to the subxiphoid region (Figure 14.16a). The ovaries cannot be visualized by transabdominal examination. Due to the extensive nature of this mass, she also exhibits obstruction and secondary hydronephrosis (Figure 14.16b,c). A CT scan is performed which shows this large cystic mass, without the ability to visualize the ovaries (Figure 14.16d). The patient undergoes a laparotomy for removal of the mass. The

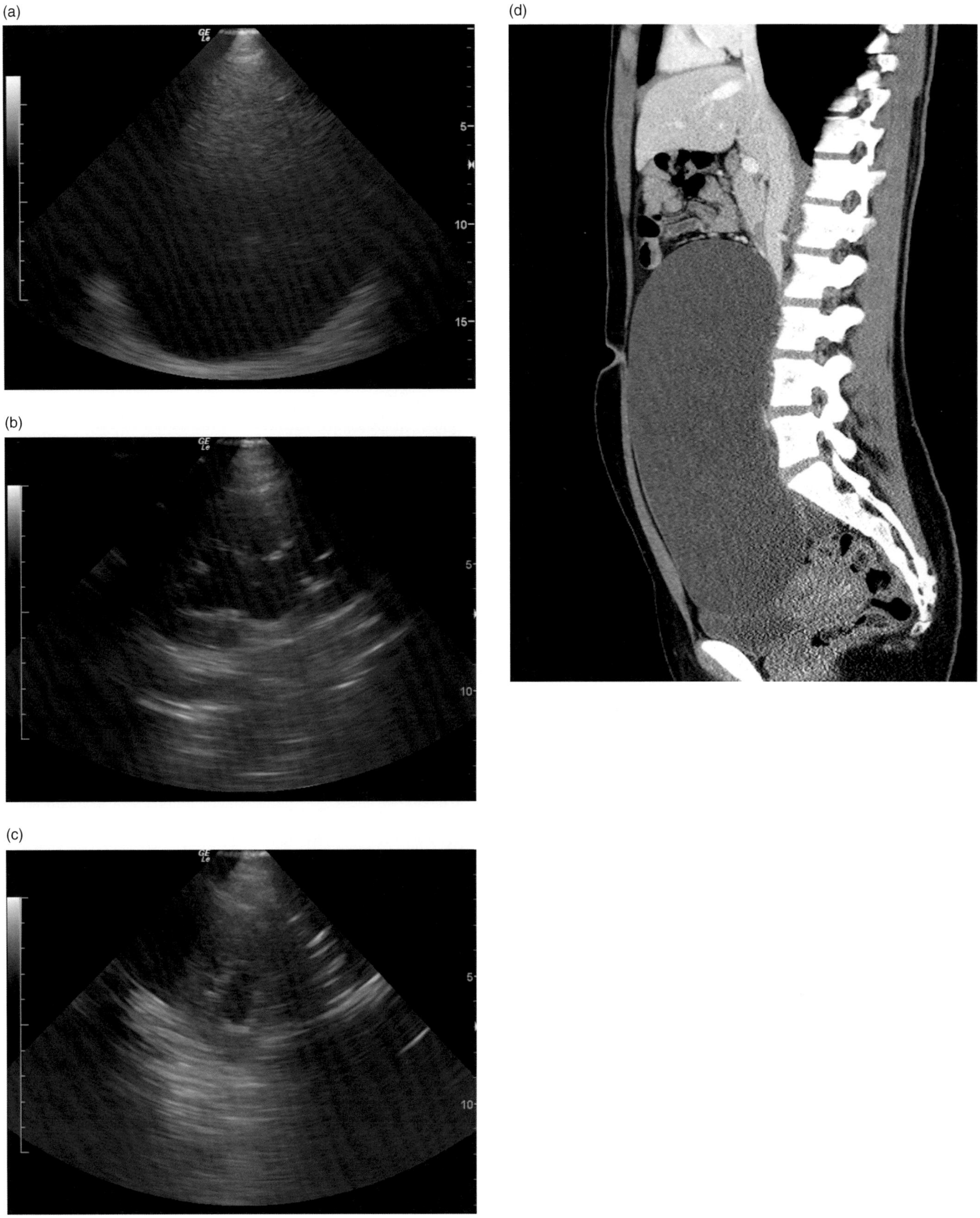

Figure 14.16 Case 3: large ovarian cyst. (a) Transverse transabdominal ultrasound of the inferior portion of this cystic mass which extended up to the patient's subxiphoid region. (b) Longitudinal view of the kidney, which shows moderate hydronephrosis. (c) Transverse view of the kidney, which shows moderate hydronephrosis. (d) A CT scan showing the extent of this large cystic mass.

pathology reveals a simple ovarian cyst, without malignancy. She undergoes a cystectomy, and has an uneventful recovery.

While adolescent females often present with abdominal pain, they uncommonly have masses as the cause of this pain. It is important to recognize that the goal of point-of-care ultrasonography is not to make a definitive diagnosis of rare entities. The goal is to enhance the clinical assessment, in order to more expeditiously manage the patient's care. In this case, the point-of-care ultrasound reveals an abnormality warranting obtaining a CT scan, additional laboratory studies, and surgical consultation. It is also important to recognize that, with large masses or cysts originating from the ovary, the ovaries are at risk of torsion. Therefore, patients with large cysts or masses presenting with an acute worsening of their pain should cause high suspicion for ovarian torsion. Even if there is normal blood flow to the affected ovary visualized on ultrasonography, a high clinical suspicion must be maintained in order to obtain time-sensitive operative intervention in order to salvage the ovary.

Summary/key points

1. The clinician can utilize ultrasound to evaluate the non-pregnant patient with gynecologic complaints. Characteristic findings of ovarian torsion, ovarian cysts, PID, TOAs, ovarian masses, and endometriomas may be appreciated.
2. Both transabdominal and transvaginal approaches to pelvic ultrasound may be performed. The technique should be chosen based upon anticipated findings and organs of interest, as well as the age and sexual maturity of the patient. Transabdominal scanning may provide a broader field of view, as well as greater depth in imaging. Transvaginal scanning offers a greater resolution and more detailed imaging of the anatomy close to the transducer.
3. Utilize a full bladder as an acoustic window in transabdominal scanning, and an empty bladder for increased comfort and visualization in transvaginal scanning.
4. Use site-specific tenderness and mobility of structures as an adjunct in determining likely pathology. Also perform an additional FAST examination when concerned for free fluid in the pelvis or abdomen.
5. Ovarian torsion cannot be fully excluded based on sonographic findings, as even vascular flow on Doppler or absence of a lead point mass may not fully rule out the condition.

Selected references

Adhikari, S., Blaivas, M., Lyon, M. (2008) Role of bedside transvaginal ultrasonography in the diagnosis of tubo-ovarian abscess in the emergency department. *J Emerg Med* **34**(4): 429–33.

Bellah, R. D., Rosenberg, H. K. (1991) Transvaginal ultrasound in a children's hospital: is it worthwhile? *Pediatr Radiol* **21**: 570–4.

Girzadas, D. V. Jr, Antonis, M. S., Zerth, H., *et al.* (2009) Hybrid simulation combining high fidelity scenario with a pelvis ultrasound task trainer enhances the training and evaluation of endovaginal ultrasound. *Acad Emerg Med* **16**(5): 429–35.

Haider, Z., Condous, G., Khalid, A., *et al.* (2006) Impact of the availability of sonography in the acute gynecology unit. *Ultrasound Obstet Gynecol* **28**: 207–13.

Jeong, Y. Y., Outwater, E. K., Kang, H. K. (2000) Imaging evaluation of ovarian masses. *Radiographics* **20**: 1445–70.

Lambert, M. J., Villa, M. (2004) Gynecologic ultrasound in emergency medicine. *Emerg Med Clin North Am* **22**: 683–96.

Lee, D. C., Swaminathan, A. K. (2011) Sensitivity of ultrasound for the diagnosis of tubo-ovarian abscess: a case report and literature review. *J Emerg Med* **40**(2): 170–5.

Servaes, S., Zurakowski, D., Laufer, M. R., *et al.* (2007) Sonographic findings of ovarian torsion in children. *Pediatr Radiol* **37**: 446–51.

Tayal, V. S., Bullard, M., Swanson, D. R., *et al.* (2008) ED endovaginal pelvic ultrasound in nonpregnant women with right lower quadrant pain. *Am J Emerg Med* **26**(1): 81–5.

Tayal, V. S., Crean, C. A., Norton, J., *et al.* (2008) Prospective comparative trial of endovaginal sonographic bimanual examination in nonpregnant women with abdominal pain with regard to body mass index classification. *J Ultrasound Med* **27**(8): 1171–7.

S3 Introduction

Stephanie J. Doniger

Procedures are performed regularly as part of the practice of emergency medicine and critical care medicine. Ultrasound has been introduced as a modality that has the potential to improve success and decrease complications of procedures.

It is important to discuss terminology, which may be applied to various procedures.

Ultrasound guidance: (direct, dynamic, real-time ultrasound) in which the needle tip is visualized in real time, throughout the puncture process and procedure.

Ultrasound assistance: (indirect, static ultrasound) ultrasound scans are performed to verify the presence and position of a suitable procedure site prior to the performance of the procedure. The actual procedure is performed without the use of ultrasound.

Single operator: (Figure S3.1) one person holds the transducer in his/her non-dominant hand, while simultaneously performing the procedure with the dominant hand.

Dual operator: one person serves as the "probe person," while the other is the "procedure person" (Figure S3.2).

Technique

Transducer selection and orientation

For the majority of procedures, a linear, high-frequency (5–10 MHz) transducer is utilized (Figure S3.3a, Table S3.1). A few procedures, such as bladder ultrasound, pericardiocentesis, paracentesis, and thoracentesis utilize a low-frequency (2–5 MHz), curvilinear or phased-array transducer (Figure S3.3b, Table S3.1). The smaller-footprint transducers are especially useful for pediatric patients.

It is also important for the operator to position him/herself with a direct line of vision for the ultrasound monitor (Figure S3.4a), and be within arms' reach to perform necessary adjustments of the ultrasound image. It is recommended to orient the probe indicator to the operator's **left**, which corresponds directly to the left-hand side of the ultrasound monitor (Figure S3.4b). This allows for ease of needle redirection when performing real-time ultrasound guided procedures. The easiest way to ensure that the transducer is oriented correctly is to perform the "indicator test," where the operator contacts one side of the transducer with gel, and looks to see if the corresponding side of the screen has an image appearing (Figure S3.4c).

Patient position and preparation

Regardless of the procedure performed, appropriate preparation is imperative. For sterile procedures, in particular, one must properly prepare the procedure site in a sterile fashion. In addition, the transducer must be prepared in order to maintain a sterile field. Transducer sterility may be attained by using commercially available sheaths (Figure S3.5). Alternatively, a sterile glove or Tegaderm® with Betadine® may be utilized when sterile sheaths are not available (Figure S3.6). When utilizing sheaths or sterile gloves, it is important to remember that ultrasound requires gel in order to allow for sound wave transmission. A layer of gel must be placed over the transducer, followed by the sterile barrier, followed by sterile gel (Figure S3.7). When utilizing Tegaderm®, only Tegaderm® directly over the transducer and Betadine® on the skin are necessary.

Adjuncts may be utilized in order to enhance visualization by ultrasound. Especially with smaller pediatric patients, many of the structures of interest are small and superficial. Commercially available stand-off pads may be utilized to increase the distance between the transducer and the structure of interest. Alternatively, saline bags, or water-filled gloves, may be utilized (Figure S3.8). For extremities, the hand or foot may be placed in a water bath (Figure S3.9a). This improves visualization, and avoids direct contact between the transducer and the affected skin (Figure S3.9b). This technique is especially helpful in the sonographic evaluation for soft tissue foreign bodies.

Ultrasound imaging

Short-axis (transverse): the structure of interest is viewed in a transverse plane, or cross-section. In the short-axis approach, the needle is oriented perpendicular to the structure of interest (Figure S3.10a,b). In the example of vascular access, a vessel is visualized in its cross-section as a circle, and only a portion of the vessel is visualized (*out-of-plane*); the needle is only visualized as it reaches the structure (Figure S3.10c). The short-axis view allows for evaluation of surrounding structures and a broad image of lateral surrounding tissue.

Pediatric Emergency and Critical Care Ultrasound, ed. Stephanie J. Doniger. Published by Cambridge University Press.

Table S3.1. Procedures with associated types of transducers used.

High-Frequency (Linear)	Low Frequency (Curvilinear or Phased Array)
Vascular access	Bladder volume, catheterization
Lumbar Puncture	Pericardiocentesis
Abscess: identification, I & D	Thoracentesis
Foreign bodies: detection, removal	Paracentesis
Fracture reduction	
Arthrocentesis	
Peripheral nerve blocks	
Airway: ETT placement, chest tubes	

Long-axis (longitudinal): the structure of interest is visualized longitudinally. The trajectory of the needle is visualized along its entire path (*in plane*). With vascular access, the needle is oriented directly under the transducer (Figure S3.11a,b). The length of the blood vessel is visualized as a tubular structure, along with the entire length of the needle entering the vessel (Figure S3.11c). The utilization of the in-plane technique may lead to higher precision, with fewer complications. However, this method is more difficult as it requires perfect orientation of the narrow ultrasound beam while maintaining the needle in the midline of the transducer axis.

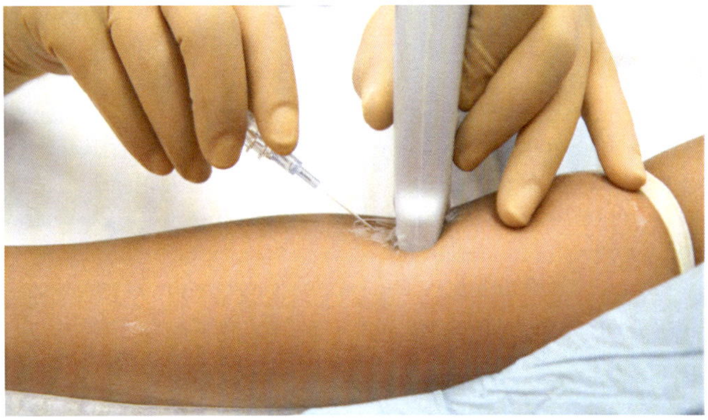

Figure S3.1 Single-operator procedural guidance. There is one operator performing ultrasonography with the non-dominant hand, while performing the procedure with the dominant hand.

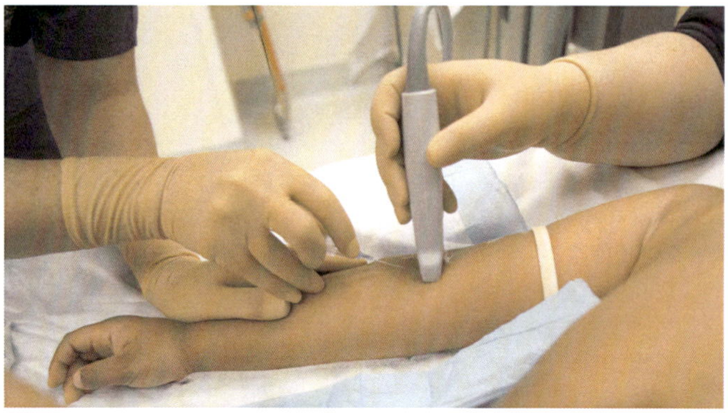

Figure S3.2 Dual-operator procedural guidance. One person performs ultrasonography and another person performs the procedure. It is important to position the machine so that both the "ultrasound person" and the "procedure person" have the ultrasound monitor within their line of vision.

(a) (b)

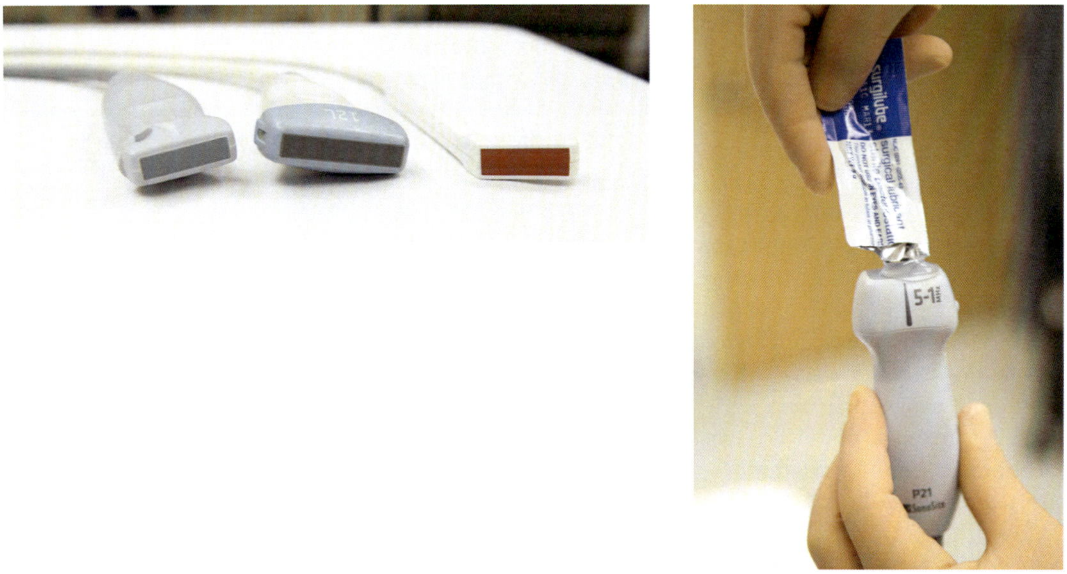

Figure S3.3 Transducers used to perform ultrasound for procedural guidance and assistance. (a) A variety of linear transducers are used to perform the majority of procedures. These high-frequency transducers are available in a variety of sizes, with different-sized footprints. One variation has a hockey-stick appearance (far right). (b) Low-frequency, phased-array transducers are used to perform bladder ultrasound, thoracentesis, pericardiocentesis, and paracentesis. Note, the sterile sheath was removed to better visualize the transducer.

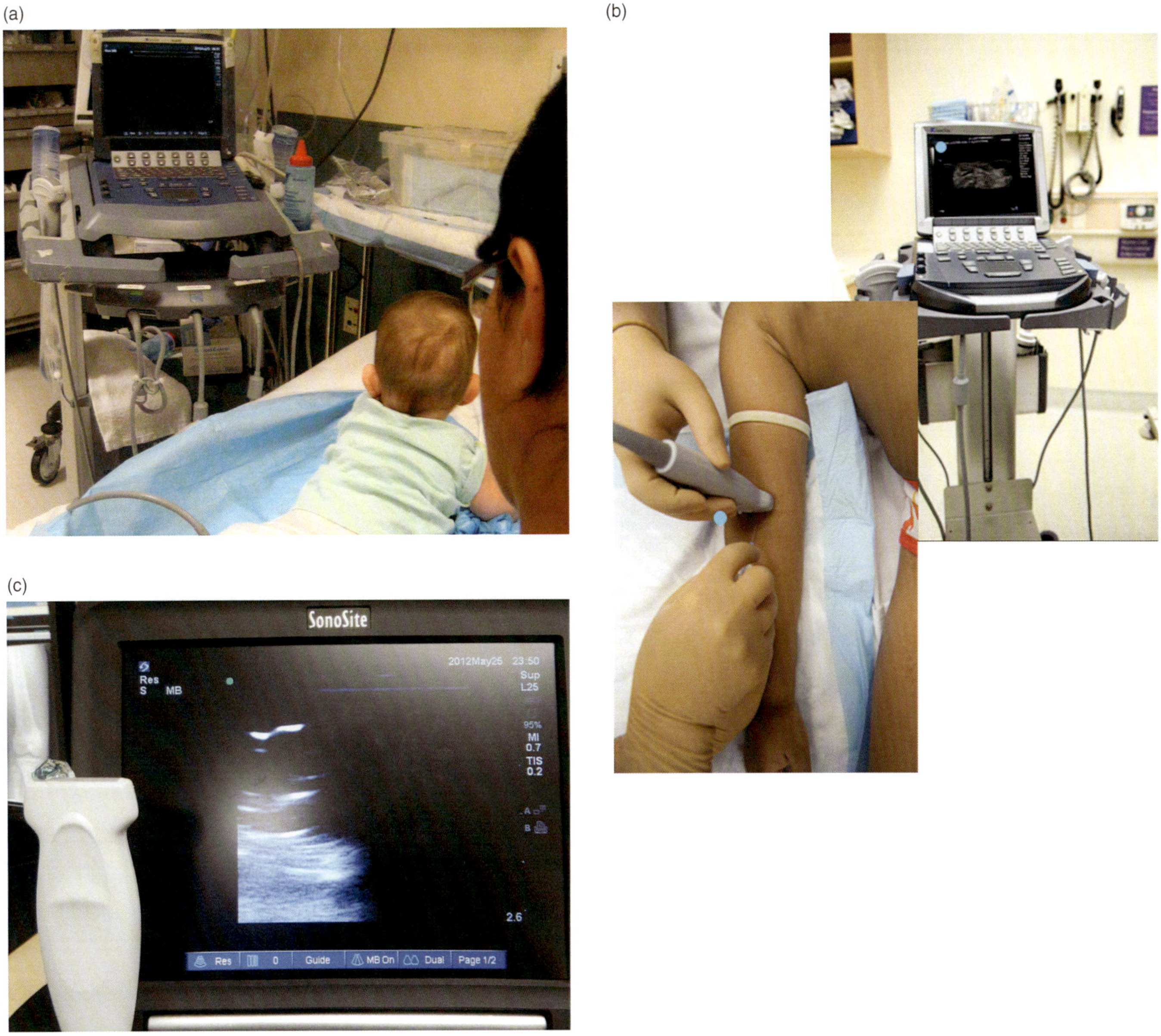

Figure S3.4 Proper transducer and machine orientation. It is important to properly position oneself prior to performing an ultrasound-guided procedure. (a) The most effective orientation is to have the machine in the direct line of vision of the operator. (b) The transducer should be oriented with the indicator to the operator's left. This directly corresponds to the left-hand side of the ultrasound image, and allows for ease of needle redirection when necessary. (c) An "indicator test" may be performed to determine which side of the transducer corresponds to which side of the ultrasound image. Gel is placed on one side of the transducer, and an image should appear on the corresponding side of the screen.

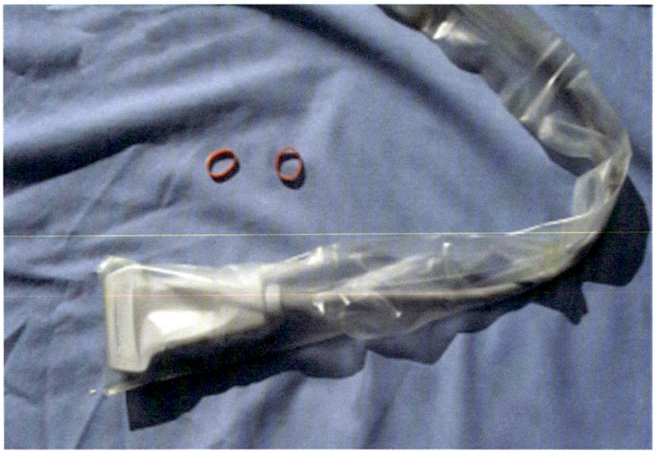

Figure S3.5 Commercially available sterile transducer sheaths. Kits include the sheath that covers the entire transducer and cord, sterile rubber bands to secure the sheath, and sterile gel.

(a) (b)

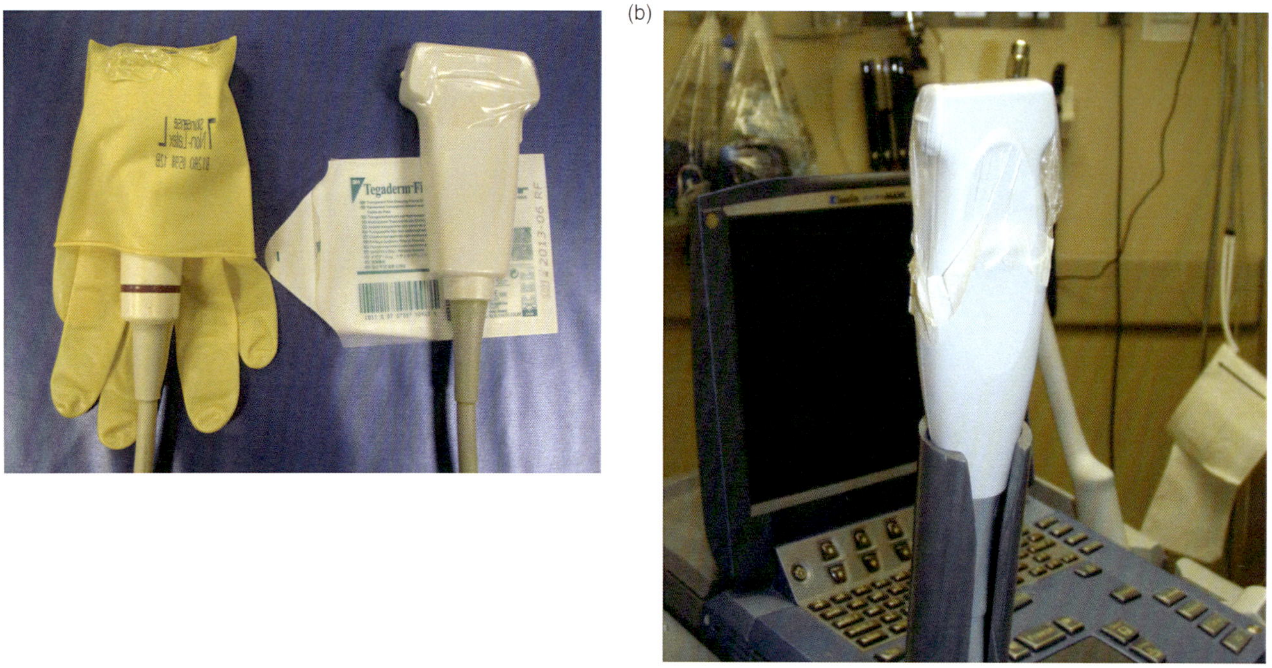

Figure S3.6 Alternative sterile transducer preparations. (a) Sterile gloves may be utilized as an alternative to commercially available transducer sheaths. A novel approach is utilizing Tegaderm® directly covering the transducer, with Betadine® as the skin preparation. Of note, with this method no gel is necessary. (b) Photograph demonstrating placing the Tegaderm® on the transducer.

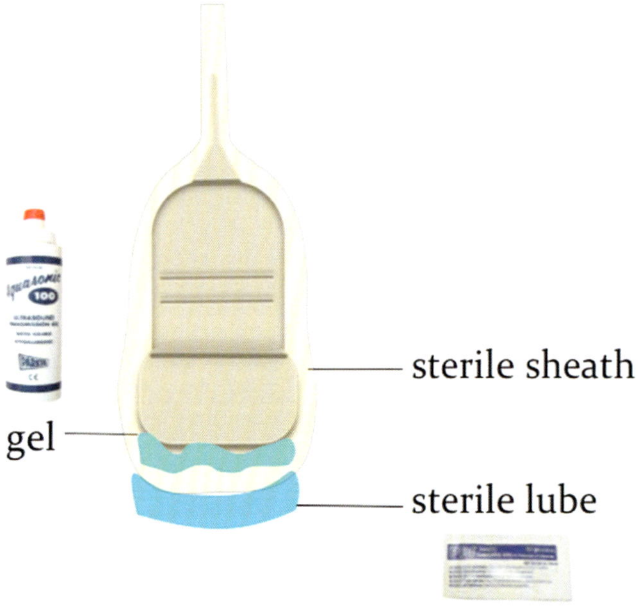

Figure S3.7 Sterile preparation of the transducer. It is important to properly prepare the transducer when performing sterile procedures. A layer of gel (non-sterile) first needs to be placed on the transducer footprint, followed by a sterile barrier (i.e. sheath or glove), and then followed by a sterile gel. *Illustration by Laura Berg.*

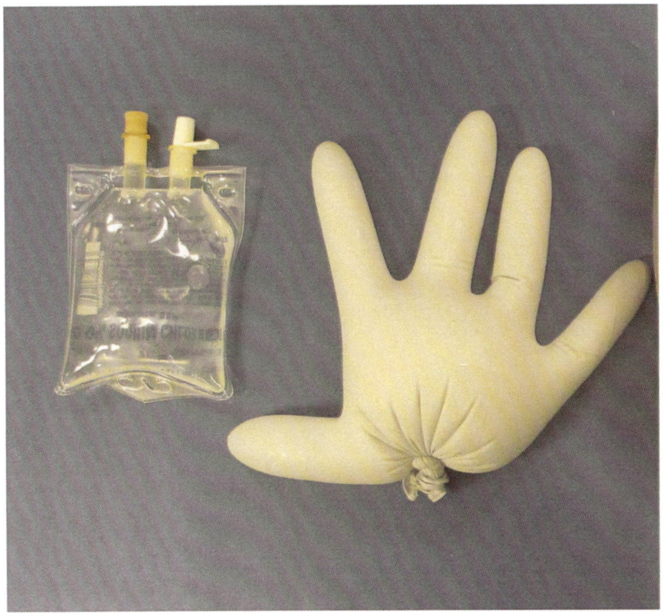

Figure S3.8 Adjunct: alternatives to stand-off pads. Water-filled gloves or saline bags are effective alternatives to commercially available stand-off pads. The water serves to enhance acoustic transmission, while the increased distance improves resolution.

Summary

It is important to recognize the limitations of ultrasound with regards to each particular procedure. All procedures are operator dependent, and require experience. In-depth discussions of the most commonly performed procedures are given in the following chapters.

(a)

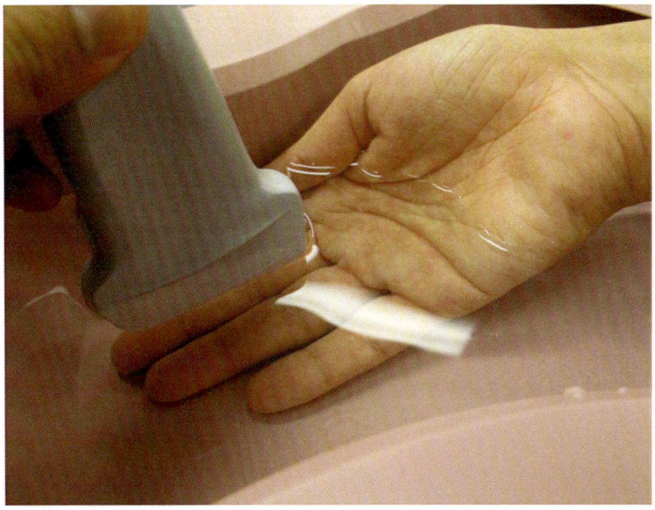

(b)

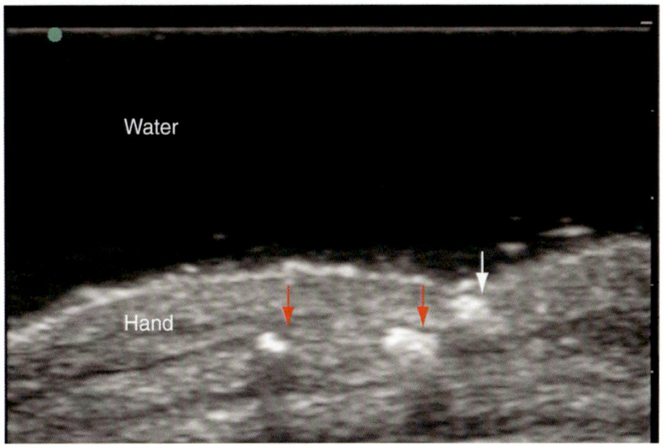

Figure S3.9 Adjunct: water bath. (a) A water bath may be utilized to improve sonographic images. The water serves to increase acoustic transmission. This may be utilized in the hands or feet, and allows the operator to avoid directly touching the affected region. (b) Ultrasound image of a patient's hand in order to identify a foreign body (arrows).

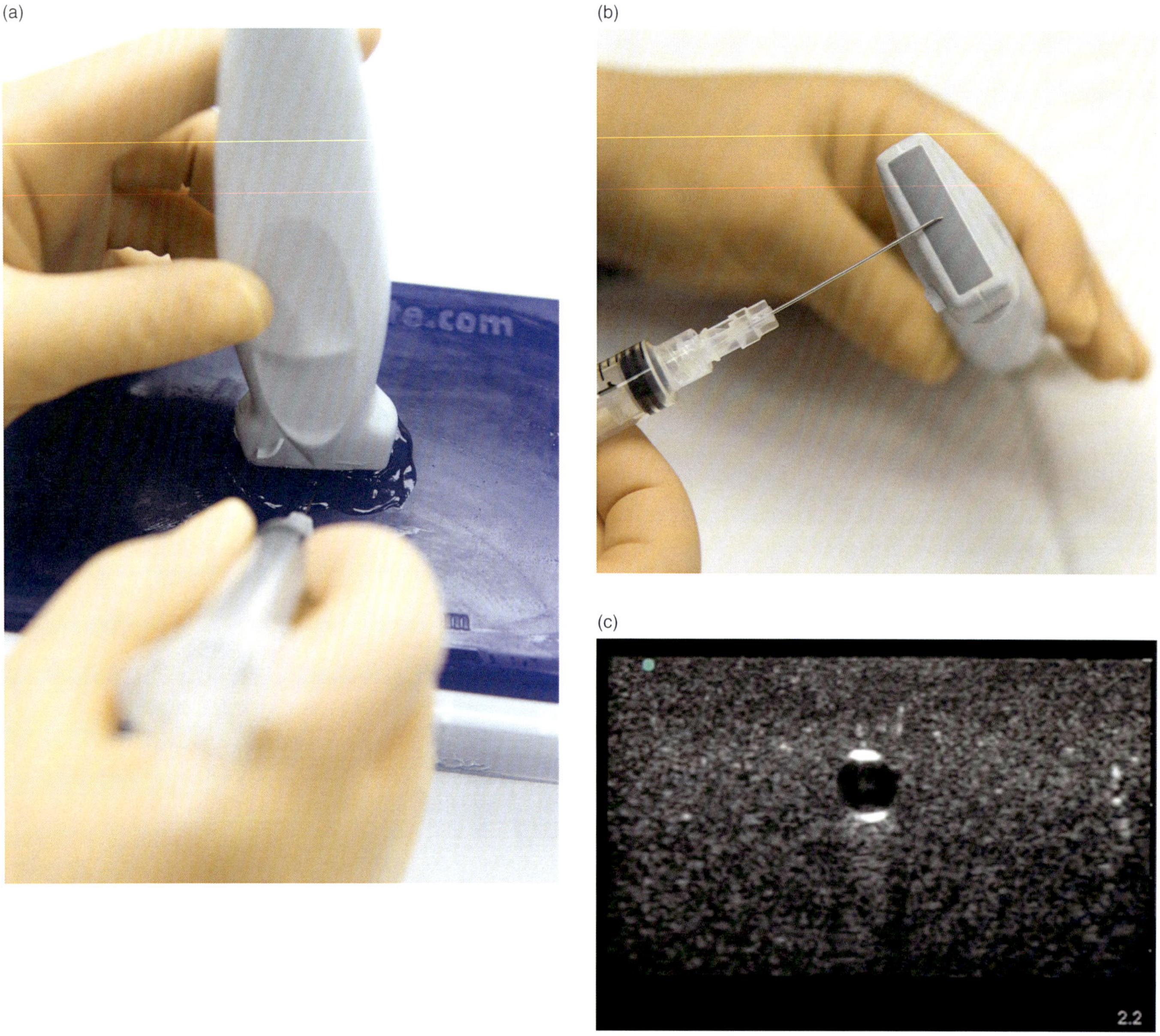

Figure S3.10 Short-axis view. (a) Positioning of the needle in a phantom model. As the needle enters, it remains perpendicular to the center of the transducer. The most common method of entry is "needle approximation." (b) The needle is oriented perpendicular to the transducer. (c) Ultrasound image of the short-axis. The blood vessel appears in cross-section, as a circle.

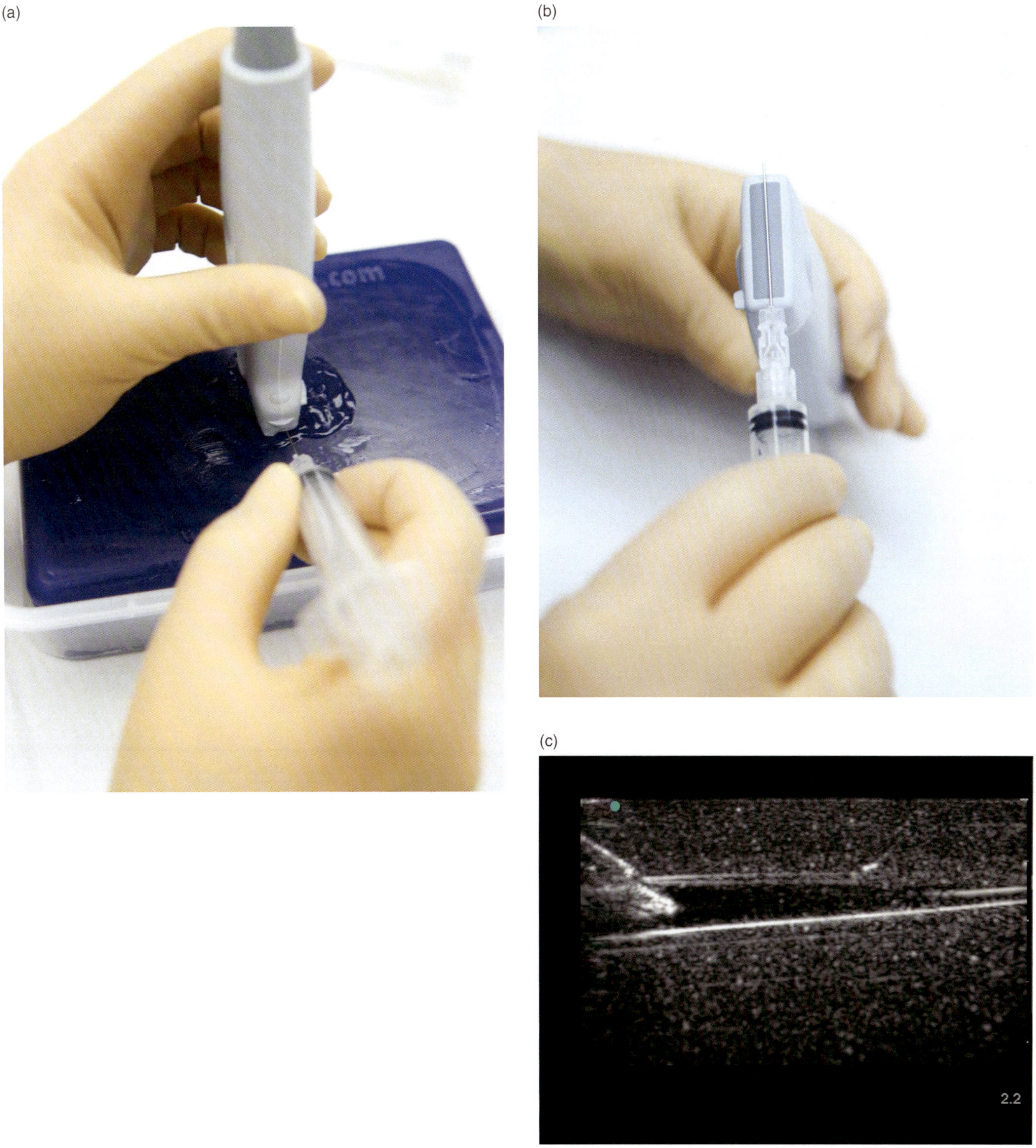

Figure S3.11 Long-axis view. (a) Positioning of the needle in a phantom. As the needle enters, it is directly adjacent to the transducer. Entrance of the needle is at the center of the shorter portion of the transducer, in the center. (b) The needle is oriented parallel to the transducer, directly beneath the length of the transducer, in the center. (c) Ultrasound image of the long-axis. The blood vessel is visualized along its length, and appears as a tube.

Selected references

Blaivas, M., Brannam, L., Fernandez, E. (2003) Short-axis versus long-axis approaches for teaching ultrasound-guided vascular access on a new inanimate model. *Acad Emerg Med* **10**: 1307–11.

Blaivas, M., Lyon, M., Brannam, L., *et al.* (2004) Waterbath evaluation technique for emergency ultrasound of painful superficial structures. *Ann Emerg Med* **22**(7):589–93.

Joshi, M., Subhan, I. (2008) A new technique for maintaining sterility in ultrasound-guided procedures. *Ann Emerg Med* **51**(4): 496.

Lamperti, M., Bodenham, A. R., Pittiruti, M., *et al.* (2012) International evidence-based recommendations on ultrasound-guided vascular access. *Intensive Care Med* **38**(7): 1105–17.

Milling, T., Holden, C., Melniker, L., *et al.* (2006) Randomized controlled trial of single-operator vs. two-operator ultrasound guidance for internal jugular venous cannulation. *Acad Emerg Med* **13**(3): 245–7.

Phelan, M., Hagerty, D. (2009) The oblique view: an alternative approach for ultrasound-guided central line placement. *J Emerg Med* **37**(4): 403–8.

Rose, J. S., Morbutas, C. M. (2008) A randomized controlled trial comparing one-operator versus two-operator technique in ultrasound-guided basilic vein cannulation. *J Emerg Med* **35**(4):431–50.

Stone, M., Moon, C., Sutijono, D., *et al.* (2010) Needle tip visualization during ultrasound-guided vascular access: short-axis vs long-axis approach. *Am J Emerg Med* **28**: 343–7.

Tirado, A., Nagdev, A., Henningsen, C., *et al.* (2013) Ultrasound-guided procedures in the emergency department – needle guidance and localization. *Emerg Med Clin North Am* **31**(1):87–115.

Tirado, A., Wu, T., Noble, V. E., *et al.* (2013) Ultrasound-guided procedures in the emergency department – diagnostic and therapeutic asset. *Emerg Med Clin North Am* **31**(1):117–49.

Chapter

15 Vascular access

Dave Spear and Stephanie J. Doniger

Objectives/indications

Children who present to the emergency department often require intravenous access (IV) as part of their treatment. It is the most common procedure performed in the emergency department, and vascular access can be a life-saving procedure for the most critically ill. Both central and peripheral venous access in adult and pediatric patients are an integral part of basic therapy in pediatric emergency medicine. Particular indications for IV placement include: intravenous fluids/hydration, antibiotics, life-saving resuscitative medications, and blood products. Those patients who are critically ill and injured are most in need of rapid vascular access.

Pediatric patients, in particular, may present challenges with intravenous access, which can be especially difficult in smaller or medically complex patients. Moreover, intravenous catheter placement in this group may require considerable time and expertise. Failure may necessitate use of alternative routes that include intraosseous needle placement, central venous cannulation, or a venous cut down. Such alternatives are more time-consuming and involve patient discomfort and the risk of complications. Intraosseous lines may be placed manually and by automated devices. While intraosseous lines may be expeditiously placed, there are potential complications of extravasation of fluid, thereby creating tissue necrosis and compartment syndrome.

Prior to the advent of ultrasonography for vascular access, venous access was limited to "palpation," "anatomic landmark," or "blind" techniques. With the development of improved technology that can be used at the bedside, ultrasound has improved success of vascular access while decreasing complications. Ultrasound guidance has been utilized by physicians, nurses, technicians, and prehospital providers to facilitate central and peripheral line placement.

Background

Point-of-care ultrasonography has been shown to facilitate central venous access in adult and pediatric patients. Compared with traditional landmark-guided approaches, ultrasound-guided central venous cannulation results in more rapid access with fewer complications, mean insertion attempts, and placement failures. The results have been so compelling that, in 1999, an Institute of Medicine report recommended ultrasound guidance as the standard of care in the placement of all central lines as a means to improve patient safety.

More recently, this technique has been applied to central lines for adults in the subclavian, internal jugular, and femoral locations. Ultrasound guidance has also been used for radial arterial catheter placement in the emergency department. When compared with blindly placed arterial catheters, ultrasound guidance required a shorter time for placement (107 vs. 314 seconds, $P = 0.0004$), fewer placement attempts (1.2 vs. 2.2, $P = 0.001$), and fewer sites (1.1 vs. 1.6, $P = 0.001$) required for successful line placement. While the majority of adult studies have focused on physician-performed vascular access, recent studies have focused on nurses and prehospital providers utilizing ultrasound for vascular access. Nurses are the primary providers of IV access in most emergency departments. Peripheral IV placement by nurses utilizing ultrasound guidance has demonstrated a high success rate and, after initial training, can redefine what nurses perceive as difficult-access patients. More recently, studies have even demonstrated that emergency department technicians can place peripheral IVs in difficult-access patients with ultrasound guidance.

The majority of pediatric studies for ultrasound-guided central line placement have focused on internal jugular and femoral routes of access. When internal jugular vein cannulation was studied in infants and children, ultrasound was seen to offer less advantage over the landmark technique in children less than 10 kg in weight and less than one year of age. More recently, ultrasound guidance has been utilized for subclavian access. Fragou *et al.* performed a large, prospective, randomized controlled trial comparing ultrasound-guided subclavian vein cannulation versus the traditional landmark method. The success of ultrasound-guidance was 100%, compared with only 87.5% in the landmark group ($P < 0.05$). Average access time and number of attempts were significantly reduced in the ultrasound group, with decreased complications (hematoma, hemothorax, pneumothorax, nerve injury, and cardiac tamponade). This technique has recently been applied to infants and children, with small studies yielding high success rates. Most recently, ultrasound-guided umbilical line catheterizations have been described in the literature (see Chapter 23).

Ultrasound guidance is especially beneficial for the subset of patients with difficult venous access. Recently, point-of-care

Pediatric Emergency and Critical Care Ultrasound, ed. Stephanie J. Doniger. Published by Cambridge University Press.

ultrasonography has been applied to vein localization and the placement of peripheral intravenous catheters in both adults and children. The majority of studies for peripheral IV placement in adults and children have focused on the antecubital region. When compared with traditional cannulation techniques, ultrasound-guided peripheral intravenous catheter placement has a greater success rate with fewer skin punctures, decreased time for intravenous catheter placement, and fewer complications. The only pediatric study, by Doniger *et al.*, showed no statistical difference in overall success rates (80% vs. 64% $P = 0.0208$), but a decreased time to placement (6.3 min vs. 14.4 min, $p = 0.001$) and decreased number of needle punctures (1 vs. 3 punctures, $P = 0.004$) and redirections (median 2 vs. median 10, $P < 0.0001$). More recently, the saphenous vein in the lower extremities has been investigated as a potential site for ultrasound-guided vascular access. In children less than three years of age, the saphenous vein was seen to be significantly larger than the hand veins (2.8 mm vs. 1.8 mm, $P < 0.0001$), and the mean depth was significantly greater than the hand veins and the antecubital veins. These early findings suggest that the saphenous vein might be viable location for ultrasound-guided peripheral IV placement.

Technique

This technique may be applied to both central and peripheral line placement. The necessary steps include:

1. Transducer selection and orientation.
2. Select the site.
3. Position the patient, the machine, and the providers.
4. Prepare the skin and transducer.
5. Image with ultrasound, distinguish artery from vein.
6. Make the puncture.
7. Confirm line placement, secure the line.

Transducer selection and orientation

Due to the physics of ultrasound imaging, higher-frequency (7 MHz or greater) transducers provide greater resolution at relatively shallow depths. This makes the high-frequency transducer the transducer of choice for vascular access procedures. Such transducers come in a variety of shapes and sizes (Figure S3.3a). Most practitioners prefer a high-frequency linear transducer with a relatively small footprint, especially for infants and small children.

When holding an ultrasound transducer on a patient, it is imperative that the transducer be positioned correctly in order to represent the correct left and right orientation on the screen (Figure S3.4). When performing ultrasound-guided vascular access, the indicator should be oriented towards the left of the person placing the line, in order to allow for easy needle redirection when needed.

Patient position and preparation

The ideal orientation is to have the screen of the ultrasound machine in the direct line of vision of the operator (Figure S3.4a). Both single- and dual-operator methods have been described. With a single operator (Figure S3.1), one person holds the transducer in his/her non-dominant hand, while the procedure is performed with the dominant hand. In the dual-operator technique (Figure S3.2), one person serves as the "probe person," while the other serves as the "IV person." With the dual-operator technique, it is often difficult to maintain sterility in the situation of central lines, and to properly position all providers in a limited space.

Various techniques may be utilized. The "static" approach is one in which the operator identifies the vein by ultrasound, marks the skin, then places the IV without further use of the ultrasound. The "dynamic" approach, or real-time guidance has been shown to be superior in success rates and allows the operator to visualize in real-time as the needle enters the vessel.

Skin preparation should be performed, and the transducer must be properly prepared in order to maintain a sterile field, which is especially important for central line placement (Figure S3.7). Whenever possible, long needles or echo-tip needles may be utilized, which may offer improved visualization and success. Tourniquets should be used for peripheral IV placement, as with traditional placement techniques.

Ultrasound imaging

Prior to choosing a vessel to cannulate, it is recommended to evaluate a number of possible sites, in order to visualize the best available vessel. This involves the identification of veins and surrounding structures such as nerves and arteries. Vessels can be visualized in the short-axis, which is a cross-section of the vessel (Figure 15.1), or long-axis, which visualizes the length of the blood vessel (Figure 15.2). Studies have shown the short-axis approach to be quicker and more accurate than the long-axis, especially with novice sonographers. In the short-axis approach, the indicator should be placed to the IV person's left (the person who is holding the IV catheter), so that any movement in the horizontal plane will parallel the visualization on the ultrasound monitor. The orientation of the indicator for the long-axis is according to the sonographer's preference. If the indicator is oriented away from the operator, the needle should come from the upper right to the lower left on the ultrasound monitor.

Once the vessel is identified, grayscale compression (gentle pressure compression) is utilized in order to distinguish veins from arteries. With gentle pressure with the transducer, veins should collapse, while arteries should stay patent (Figure 15.3). This is most easily performed in the short-axis view of the blood vessel. It is important to note that with sufficient pressure some arteries will collapse, especially with smaller-diameter vessels and in smaller infants/children. Another means by which one can distinguish artery from vein is color Doppler, which shows constant flow through a vein, compared with the pulsations from an artery.

Ultrasound-guided procedure

Long-axis (in-plane) approach

The needle is oriented parallel to the long-axis of the transducer (Figure 15.2). The needle is immediately adjacent to the center of the smaller width of the transducer. It is important to note the orientation of the probe indicator. If the

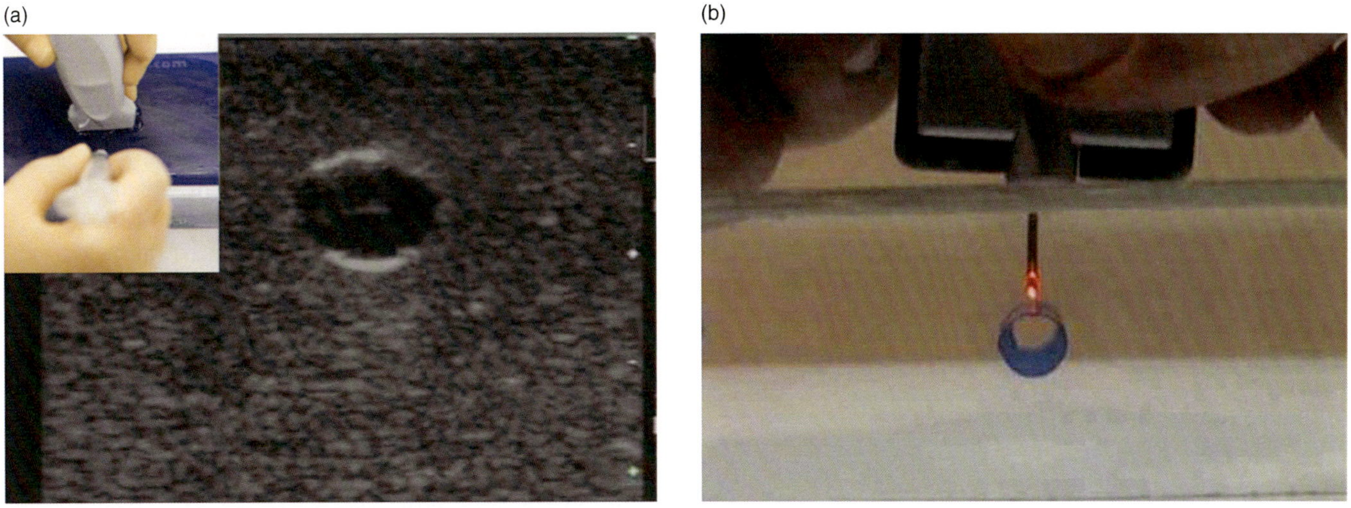

Figure 15.1 Short-axis view in a phantom model. (a) This is a short-axis view with picture-in-picture of a phantom gel being cannulated. On the ultrasound image, the vessel appears as a circle in cross-section. The needle is oriented perpendicular to the transducer. (b) Demonstration of the needle path in a phantom vessel.

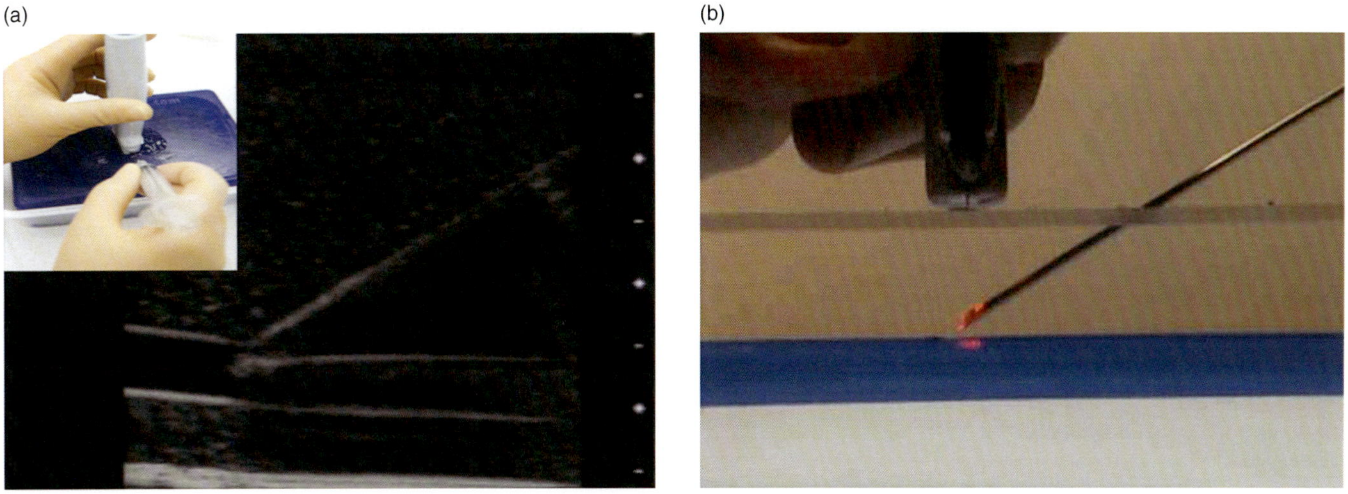

Figure 15.2 Long-axis view in a phantom model. (a) This is a long-axis view with picture-in-picture of a phantom gel being cannulated. The needle tip appears at the right upper portion of the ultrasound image. The needle tip is then tracked as it follows through the tissue down to the vessel which appears as a tubular structure. The needle is oriented parallel to the transducer. (b) Demonstration of the needle path in a phantom vessel.

indicator is oriented towards the operator, the needle will be visualized as entering the left-hand side of the ultrasound image.

Short-axis (out-of-plane) approach: approximating needle entry

In the short-axis approach, one must approximate needle entry (Figure 15.4). Once the vessel is identified on the ultrasound image, the depth can be readily determined by the markings on the right-hand side of the image. In utilizing the Pythagorean theorem, the depth should equal the distance away from the transducer:

$$\mathbf{a}^2 + \mathbf{b}^2 = \mathbf{c}^2$$

It is important to note that this is only true if the needle is at a 45° angle to the skin. Errors in needle placement may lead to under- or over-estimation of the target structure (Figure 15.5). Needle redirections may be performed under real-time guidance. Limitations are that the needle is not visualized until it actually enters the vessel. The needle tip, or ring-down artifact, will only be visualized as it arrives at and penetrates the targeted structure, thereby being "out of plane."

Short-axis approach: following the tip

Some practitioners feel uncomfortable not being able to visualize the needle tip until it reaches the target. Therefore, a new method was developed called "following the tip." The needle is oriented in the short-axis, or perpendicular to the transducer. The needle enters the skin immediately adjacent to the transducer (Figure 15.6a). As the needle/catheter is advanced, the transducer is moved away from the operator at the same velocity (Figure 15.6b). Therefore, the ultrasound beam tracks the needle tip throughout its course, until it reaches the target. It is important to note that this method requires significant manual dexterity and presumably more practice than the other methods.

The oblique approach

This is a novel method that is a combination of the short-axis and long-axis views for vessel cannulation (Figure 15.7). The vessel is first identified in the short-axis, and then the transducer is rotated almost midway between the short-axis and long-axis. Vessels appear as slightly elongated, and the needle is visualized along its entire path of entry. Further research needs to be performed regarding the success of the oblique method in comparison to the other, well-established techniques.

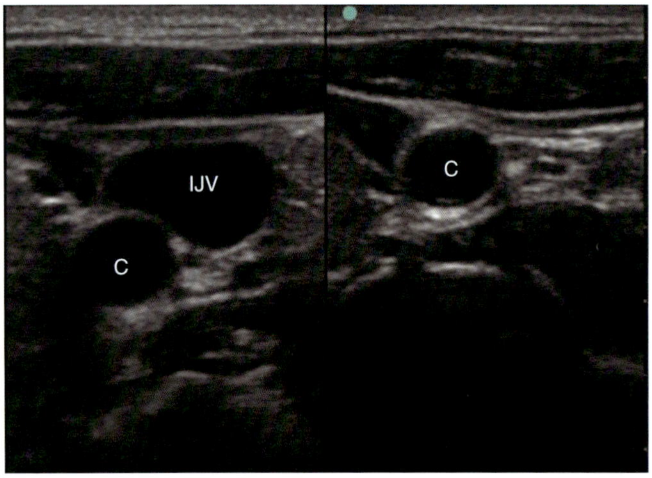

Figure 15.3 Graded compression. Gentle pressure is applied with the transducer to distinguish arteries from veins. This split-screen image shows the internal jugular vein (IJV) and carotid artery (C) on the left, precompression. On the right, post-compression image shows the internal jugular vein collapsed and not visible, while the thicker-walled carotid (C) stays patent.

Confirmation of placement, securing the line

Prior to penetrating the blood vessel, one may visualize "tenting of the blood vessel" (Figure 15.8a) and the "ring-down" artifact (Figure 15.8b) of the needle as it enters the vessel lumen. Blood vessel cannulation may be confirmed by visualizing needle placement in two planes, the visualization of a blood flash in the catheter, and the ability to flush saline. Once this occurs, ultrasonography may be discontinued and the catheter secured. Once the needle tip is in the vessel, the needle must be advanced far enough such that the catheter is in the vessel. Once this position is obtained, the catheter can be moved and advanced forward successfully.

In the traditional "landmark" or "blind" technique of central line placement, it is imperative that the syringe be aspirated during the time of needle advancement into the vein. Having blood returning into the syringe denotes successful cannulation of the central vein. By contrast, with ultrasound guidance, a syringe does not necessarily even need to be attached to the needle.

It is important to note that, since IV placement occurs at a 45° angle in the needle-approximation technique, smaller-gauge catheters have the potential to kink. In order to maintain the angle of entry, one may prop the catheter hub with 2″×2″ gauze prior to securing the catheter against the skin.

Training and education

The dynamic or real-time ultrasound guidance involves a steep learning curve and multiple steps to become proficient in it. The reward of learning the procedure is in the precision that it provides in guiding a needle into the desired location. Commercially available phantom models simulate blood vessels in order to teach hands-on vascular access (Figure 15.9a,b), prior to attempting to place the IV in a patient. Other less-expensive, home-made phantoms may be prepared which are

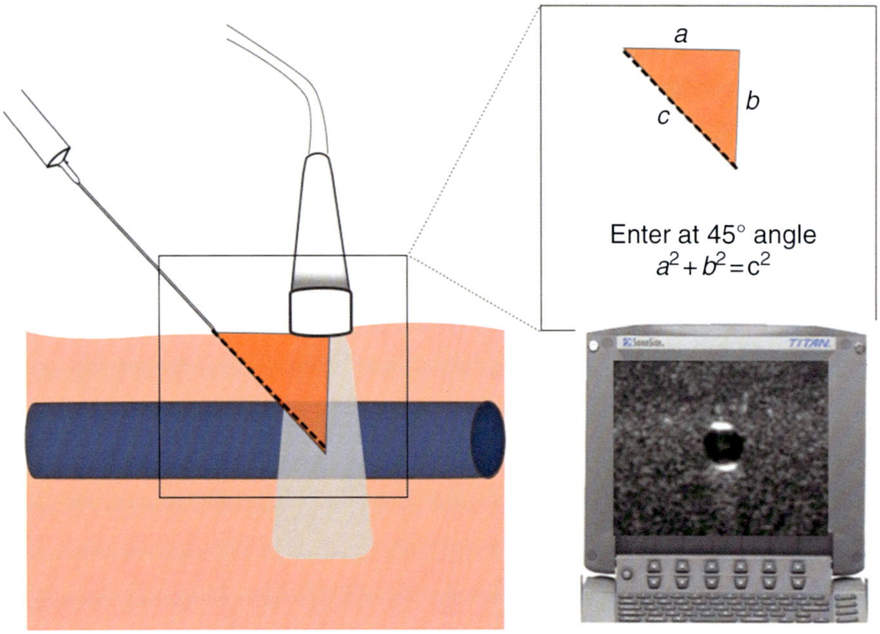

Figure 15.4 Approximating needle entry. In the short-axis plane, the needle enters at a 45° angle to the skin, at a distance away from the transducer that equals the depth of the target structure. This is true because of the Pythagorean theorem ($a^2 + b^2 = c^2$). Depth can be determined from the depth markers on the right side of the ultrasound image (arrow).

effective as well (Figure 15.9c). It has been suggested that when comparing the different approaches to ultrasound-guided vascular access, the short-axis (out-of-plane) approach is the easiest to teach and learn.

Specific scanning techniques

Femoral vein

The femoral vein is one of the preferred sites for central venous cannulation in the cardiac arrest/CPR situation.

Anatomy

In most patients, the femoral nerve is lateral to the femoral artery, and the femoral vein medial to the artery (Figure 15.10a). However, it has been shown by ultrasound that there are variations in the anatomic relationship of the femoral vein and artery.

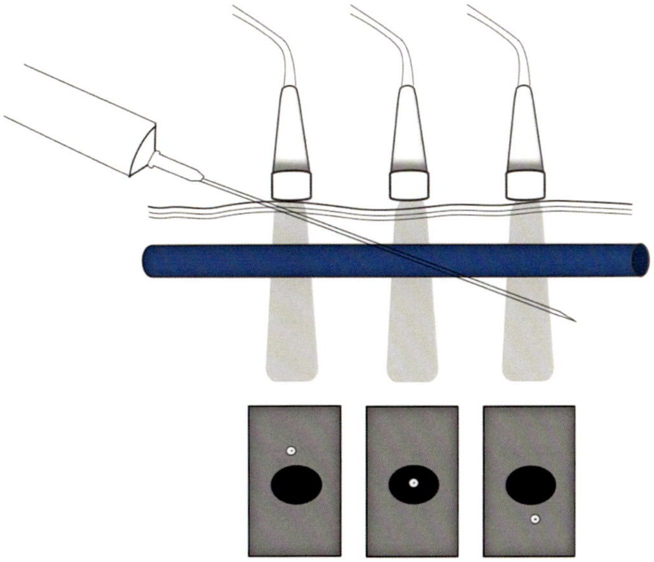

Figure 15.5 Errors in needle placement. If the needle is placed too close to the transducer, the needle will be above the target vessel. In contrast, if the needle is placed too far away from the transducer, the needle will be below the target vessel. *Illustration by Laura Berg, MD.*

Technique

For femoral access, the transducer should be placed in the inguinal region (Figure 15.10b). In order to obtain the short-axis view, the transducer should be oriented with the indicator towards the proceduralist's left side (Figure 15.10c,d). In the majority of patients, the femoral artery will lie to the left of the femoral vein. However, it is important to interrogate both the patient's right and left sides since there is anatomic variation with regards to the relationship between femoral artery and vein. In order to obtain the long-axis view, the transducer should be oriented with the indicator towards the patient's head (Figure 15.10f,g).

Subclavian vein

The subclavian vein is the preferred site for central venous cannulation for sepsis, since the femoral site is more at risk for infection. The subclavian vein is often the preferred site of central line placement in children, due to space constraints.

Anatomy

The axillary vein courses through the pectoralis muscle in a medial and superior direction. Once the vein crosses below the clavicle it is known as the subclavian vein (Figure 15.11a).

Technique

The subclavian line placement has been recently performed with ultrasound guidance, but this location has some limitations. Due to the density of bone, there is a shadow on ultrasound, which prevents the operator from seeing the entire path of the needle. Furthermore, since the approach to subclavian access is a superficial orientation of the needle, it is recommended to perform the procedure in the long-axis view (Figure 15.11b,d). It also seems to be preferred in children, due to space constraints. Both supraclavicular and

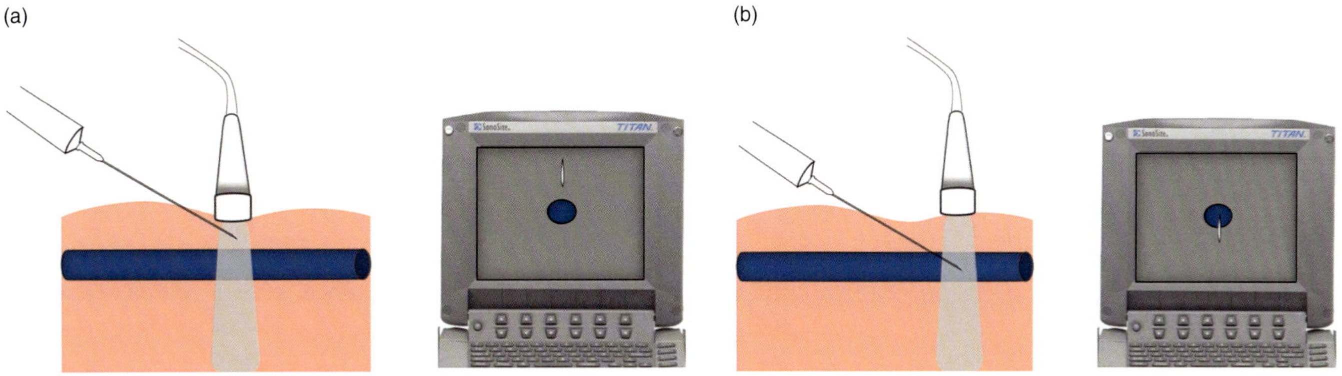

Figure 15.6 "Following the tip." The needle is oriented perpendicular to the transducer, immediately adjacent to its center. The corresponding ultrasound image is a cross-section of the targeted vessel, with the needle tip above it (a). As the needle is advanced, the transducer is moved away from the operator at the same velocity. The corresponding ultrasound image ultimately shows the needle tip penetrating the target vessel (b). In this approach, the needle tip is visualized along its entire path, in the short-axis view. *Illustration by Laura Berg, MD.*

infraclavicular approaches have been described (Figure 15.11b). A suggested approach is:

1. Pre-procedural ultrasound scanning: obtain both supraclavicular and infraclavicular views, identify the axillary and subclavian veins, and evaluate for patency; identify surrounding structures.
2. Infraclavicular approach: identify the subclavian vein in the long-axis, and utilize Doppler for confirmation. Imaging in the long axis should be performed along the imaging path of the needle to the vein, as the angled path of the needle is towards the lung.
3. Advance the needle slowly so that its trajectory and/or tip can be detected superficially. Advance the needle in real time in the longitudinal axis, in the direction of the acoustic shadow from the thoracic rib. The needle enters the vessel either at the level of the axillary vein or where it continues medially as the subclavian vein. The angle of penetration and the course of the needle may be adjusted according to the patient.
4. Advancement of the guidewire according to the Seldinger technique.
5. Post-procedure scanning of the internal jugular vein and contralateral subclavian vein to identify malpositioning. Also perform lung scanning to evaluate for pneumothoraces.

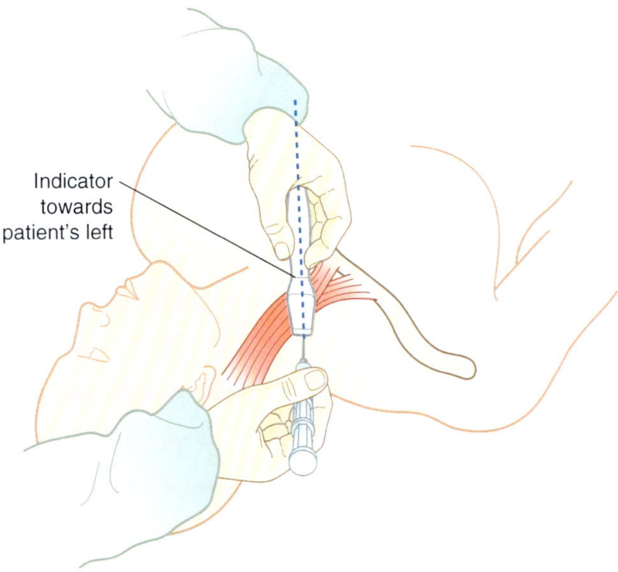

Figure 15.7 The oblique approach. The vessel is first identified in the short-axis. The transducer is then rotated midway between short-axis and long-axis (rotation of 45°). *Artwork created by Emily Evans © Cambridge University Press.*

Internal jugular vein

Anatomy

The internal jugular vein lies lateral to the carotid artery (Figure 15.12a). However, there are anatomic variations including the vein being directly anterior to the carotid artery (Figure 15.12b). Because of these variations, it is especially important to utilize ultrasound prior to placing a central line or with real-time guidance during the procedure.

Technique

In order to place an internal jugular line, the patient should be in the Trendelenburg position, and the operator should be at the head of the patient's bed (Figure 15.13a).

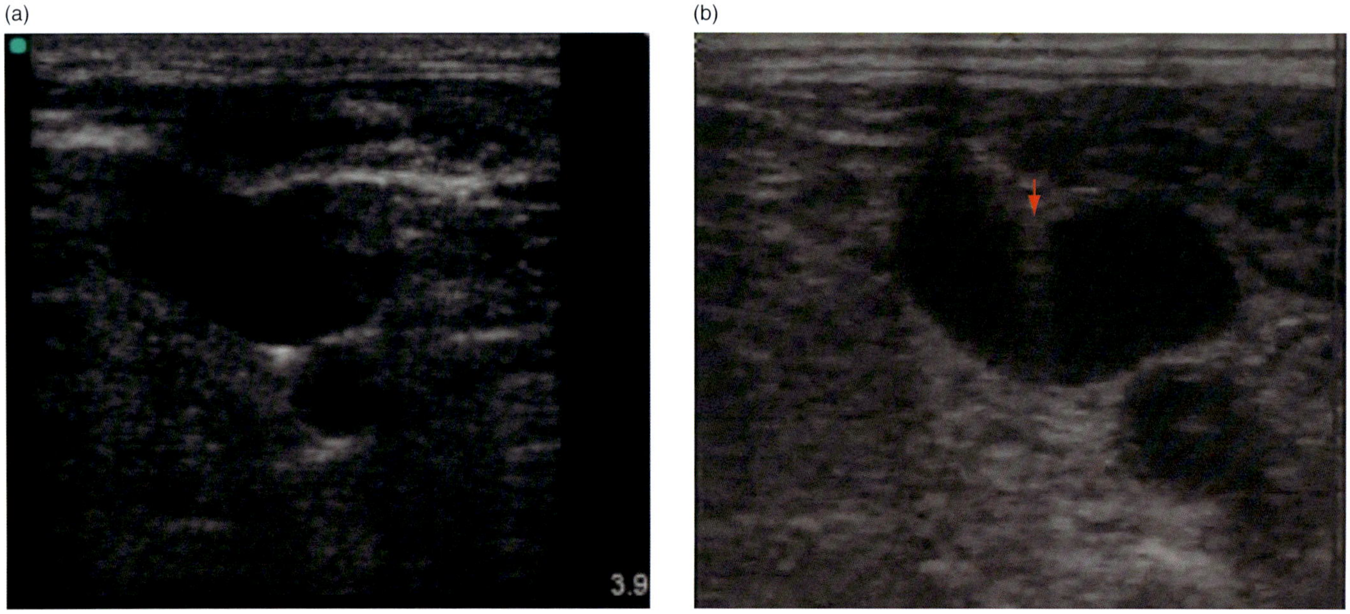

Figure 15.8 Short-axis confirmation of line placement. (a) Prior to penetration of the blood vessel, the vessel exhibits deformation, or "tenting," as is evident in this ultrasound image of an IJ line placement. (b) Once the needle enters the blood vessel, one can visualize the needle tip and the "ring-down" artifact (arrow) that arises from the metal of the needle.

Since this is opposite to general positioning, the probe indicator should be oriented towards the operator's left, in order to correlate with the left-hand side of the ultrasound monitor. In the short-axis view, the left-hand side of the monitor should correlate with the patient's left, and the right-hand side of the monitor should correlate with the patient's right (Figure 15.13b,c). When rotating the transducer to obtain the long-axis view, the operator should direct the probe indicator towards the patient's head (Figure 15.13d,e). Therefore, the left-hand side of the ultrasound image should correlate with the patient's head, and the right-hand side of the image should correlate with the feet, respectively.

Gentle compression may be utilized to distinguish the internal jugular from the carotid artery (Figure 15.3). Additionally, having the patient perform a Valsalva maneuver should increase

(a)

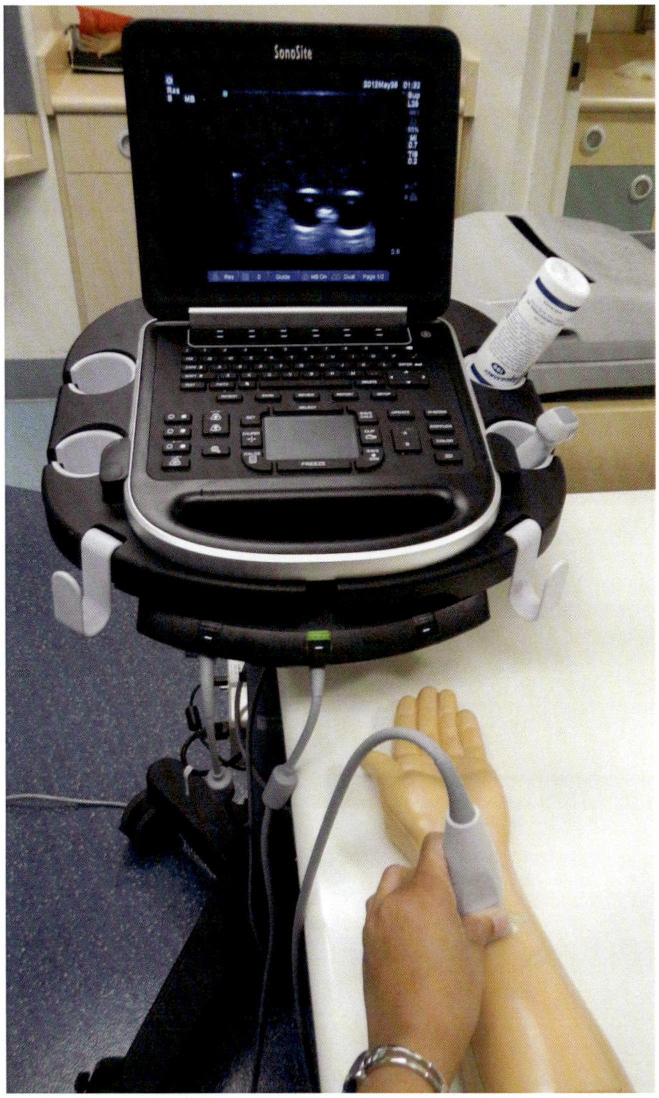

(b)

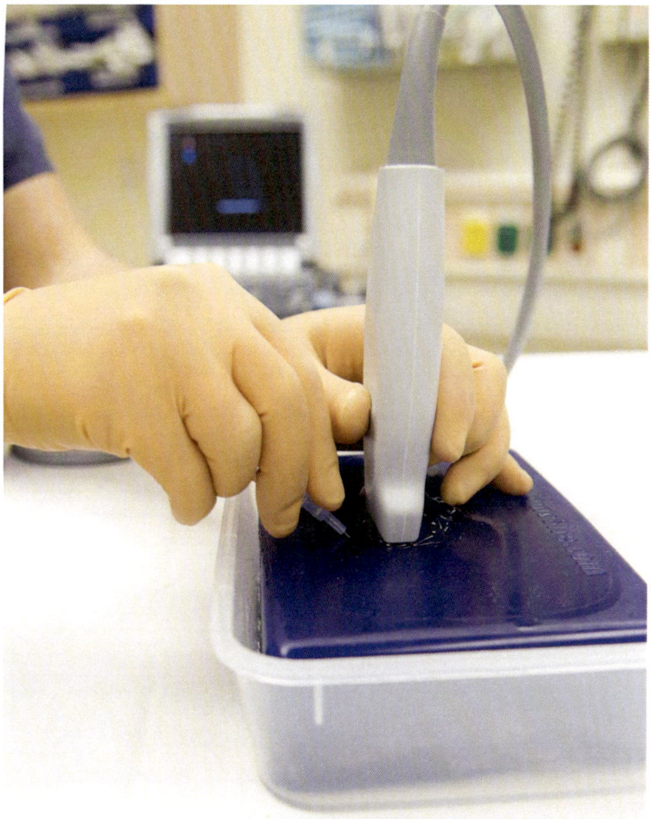

(c)

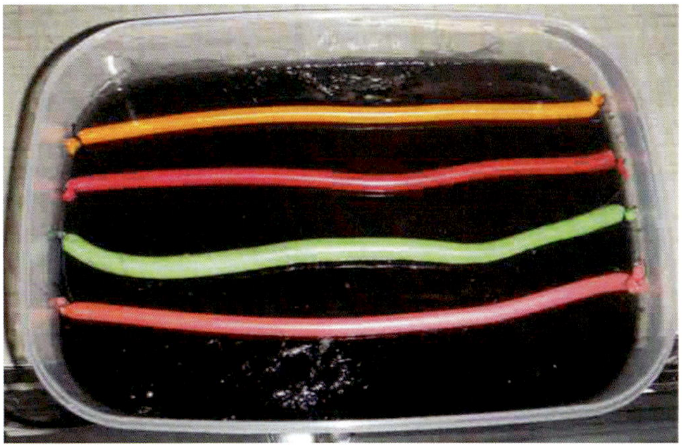

Figure 15.9 Phantoms for vascular access instruction. (a, b) Commercially available phantoms. (c) A home-made version of a training phantom. This particular version consists of store-bought gelatin with toy balloons filled with colored liquid. When the gel is chilled in the refrigerator, the balloons are suspended in the center of the gelatin-filled container.

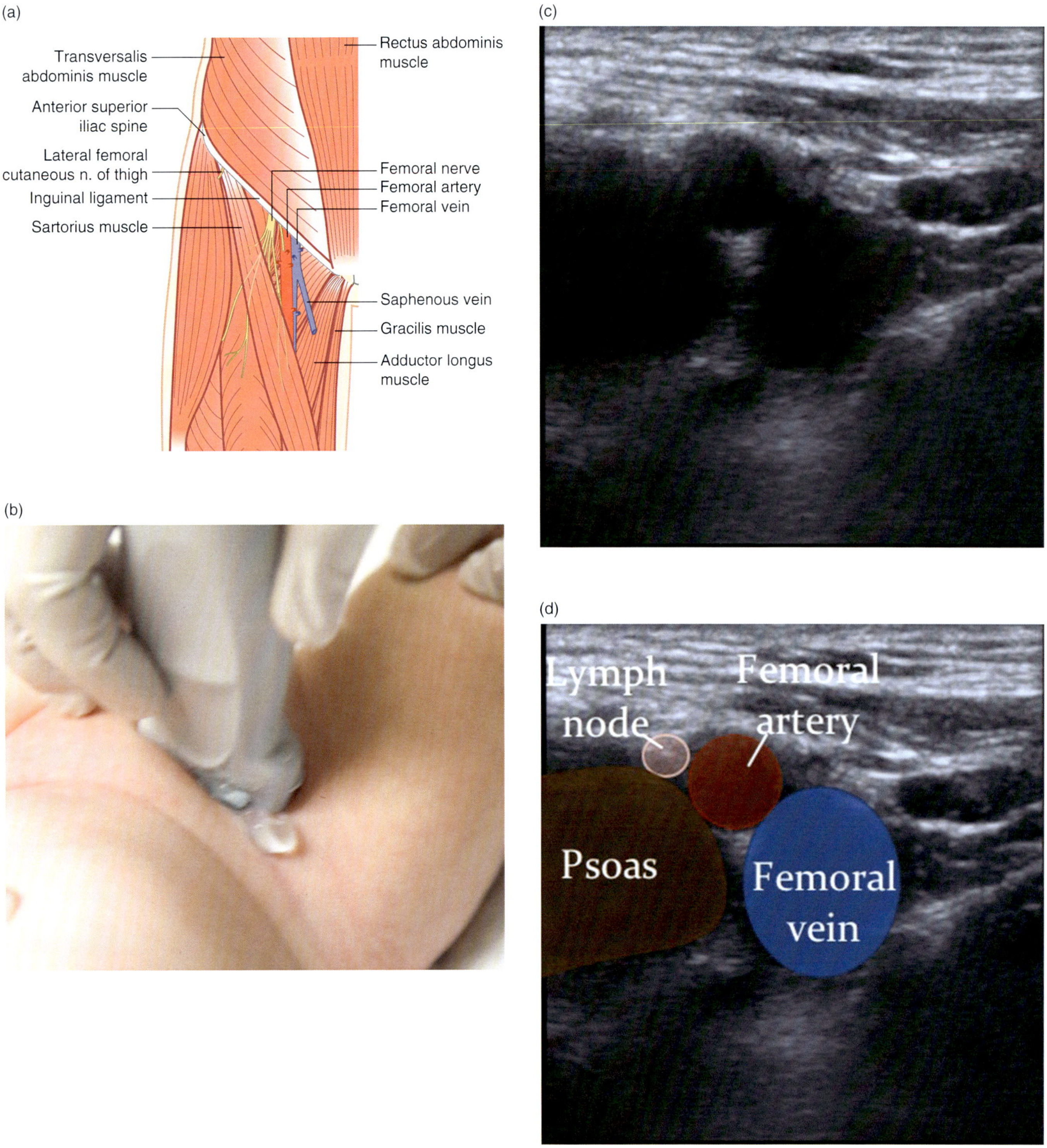

Figure 15.10 Femoral vein. (a) Femoral vein anatomy. The femoral vein is larger in diameter than the artery, and typically lies medial to the femoral artery. *Artwork created by Emily Evans © Cambridge University Press.* (b) Transducer placement in the inguinal region for femoral vein access. The leg may be flexed forward or held in extension to improve visualization. Note that the sterile preparation was removed in order to demonstrate proper transducer placement. (c) Ultrasound image of the short-axis view of the femoral vessels. (d) Associated structures visualized by ultrasound in the short-axis view, including the psoas muscle and the femoral nerve, femoral artery, and femoral nerve. (e) Femoral vessels with color Doppler. (f) Ultrasound image of the long-axis view of the femoral vein. (g) Associated structures visualized by ultrasound in the long-axis view. *Illustration by Laura Berg, MD.*

(e)

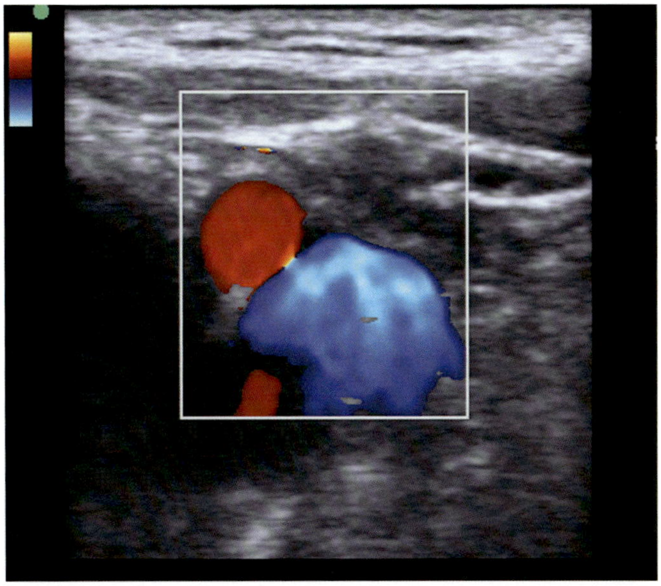

(f)

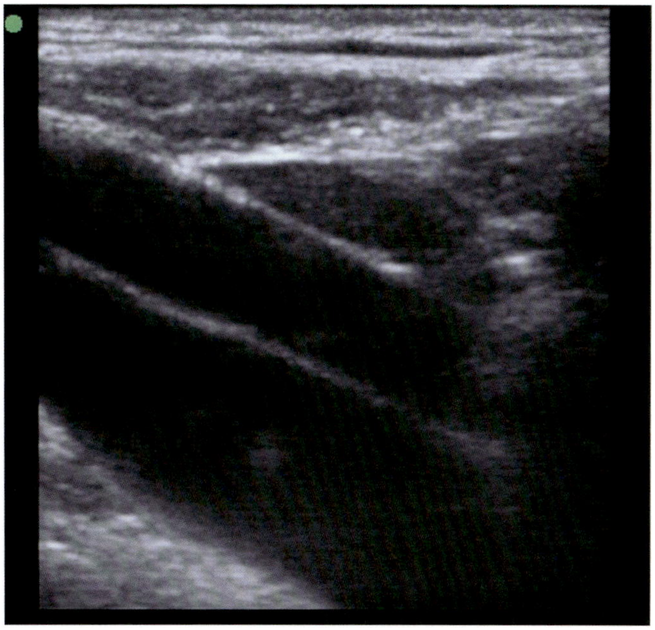

(g)

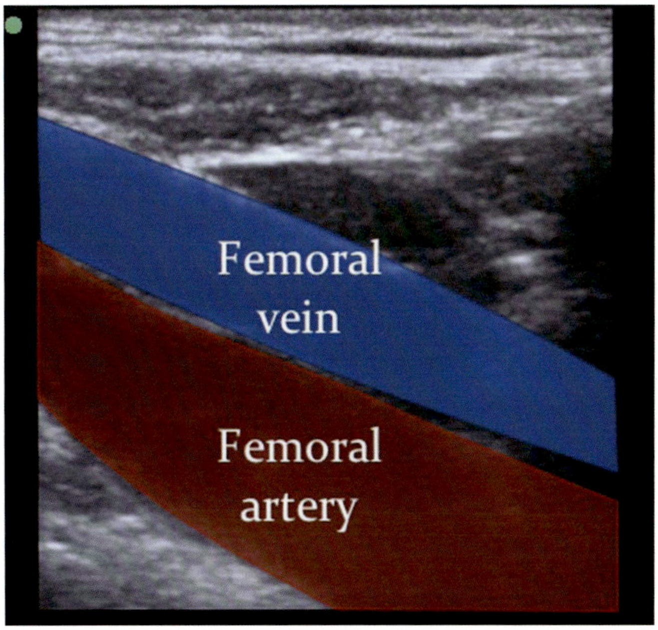

Figure 15.10 (cont.)

the size of the internal jugular vein, due to the change in pressure. Note that, when using color Doppler, the direction of blood flow may reverse with the Valsalva maneuver.

Antecubital region (peripheral IVs, PICC lines)

The antecubital region, in particular, has several potential sites for vascular access. The superficial and deep antecubital veins are ideal for ultrasound-guided peripheral line placement. In the upper arm, the deep vessels are often accessed as peripherally inserted central catheters (PICCs).

Anatomy

These include cephalic, basilic, and brachial veins (Figure 15.14a). It is important to note that nerves course through the arm region.The upper medial arm is an ideal site for PICCs.

Technique

The same principles are utilized as for ultrasound-guided central line placement. However, peripheral vessels tend to be much more superficial and small, when compared to vessels utilized for central line placement. It is important to recognize surrounding structures such as nerves and arteries, which should be avoided. These may be especially small and superficial in smaller children and infants. The majority of vessels are located at depths between 0.25 and 0.5 cm in children (Figure 15.14b).

Saphenous (peripheral IVs)

Anatomy

The Saphenous vein is another potential location for ultrasound-guided IV placement. The saphenous vein lies anterior to the medial malleolus. Its course is relatively straight (Figure 15.15a). Neither the dorsalis pedis nor the posterior tibialis artery are in close proximity to the saphenous vein. Therefore, arterial puncture is unlikely.

Technique

A linear transducer is placed anterior and superior to the medial malleolus (Figure 15.15b). On the ultrasound image, the saphenous vein may be visualized just anterior to the medial malleolus (Figure 15.15c).

Arterial lines

Arterial line placement may be required in critically ill patients, in order to monitor blood pressure and provide frequent blood gas measurements. Arterial lines are generally placed at the wrist by palpating the radial artery. Arterial line placement can be an especially challenging procedure in small, pediatric patients.

Anatomy

The radial artery can be seen in the distal forearm, the most common location for placing an arterial line (Figure 15.16a).

Technique

The transducer is applied to the radial aspect of the distal forearm (Figure 15.16b). Grayscale ultrasonography is utilized in order to locate the radial artery. The radial artery is identified by the lack of compressibility and visible pulsations (Figure 15.16c). Color Doppler may also be utilized in order to further identify the radial artery. The catheter is placed either by the short-axis (out-of-plane), or long-axis (in-plane) technique.

(a)

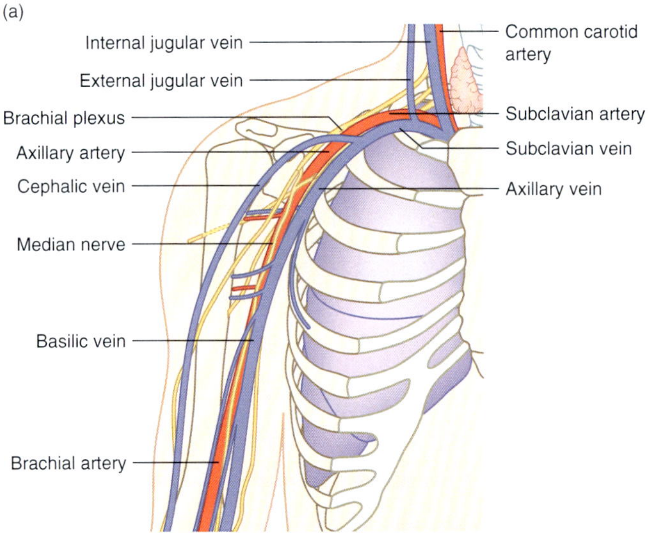

(b)

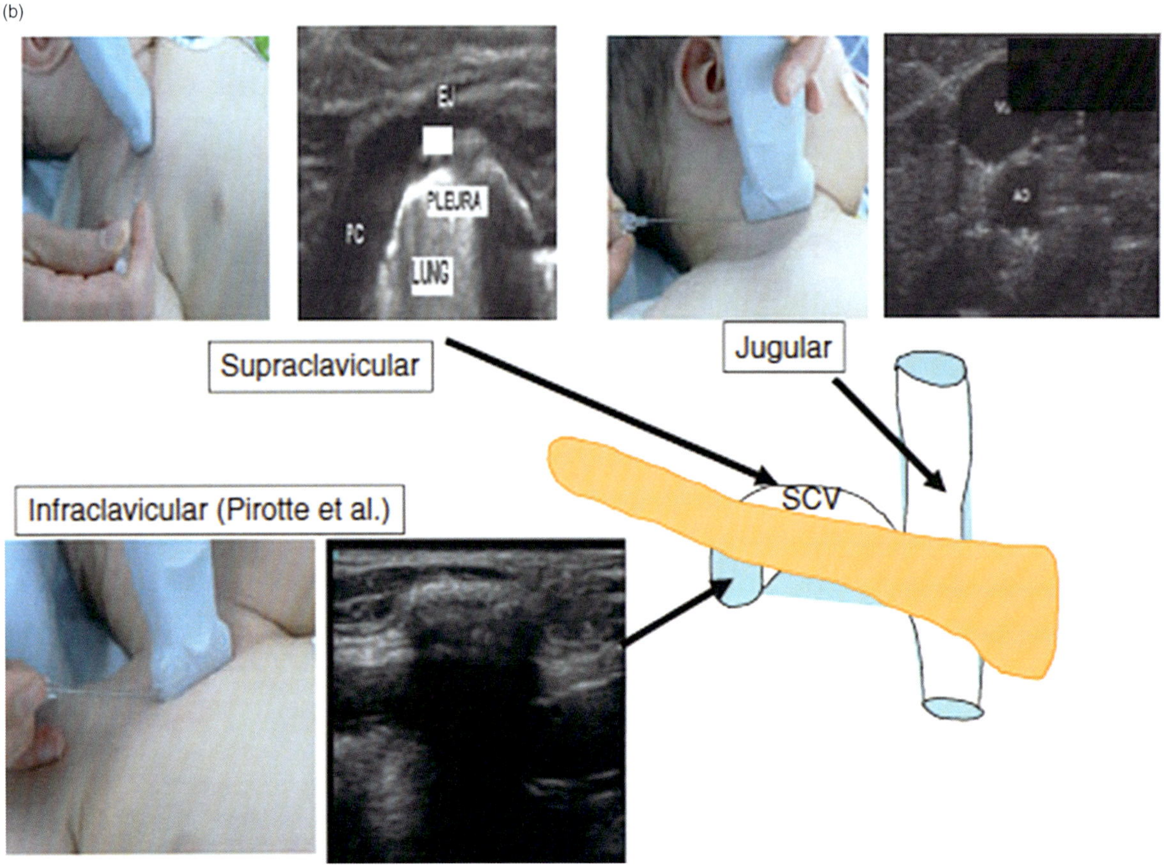

Figure 15.11 Subclavian vein. (a) Subclavian vein anatomy. *Artwork created by Emily Evans © Cambridge University Press.* (b) Illustration of different approaches of subclavian line placement, including supraclavicular and infraclavicular approaches. Rhondali, O., Attof, R., Combet, S., *et al.* (2011) Ultrasound-guided subclavian vein cannulation in infants: supraclavicular approach. *Pediatr Anesthes* **21**(11):1136–41. (c) The ultrasound image of the short-axis view of the subclavian vein (SCV) with adjacent carotid artery (C), clavicle (arrowhead), and posterior shadowing. (d) The ultrasound image of the long-axis view of the subclavian vein. Associated structures visualized in the long-axis view include the clavicle (arrowhead) with posterior shadowing, and the needle (arrows) as it enters the subclavian vein. *Ultrasound images courtesy of David J. Wallace, MD MPH RDMS.*

(c) (d)

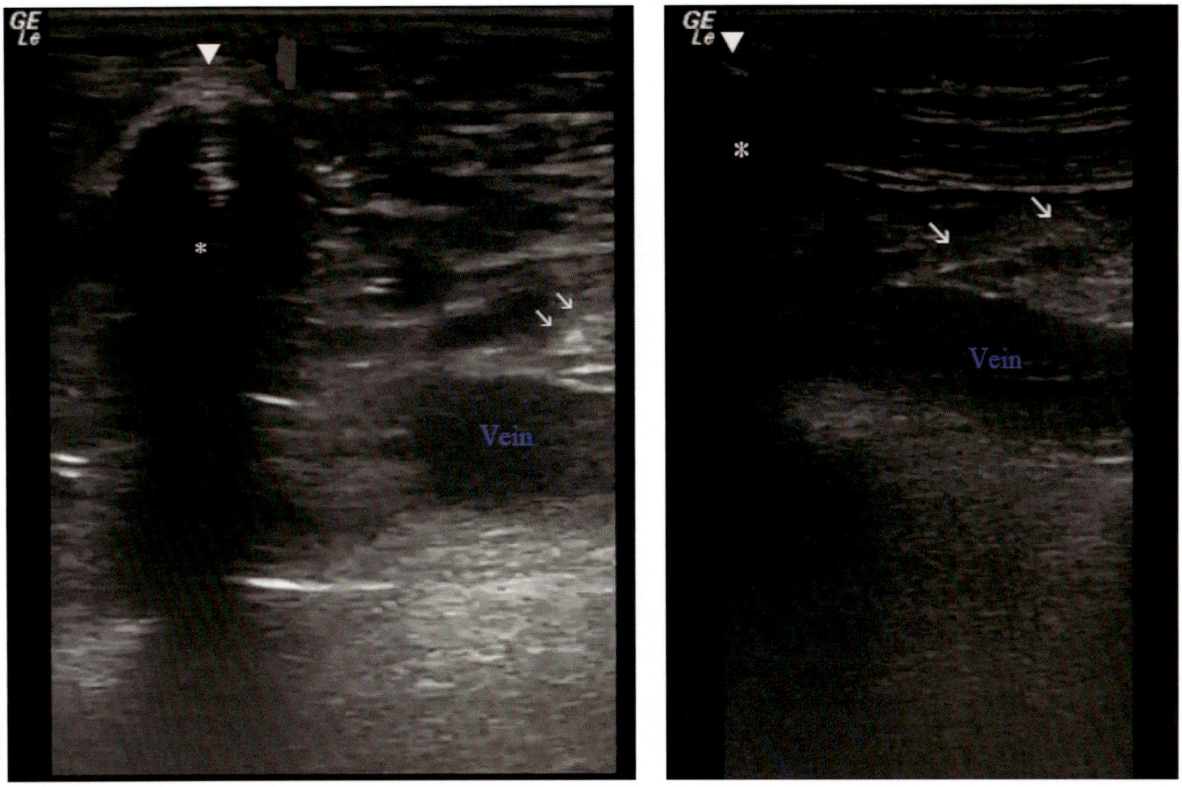

Figure 15.11 (cont.)

(a)

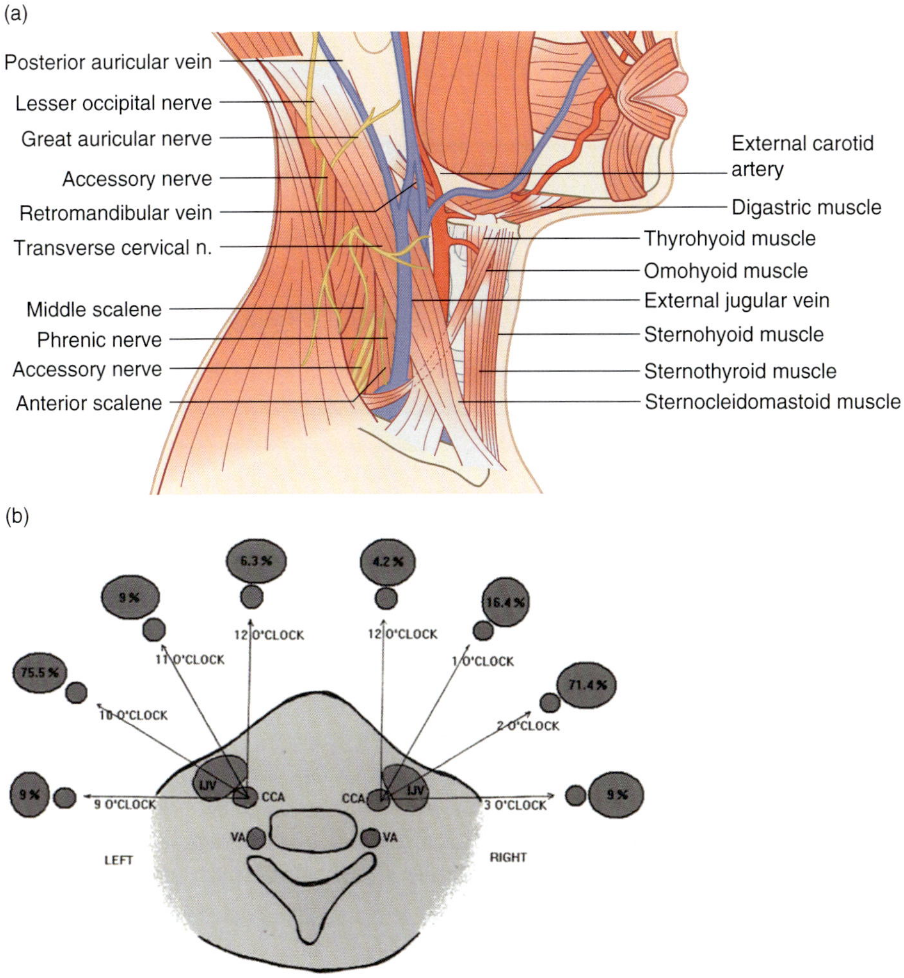

Figure 15.12 Internal jugular vein. (a) Internal jugular vein anatomy. *Artwork created by Emily Evans © Cambridge University Press.* (b) Anatomic variations of the internal jugular vein (IJV) in relation to the carotid artery (C).VA, vertebral artery. Turba, U.C., Uflacker, R., Hannegan, C.H., *et al.* (2005) Anatomic relationship of the internal jugular vein and the common carotid artery applied to percutaneous transjugular procedures. *Cardrovasc Intervent Radiol* **28**:303–06.

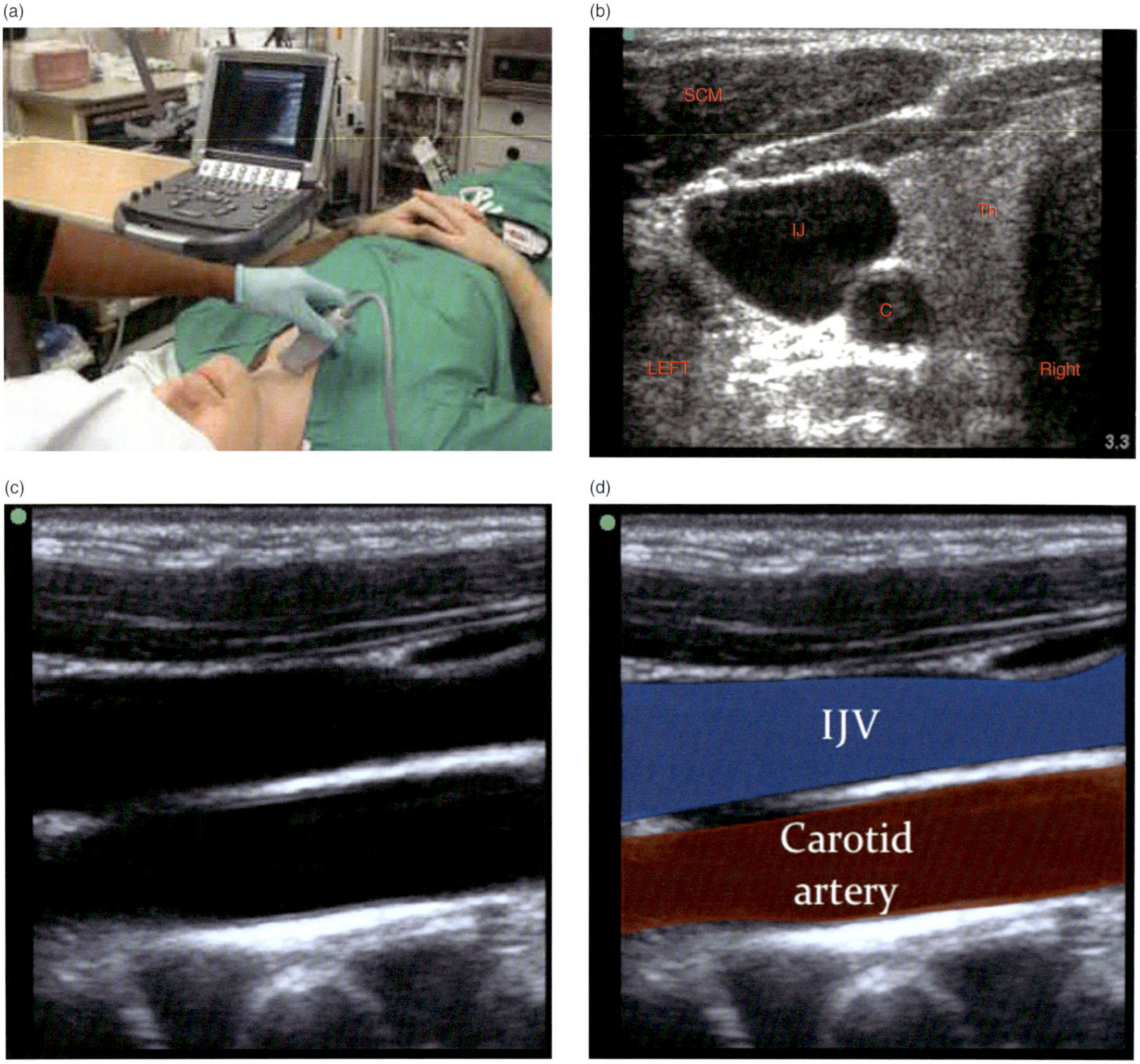

Figure 15.13 Internal jugular vein. (a) Transducer positioning for internal jugular placement. Note, the sonographer is standing at the patient's head. (b) Ultrasound image of the short-axis view with important structures noted: the sternocleido mastoid muscle (SCM), internal jugular vein (IJV), carotid artery (C) and thyroid (Th). (c) Ultrasound image of the long-axis view. (d) Associated structures visualized in the long-axis view. *Illustration by Laura Berg, MD.*

Intraosseus lines

Intraosseous lines may be required in critically ill patients. They can be expeditiously placed, especially with newer techniques of intraosseous placement such as the Easy-IO™ gun. They provide rapid central line access for the administration of life-saving medications, blood products, and intravenous fluids. Traditional methods of intraosseous needle placement confirmation, including aspiration of bone marrow, blood visualization at the needle tip, the needle standing firmly upright, or the infusion of fluid without soft tissue infiltration, are unreliable.

Anatomy

The most common location for placing an intraosseous line in children is at the tibia, below the tibial tuberosity (Figure 15.17a).

Technique

A high-frequency (5–10 MHz), linear transducer is oriented both parallel to the bone and perpendicular (Figure 15.17b). Doppler ultrasound can further assist in determining whether an intraosseous needle is placed correctly in the intraosseous space (Figure 15.17c) rather than in the soft tissue (Figure 15.17d).

Scanning tips

Pitfalls

- Regardless of whether ultrasound visualization is utilized, one may encounter the same difficulties as with traditional line: valves are still present, and vessels still collapse and roll.
- The operator should confirm catheter placement in two views, and use long catheters whenever possible.
- In placement of central and peripheral IV catheters, inadvertent nerve contact or aterial cannulation may occur. Once recognized, the catheter should immediately be removed.
- When placing a line by the "approximating needle entry" technique, errors in placement may occur (Figure 15.5).
- Small children pose particular challenges. Their vessels may be especially small and superficial, limiting resolution of ultrasound and limiting which catheters may be used. It is especially challenging to immobilize the extremities in order to facilitate ultrasound guidance.
- Whenever possible, one may utilize an additional staff person to immobilize the extremity, or use arm boards and papooses.

Tips to improve scanning

✓ While attempting ultrasound-guided vascular access, it is often difficult to ascertain the positioning of the needle tip. One may give the needle "a wiggle," moving the needle in and out by a millimeter or so. In doing so,

(a)

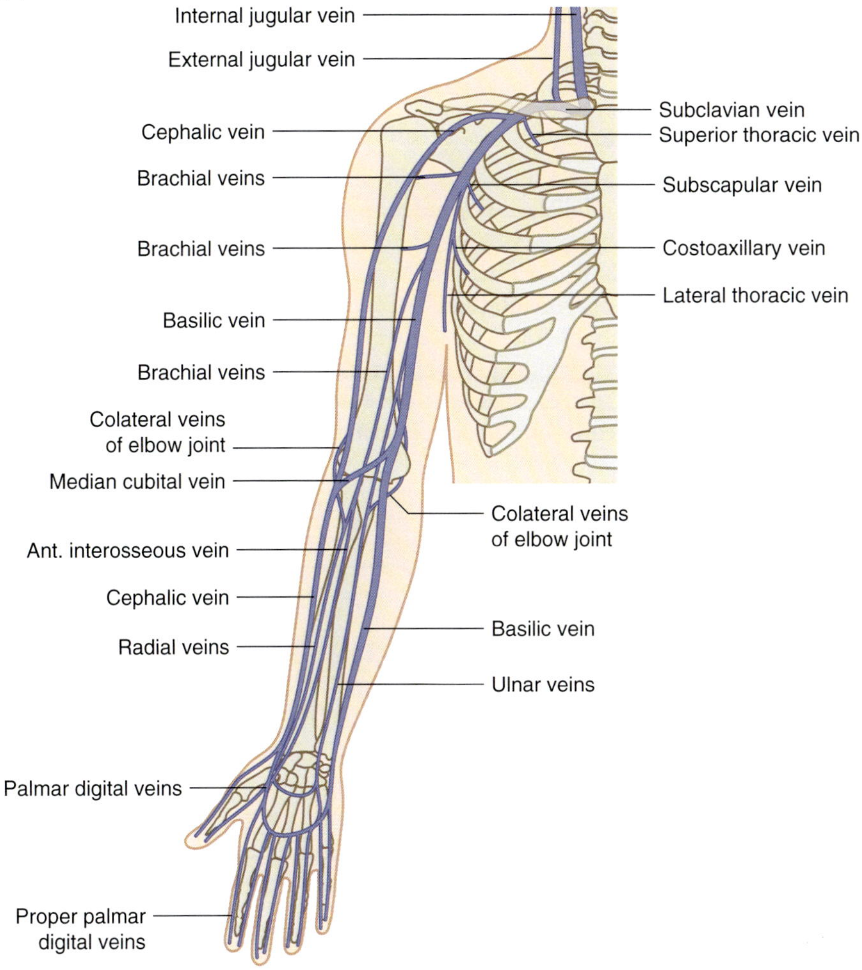

Figure 15.14 Peripheral veins: antecubital region. For peripheral IV placement and PICC lines. (a) Peripheral vein anatomy in the antecubital region. *Artwork created by Emily Evans © Cambridge University Press.* (b) Transducer placement in the antecubital region. (c) Ultrasound image of vessels in the antecubital region, in the short-axis view, with arteries (A) and veins (V). (d) After graded compression, the arteries (A) stay patent, while the veins (V) collapse.

(b)

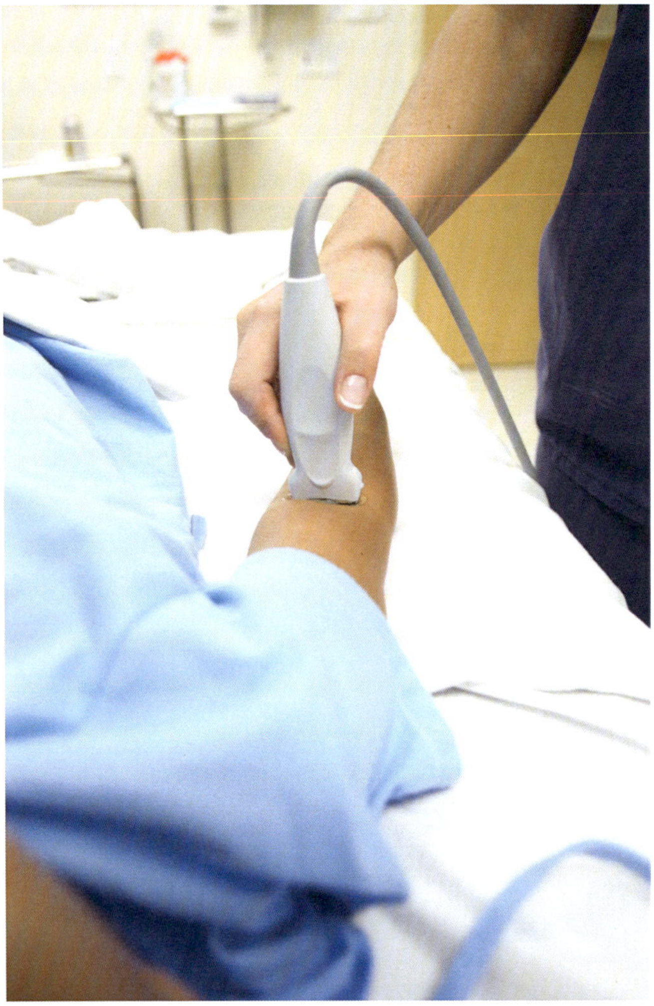

the needle tip can be seen coming in and out of the transducer beam. During this process, the transducer is held completely still. In some patients, you cannot see the needle tip itself, but you may only see movement of the tissue.

- ✓ It is important to choose the IV catheter carefully. A catheter that is too small (i.e. 24g) may bend or "kink," especially when entering a vessel at 40–45°. In contrast, a larger gauge catheter (i.e. 16–18g) may be too large for the targeted vessel. It may either not be able to cannulate the vessel, or lead to thrombosis.
- ✓ There are special echo-tip needles which may enhance visualization on ultrasound. In addition, there are extra long catheters which are more amenable to catheterizing deep vessels.
- ✓ Occasionally with peripheral IV placement, you may not visualize a flash of blood in the catheter hub. In these situations, it is crucial to confirm intravascular placement by scanning in another plane and then flushing the line with saline.

Case

1. JM is a seven-year-old with a history of renal failure, and dialysis dependence. He has frequented the emergency department and has a history of extremely difficult IV access. On his last visit to the emergency department, there were numerous failed attempts at peripheral IV placement, warranting him to have a central line placed in order to receive IV antibiotics. On presentation to the emergency department, he is febrile and toxic appearing, but has stable vital signs.

(c)

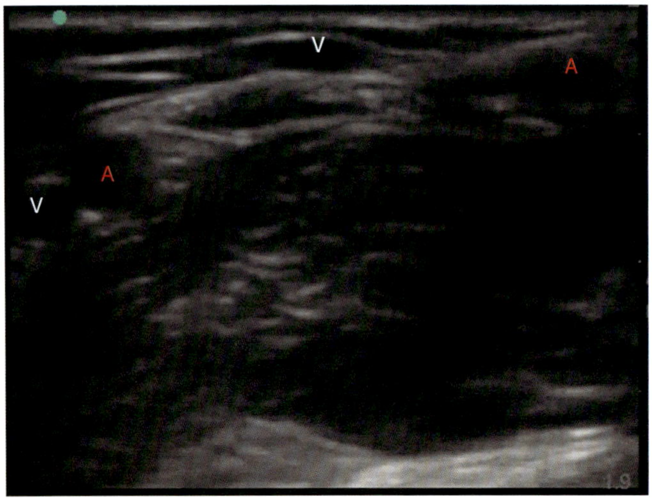

(d)

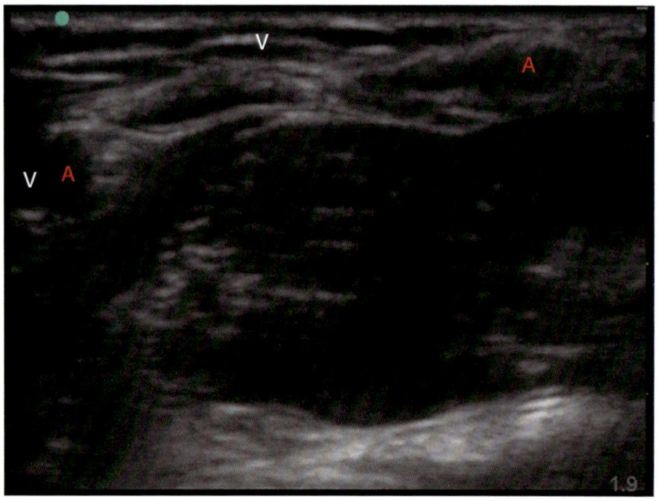

Figure 15.14 (cont.)

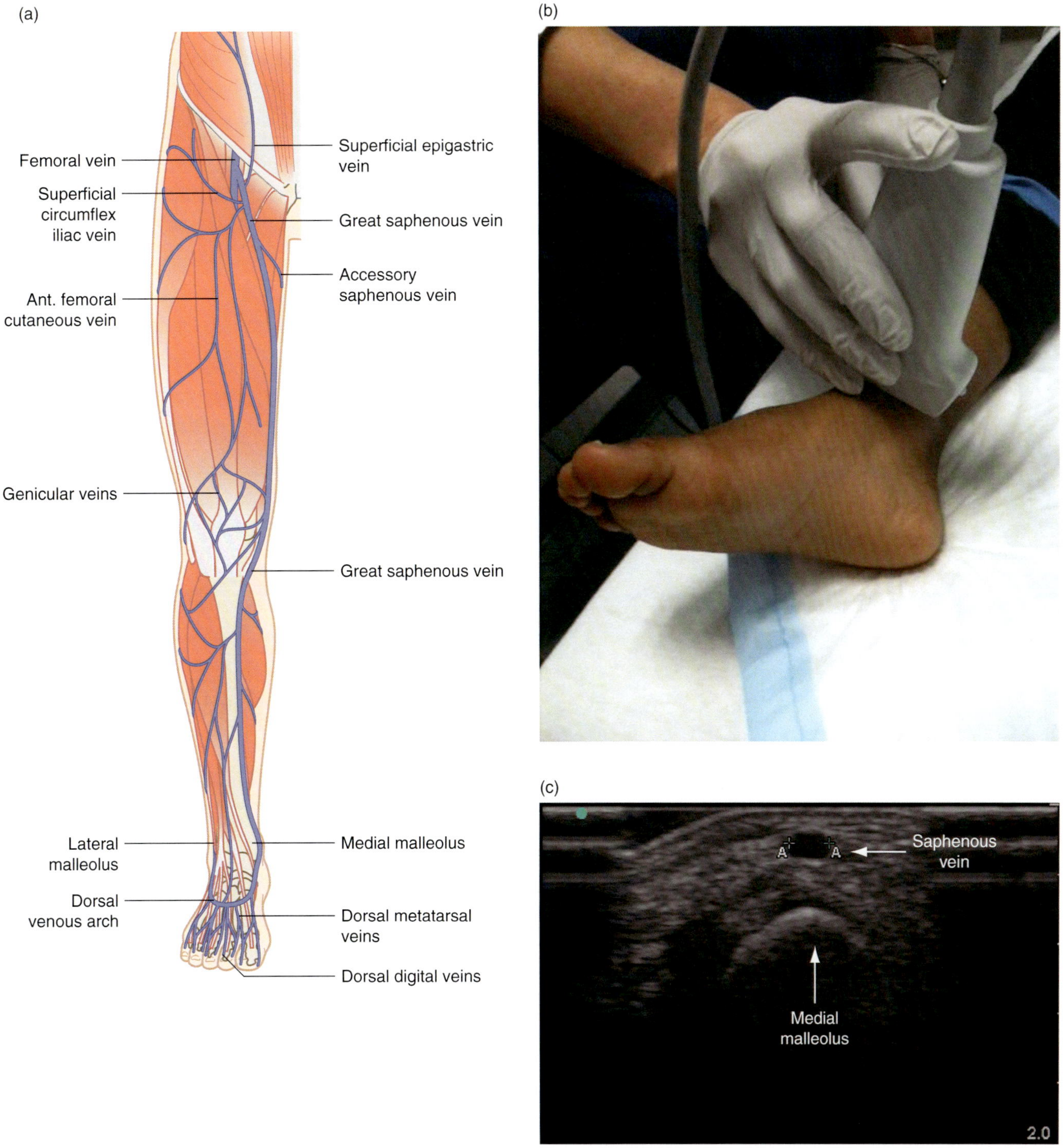

Figure 15.15 Peripheral veins: the saphenous vein for vascular access. (a) Anatomy of the saphenous vein. *Artwork created by Emily Evans © Cambridge University Press.* (b) Transducer placement for visualization of the saphenous vein. (c) Ultrasound image of the saphenous vein, which is anterior to the medial malleolus.

On physical examination, no adequate blood vessels are visualized or palpated for vascular access by traditional methods. Therefore, a peripheral IV is placed with ultrasound guidance, and dual-operator method. The IV is successfully placed on the first attempt, with only two needle redirections. The child and family are extremely pleased, and ask for ultrasound guidance immediately after arriving to the emergency department on a subsequent visit. This demonstrates the utility of ultrasound guidance on peripheral IV placement in

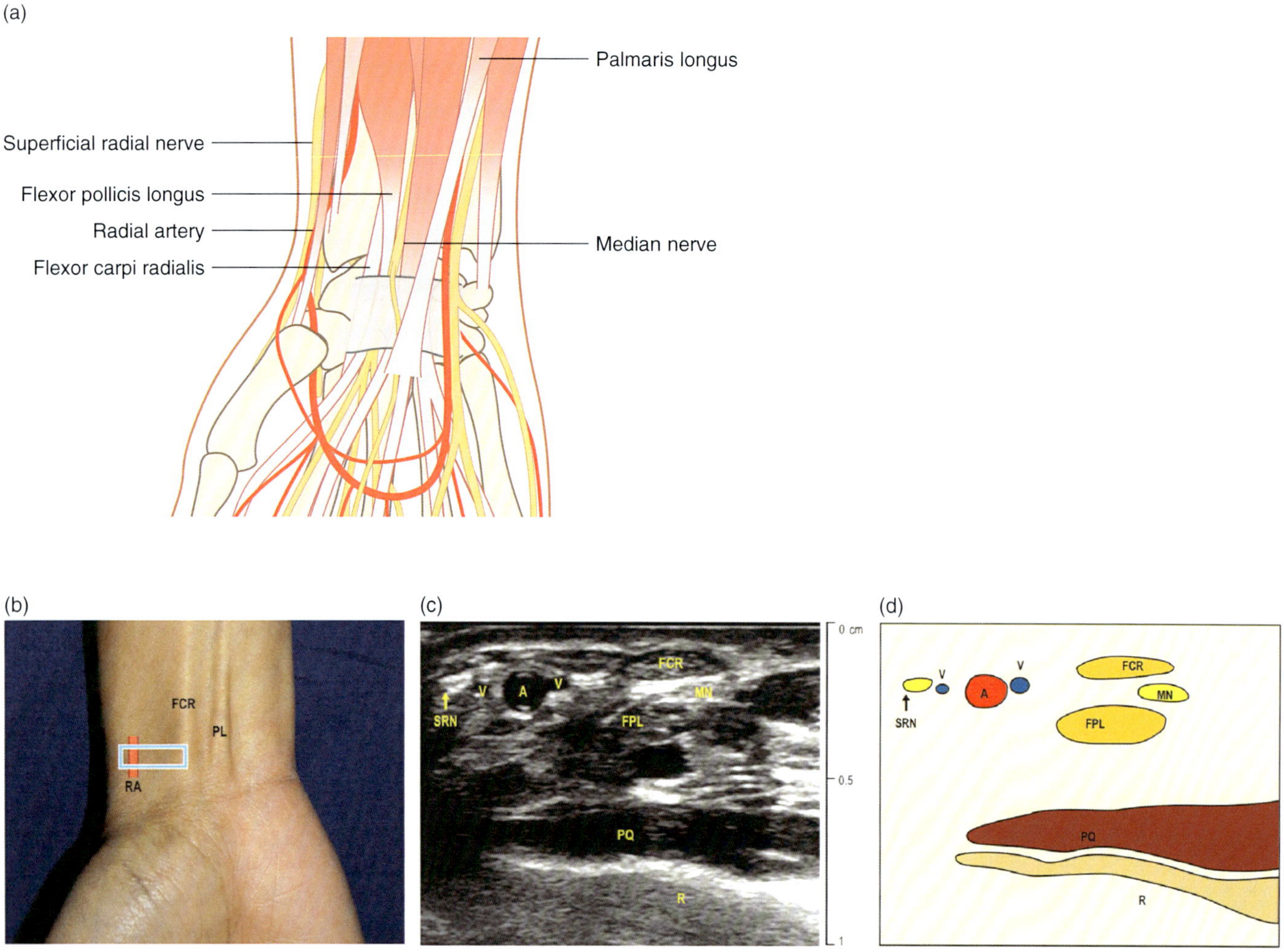

Figure 15.16 Radial artery for vascular access. (a) Anatomy. *Artwork created by Emily Evans © Cambridge University Press.* (b) Transducer positioning. Important structures are the radial artery (RA), and the flexor carpi radialis (FCR) and palmaris longus (PL) tendons. The transducer placement is represented by a blue box. (c) Ultrasound image. (d) Corresponding illustration depicting important structures: radial artery (A), radius (R), fexor carpi radialis (FCR), and median nerve (MN). Images for Figure 15.16 b, c, and d: Copyright Lin, M. Jones, A. Gaur and A. Ahmed. *Artwork created by Emily Evans.* Sonoanatomy for Anaesthetists, 2012.

children with difficult access. This technique has been shown to have great success rates, with less time to placement fewer needle redirections, all of which can be painful for pediatric patients.

Summary/key points

1. Ultrasound-guided vascular access may be utilized by physicians, nurses, and prehospital providers with appropriate training. The single-operator and dual-operator methods may be utilized.
2. In 1999, an Institute of Medicine report recommended ultrasound guidance as the standard of care in the placement of all central lines, as a means to improve patient safety.
3. Linear, high-frequency transducers are utilized for vascular access. It is important to identify landmarks and avoid surrounding structures such as arteries and nerves.
4. Ultrasound-assisted vascular access involves identifying the target blood vessel by ultrasound and marking the skin. Ultrasound-guided vascular access involves real-time visualization during the line placement.
5. Methods of line placement include (1) the in-plane (long-axis) approach, (2) the out-of-plane (short-axis) approach of approximating needle entry, and (3) "following the tip." A new alternative method is an oblique approach.

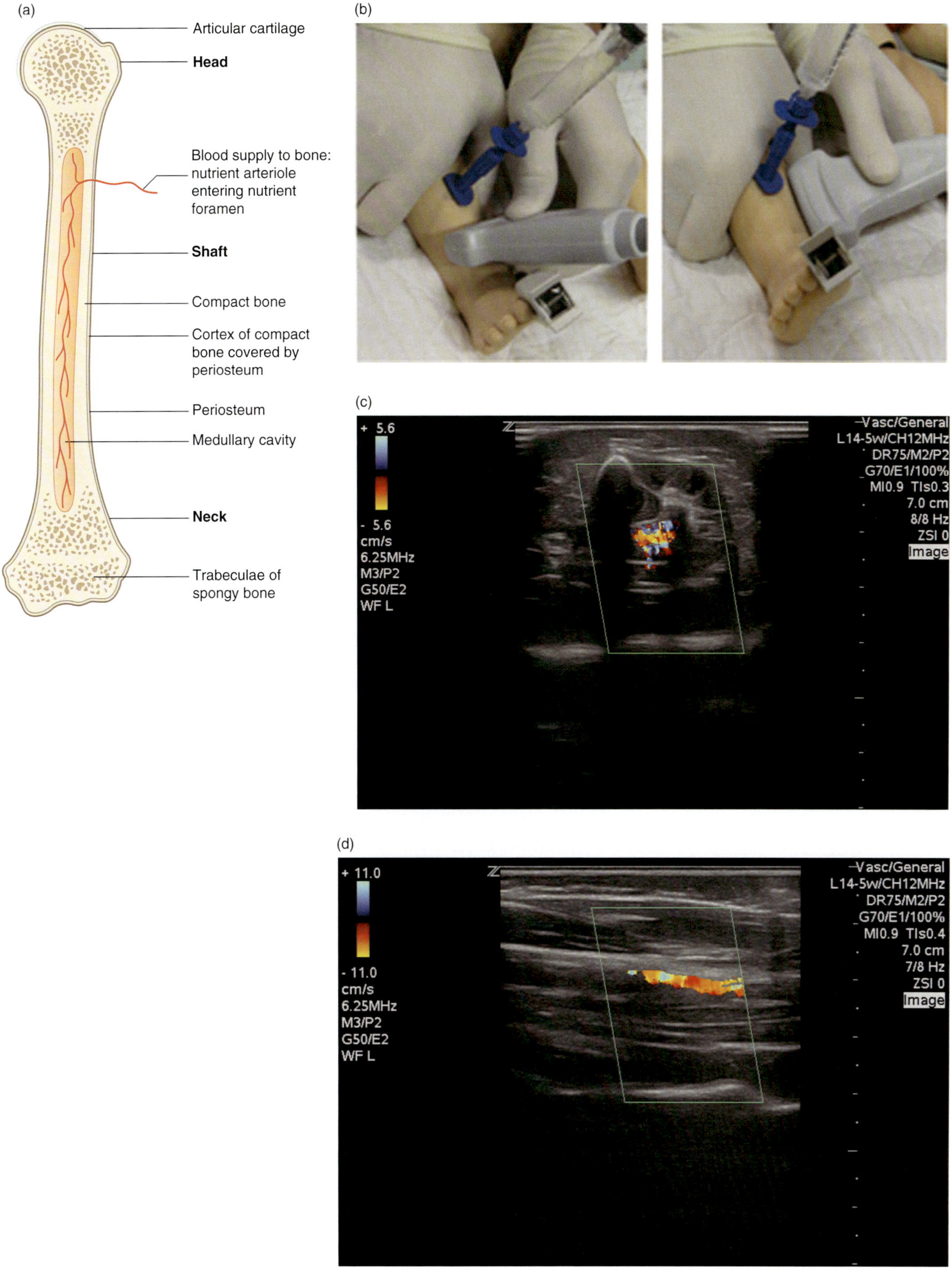

Figure 15.17 Intraosseous lines for vascular access. (a) Anatomy of the bone *Artwork created by Emily Evans © Cambridge University Press*. (b) Transducer placement with the transducer in relation to the intraosseous needle with the short-axis (left) and long-axis (right). *Photos courtesy of Jim Tsung, MD*. (c) Ultrasound image (short-axis) with Doppler confirming correct intraosseous placement in a chicken model. (d) Ultrasound image (long-axis) with correct intraosseous placement. (e) Ultrasound image (short-axis) with Doppler showing failure to place within the bone, and extravasation of fluid into surrounding tissues. (f) Ultrasound image (long-axis) showing incorrect placement. *Ultrasound images courtesy of Jason W. Fischer, MD MSc.*

(e)

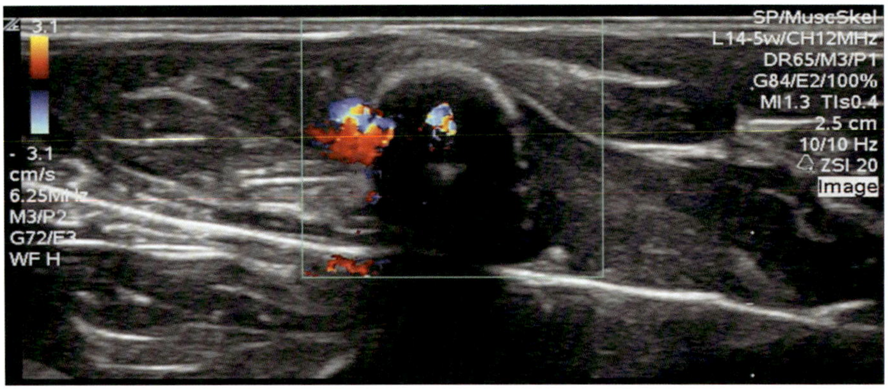

(f)

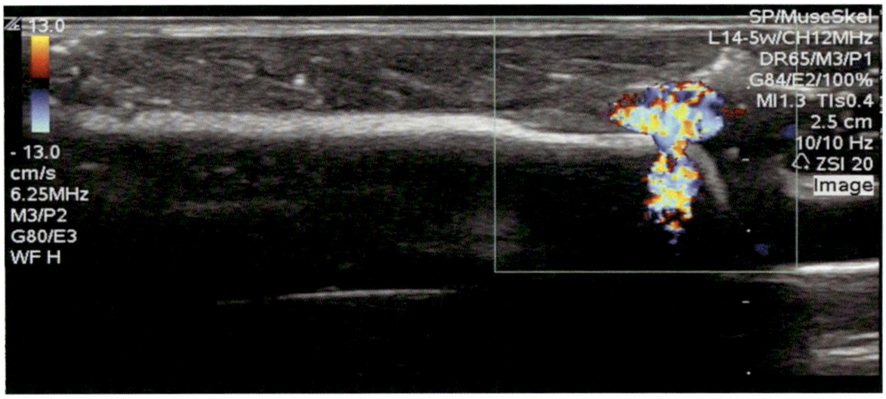

Figure 15.17 (cont.)

Selected references

Doniger, S., Ishimine, P., Fox, J. C., Kanegaye, J. T. (2009) Randomized controlled trial of ultrasound-guided peripheral intravenous catheter placement versus traditional techniques in difficult-access pediatric patients. *Pediatr Emerg Care* **25**(3): 154–9.

Fragou, M., Gravvanis, A., Dimitriou, V., *et al.* (2011) Real-time ultrasound-guided subclavian vein cannulation versus the landmark method in critical care patients: a prospective randomized study. *Crit Care Med* **39**(7): 1607–12.

Heinrichs, J., Fritze, Z., Vendermeerm, B., *et al.* (2013) Ultrasonographically guided peripheral intravenous cannulation of children and adults: a systematic review and meta-analysis. *Ann Emerg Med* **61**(4):444–54

Hind, D., Calvert, N., McWilliams, R., *et al.* (2003) Ultrasonic locating devices for central venous cannulation: meta-analysis. *BMJ* **327**: 361–7.

Lamperti, M., Bodenham, A. R., Pittirutti, M., *et al.* (2012) International evidence-based recommendations on ultrasound-guided vascular access. *Intensive Care Med* **38**(7): 1105–17.

Panebianco, N. L., Fredette, J. M., Szyid, D., *et al.* (2009) What you see (sonographically) is what you get: vein and patient characteristics associated with successful ultrasound-guided peripheral intravenous placement in patients with difficult access. *Acad Emerg Med* **16**(12): 1298–303.

Phelan, M., Hagerty, D. (2009) The oblique view: an alternative approach for ultrasound-guided central line placement. *J Emerg Med* **37**(4): 403–8.

Riera, A., Langhan, M., Northrup, V., *et al.* (2011) Remember the saphenous: ultrasound evaluation and intravenous site selection of peripheral veins in young children. *Pediatr Emerg Care* **27** (12): 1–5.

Shiver, S., Blaivas, M., Lyon, M. (2006) A prospective comparison of ultrasound-guided and blindly placed radial arterial catheters. *Acad Emerg Med* **13**(12): 1275–9.

Tsung, J. W., Blaivas, M., Stone, M. B. (2009) Feasibility of point-of-care colour Doppler ultrasound confirmation of intraosseous needle placement during resuscitation. *Resuscitation* **80**: 665–8.

Chapter 16

Bladder ultrasound for catheterization and suprapubic aspiration

Alexander C. Arroyo

Objectives/indications

The collection of a urine specimen from an infant is one of the most common procedures performed in the pediatric emergency department. Every practitioner has been in the situation where a catheter is placed in an infant and no urine is returned. The result is recatheterization, which becomes stressful for the parents, the staff, and, most of all, the child. Point-of-care ultrasound may be utilized prior to catheterization, in order to ensure an adequate amount of urine and to avoid the need for recatheterization. In addition, the bladder volume may be calculated, and may serve as an adjunct to performing bladder catheterization and suprapubic aspiration.

Frequently, a sterile urine sample is required to assess if a child has a urinary tract infection. Properly collected "clean catch" urine samples are acceptable in patients who are toilet trained, which is usually above two years of age. Alternatively, those patients who cannot provide reliable clean-catch urine samples may require bladder catheterization or aspiration. A urine bag specimen for culture should be avoided due to their unreliability and high incidence of contamination from surrounding skin flora. For most patients, catheterization will be adequate for a urine sample. Occasionally however, suprapubic aspiration may be preferred or required with the following conditions: phimosis, labial adhesions, severe urethral strictures, severe hypospadias, and urethral trauma. Suprapubic bladder aspiration is rarely performed on adult patients. Contraindications to suprapubic aspiration are bleeding diatheses, abdominal wall infections, and congenital anatomic abnormalities of the gut or genitourinary tract.

The determination of the amount of urine in the bladder can be helpful prior to suprapubic aspiration or catheterization. This volume calculation can also serve to assess how much urine remains after voiding, which is known as a post-void residual. Normally after voiding the bladder is completely empty and often not seen with ultrasound. Conditions that cause urinary retention lead to large post-void residuals. In older adults, urinary incontinence, urinary tract infections, neoplasms, prostatic hypertrophy, and cystoceles may lead to large amounts of urine being left in the bladder. In children, causes include neurogenic bladder, severe constipation, urinary tract infection, neoplasms, and benign obstructing lesions.

Background

Several years ago, suprapubic aspiration was the standard procedure for obtaining urine specimens. The failure rate of blind suprapubic aspiration was 8% or higher. Ultrasound was introduced nearly 40 years ago to confirm adequate urine volume prior to bladder aspiration, and to guide the needle during the procedure. One randomized trial of ultrasound prior to aspiration showed that the ultrasound group had successful collection in 79% of attempts compared with 52% where no ultrasound was utilized ($P = 0.04$). Another study demonstrated a first-attempt success rate of 100% with ultrasound guidance, when compared to 36% without ultrasound. Other studies showed similar results, with fewer needle punctures required in the ultrasound group. Real-time, ultrasound-guided suprapubic aspiration has been shown to be even more successful, when compared with blind suprapubic aspiration.

More recently, ultrasound evaluation has been performed prior to urethral catheterization in order to assess for the presence of adequate urine. Chen *et al.* showed that ultrasound improves overall success of catheterization on the first attempt from 72 to 96%. Successful catheterization was obtained on the first attempt in 94% in the ultrasound group, compared to 68% without ultrasound.

This technology has also been expanded to included nurse-performed ultrasonography prior to bladder catheterization. In one study, first-attempt success rates were higher in the ultrasound group: 92% compared with 67% in the group without ultrasound ($P = 0.003$). However, the time to collect the specimen was slightly longer in the ultrasound group (12 vs. 28 minutes; $P < 0.001$). Most recently, automated bladder scan devices have been investigated, but demonstrated poor repeatability and accuracy in bladder volume measurements when compared to point-of-care ultrasound.

Based on these studies, ultrasound assessment prior to bladder catheterization or aspiration should become the standard of care, for obvious reasons. Both ultrasound assistance and ultrasound guidance improve success of suprapubic aspiration and catheterization.

Anatomy

The urinary bladder is a hollow, muscular, elastic organ responsible for collecting urine from the kidneys. Urine exits the bladder via the urethra. In children younger than two years of age, the bladder is actually more of an intra-abdominal organ, placing it in

Pediatric Emergency and Critical Care Ultrasound, ed. Stephanie J. Doniger. Published by Cambridge University Press.

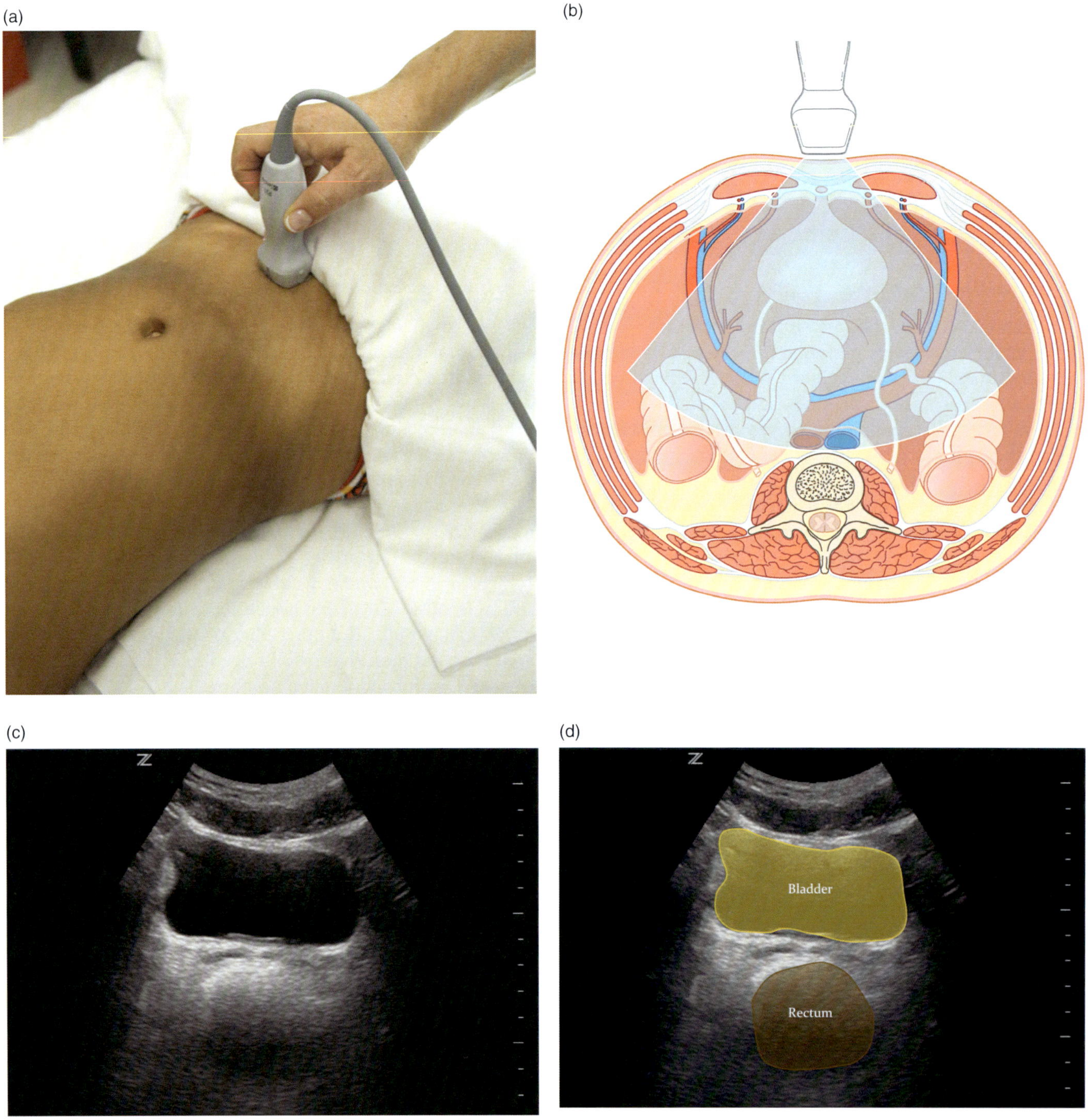

Figure 16.1 Bladder imaging, transverse view. (a) Transducer placement with the indicator oriented towards the patient's right side. (b) Anatomy, depicting the bladder and rectum. (c) Transverse ultrasound image of the bladder. Of note, it is important to angle the image beam down into the pelvis to obtain a proper image. (d) Corresponding illustration depicting major structures visualized including bladder and rectum. *Illustration by Laura Berg, MD.*

the perfect location for suprapubic aspiration. As children become older, the bladder moves inferiorly into the pelvis. The symphysis pubis, rectus muscle, uterus in females, and intestines are the other pertinent anatomic structure in this region (Figures 16.1b and 16.2b).

Technique

Transducer selection and orientation

A curvilinear transducer with an effective frequency of 2–5 MHz is used to visualize the bladder (Figure S3.3b). The bladder is imaged in two planes: transverse, with the indicator oriented towards the patient's right (Figure 16.1a), and sagittal, with the indicator oriented towards the patient's head (Figure 16.2a).

Patient position and preparation

For the point-of-care bladder ultrasound evaluation, the patient should be lying supine. When considering a suprapubic aspiration or catheterization, appropriate preparation must be performed, including the sterile preparation of the transducer (Figures S3.5–7), and of the patient's skin. It is

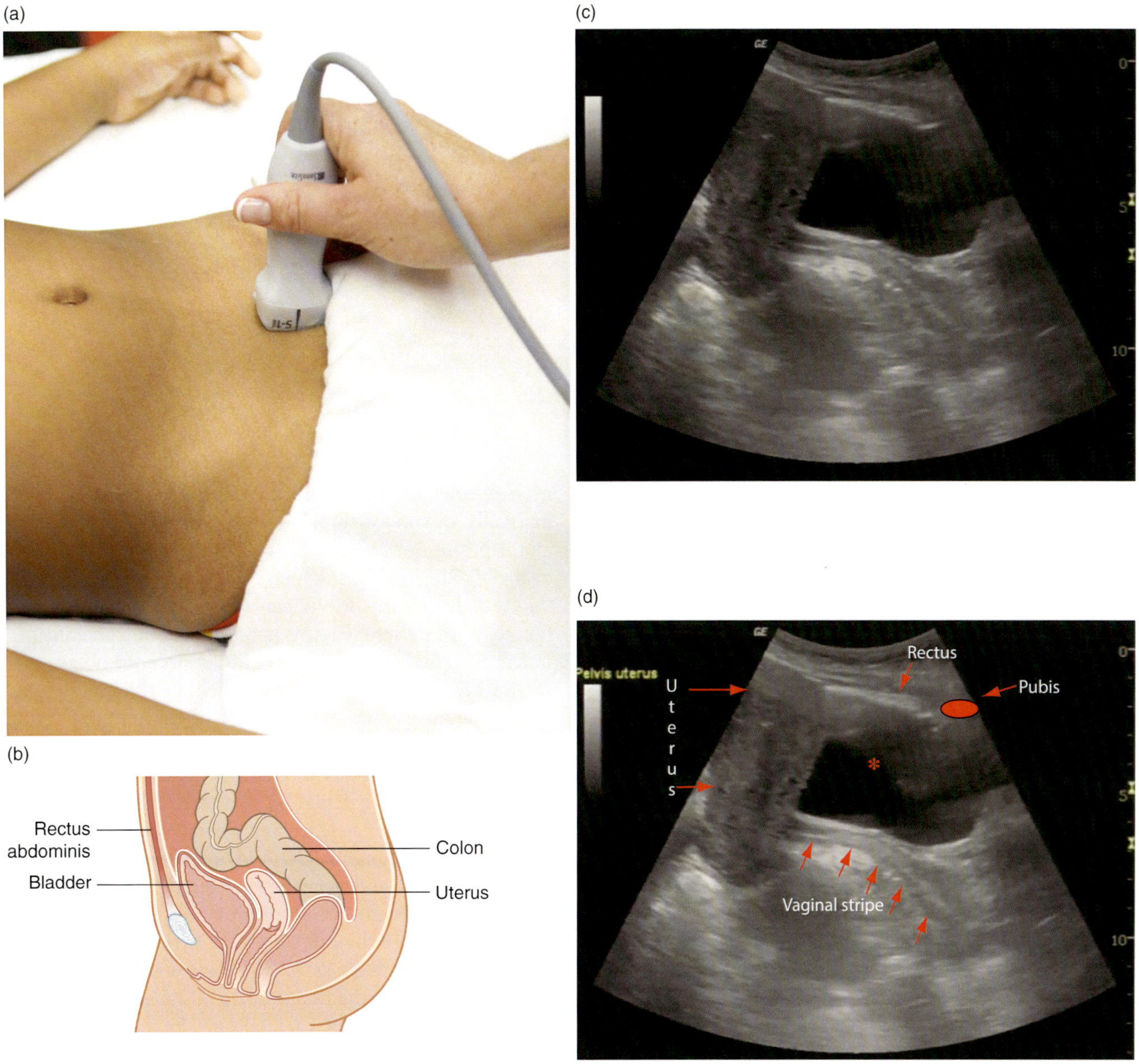

Figure 16.2 Bladder imaging, sagittal view. (a) Transducer placement with the indicator oriented towards the patient's head. (b) Anatomy, showing the bladder, rectum, and uterus in a female patient. *Artwork created by Emily Evans © Cambridge University Press.* (c) Sagittal ultrasound image of the bladder. (d) Structures visualized: the bladder (*), pubis, uterus, vaginal stripe (arrows), and rectus muscle.

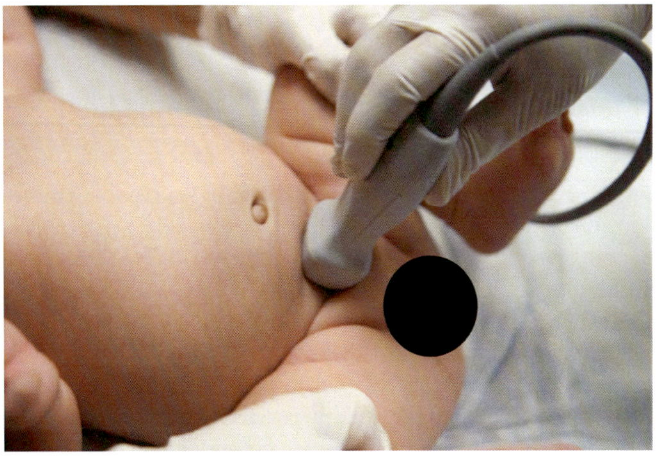

Figure 16.3 Proper frog-leg positioning of a patient for bladder catheterization and suprapubic aspiration.

important to appropriately restrain the child, holding him/her in a frog-leg position (Figure 16.3).

Ultrasound imaging

First, locate the pubic symphysis by manual palpation of the lower abdomen. Place the transducer midline, immediately superior to the pubic symphysis. Then, gently push down and slowly angle the transducer towards the patient's feet, directing the beam into the pelvis (Figure 16.1a).

When full, the bladder should appear on screen as a trapezoidal anechoic structure with a surrounding thin, smooth, echogenic wall (Figures 16.1c,d and 16.2c,d). Once the transverse view is obtained, rotate the transducer clockwise 90°, with the indicator oriented towards the patient's head in order to obtain the sagittal view. Again, push down gently and slowly

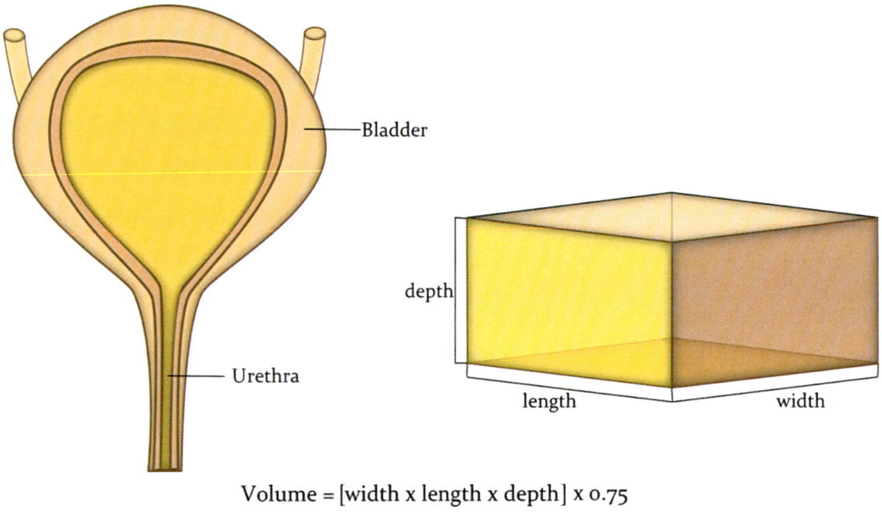

Figure 16.4 **Calculation of bladder volume.** An estimate of bladder volume may be calculated using the formula for a cube. However, since the bladder is more similar in shape to a sphere, a correction factor of 0.75 needs to be incorporated into the formula. Bladder volume = ([width x length x depth] x 0.75). This formula has been shown to correlate well with volumes obtained from catheterized specimens.

angle the transducer slightly into the pelvis, pointing the beam towards the feet (Figure 16.2a). The bladder should be easily visualized when full. In contrast, an empty bladder may be difficult to visualize. The importance of obtaining two views of the bladder (transverse and sagittal) cannot be emphasized enough. However, the order in which these two views are obtained is up to the operator's preference.

Ultrasound-guided procedure

Place the curvilinear or phased-array transducer just above the symphysis pubis and obtain both the transverse and sagittal views of the bladder. One may calculate bladder volume manually or as part of the machine's calculation software. Alternatively, a novel single measurement has been utilized. Witt *et al.* utilized a single measurement of the transverse bladder diameter of greater than 2 cm as correlating with a sufficient volume for catheterization.

The formula for the calculation of bladder volume was derived from estimation.

$$\text{Bladder volume} = ([\text{width} \times \text{length} \times \text{depth}] \times 0.75)$$

One may assume that the bladder is similar to a sphere or a rectangle. Patients show variation in the shape of their bladder. Further, bladders with smaller volumes assume a trapezoidal shape, while those with larger volumes assume a more spherical shape. Therefore, the formula obtained takes into account these features with a correction factor of 0.75 (Figure 16.4). Note that different references use a slightly different correction factor, but the correction factor of 0.75 is the most widely used. Utilizing this formula correlates well with catheterized specimens. Of note, it is important to obtain measurements in centimeters, since the resulting cubic centimeters (cm^3) are equivalent to milliliters (mL). This can be compared to the volume of urine expected for a particular age calculated by the equation:

$$([\text{age in years} + 2] \times 30\,\text{cm}^3)$$

Any volume greater than 3 cm^3 will usually be adequate for specimen collection in 98% of catheterized patients.

There are two methods of calculating the bladder volume: manually or via the machine's automated calculation.

1. **Manual calculations:** to calculate bladder volume manually, obtain the three measurements of width, height, and depth in centimeters. First, obtain the transverse view of the bladder. Freeze the image, and measure the width (left to right) where the bladder is its largest, and the height (anterior–posterior) (Figure 16.5a). Then, unfreeze the image and rotate the transducer 90° in order to obtain the sagittal view. Freeze the image, and obtain the last remaining measurement, which will be the depth (Figure 16.5b).
2. **Automated calculations:** ultrasound machines have automated volume calculation software. Volume is calculated with the measurements height, width, and depth, as with the manual method described. First freeze a transverse image and measure the height (Figure 16.6a) and the width (Figure 16.6b). Input and save each measurement into the calculation. Un-freeze the image, and rotate the transducer 90° to obtain a sagittal view of the bladder. Freeze the image again and measure the depth and input into the calculation. The machine will calculate a resulting number, which will represent the total bladder volume in cubic centimeters (Figure 16.6c). One cubic centimeter is equivalent to one milliliter (mL).

Specific scanning techniques

Ultrasound assistance for suprapubic aspiration and bladder catheterization

Ultrasound can be an invaluable tool prior to suprapubic aspiration and bladder catheterization, in order to assess if a patient has enough urine for collection. The procedure is easily learned and will lead to fewer collection failures when used. Place the curvilinear transducer just above the symphysis pubis and obtain both the transverse and sagittal views of the bladder. One may then calculate bladder volume manually or as part of the machine's calculation software. If the volume is determined to be adequate (greater than 3 cm^3 will be adequate for specimen collection in

(a) (b)

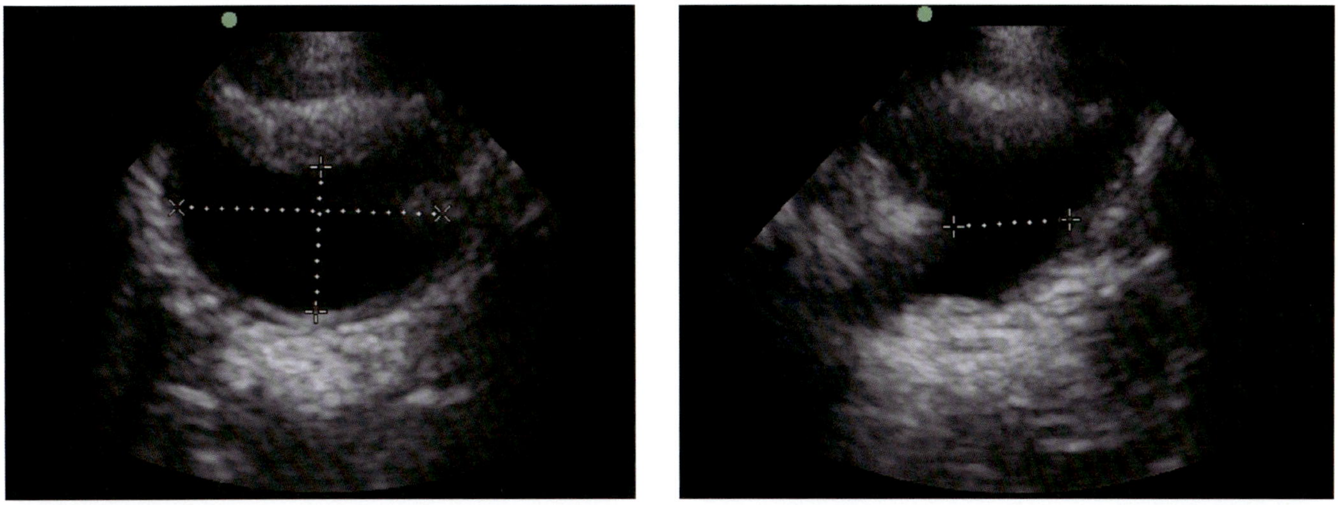

Figure 16.5 **Bladder volume** is calculated by making three measurements: width, height, and depth. (a) First the transverse image of the bladder is obtained (with the indicator oriented towards the patient's right) and its height and width are measured. (b) The transducer is rotated with the indicator positioned towards the patient's head. The additional measurement of depth may be obtained. Of note, some machines have automated programs, which will calculate the bladder volume when the operator inputs these measurements.

98% of catheterized patients), proceed with the catheterization. If there is an insufficient amount of urine, hydrate the patient and return in 30 minutes to rescan the bladder.

Ultrasound guidance for suprapubic aspiration

It is recommended to perform an initial ultrasound scan in order to confirm an adequate amount of urine is present prior to initiating the procedure. In order to attain appropriate dermal anesthesia, lidocaine/prilocaine topical cream may be applied, followed by an injection of 1% lidocaine with epinephrine above the symphysis pubis. The procedure may be performed with a single-operator or dual-operator approach (Figures S3.1, S3.2).

First, place the transducer on the abdomen with the indicator oriented towards the patient's right, and locate the maximum diameter of the bladder in the transverse view (Figure 16.1a). Then, palpate the symphysis pubis and keep one or two fingertips on it, while pulling down on the skin to create tension. Some practitioners advocate applying pressure to the base of the penis in boys or to the urethral meatus in girls in order to prevent urination while performing the procedure. Next, using a sterile 5 mL syringe, with a 22- or 23-gauge, with a 1.5 inch needle attached, puncture the skin 1–2 cm above the symphysis pubis. Aim the needle cephalad at a 10–20° angle from the vertical axis while applying gentle negative pressure on the syringe plunger (Figure 16.7a). Of note, the depth markers on the right side of the screen will guide how far the needle must be inserted to obtain urine. The needle should be visualized on screen as a thin, linear, hyperechoic structure, and directed into the bladder (Figure 16.7b). If the needle is in the anechoic bladder, urine should easily be aspirated into the syringe. If not, slightly withdraw the needle without actually removing it from the abdominal wall, and redirect it to attempt re-insertion and aspiration. Once the urine sample is obtained, remove the needle and place the urine in a sterile container. Finally, clean the skin and place a bandage over the insertion site.

Ultrasound guidance for bladder catheterization

If desired, the catheter can be observed entering the bladder by holding the transducer in the sagittal plane on the patient while performing the catheterization. The catheter will appear as two hyperechoic parallel lines with an anechoic center (Figure 16.8). This is particularly helpful when the location of catheter placement is in question.

Scanning tips

Pitfalls

- When performing bladder ultrasound, dark shadowing will frequently show up on the right side of the screen in this orientation (Figure 16.9). This can occur for several different reasons: the lower portion of the transducer may be on top of the bony pubic symphysis thereby creating a shadow, the lower portion of the transducer has been slightly lifted off the patient, or there is insufficient gel on that portion of the transducer. Try repositioning the transducer and applying sufficient gel in order to obtain better images.
- A collapsed bladder may not be able to be identified by ultrasound examination (Figure 16.10).
- Bladder volume measurement is merely an estimate of bladder volume. At small bladder volumes, the bladder has a trapezoidal shape, rather than that of a sphere, when it is full. There is no clear lower volume limit for when catheterization will yield urine. Always ensure that the bladder has sufficient urine volume prior to aspiration or catheterization.

(a)

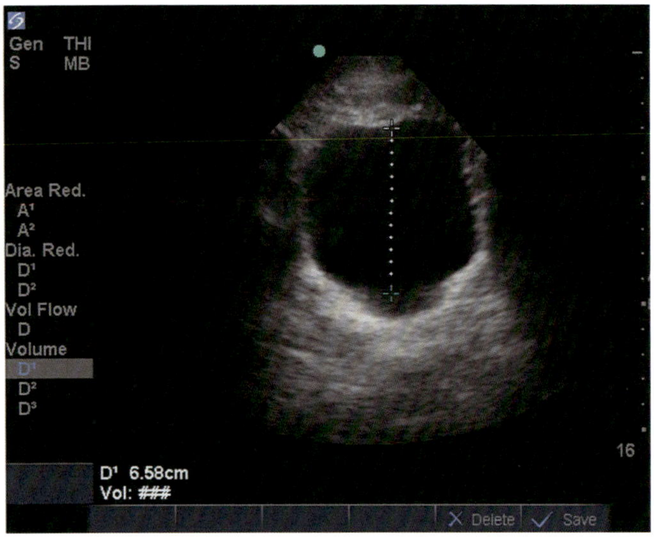

(b)

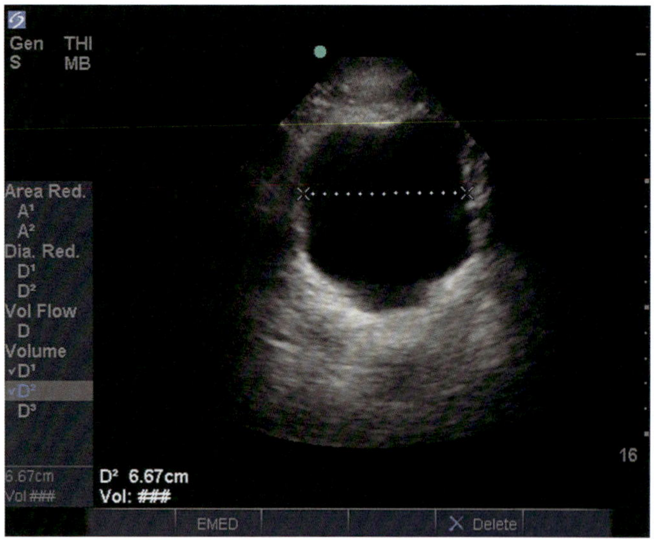

(c)

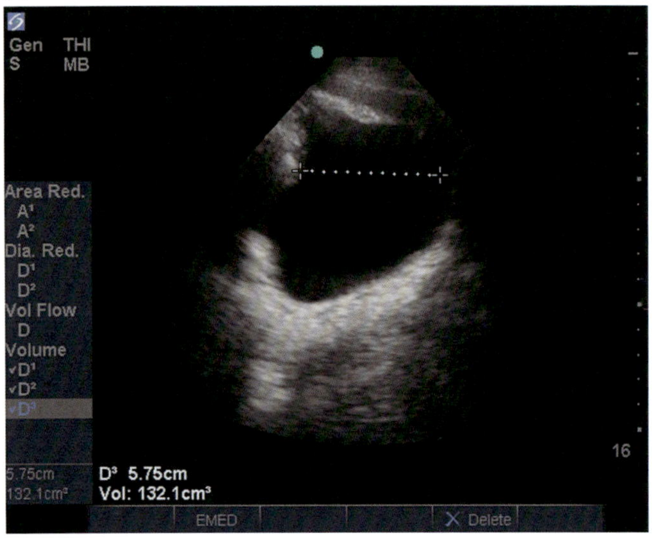

Figure 16.6 Automated bladder volume calculations. This is an example of the automated software in the Sonosite™ machine. First obtain the transverse view, and input (a) the height (D^1) and (b) the width (D^2) measurements. Then, rotate the transducer to obtain the sagittal view. (c) Measure the depth (D^3) and input into the formula. The result (vol) will be the calculated volume, with automatic consideration of the correction factor.

- Complications that arise from performing a suprapubic bladder aspiration include micro-hematuria, and inadvertent bowel puncture. Visualization by ultrasound decreases these complications. Other infrequent complications include infection or the development of a hematoma.
- There are other anechoic, fluid-filled structures that may be mistaken for the bladder on ultrasound. An example is an ovarian cyst, which may be inadvertently punctured (Figure 16.11).

Tips to improve scanning

✓ Ensure that what you are identifying as the bladder is in fact the bladder. Scan it in both transverse and sagittal planes, looking for the classic appearance of the bladder.

✓ Fluid-filled bowel can mimic the bladder; watching for the presence of peristalsis in bowel distinguishes the two. In the sagittal orientation, make sure the lower portion of the transducer is touching the patient during the scan.

✓ While performing catheterization and suprapubic aspiration, sufficient analgesia will decrease patient movement, improve comfort, and improve success of the procedure. Topical creams and local anesthetic injections may also be used.

Cases

1. A six-year-old male is intubated in the pediatric intensive care unit (PICU) for septic shock. A Foley catheter is placed in order to monitor urine output. After two days, the

(a)

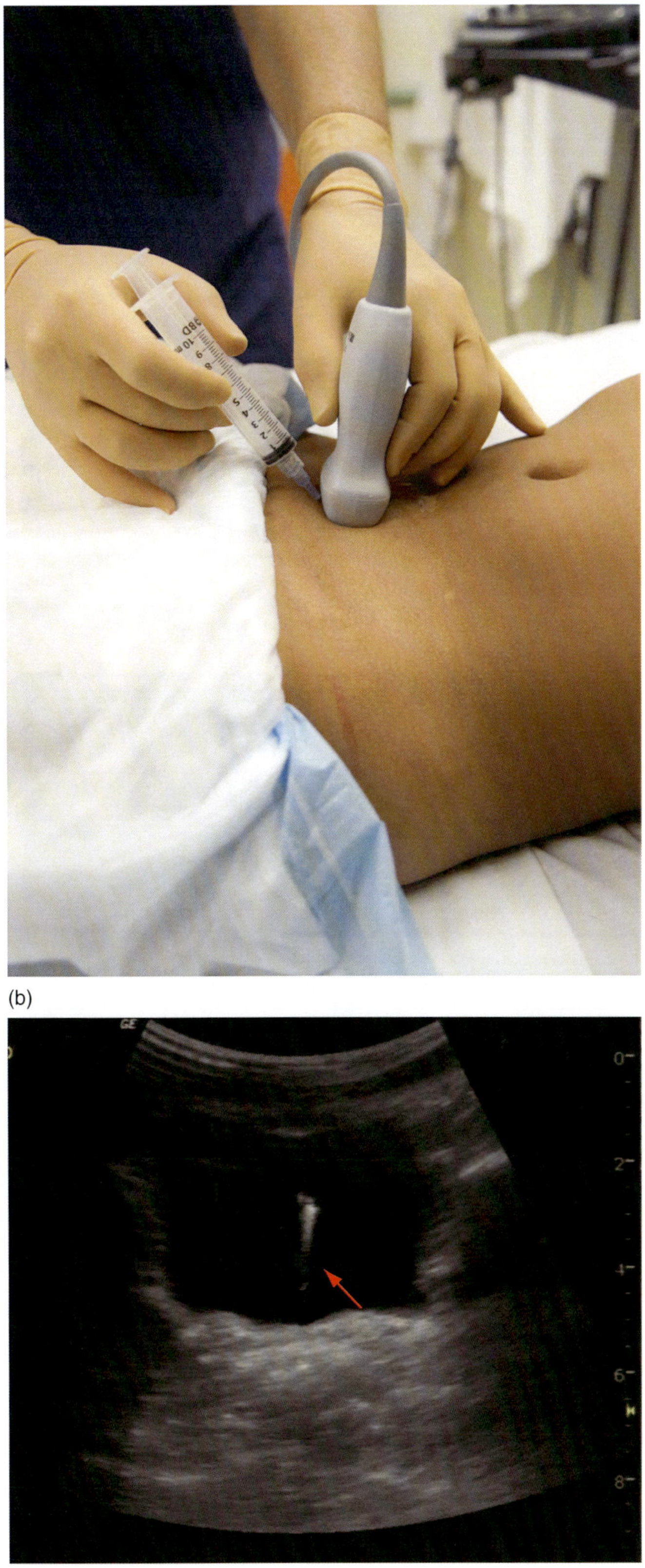

Figure 16.7 Suprapubic bladder aspiration. (a) The angle and position of needle insertion for suprapubic bladder aspiration (sterile drape and sterile probe cover omitted for illustration purposes). (b) This transverse image demonstrates visualization of a needle in the bladder during suprapubic bladder aspiration. The needle appears hyperechoic with a "ring-down" artifact (arrow).

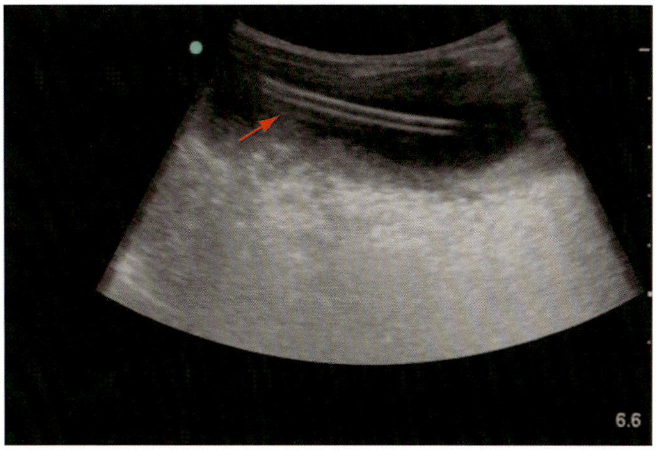

Figure 16.8 Catheter. Sagittal ultrasound view of the bladder, with visualization of an 8-French catheter in its long-axis. The catheter (arrow) appears as two hyperechoic lines, with an anechoic lumen. *Image courtesy of Sharon Yellin, MD.*

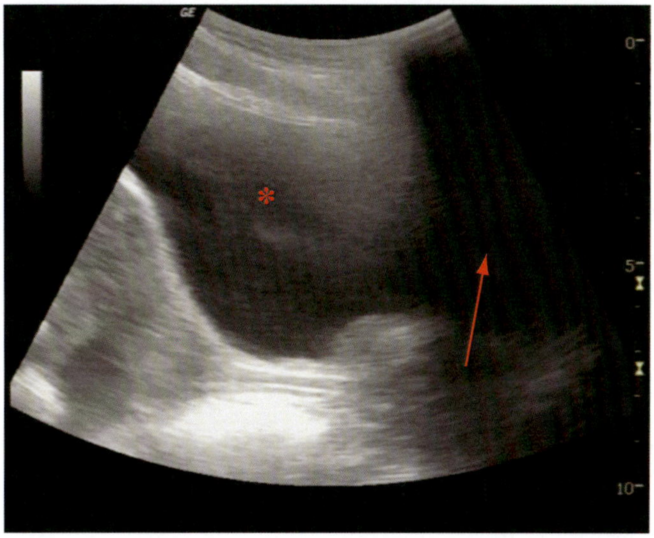

Figure 16.9 Sagittal image of the bladder (*) demonstrating shadowing (arrow), which represents the failure of the transducer to directly contact the skin, or insufficient gel.

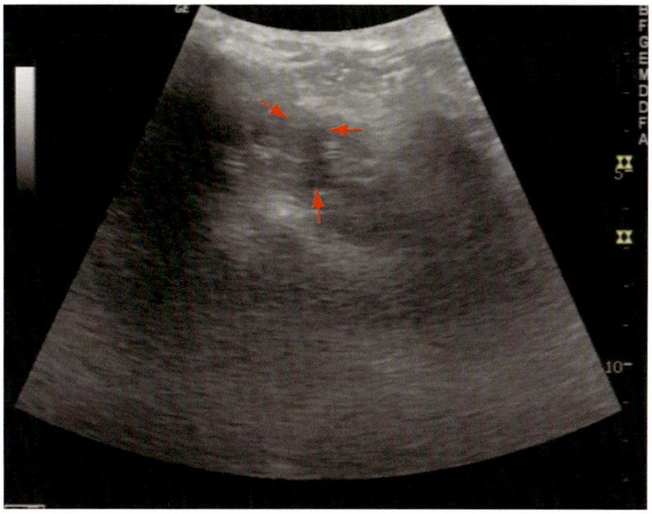

Figure 16.10 Empty bladder. This ultrasound image demonstrates the typical appearance of a bladder after voiding (arrows), which can be difficult to see. This patient has insufficient volume for catheterization and should be hydrated and rescanned again in 30 to 60 minutes.

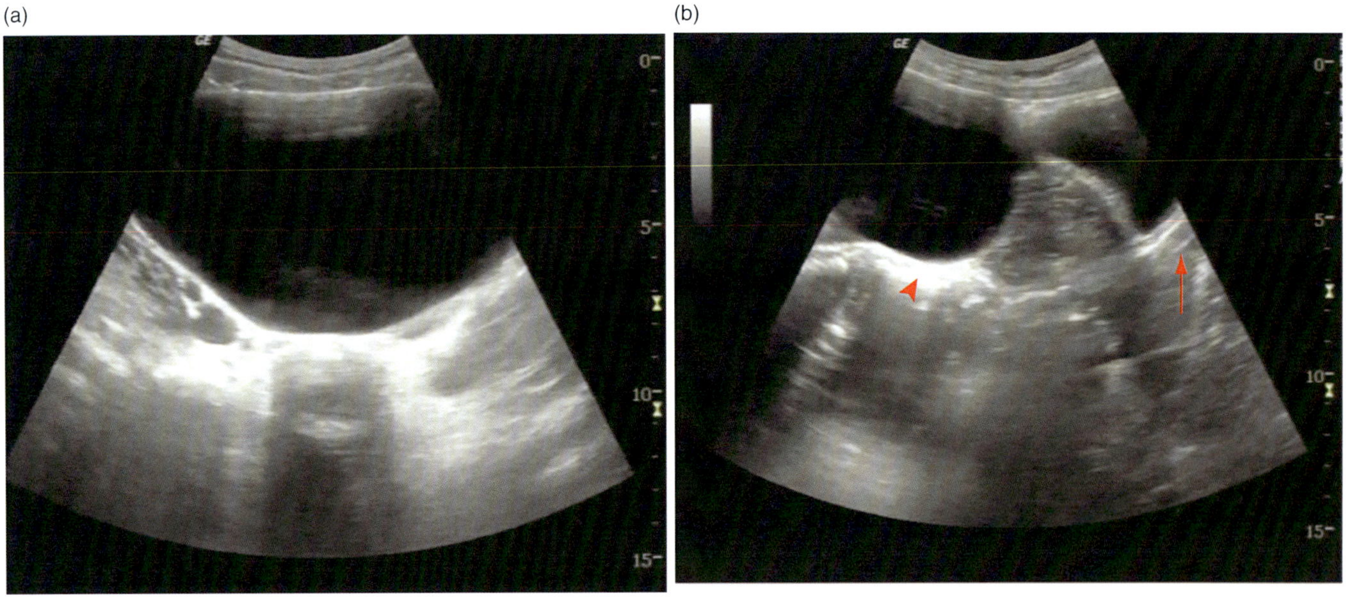

Figure 16.11 Ovarian cyst mimicking the bladder. (a) An anechoic, thin-walled, cyst-like structure that appears to be the bladder in transverse ultrasound. This structure is actually a large ovarian cyst. (b) A sagittal image of the same patient showing the true bladder (arrow) and the ovarian cyst (arrowhead).

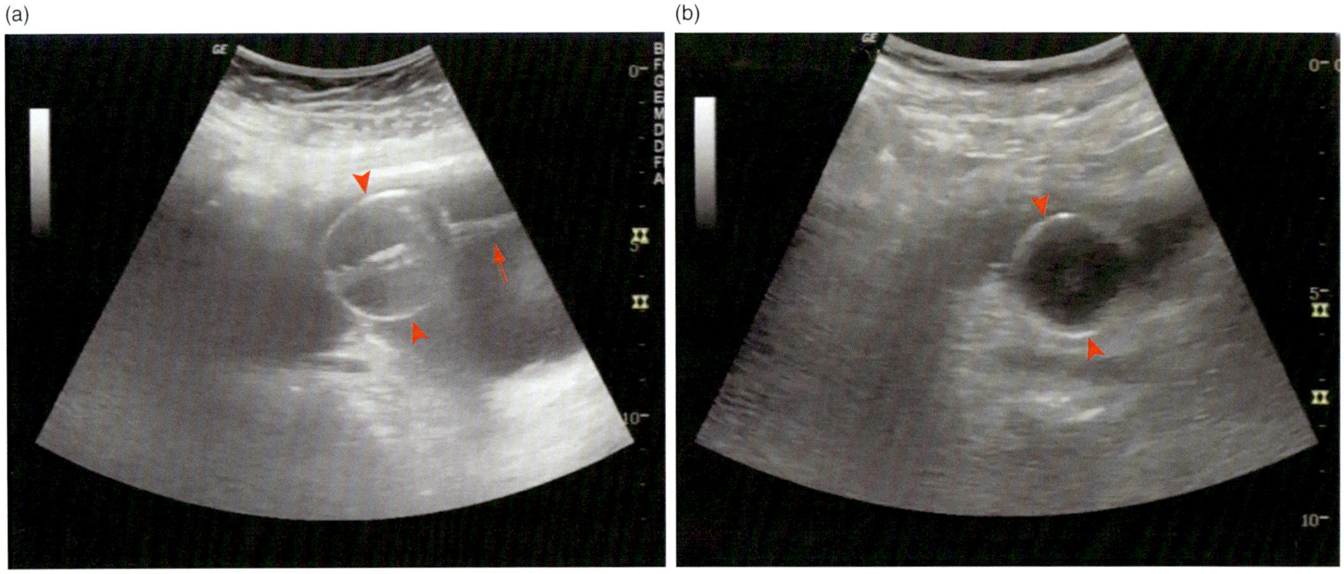

Figure 16.12 Foley catheter. Ultrasound image of a Foley catheter in the bladder. If the Foley is working properly, the bladder will have little or no urine in it. (a) A sagittal image of the Foley catheter balloon (arrowheads) and the distal end of the catheter tubing (arrow). (b) A transverse image of a Foley catheter balloon (arrowheads) inflated in the bladder.

nursing staff raise a concern that the Foley is not in place because it has stopped draining urine. An ultrasound of the patient's bladder is performed (Figure 16.12), confirming the placement of the catheter within a full bladder. As a result, the Foley is flushed and urine subsequently begins to drain.

Foley catheter balloons are easily seen on ultrasound of the bladder as a perfectly round anechoic structure with hyperechoic walls. If visualized in the sagittal plane, the hollow tubing can also be seen on both sides of the balloon. Ultrasound can confirm the proper placement of urinary catheters within the bladder. Properly functioning Foley catheters should have the bladder collapsed around the Foley. When a full bladder is visualized around a Foley catheter, the catheter is not functioning properly and should be flushed.

2. An 18-day-old female presents to the emergency department with a fever of 38.3 °C. Prior to urine catheterization, you perform an ultrasound to confirm the presence of urine (Figure 16.10). This image demonstrates insufficient volume for catheterization. Therefore, the patient is hydrated for 60 minutes and then rescanned. Once the bladder volume is sufficient, catheterization is performed and is successful on the first attempt. It is important to emphasize that when insufficient bladder volume is visualized on point-of-care ultrasound, the

provider should wait 30–60 minutes, prior to attempting catheterization, in order no improve success.

3. A six-month-old female presents with three days of fever to 40.1 °C. On inspection of her vagina, she has labial adhesions, which obscure the urethra. An ultrasound-guided suprapubic bladder aspiration is chosen as the best course of action to collect urine (Figure 16.7b). The transverse image shows a needle in the bladder with ring-down artifact. Urine is successfully obtained.

   While uncommonly performed, suprapubic aspiration may be indicated in certain situations, such as labial adhesions. Point-of-care ultrasound can directly visualize the needle entering the bladder, thereby reducing complications associated with the procedure.

Summary/key points

Though transurethral catheterization has moved us away from the more invasive suprapubic bladder aspiration, it still remains the method of obtaining urine samples to ensure the most sterile urine sample, and is the preferred method in certain circumstances. Using ultrasound to confirm adequate volume of urine prior to collection gives a near 100% success rate, and should always be performed. Other key points to keep in mind are:

1. Utilize a low-frequency 2–5 MHz transducer, and always obtain both sagittal and transverse views of the bladder.
2. In order to calculate bladder volume, measure the width and height in the transverse view, and the depth in the sagittal view in centimeters. Then multiply Height × Width × Depth × 0.75 to get bladder volume in cm^3 mL.
3. Large bladder diameters lead to more successful collection of urine either by aspiration or catheterization. A volume of greater than 3 mL will yield sufficient urine for catheterization or suprapubic aspiration. Alternatively, a single transverse diameter measurement of >2.5 cm will yield a 90% success rate for obtaining urine.
4. If the bladder does not have sufficient urine for collection, wait 30–60 minutes while hydrating and then rescan the patient.
5. Suprapubic aspiration should be performed in patients with the following conditions: phimosis, labial adhesions, severe urethral strictures, severe hypospadias, and urethral trauma. Avoid complications by utilizing ultrasound assistance or ultrasound guidance.

Selected references

Baumann, B. M., McCans, K., Stahmer, S. A., *et al.* (2008) Volumetric bladder ultrasound performed by trained nurses increases catheterization success in pediatric patients. *Am J Emerg Med* **26**(1): 18–23.

Bevan, C., Buntsma, D., Stock, A., *et al.* (2011) Assessing bladder volumes in young children prior to instrumentation: accuracy of an automated ultrasound device compared to real-time ultrasound. *Acad Emerg Med* **18**: 816–21.

Bih, L. I., Ho, C. C., Tsai, S. J., *et al.* (1998) Bladder shape impact on the accuracy of ultrasonic estimation of bladder volume. *Arch Phys Med Rehabil* **79**: 1553–6.

Chan, H. (1993) Noninvasive bladder volume measurement. *J Neurosci Nurs* **25**: 309.

Chen, L., Hsiao, A. L., Moore, C. L., *et al.* (2005) Utility of bedside ultrasound before urethral catheterization in young children. *Pediatrics* **115**: 108–11.

García-Nieto, V., Navarro, J. F., Sánchez-Almeida, E., García-García, M. (1997) Standards for ultrasound guidance of suprapubic bladder aspiration. *Pediatr Nephrol* **11**(5): 607–9.

Gochman, R. F., Karasic, R. B., Heller, M. B. (1991) Use of portable ultrasound to assist urine collection by suprapubic aspiration. *Ann Emerg Med* **20**: 631–5.

Goldberg, B. B., Meyer, H. (1973) Ultrasonically guided suprapubic urinary bladder aspiration. *Pediatrics* **51**: 70–4.

Kiernan, S. C., Pinckert, T. L., Kezler, M. (1993) Ultrasound guidance of suprapubic bladder aspiration in neonates. *J Pediatr* **123**: 789–91.

Witt, M., Baumann, B. M., McCans, K. (2005) Bladder ultrasound increases catheterization success in pediatric patients. *Acad Emerg Med* **12**(4): 371–4.

Chapter

17

Ultrasound-guided lumbar puncture

Alyssa Abo

Objectives/indications

In 1891, Quinke performed the first diagnostic lumbar puncture. Now, over a century later, the procedure remains an integral part of medical decision-making in the acute care setting. In the pediatric emergency department, in particular, lumbar punctures are routinely performed in order to evaluate for infectious and neurologic processes. The use of ultrasound for the identification of landmarks was first described in 1971.

The objective of the lumbar puncture, or spinal tap, is to obtain cerebrospinal fluid (CSF) by inserting a styletted needle in between the spinous processes into the subarachnoid space. This is generally performed in the L4–5 interspinous space. The blind approach estimates the location of this space by Tuffier's line, an imaginary line, which connects the two iliac crests. While lumbar punctures are commonly performed, they pose challenges even for the most experienced of physicians. Pre-puncture challenges are often associated with identifying the appropriate landmarks, either in neonates where the interspinous spaces are small, or in obese children where the bony landmarks are obscured. Failed lumbar punctures, where no cerebrospinal fluid is obtained, pose another challenge and may result in a referral to interventional radiology.

When performing a lumbar puncture, clinicians may be most interested in identifying the bony landmarks and interspinous spaces. Current literature suggests that ultrasound has capabilities beyond this. Ultrasound has the potential to assist in these difficult situations, identify bony landmarks, and provide procedural guidance.

Background

Point-of-care ultrasound has been recently introduced into the adult emergency department as an adjunct to lumbar punctures. In the adult literature, there is evidence to support ultrasound for lumbar punctures, especially for obese patients. In 2005, Peterson *et al.* reported the use of point-of-care ultrasound in the adult emergency department for difficult lumbar punctures. Subsequent studies have demonstrated the ability of emergency physicians to sonographically locate anatomical landmarks, in a timely fashion. Also, in a prospective observational study, Ferre *et al.* showed that the pre-puncture distance to the dura, as measured by ultrasound, strongly correlated with depth of the spinal needle insertion. Moreover, in a prospective randomized trial of ultrasound versus palpation in identifying landmarks for lumbar punctures, Nomura *et al.* showed that ultrasound reduced the number of failed lumbar puncture attempts in all patients and improved the ease with which the procedure was performed in obese patients.

To date, there is a paucity of literature pertaining specifically to point-of-care ultrasound in the pediatric emergency department for ultrasound-assisted or ultrasound-guided lumbar punctures. Fortunately, neuroaxial ultrasonic imaging has been investigated by other disciplines including pediatric radiology and pediatric anesthesiology. Pediatric anesthesiologists have evaluated the role of ultrasound, as it relates to spinal anesthesia, particularly in the placement of epidural catheters. Ultrasound has been shown to be reliable in identifying the distance to the epidural space, and overall improved safety and efficacy, as ultrasound enables visual verification of spinal anesthesia and catheter placement with fewer bony contacts. In addition, pediatric radiologists have utilized ultrasound as a first-line imaging modality in infants after failed lumbar punctures. The main focus of the radiologist-performed ultrasonography was to evaluate the CSF below the conus medullaris and to assess for intrathecal and epidural blood collections. The ultrasound guided the radiologists' decision on whether to proceed with the lumbar puncture, or to defer the image-guided lumbar puncture. In addition, several studies have investigated the level of the conus medullaris sonographically in infants and children. The literature suggests that, in healthy children, with normal anatomy, the average level of the conus medullaris is actually L1/L2, with a range from T10 to L3. This data supports the current clinical practice of performing lumbar punctures in the L4–5 space, but raises the possibility of performing lumbar punctures in the L2–3 interspinous space, if clinicians could confidently identify the conus medullaris and cauda equina.

Within the scope of pediatric emergency medicine, there are recent published data to support ultrasound as an adjunct in assessing the size of the interspinous space, with sitting and flexing the hips providing the largest interspinous space. Furthermore, Abo *et al.* demonstrated that neck flexion does not affect the interspinous space. It has been well established

Pediatric Emergency and Critical Care Ultrasound, ed. Stephanie J. Doniger. Published by Cambridge University Press.

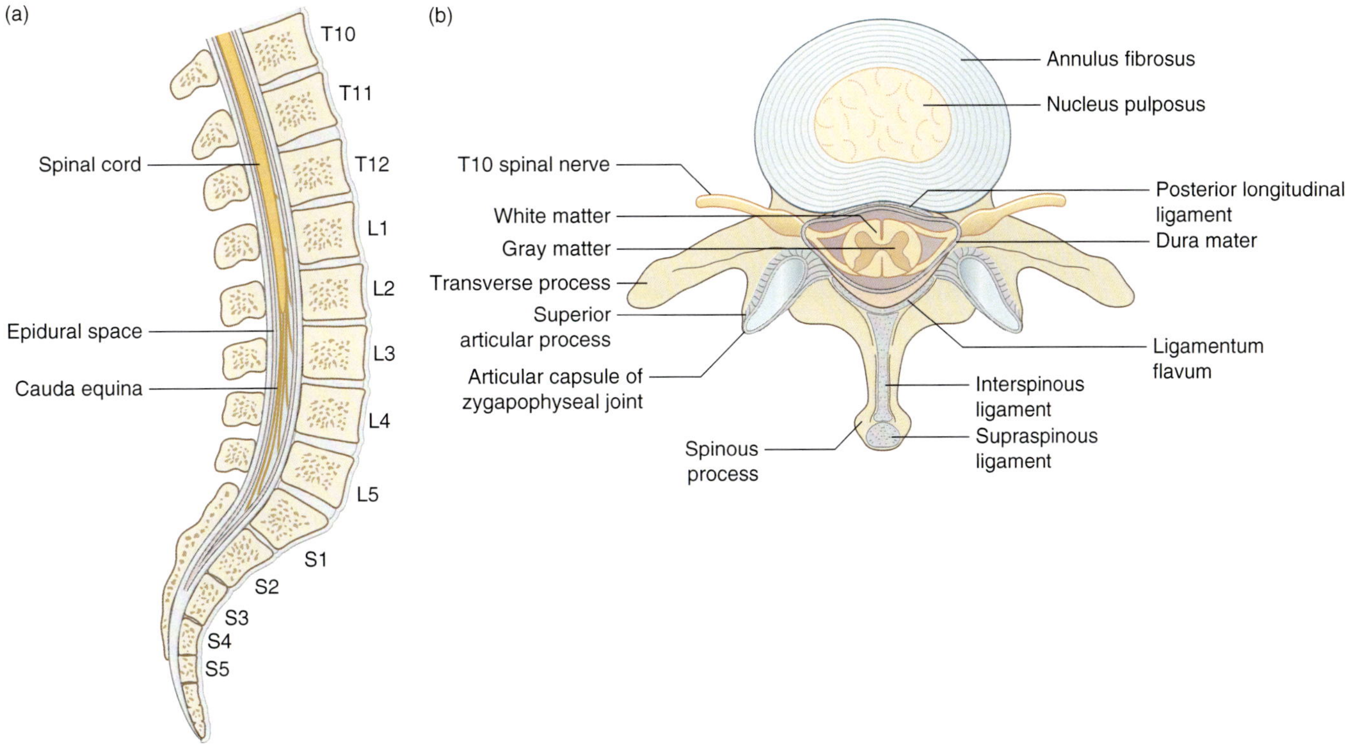

Figure 17.1 **Anatomy of the lumbosacral spine**. *Artwork created by Emily Evans © Cambridge University Press.*

that neck flexion in neonates can lead to hypoxia. Therefore, neonates should be held by their shoulders in the lateral recumbent position or alternatively in the seated position. The lateral recumbent positioning may also lead to the acute decompensation of critically ill infants. More recently, Cadigan *et al.* compared the interspinous distance between the lateral recumbent position and a spine-neutral position. Results showed that, while the tight lateral decubitus position increases the space between the lumbar spinous processes, a spine-neutral positioning might actually provide enough space. To date, there are no data regarding lumbar punctures in the spine neutral positioning. It has been suggested, however, that the angle of insertion of the needle may be more acute than that of older children.

With regard to ultrasound as an adjunct to performing pediatric lumbar punctures, there are currently no data demonstrating whether ultrasound improves safety or efficacy of lumbar punctures in the emergency department. More studies need to be performed in order to assess this.

Anatomy

In order to obtain CSF during a lumbar puncture, the needle traverses several anatomical layers to reach the subarachnoid space, including the supraspinous and interspinous ligaments, ligamentum flavum, dura, and arachnoid. The needle is inserted at the level of the cauda equina, so as to avoid contact with the conus medullaris, the inferior portion of the spinal cord (Figure 17.1). It is widely accepted that, in neonates, the conus medullaris approximates the L3 vertebrae and that by one year of age it ascends, as the vertebral column grows, to L1–2, where it remains through adulthood. Thus, lumbar punctures are performed at the L3–4 or L4–5 interspaces. When performing the procedure via the "blind technique," the level of the L4 vertebrae is estimated clinically by palpating the posterior spinous process that is intersected by Tuffier's line, an imaginary line between the two posterior superior iliac crests (Figure 17.2).

Technique

Transducer selection and orientation

A linear-array transducer (5–10 MHz) is the preferred transducer for performing ultrasound-assisted lumbar punctures, providing superior resolution at shallow depths (Figure S3.3a). In neonates, the pediatric linear transducer, or "hockey stick," is appropriate but may be too small for older children. In obese patients, the curvilinear transducer may provide additional resolution of deeper structures and should be considered as an alternative to the linear transducer (Figure S3.3b).

Ultrasound images should be obtained in two views: in the longitudinal and transverse planes. The longitudinal plane includes two approaches: the median and paramedian approaches. In the median longitudinal approach, the transducer is placed directly over the posterior spinous processes. In the paramedian longitudinal approach, the transducer is off midline; therefore, there is less interference from the spinous processes, providing a better acoustic window. In addition, the paramedian approach allows for a more clear distinction between the ligamentum flavum and the dura mater.

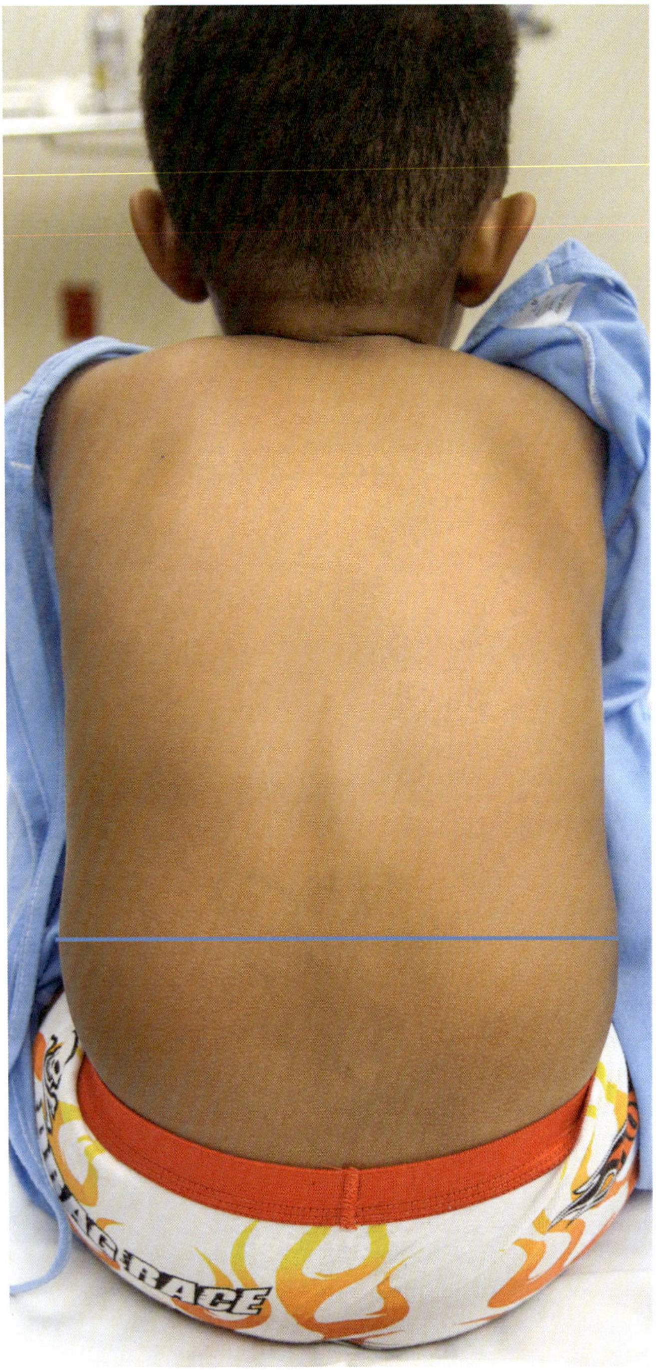

Figure 17.2 Tuffier's line. The imaginary line that connects the right and left iliac crests. This line estimates the location for L4–5, which is the ideal location for a lumbar puncture to be performed by traditional methods.

Patient position and preparation

There are two generally accepted positions for performing ultrasound-guided lumbar punctures. Patients may either be seated upright (Figure 17.3a), or placed in a lateral recumbent position (Figure 17.3b). In both positions, hip flexion will increase the interspinous spaces. Contrary to what was previously thought, neck flexion actually does not affect the interspinous spaces, and should be avoided. For infants in the seated position, rolling a small towel and placing it under the knees may achieve hip flexion. In the lateral recumbent position, the knees should be drawn up to the chest and the shoulders rotated forward.

Ultrasound imaging

Ultrasound can identify a number of anatomical structures of the pediatric spine. If the clinician is identifying solely the bony landmarks and the interspinous spaces, a shallow depth of a few centimeters is sufficient. For identification of the dura and deeper structures, the depth will need to be increased in order to allow for better visualization. The posterior spinous processes are covered by continuous layers of hyperechoic skin, hypoechoic subcutaneous tissue, and a hyperechoic layer of the thoracolumbar fascia and the supraspinal ligament. To identify the specific lumbar vertebra, the transducer can be moved inferiorly to the sacrum and upward towards L5. Sonographically, the supraspinous ligament will pass over L5 and then curve inferiorly in order to insert onto the sacrum.

When performing a sonographic evaluation of the spine and spinal cord, both transverse and longitudinal views should be obtained. The transducer should be oriented perpendicular to the spine (Figure 17.4a) in order to obtain the short-axis or transverse view of the spinal cord (Figure 17.4b,c). In order to obtain the longitudinal, or long-axis view of the spinal cord, the transducer should be oriented parallel to the spine (Figure 17.5a). There are two methods of obtaining the longitudinal view – the midline sagittal plane, and the paramedian plane (off midline). In the midline sagittal plane, the spinous processes are discrete, hyperechoic, curved lines that are separated by an echogenic interspinous spaces. The posterior vertebral column is shaped like a "Y," where the laminae are the arms of the "Y" and join to form the posterior spinous process (Figure 17.5b,c). In the paramedian plane (off midline), more anatomic elements are seen (Figure 17.6a,b). There is a small window between the spinous processes, and the acoustic shadow resulting from bone represents the lamina, rather than the posterior spinous process. Deeper in the interspinous space there is a hyperechoic line representing the ligamentum flavum and dura mater, separated by the epidural space (Figure 17.6c). Of note, it may be difficult to distinguish the ligamentum flavum and dura mater; however, sonographically the dura will predominate. Below the dura is the hypoechoic subarachnoid space.

The ability to sonographically visualize detailed spinal anatomy in neonates and infants is unique because the posterior vertebral column is mostly cartilaginous, allowing for ultrasound beam penetration. Ossification of the posterior vertebral column begins at approximately three to four months of age. However, in young children the vertebral column is still largely cartilaginous, allowing for less shadowing and better visualization than older children. The neonatal spine is a hypoechoic, tubular structure with hyperechoic walls (pia mater) and a hyperechoic center, the median sulcus. The cord is surrounded by hypoechoic subarachnoid space bounded by the thecal sac, with hyperechoic walls. The caudal spinal cord becomes the conus medullaris and then the filum terminale, a thin hyperechoic structure less than 2 mm. The

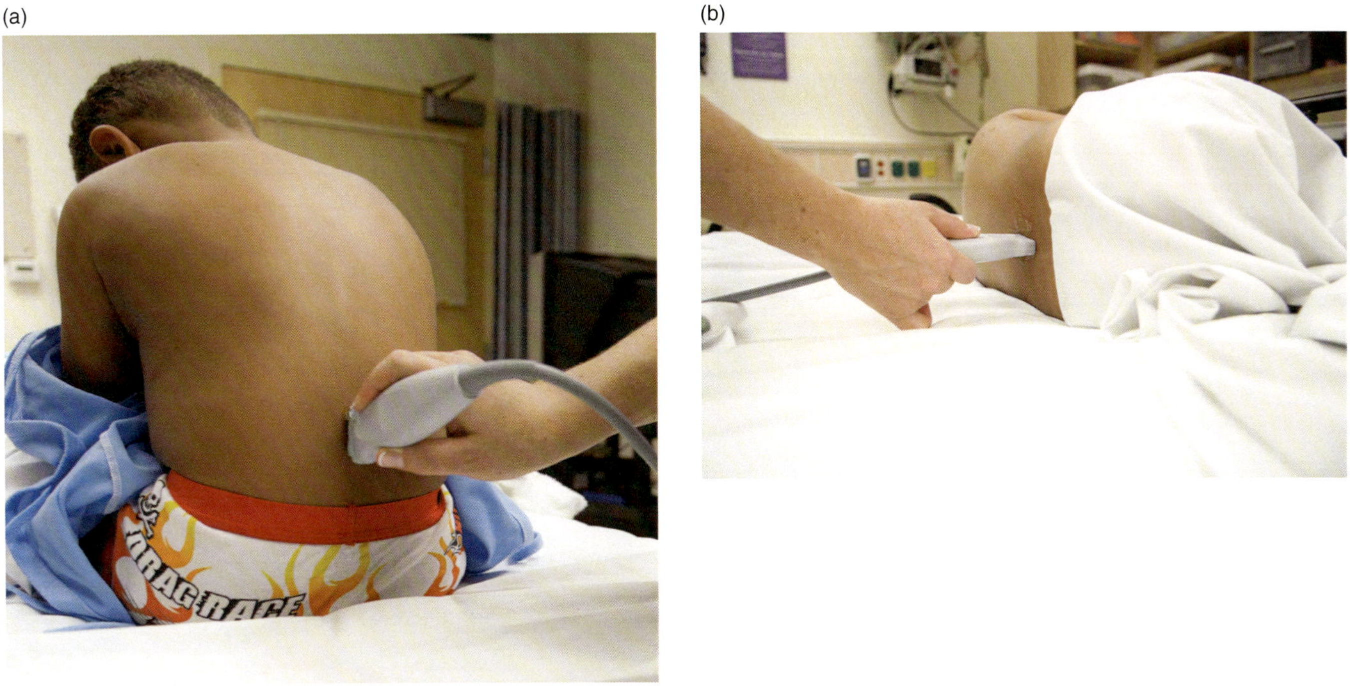

Figure 17.3 Positioning for ultrasound-guided lumbar punctures. (a) Seated positioning for ultrasound-guided lumbar puncture. (b) Lateral recumbent positioning for ultrasound-guided lumbar puncture.

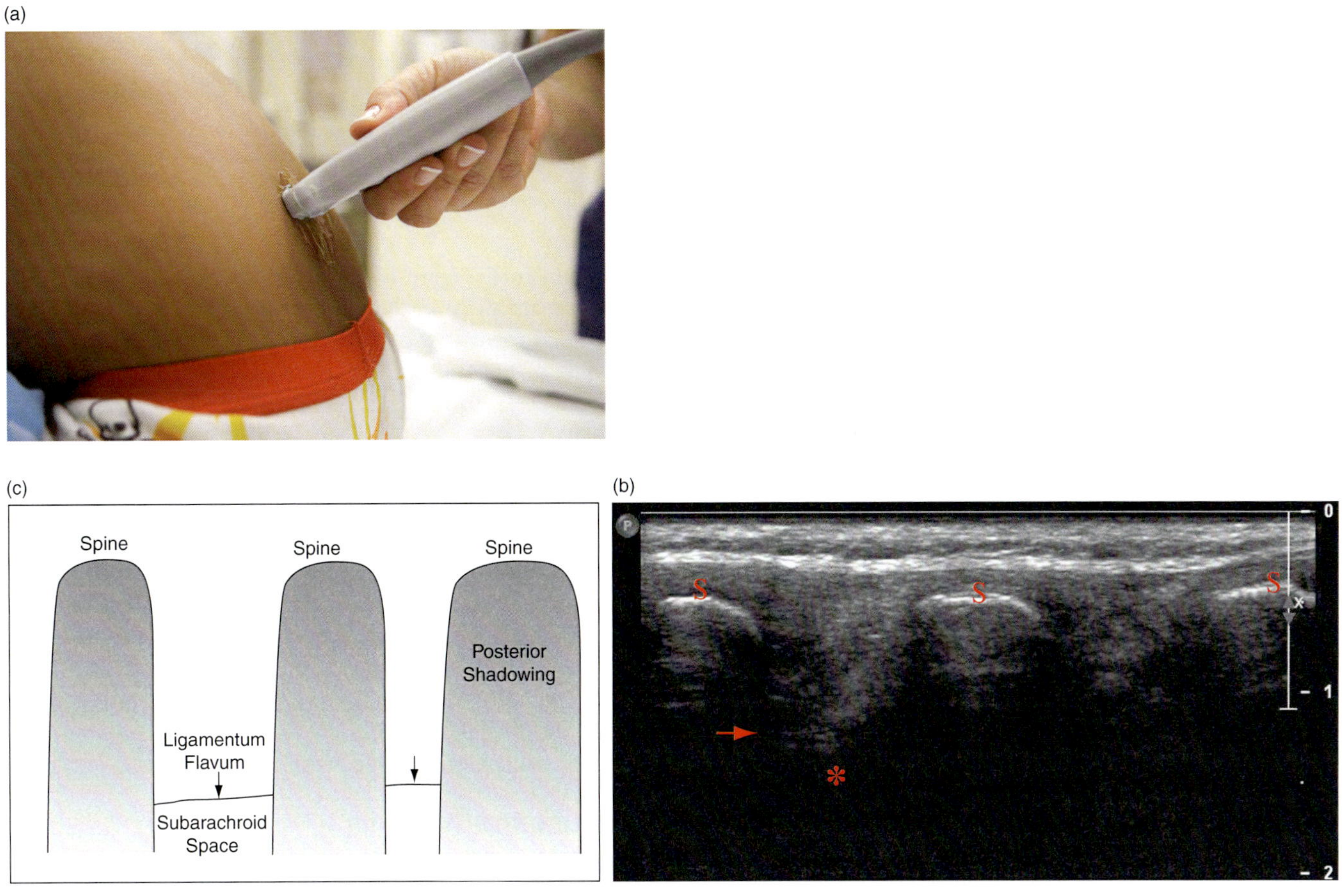

Figure 17.4 Spinal imaging, transverse view. (a) Transducer placement perpendicular to the spine. (b) Ultrasound of the transverse spine. Structures visualized by ultrasound include the spine (S) with posterior shadowing, the dura mater/ ligamentum flavum (arrow), and the subarachnoid space (*). (c) Illustration depicting these structures. *Ultrasound image courtesy of Brian Coley, MD.*

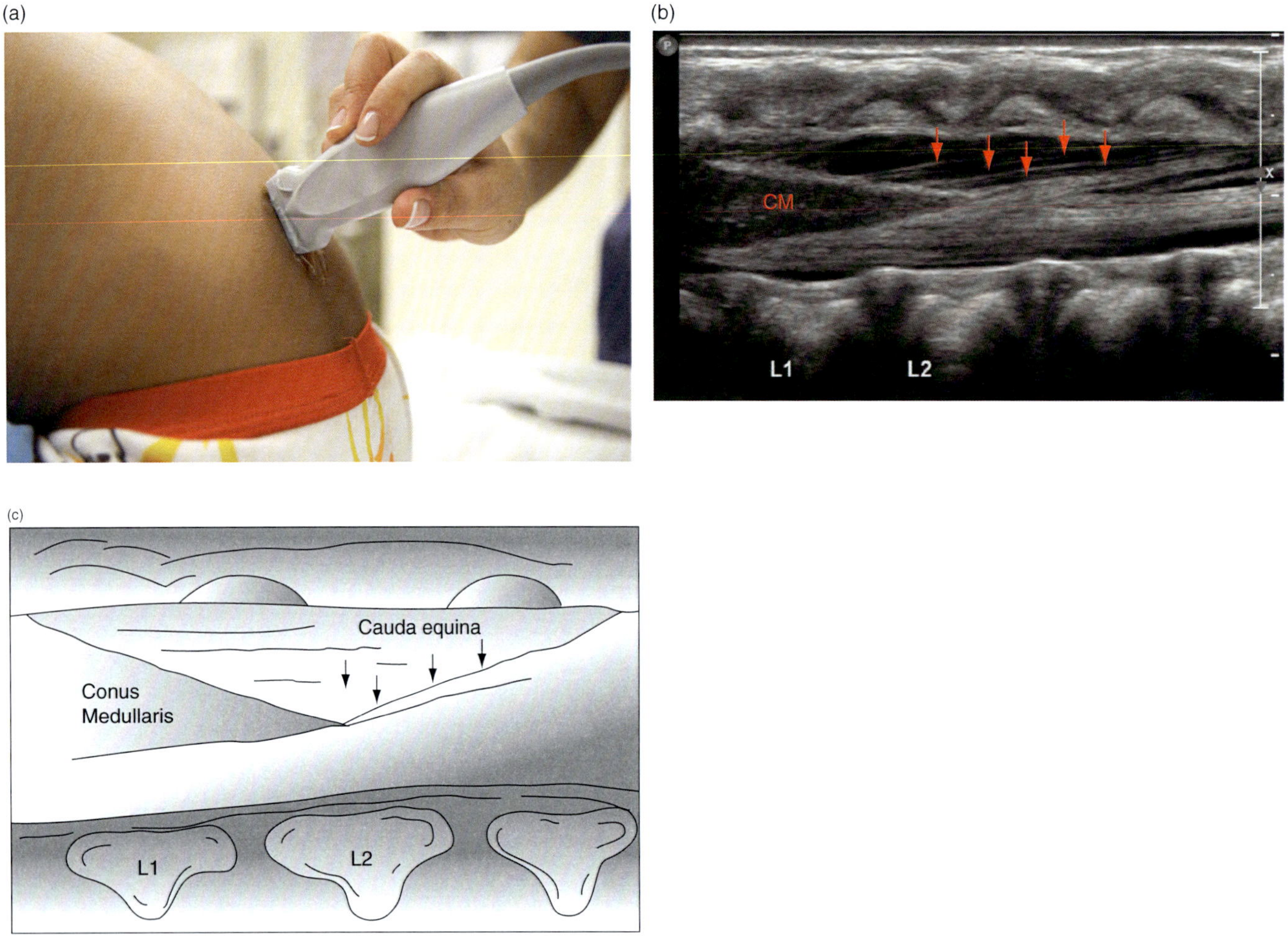

Figure 17.5 Spinal imaging, longitudinal view. (a) Transducer placement parallel to the spine. (b) Ultrasound of the longitudinal spine. Structures visualized by ultrasound. The conus medullaris (CM) and the cauda equina (arrows) can be easily visualized in this image. *Ultrasound image courtesy of Brian Coley, MD.* (c) Illustration depicting these structures.

cauda equina is represented as linear echogenic lines around the filum terminale (Figures 17.6, 17.7).

Ultrasound-guided procedure

Ultrasound may be utilized to augment lumbar punctures, either by static (ultrasound-assisted), or dynamic (ultrasound-guided) techniques. However, at the present time, there are no studies to suggest which method is preferred. Ultrasound evaluation may help in determining the depth, direction, and angulation of the needle placement.

In the static method, the interspinous space for lumbar puncture is identified and marked on the patient's skin. There are various ways to mark the skin. Possibilities include outlining the posterior spinous processes on the skin, noting the interspinous spaces in between. A vertical line may be drawn parallel to the thecal sac, and a horizontal line can be drawn to identify Tuffier's line. The point of intersection is where the spinal needle is inserted. Another technique involves placing paperclips under the ultrasound transducer, in order to identify where to insert the needle. The paperclip will produce a reverberation artifact, allowing the sonographer to mark the skin with an "X" and subsequently place the needle there for the lumbar puncture (Figure 17.8). In the dynamic approach, clinicians can place the transducer in the paramedian longitudinal position and identify the needle as it enters the subarachnoid space (Figure 17.9).

Scanning tips

Pitfalls

- An incorrect needle trajectory may be misleading and make performing a lumbar puncture more difficult. Therefore, the sonographer should scan thoroughly and obtain images in more than one plane.
- Another potential challenge is obesity and the ability to visualize anatomic landmarks sonographically. Using a curvilinear transducer may provide better resolution of deeper structures in larger patients.

Tips to improve scanning

✓ For infants in the seated position, placing a small, rolled towel under the knees may provide adequate hip flexion.

✓ Ultrasound should be performed in both the transverse and longitudinal views. The two longitudinal views include the

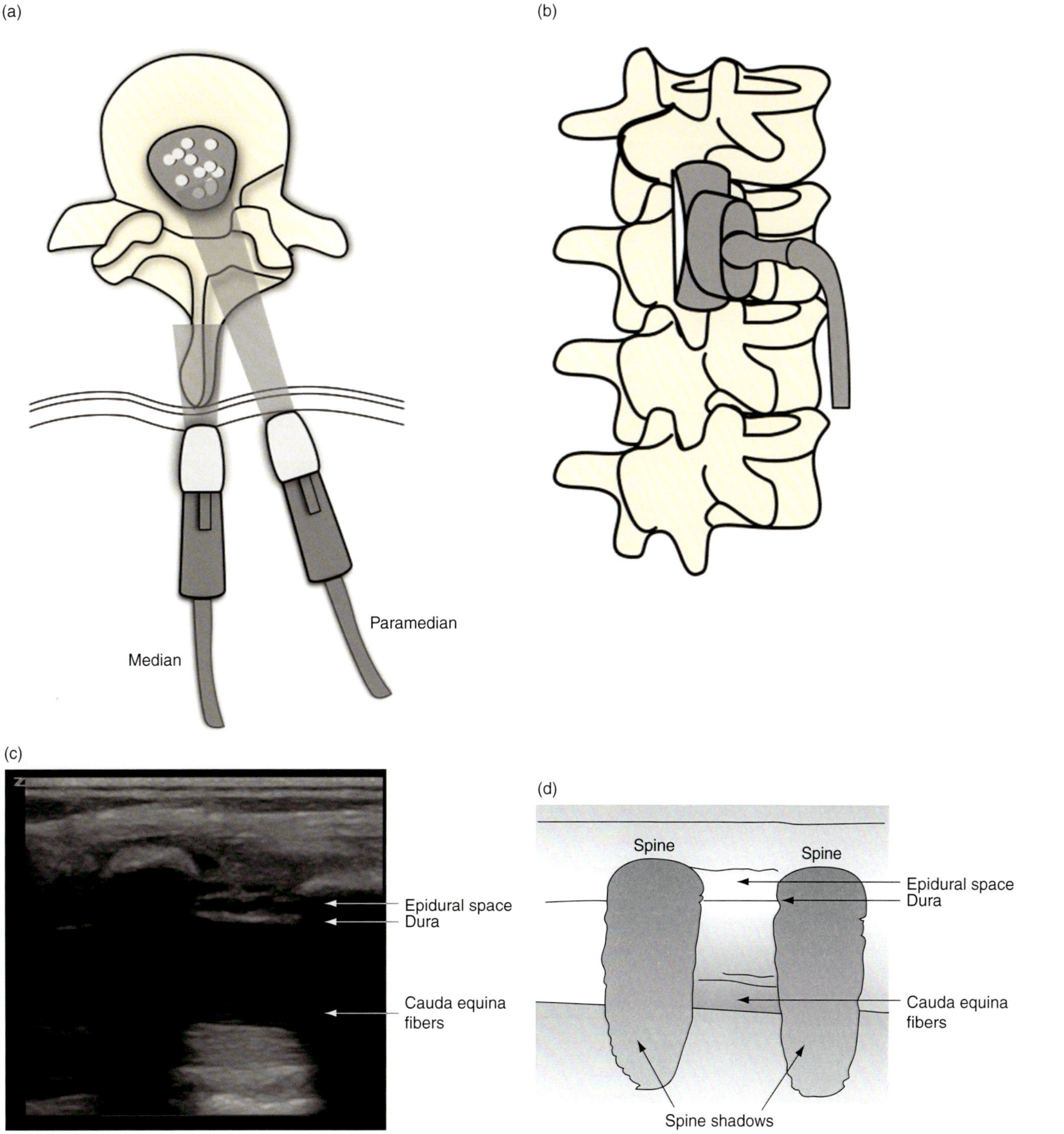

Figure 17.6 Spinal imaging, longitudinal (median and paramedian) views. (a) Vertebral body illustration of both the median and paramedian transducer placements. (b) Spinal anatomy illustration with median and paramedian approaches. (c) Ultrasound image of the paramedian transducer orientation. (d) Illustration depicting the structures visualized by ultrasound.

midline sagittal plane, and the paramedian plane. The paramedian plane causes less interference and improved visualization when compared to the midline sagittal plane.

✓ For identifying bony landmarks and the interspinous space, a shallow depth of a few centimeters is sufficient. However, for the identification of the dura and deeper structures, the depth will need to be increased.

✓ A useful technique for skin marking, prior to lumbar puncture, involves identifying the ideal interspinous location, then placing paperclips under the ultrasound transducer. The paperclip will produce a reverberation artifact, allowing the sonographer to then mark the skin with an “X” prior to needle puncture.

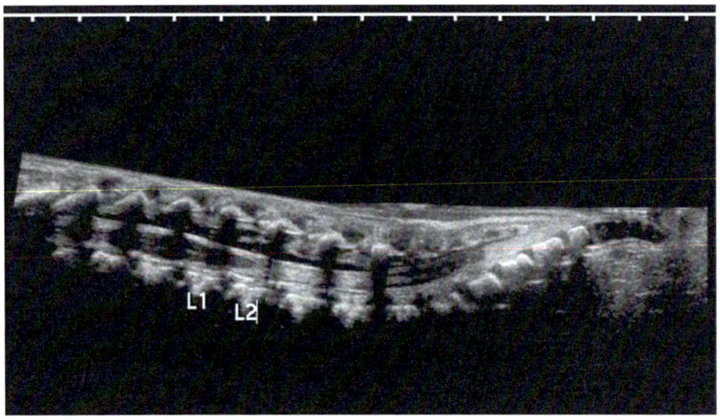

Figure 17.7 Extended field of view (EFOV) ultrasound of the spine. This demonstrates the length of the lumbosacral spine. Though this technique is not traditionally utilized in the emergency department, it allows for orientation and demonstration of anatomical structures. *Image courtesy of Brian Coley, MD.*

Cases

1. A four-month-old infant presents to the emergency department with irritability, and a fever to 39 °C rectally for four hours. On examination, the patient is febrile and toxic appearing. Given the child's age and risk for sepsis, the decision is made to perform a lumbar puncture in order to evaluate for meningitis. The resident performs two unsuccessful attempts, and calls the attending physician for assistance; the attending is unable to obtain CSF on an additional attempt. Therefore, the physician positions the child in a seated position. A point-of-care ultrasound is performed, the spinous processes are identified, and the largest interspinous space is identified at L4–5, well below the conus medullaris (Figure 17.10). The skin is marked. The physician then performs the lumbar

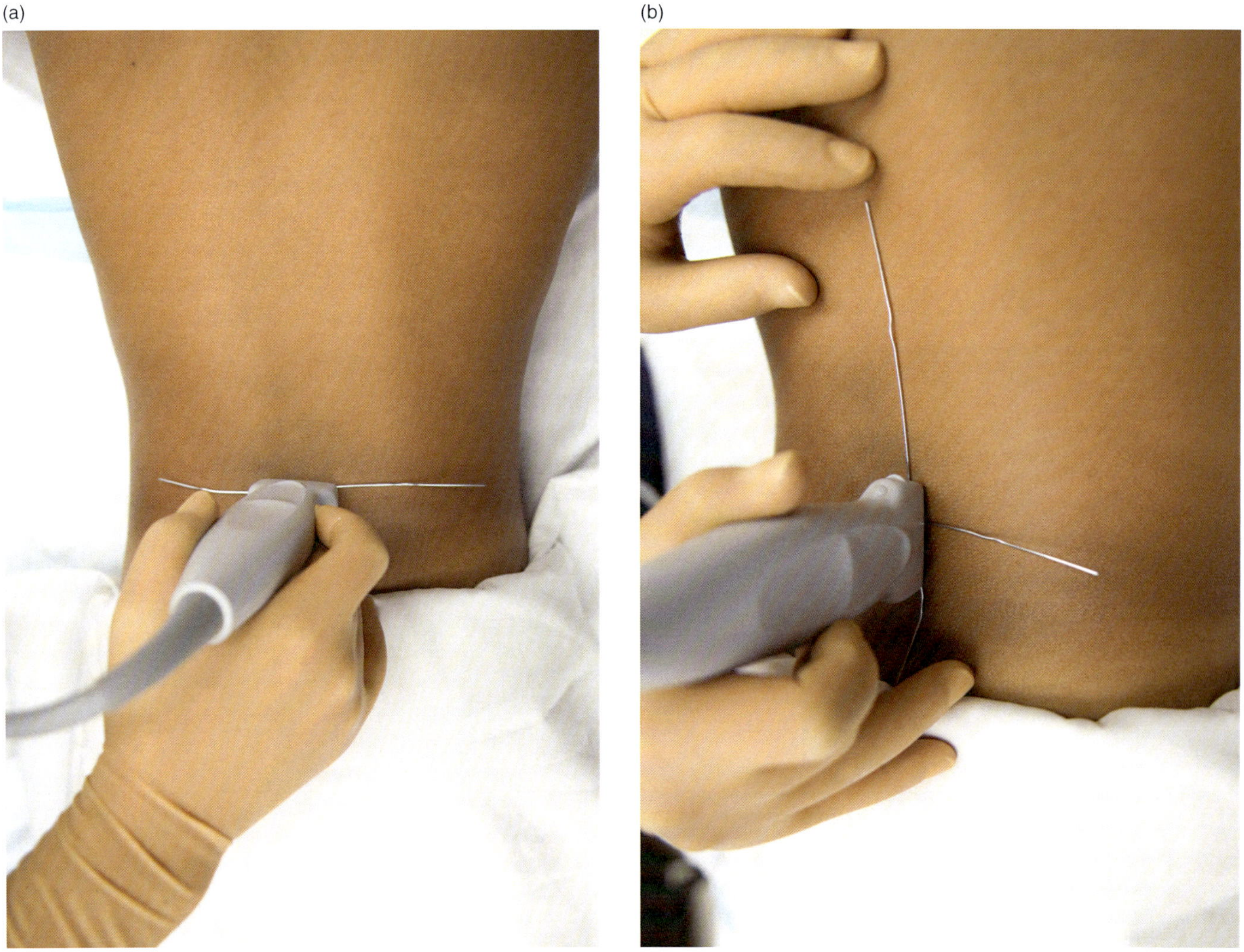

Figure 17.8 Static marking of the skin prior to lumbar puncture. In this technique, a paperclip is utilized in order to demarcate both transverse and longitudinal planes. (a) First, the transverse view is obtained, and a paperclip is centered under the transducer. (b) The longitudinal view is then obtained and a second paperclip is placed underneath the transducer. Finally the place where the two paperclips intersect is the ideal location for the needle puncture.

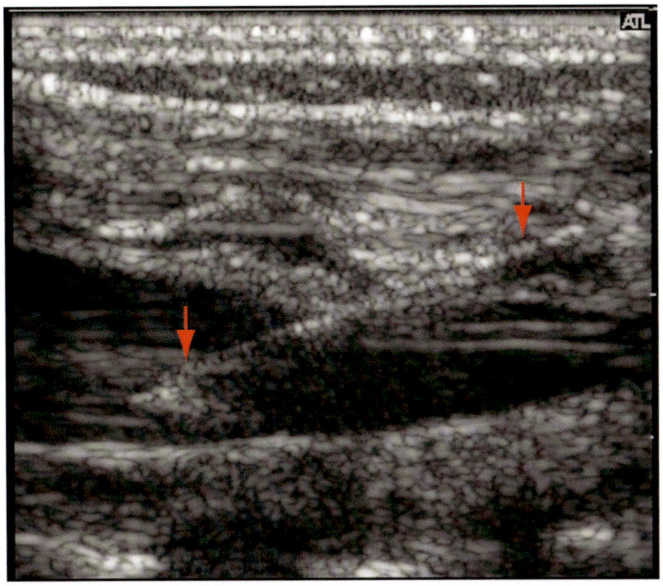

Figure 17.9 Real-time ultrasound visualization for lumbar puncture. In this longitudinal view, the hyperechoic needle (arrows) is easily visualized as entering into the subarachnoid space. *Image courtesy of Brian Coley, MD.*

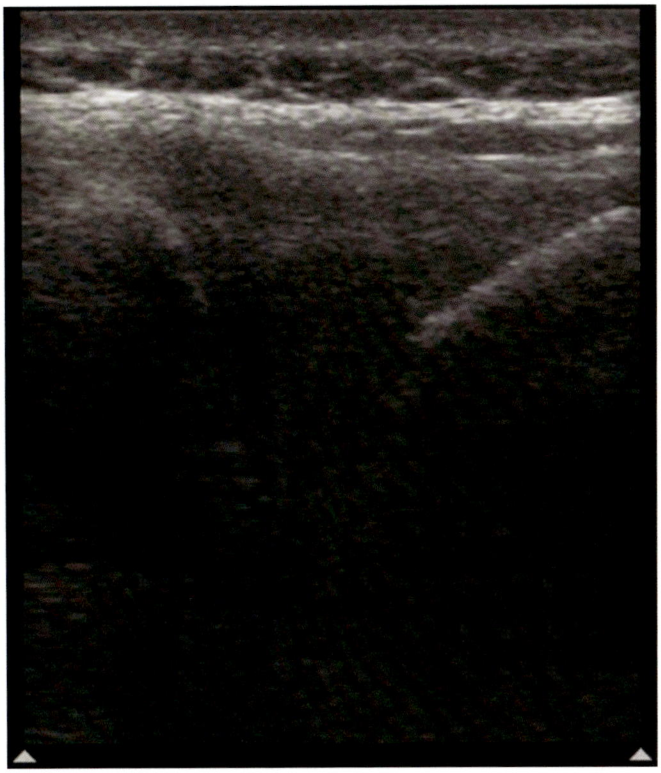

Figure 17.11 Case 2: obese child. Ultrasound was performed in order to identify spinous processes and interspinous spaces, in order to perform a lumbar puncture.

puncture and successfully obtains CSF. The infant is admitted to the hospital on empiric antibiotics.

This case highlights the utility of ultrasound in determining the ideal location for performing a lumbar puncture. The largest interspinous space may be identified, especially in those cases where prior attempts have been unsuccessful.

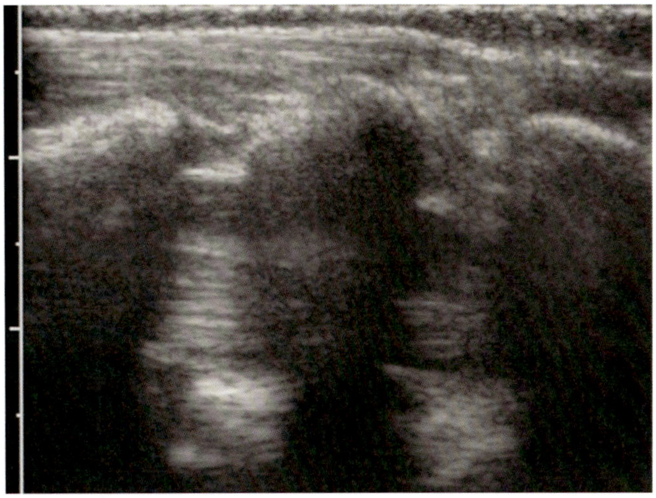

Figure 17.10 Case 1: baby. This case demonstrates visualization of the longitudinal view of the lumbar spine. *Image courtesy of Brian Coley, MD.*

2. A 14-year-old, morbidly obese male presents to the emergency department with fever, a stiff neck, and vomiting for the past day. On physical examination, he is toxic appearing, febrile, and exhibits meningismus. Due to the high suspicion for bacterial meningitis, it is decided to perform a lumbar puncture. However, when the PEM attending physician attempts to palpate the iliac crests in order to estimate the L4–5 interspinous space, she is unable to palpate the iliac crests or spinous processes due to the patient's body habitus. Therefore, ultrasound is performed in in order to identify bony landmarks (Figure 17.11). The ideal interspinous space is located, the depth is measured, and the skin is marked. The physician then performs the lumbar puncture, successfully obtaining CSF on the first attempt. There are no complications, and the child is admitted with IV antibiotics. The CSF culture is positive for meningococcus. The child receives a prolonged course of IV antibiotics, and recovers uneventfully.

   This case demonstrates the utility of ultrasound for identifying anatomical landmarks that cannot be palpated in obese patients. It is important to note that occasionally a lower frequency transducer may need to be utilized, since the linear transducer has a limitation in its penetration.

Summary/key points

1. Ultrasound has the potential to be useful in pediatric lumbar punctures, especially for neonates and obese children. Since there is a paucity of research dedicated to ultrasound-assisted and ultrasound-guided lumbar punctures in the pediatric emergency department, more research needs to be performed in order to appropriately assess its utility and effect on clinical practice.
2. Generally accepted positionings for children during a lumbar puncture are the lateral recumbent positioning and upright seated position. Ultrasound-guided lumbar

puncture should be performed in both the transverse and longitudinal views. The longitudinal view may be obtained by the median or paramedian approach.

3. A linear, high-frequency transducer is generally used for assessing the lumbar spine. However, a lower-frequency transducer may be necessary in larger, obese patients.
4. Ultrasound can identify the superficial anatomical landmarks including the spinous processes and interspinous spaces. Ultrasound can also identify deeper structures, such as the dura mater, which may guide the clinician in how far to insert the spinal needle.
5. Ultrasound can be used in a static technique, in which structures are identified by ultrasound, and the skin is marked prior to the procedure. Alternatively, the dynamic technique offers real-time visualization of the needle during the lumbar puncture.

Selected references

Abo, A., Chen, L., Johnston, P., *et al.* (2010) Positioning for lumbar puncture in children evaluated by bedside ultrasound. *Pediatrics* **125**: e1149–53.

Bruccoleri, R. E., Chen, L. (2011) Needle-entry angle for lumbar puncture in children as determined by using ultrasonography. *Pediatrics* **127**: e921.

Cadigan, B. A., Cydulka, R. K., Werner, S. L., *et al.* (2011) Evaluating infant positioning for lumbar puncture using sonographic measurements. *Acad Emerg Med* **18**: 215–18.

Coley, B. D., Shiels, W. E., Hogan, M. J. (2001) Diagnostic and interventional ultrasonography in neonatal and infant lumbar puncture. *Pediatr Radiol* **31**: 399–402.

Dick, E. A., Patel, K., Owens, C. M., *et al.* (2002) Spinal ultrasound in infants. *Br J Radiol* **75**: 384–92.

Ferre, R. M., Sweeney, T. W., Strout, T. D. (2009) Ultrasound identification of landmarks preceding lumbar puncture: a pilot study. *Emerg Med J* **26**: 276–7.

Marhofer, P., Bosenberg, A., Sitzwohl, C., *et al.* (2005) Pilot study of neuraxial imaging by ultrasound in infants and children. *Paediatr Anaesth* **15**: 671–6.

Nomura, J. T., Leech, S. J., Shenbagamurthi, S., *et al.* (2007) A randomized controlled trial of ultrasound-assisted lumbar puncture. *J Ultrasound Med* **26**: 1341–8.

Tsui, B. C., Suresh, S. (2010) Ultrasound imaging for regional anesthesia in infants, children, and adolescents: a review of current literature and its application in the practice of neuraxial blocks. *Anesthesiology* **112**: 719–28.

Whitty, R., Moore, M., Macarthur, A. (2008) Identification of the lumbar interspinous spaces: palpation versus ultrasound. *Anesth Analg* **106**: 538–40.

Chapter 18

Soft tissue applications

Daniela Ramirez-Schrempp and Andrew S. Liteplo

Objectives/indications

Ultrasound is a valuable tool in the evaluation and management of soft tissue in pediatrics: for infections and wounds with suspected retained foreign bodies. It is a safe and inexpensive modality that is rapid, repeatable, non-invasive, and can be performed at the bedside.

An accurate diagnosis is needed when evaluating soft tissue infections, as the treatment differs. Clinical differentiation of cellulitis from abscess is sometimes challenging, as they may present with similar symptoms and clinical findings. The benefits of ultrasound visualization are numerous: ultrasound has a high sensitivity and specificity for detecting subcutaneous fluid, provides real-time guidance for fluid drainage, determines the precise measurements of the size and depth of an abscess, demonstrates the absence of vascular flow, and shows the proximity to other structures such as vessels, tendons, and nerves. Armed with this knowledge, a healthcare provider can make more accurate diagnoses and treatment decisions, and more precise incisions and needle aspirations, resulting in better care for the patient.

Ultrasound can also help in the detection of foreign bodies in the soft tissue. Missed foreign bodies are a frequent cause of inadequate wound healing or infection. It is also a common cause of litigation against emergency physicians. The clinical diagnosis of a foreign body may be difficult, especially in a pediatric patient. A plain radiograph is usually an adequate screening tool to assess for the presence of radiopaque foreign bodies. However, radiographs have a poor sensitivity in detecting radiolucent foreign bodies such as wood, plastic, or thorns. MRIs are considered very accurate at detecting foreign bodies, but are expensive, have limited availability, and are especially challenging in uncooperative children. Growing literature supports the use of ultrasound as the imaging modality of choice in the evaluation of suspected radiolucent and radio-opaque foreign bodies. In addition to detecting foreign bodies, it may serve as an adjunct for the procedural removal of them.

Background

There are a few landmark studies in the adult emergency medicine literature showing the benefits of real-time ultrasound for management of soft tissue infections. Squire *et al.* performed a prospective observational study which showed that ultrasound was superior to clinical examination alone, with higher sensitivity (98 vs. 86%), specificity (88 vs. 70%), PPV (93 vs. 81%), and NPV (97 vs. 77%). This superiority was despite the fact that the physicians had limited experience with ultrasound for soft tissue infections. In another study, Tayal *et al.* evaluated the effect of point-of-care ultrasound on the management of patients with soft tissue infections without obvious signs of an abscess. Overall, ultrasound changed the patients' management in approximately half of patients in the emergency department with clinical cellulitis, and prevented unnecessary invasive procedures.

There is limited literature on point-of-care ultrasound in pediatric soft tissue infections. A recent study by Sivitz *et al.* showed similar results to the previous adult studies in the diagnosis of soft tissue infections in children. In this prospective observational series, ultrasound was superior to clinical assessment, with a higher sensitivity (90 vs. 75%), and specificity (83 vs. 80%), when compared to the gold standard of obtaining pus on incision and drainage. Ultrasound changed management in 22% of cases by detecting subclinical abscesses or by avoiding unnecessary invasive procedures.

Point-of-care ultrasound for foreign-body detection and removal has also been described in the adult literature. There is growing evidence supporting the use of ultrasound as the primary imaging modality. The majority of studies investigating the detection of foreign bodies have used animal or inanimate objects to simulate human tissue. Sensitivities and specificities for detecting foreign bodies by ultrasound vary depending on the material used, the size of the foreign bodies, and the operator's experience, and range from 43 to 98% and 59 to 98%, respectively. Orlinsky *et al.* compared the accuracy of ultrasound in the detection of foreign bodies when performed by novice emergency physicians, attending radiologists, and experienced sonographers. They found an overall sensitivity of 79% and specificity of 86%. There was no statistically significant difference in accuracy among the three groups. Together, these studies suggest that ultrasound is a reliable means by which to assess soft tissue for the presence of foreign bodies, even in the hands of novice sonographers. Its role is even more significant in the identification of wood, plastic, or other radiolucent foreign bodies, where the sensitivity of radiography is poor.

Similarly, ultrasound has been shown to be helpful in the detection of soft tissue foreign bodies in children. Friedman

Pediatric Emergency and Critical Care Ultrasound, ed. Stephanie J. Doniger. Published by Cambridge University Press.

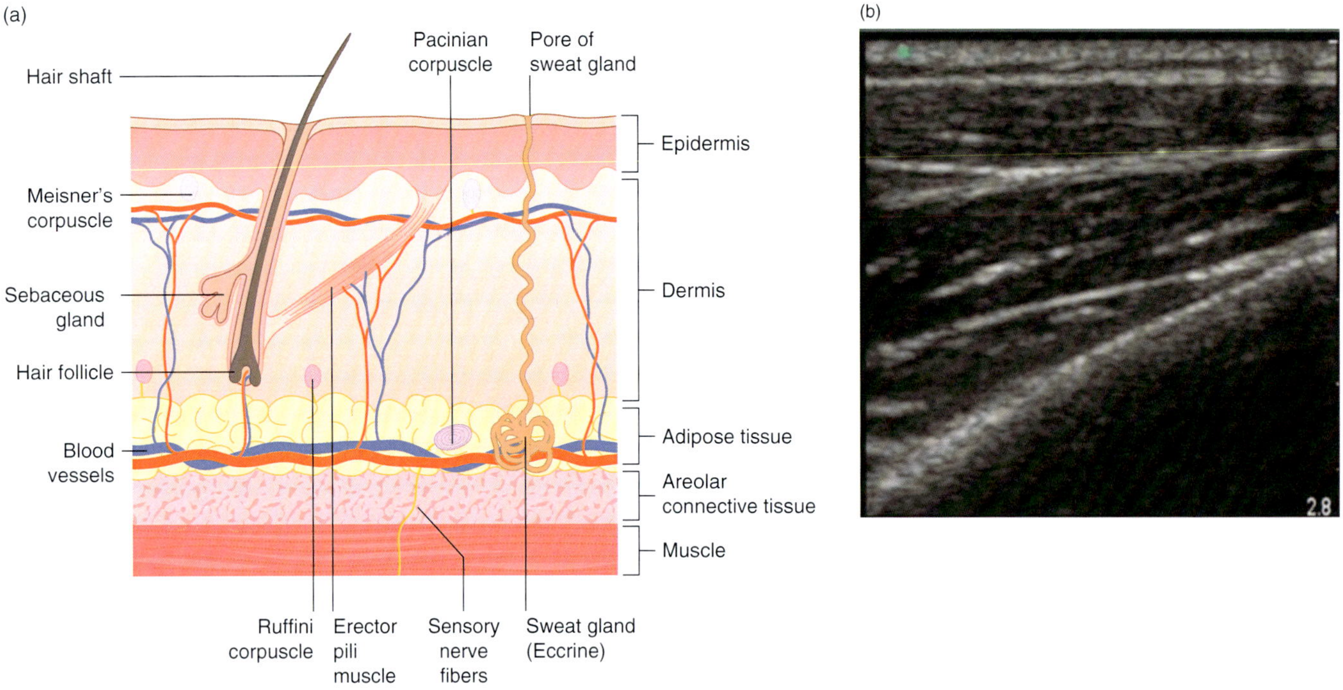

Figure 18.1 Anatomy of the skin. Normal layers of skin include the epidermis, dermis, subcutaneous, and muscular layers. *Artwork created by Emily Evans © Cambridge University Press.*

et al. performed a prospective study, comparing ultrasound with conventional radiographs in the identification of foreign bodies. The gold standard was the retrieval of a foreign body from the wound. Ultrasound was superior to conventional radiographs, with a higher sensitivity (67 vs. 58%) and a higher specificity (97 vs. 90%). When ultrasound was combined with the patient perception of a foreign body in the wound, the sensitivity rose to 89%, but specificity decreased to 77%.

Anatomy

Normal skin is comprised of well-organized layers including the epidermis, dermis, subcutaneous, and muscle layers (Figure 18.1a).

Technique

Transducer selection and preparation

High-frequency (5–10 MHz or higher), linear-array transducers are the best option for the assessment of superficial structures. These transducers have excellent resolution for superficial areas, but are limited in penetration. If there is a need for deeper assessment, a transducer with a lower frequency should be utilized. Alternatively, a curvilinear or endocavitary transducer may be substituted for the assessment of superficial areas. These have the advantage of having a rounded footprint, which might have better skin contact with concave skin surfaces such as webspaces or intergluteal folds.

It is crucial to clean the transducer with an appropriate disinfectant to avoid any possible transmission of pathogens. The transducer needs to be cleaned before and after its use. If the skin is not intact, for example in the case of an open wound or draining lesion, the transducer should be prepared in a sterile fashion (Figures S3.5–7).

Patient position and preparation

Imaging should be acquired prior to the irrigation of the wound, as the introduction of air bubbles could obscure the image. Skin infections and wounds with concern for retained foreign bodies are usually painful, so it is important to take all measures to minimize the patient's discomfort during the ultrasound examination. This will also help in acquiring optimal images. The region of interest might be prepared with topical anesthetic so that the contact with the transducer is better tolerated. When appropriate, the use of a water bath or stand-off pad can also minimize pressure on the affected area. Having the region of interest fully exposed and easily accessible to the ultrasonographer will facilitate complete scanning. Preparing the (normal) contralateral side is also helpful, as it can be used as a control, and subtle changes will become more noticeable.

Ultrasound imaging

The transducer should be held perpendicular to the skin. The depth should be adjusted, so that the region of interest is in the center of the ultrasound image. A minimal amount of pressure should be used in order to avoid possible collapse of an overlying blood vessel.

The region of interest should always be scanned in two orthogonal planes in order to appropriately assess the size and shape of the area of interest and surrounding structures. It is useful to start to scan from unaffected tissue and more towards the affected tissue. Additionally, if applicable, the affected area should be compared to the corresponding normal contralateral part of the body, to appreciate differences between the healthy tissue and the affected side. This is especially important in subtle cases.

On ultrasound, soft tissue has a very organized pattern on ultrasound (Figure 18.1b). The dermis and epidermis appear as a single echogenic and bright layer relative to the subcutaneous tissue, which is mainly comprised of fat. Subcutaneous fat appears hypoechoic, in a reticular pattern. Some thin echogenic tracts of connective tissue can usually be seen crossing the subcutaneous tissue. The thickness of this layer varies greatly depending on the region of the body and the body habitus of the person.

Deeper structures are also visible on ultrasound, and are important to identify so as to avoid them during incision and drainage (Figure 18.2). Muscular fascia appears as thin, bright, hyperechoic layers superficial to the muscular planes. When viewed in the long-axis, muscles have a characteristic striated appearance. When viewed in the short-axis, muscles have a characteristic speckled appearance. In addition, tendons may be visualized, and appear echogenic, finely striated, and can be observed to move when the patient moves the corresponding joint. Further, blood vessels appear as anechoic, linear or circular structures, depending on probe orientation. It is important to use minimal pressure when assessing the area of incision, as overlying veins could collapse and go unnoticed. Arteries have thicker walls, are pulsatile, and require a larger force to be compressed. Finally, depending on the area that has been scanned and the depth that is required, bone might be also visualized. It has a characteristic bright, echogenic cortex, with posterior shadowing.

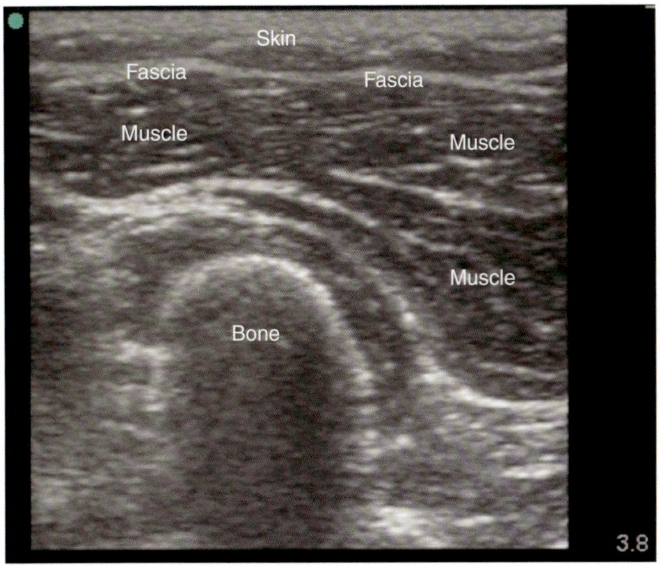

Figure 18.2 Normal soft tissue layers on ultrasonography. The skin and fascia can be visualized superficially. The muscle is seen as striated, with hyperechoic connective tissue running among the fibers. Deep to these layers, a bone is seen, with its characteristic posterior shadowing.

Specific scanning techniques

Cellulitis vs. abscess

Cellulitis is an infection of the skin and subcutaneous tissues. There is a spectrum of sonographic appearances, and findings that are nonspecific. Sonographic findings arise from the accumulation of fluid and swelling of the subcutaneous tissue. When compared to the normal contralateral side (Figure 18.3a), there is initial thickening of the subcutaneous tissue layer visualized on ultrasound (Figure 18.3b). As it progresses, there is disruption of the normal soft tissue architecture and develops disarray in the subcutaneous tissue (Figure 18.4a). On ultrasound, the intracellular edema appears as hypoechoic or anechoic strands which randomly traverse the subcutaneous fat and cause increased separation of the fat globules (Figure 18.4b). This is called "cobblestoning," as its pattern resembles that of a cobblestoned street (Figure 18.4c). There is also some posterior enhancement artifact as ultrasound passes through the fluid, which makes the fat appear

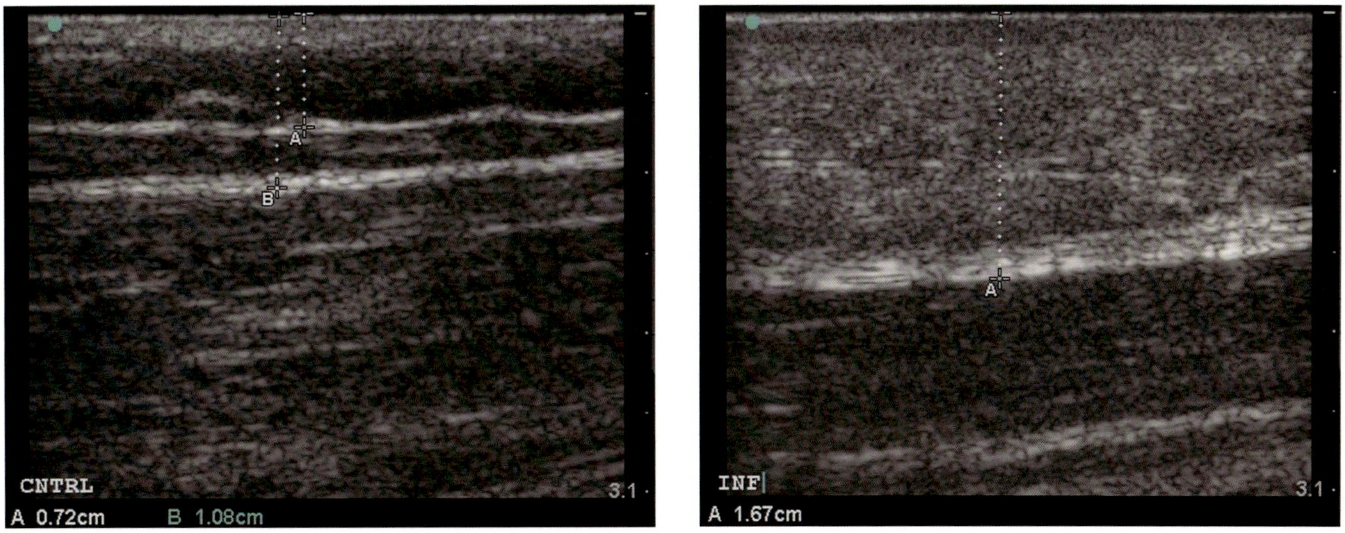

Figure 18.3 Cellulitis. (a) Normal soft tissue thickness is measured from the skin surface to the pre-muscular fascia; here it is measured at 1.08 cm. (b) In early cellulitis, the thickness of the soft tissue is increased and hyperechoic, measured here at 1.67 cm. It is thicker than the normal, contralateral side.

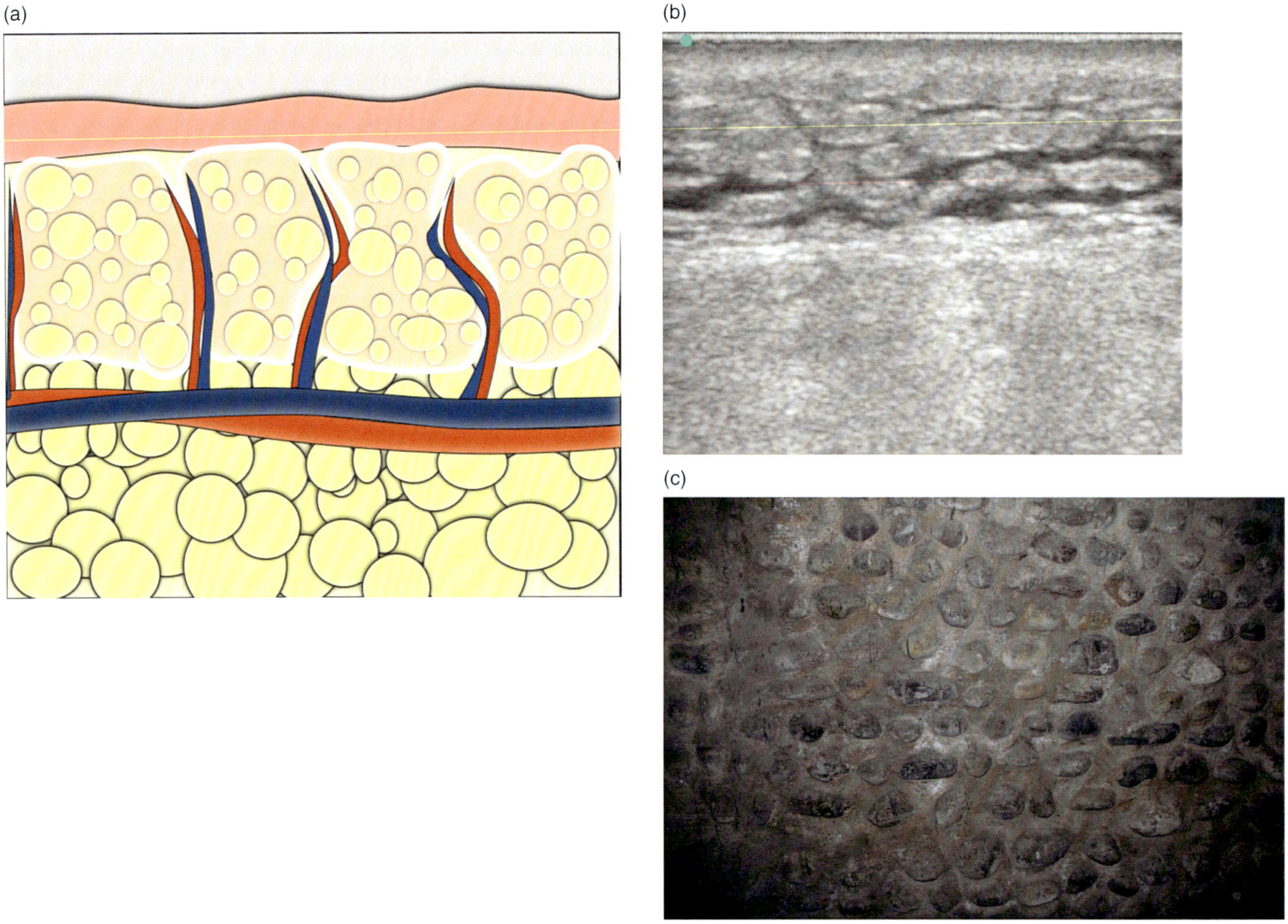

Figure 18.4 **Cellulitis.** (a) Illustration of the development of lobules and intracellular edema seen in cellulitis. (b) Ultrasound image of cellulitis demonstrates this classic "cobblestoning" pattern, in which subcutaneous edema is seen as hypoechoic stranding within the soft tissue and surrounding the fat globules. (c) Resemblance to cobblestones.

hyperechoic when compared to the contralateral side. As cellulitis progresses, there is extravasation of inflammatory fluid from the vessels, and occasionally a layer of pre-fascial fluid will accumulate. A thick layer of pre-fascial fluid of greater than 4 mm has been described in necrotizing fasciitis, and if seen should raise the suspicion for this disease.

Abscesses have a highly variable appearance on ultrasound (Figure 18.5). Their usual sonographic appearance is an anechoic or hypoechoic spherical or elliptical-shaped collection of fluid. The margins may be outlined by an echogenic rim or blend in with the surrounding tissue, with posterior acoustic enhancement. The surrounding tissues may appear hyperechoic. Within the abscess, there are variable amounts of internal echoes, ranging from none to a frankly heterogeneic collection of fluid. The ability to induce visible motion of abscess contents with gentle compression of the transducer will also help with the diagnosis. This is especially helpful when the suspected fluid is isoechoic or hyperechoic to the surrounding tissue. When compression causes movement of this material, it is called a positive "squish sign," which means that the material is likely to be fluid and therefore susceptible to drainage (Figure 18.6). If available, color flow or Doppler may also be used to confirm that the structure is not vascular, as no color flow or Doppler waveform should be seen in an abscess. This can also be helpful in differentiating a lymph node from an abscess, as flow within a central vessel of a lymph node can sometimes be seen.

Foreign-body detection

The sonographic appearance of foreign bodies varies greatly by material, size, and duration of time they have been embedded in the soft tissue. Generally, foreign bodies are hyperechoic and interrupt the well-organized structure of the soft tissue. Wood, glass, plastic, metal, and gravel will all appear hyperechoic when compared with the surrounding tissue (Figure 18.7). If ever in doubt, the normal contralateral side of the body can be scanned for comparison.

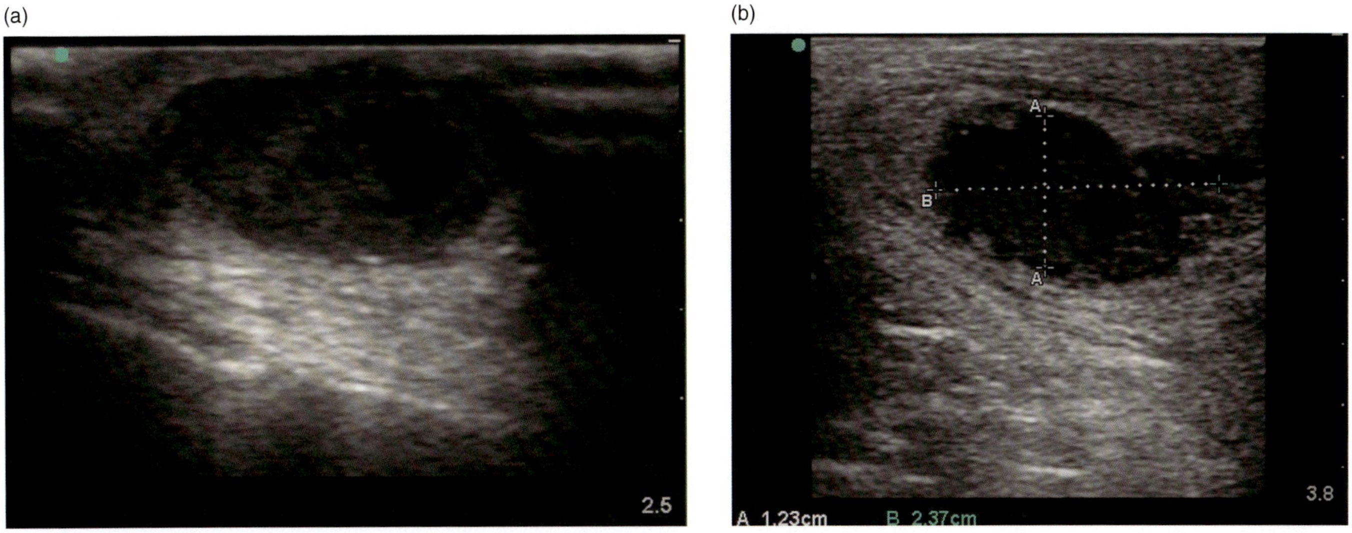

Figure 18.5 **Abscesses.** (a) An abscess with both anechoic fluid and isoechoic debris. Note also its extension to the surface that is often seen. This is an optimal location for incision and drainage. (b) An abscess with hypoechoic debris, and thick isoechoic walls.

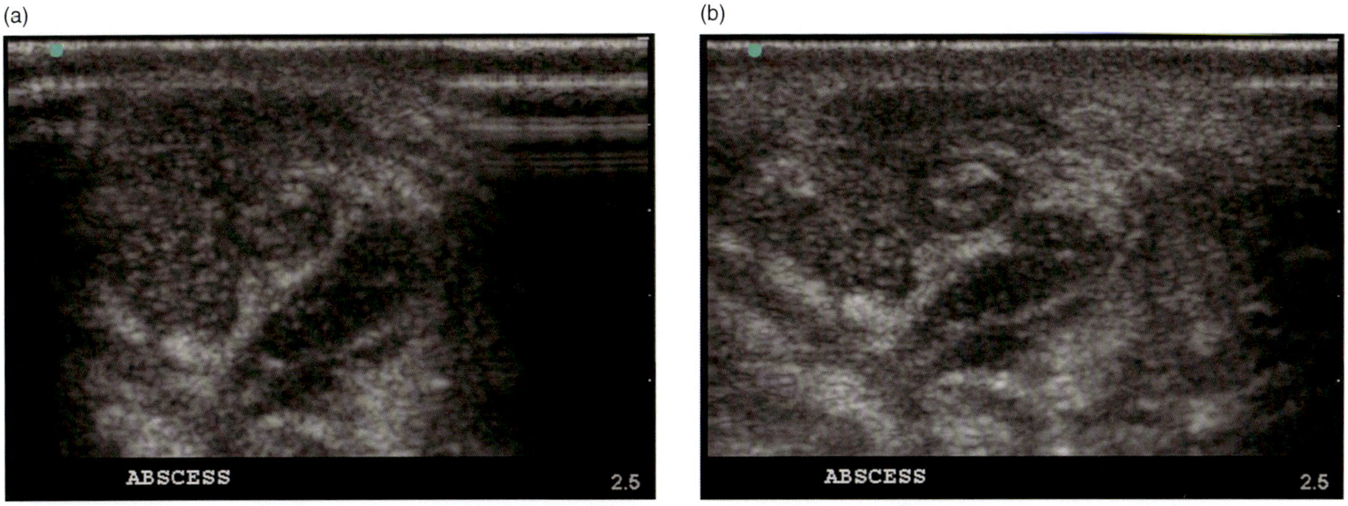

Figure 18.6 **The "squish sign."** (a) A superficial abscess in the antecubital fossa of an intravenous drug user. In the center is a clotted vein, consistent with superficial thrombophlebitis. Surrounding the vein anteriorly and medially (to the left of the screen) is an isoechoic fluid collection. It is not obvious that this is fluid until (b) the abscess is compressed and the size and shape of the fluid changes. This is known as a positive "squish sign."

Foreign bodies are recognizable by their associated sonographic artifacts. Often, the actual foreign body is not visualized, but the presence of such artifacts may be the only clue to the location of the foreign body. A common artifact is posterior shadowing from dense structures. This occurs because the surface of the foreign body is so echo-reflective that no ultrasound beams pass through, and hence no ultrasound image is generated deep to the foreign body. This is often seen in small stones or gravel, but can also be seen in wood or plastic, but typically to a lesser degree. Metal (and occasionally plastic) may have a characteristic "reverberation" artifact, which appears as multiple, hyperechoic, parallel, regularly spaced lines, deep to the foreign body. Glass foreign bodies can cause a variety of artifacts, according to its orientation, size, and composition. These include "posterior shadowing," "scattering," "reverberation," or "ring-down" artifacts (see Chapter 1). Finally, when a retained foreign body has been present in the soft tissue for some time, a hypoechoic ring may surround it. This "halo" represents inflammatory and granulation tissue.

Procedural guidance

Incision and drainage

In addition to confirming the presence of a drainable fluid collection, ultrasound can assist with the drainage procedure itself. Sonographic guidance for incision and drainage can be performed either statically or dynamically. There are no studies comparing dynamic vs. static guidance for drainage of abscesses. In practice, the static technique, which is easier as it requires less hand–eye coordination, is usually adequate as abscesses are frequently large and non-mobile. However, if

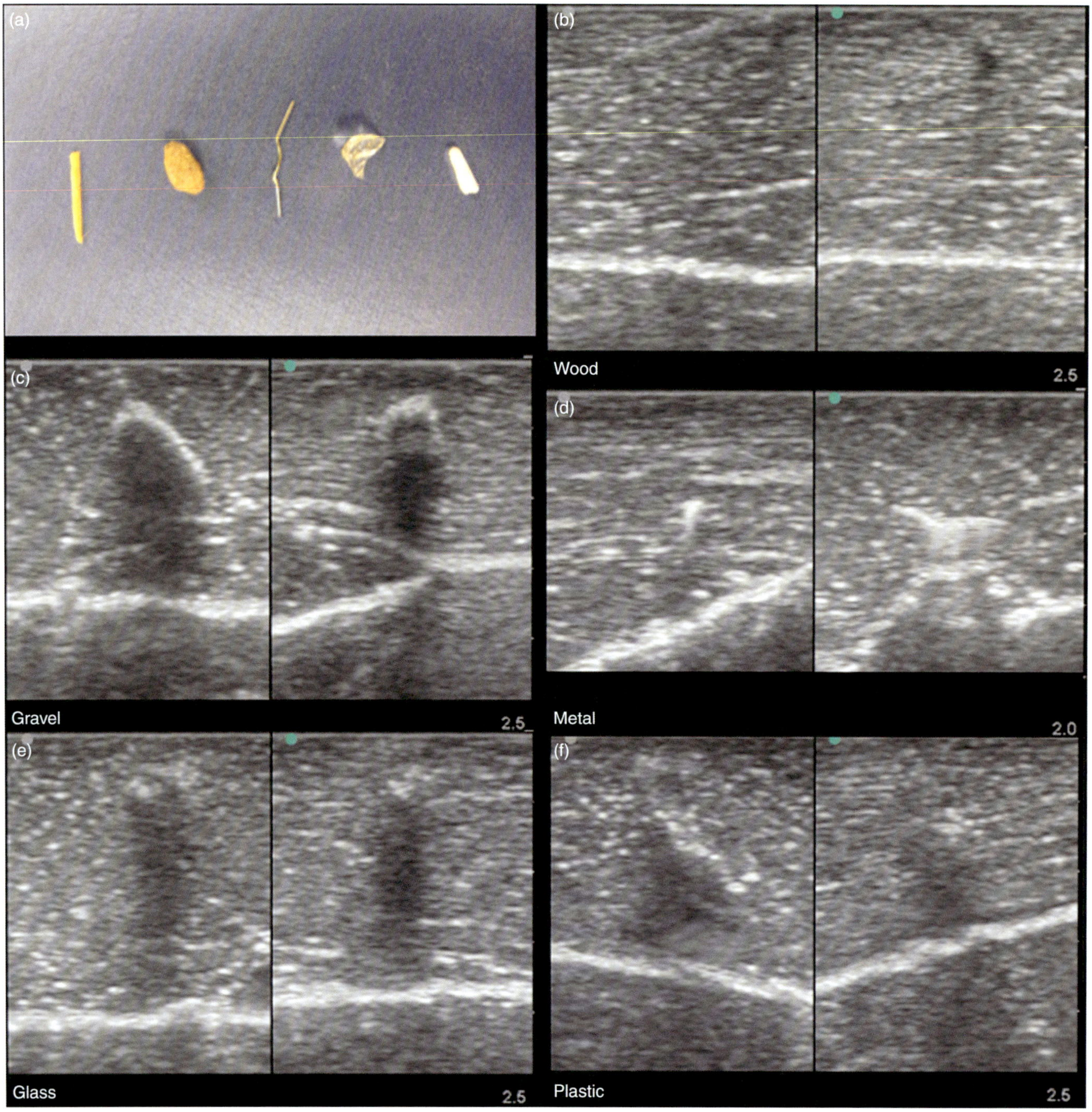

Figure 18.7 Foreign bodies. (a) From left to right: wood, gravel, metal, glass, and plastic. For size comparison, the metal object is a paper staple. These were inserted into a chicken thigh and scanned in two planes. (b) The wooden object is the most difficult to detect in this case, as it casts only a small shadow in one view and none in the other. (c) The gravel has a characteristic shadowing artifact, as do the glass (e) and plastic (f) to a lesser degree. (d) The metal has a classic reverberation artifact, detected as multiple parallel hyperechoic lines inferior to the object.

the target is small or the child is likely to move, dynamic guidance may be advantageous.

In the static technique, the abscess is visualized in two orthogonal planes and the largest pocket of mobile fluid is identified. It is important to carefully identify the location, size, and shape of the abscess (Figure 18.8). In addition, critical surrounding structures such as vessels, nerves, and tendons should be identified and avoided. Once the abscess and surrounding structures are identified, it is useful to measure the distance from the skin to the fluid, as this will guide the proceduralist on how deep to incise. The skin is marked with a pen or marker, the ultrasound is put away, and the incision and drainage is performed as usual. Once drainage is completed, the ultrasound can be repeated to assure that no fluid remains. This can be especially helpful when the abscess is loculated and separate fluid pockets remain walled-off.

In addition, real-time ultrasound guidance may be utilized for incision and drainage. The sterilely prepared transducer is used to

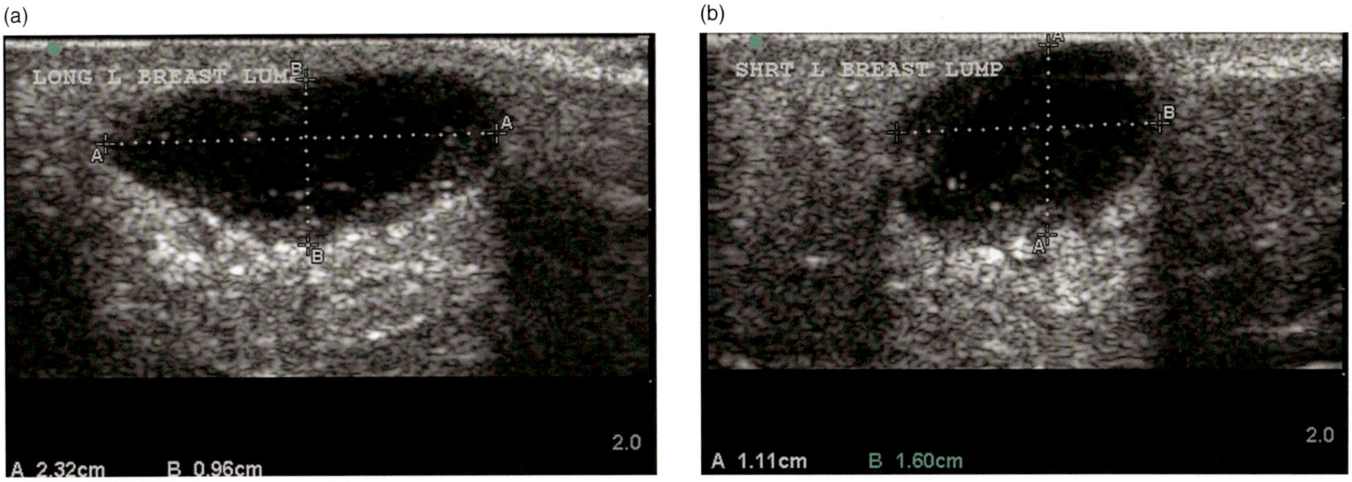

Figure 18.8 Abscess scanning and measurements. An elliptical superficial abscess in (a) its long-axis and (b) its short-axis. The interior is mostly anechoic and hypoechoic, with some hyperechoic spicules internally. Note the posterior acoustic enhancement seen in both long and short axes. Scanning in two orthogonal planes is important to confirm that the structure is not vascular.

visualize the abscess in real time, and guide the needle or scalpel as needed. Depth and gain are adjusted in advance of the procedure. The largest pocket of fluid should be centered in the middle of the screen and the transducer held steady in the non-dominant hand (single-operator), or by a second person (dual-operator), when available. It is helpful to stabilize the hand by resting your wrist or fourth and fifth fingers on the patient's skin so that the only point of contact between you and the patient is not the slippery probe–gel–skin interface. The dominant hand holds the scalpel and incises underneath the middle of the transducer. As in the static technique, once the abscess is reached and pus is expressed, the transducer can be put away and the procedure carried out as usual.

Foreign-body removal

Ultrasound-guidance serves as a very useful adjunct for foreign-body removal. Ultrasound imaging may accurately identify the foreign body's location, size, depth, orientation, and relationship to other structures (Figure 18.9). Both static ultrasound assistance and real-time ultrasound guidance may be utilized. Static assistance is helpful when the target is large, but in general lacks the precision needed to locate and remove most foreign bodies, which tend to be very small.

First, the location and orientation of the foreign body is identified. If air is present inside of a wound, it may be difficult to visualize the foreign body, since air causes scattering of the ultrasound beams. In this case, slight compression may alleviate the problem. Alternatively, air can be minimized or eliminated by filling the wound with sterile surgical gel or using a water bath, when appropriate. The foreign body should be scanned in two orthogonal planes in order to determine its shape and orientation. The transducer should then be rotated so that the foreign body is seen in its longest axis. Linear foreign bodies such as splinters or needles are best removed in the plane of their longest axis to minimize tissue disruption.

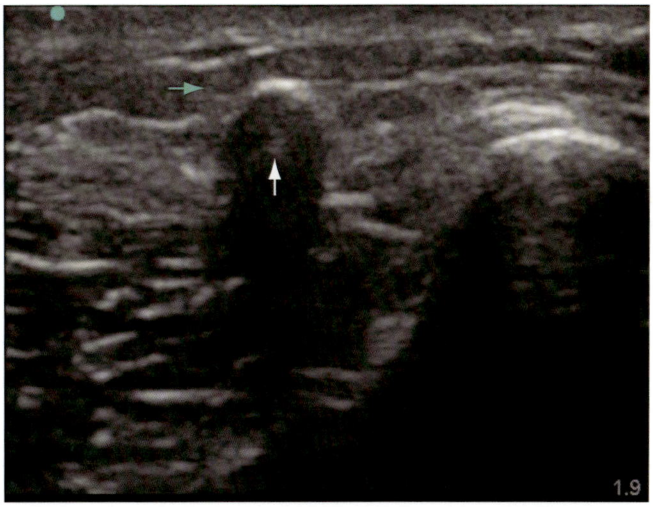

Figure 18.9 Metallic foreign body: BB pellet. This is a metallic BB embedded in a child's leg (blue arrow), which exhibits posterior shadowing and the "ring-down" artifact (white arrow). Surrounding structures may be visualized, including the tibia bone on the right side of the image.

Once visualized, an anesthetic may be applied. A topical anesthetic such as EMLA® or ELA-max may be appropriate for superficial procedures. Subcutaneous anesthesia, however, has the added benefit not only of relieving the pain associated with the procedure itself, but also of facilitating removal through a process known as "hydrodissection." With the foreign body visualized in the longitudinal orientation, a small (25- or 27-gauge) needle is inserted at an angle and depth sufficient to reach the foreign body. Sometimes this is best accomplished in the long-axis view. Once reached, lidocaine is infiltrated directly around the foreign body; the lidocaine itself dissects and loosens the foreign body from the surrounding tissue, making removal easier. On ultrasound, this appears like a dark anechoic halo forming around the foreign body (Figure 18.10).

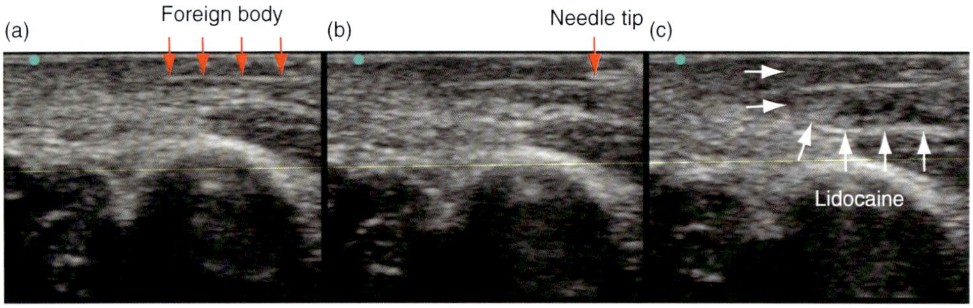

Figure 18.10 Hydrodissection technique. (a) A wooden splinter in a forearm is seen in its long-axis as a hyperechoic, linear foreign body without posterior shadowing. (b) A 25-gauge needle is seen entering from the right side of the screen, parallel to the foreign body and transducer. A small amount of lidocaine is visible as a hypoechoic halo around the splinter. (c) More lidocaine has been injected, providing analgesia and loosening the splinter from the soft tissue.

Once properly anesthetized, an incision is made directly over the object. It is ideal for the incision to be parallel to the longest axis of the foreign body. A "finder needle" can be inserted first until the foreign body is felt (or seen to be touching the object on ultrasound), then the scalpel used to cut down along the needle. Once visualized, the foreign body may be removed with forceps and the incision closed with sutures, if appropriate.

Scanning tips

Pitfalls

- As with all ultrasound applications, soft tissue ultrasound is operator dependent. Proper training is necessary before decisions should be made based on ultrasound findings. It is also important to incorporate ultrasound findings with the clinical scenario and physician examination.
- It is important to remember that the spectrum of soft tissue infections extends beyond cellulitis and abscesses. Necrotizing fasciitis has a sonographic appearance similar to cellulitis, and should not be ruled out on ultrasound alone. A high clinical suspicion is necessary, as emergent treatment is imperative. Also, air seen within the soft tissue can suggest gas gangrene. This appears sonographically as shadowing or scattering of ultrasound beams within the soft tissue.
- The absence of an anechoic fluid collection does not entirely rule out the presence of an abscess. It is possible to miss an abscess, especially when it is isoechoic to the surrounding tissue. In these cases, assessing for a "squish sign" or for posterior enhancement can be helpful. In some cases, interconnected bands of fluid, as seen in prominent cellulitis, can be confused with atypically shaped or pointed abscesses.
- It is easy to miss small foreign bodies, or mistake normal hyperechoic structures such as muscle fibers, cartilage, small bones (i.e. sesamoid), or air within a wound for foreign bodies. Radiography still has a role, especially when a suspected foreign body is known to be radiopaque. If there is a high clinical suspicion for the presence of a foreign body but none is seen on ultrasound, additional imaging or consultation may be required.

Tips to improve scanning

- ✓ Be familiar with normal anatomy. It is easier to identify pathology when you know what you are looking at.
- ✓ Make sure that both you and your patient are comfortable. You will acquire better images.
- ✓ Use plenty of gel and a minimal amount of pressure in order to minimize pain. Use scanning adjuncts whenever possible, such as a water bath or stand-off pads.
- ✓ Scan the contralateral part of the body for comparison.
- ✓ "Squish" the soft tissue – movement of isoechoic fluid may be your only clue to the presence of a fluid collection.
- ✓ Anchor the wrist or pinky of your scanning hand on the patient to minimize unwanted movements of the transducer. Perform ultrasound scanning with your non-dominant hand, and the procedure with your dominant hand.

Cases

1. A three-year-old boy is referred by his primary care physician to the emergency department, for concern of an abscess that may require conscious sedation in order to be drained. He has a three-day history of redness over his right thigh, and tactile fevers. He has no past medical history, but his mother has had multiple abscesses in the past. On examination, he is non-toxic appearing and afebrile. He has a 4 × 6 cm area of induration over his right thigh that is exquisitely tender to palpation. It has a central white lesion that is draining a small amount of yellow material. A point-of-care ultrasound is performed with a stand-off pad and copious amount of warm gel, revealing "cobblestoning" without a fluid collection (Figure 18.11). A culture is taken from the small amount of purulent material, and he is started on oral clindamycin. He does not require sedation or intervention. After three days, he has a follow-up visit at his primary care physician,

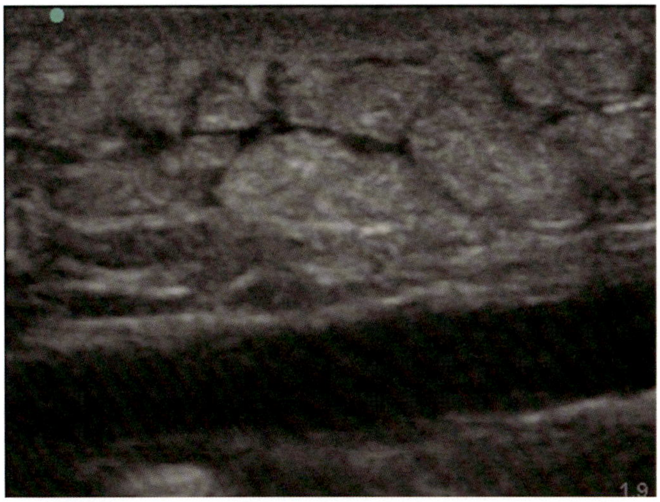

Figure 18.11 **Case 1: cellulitis.** Cobblestoning can be appreciated, without the presence of the anechoic fluid collection of an abscess.

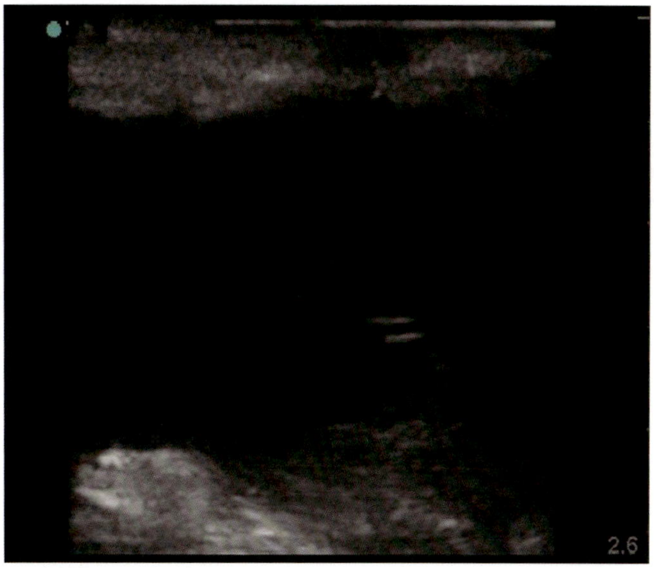

Figure 18.12 **Case 2: abscess.** The large anechoic abscess is visualized at the sacral region. Also note hypoechoic densities within the abscess.

and his cellulitis shows marked improvement. The culture grows methicillin-resistant *Staphylococcus aureus* (MRSA). This case demonstrates the utility of soft tissue ultra-sound in distinguishing between cellulitis and an abscess. In this particular case, as a result of the absence of an abscess, the patient was spared an unnecessary procedure and sedation.

2. A 16-year-old female presents to the emergency department with significant pain over her sacral area for the last four days. She states that she fell over a week ago onto her buttocks, and is concerned she "broke something." She has no significant past medical history, including no prior skin infections. On examination she exhibits tenderness to palpation in the region over her sacrum, at the buttock crease. No fluctuance or induration is appreciated. The overlying skin is intact and shows no erythema. A point-of-care ultrasound reveals a 2 × 3.5 cm collection of fluid (Figure 18.12), consistent with an infected pilonidal cyst. Incision and drainage is performed, and packing is placed inside the abscess cavity. In contrast to the previous case, this patient has an abscess on ultrasound, which warrants an incision and drainage. Ultrasound can be particularly helpful in situations where the clinical examination is unclear as to whether an abscess is present or not.
3. An eight-year-old boy presents to the emergency department one day after he fell against a wooden dresser. He is unsure whether a fragment of the dresser penetrated beneath his fingernail. On examination, he has significant discomfort and is unable to flex his finger secondary to pain. There is a slight discoloration of his nail (Figure 18.13a). An X-ray is performed that shows no evidence of a foreign body. Despite the negative X-ray, an ultrasound is performed, given the degree of pain and persistent concern for the presence of a foreign body. It reveals a 2 cm hyperechoic foreign body beneath the fingernail, extending proximally past the eponychium (Figure 18.13b). The exact area to be incised is identified and infiltrated with lidocaine under ultrasound guidance. A portion of the nail is removed, in order to to retrieve the splinter (Figure 18.13c).

   This case highlights the utility of ultrasound in the detection of a foreign body. Additionally, an ultrasound may be repeated following foreign body removal, to ensure that the foreign body has been removed in its entirety.

Summary/key points

1. Ultrasound is sensitive and specific in the assessment of soft tissue infections and suspected superficial foreign bodies.
2. Ultrasound is superior to clinical evaluation alone, in the differentiation of cellulitis from abscess, and frequently changes management decisions.
3. Ultrasound is the imaging modality of choice for both radiolucent and radiopaque foreign bodies.
4. Scanning adjuncts such as a stand-off pads or a water bath can greatly assist in the scanning of pediatric patients, in improving visualization of structures, and enhancing patient comfort.
5. Ultrasound facilitates procedural guidance for abscess incision and drainage, and for foreign-body removal.

(a)

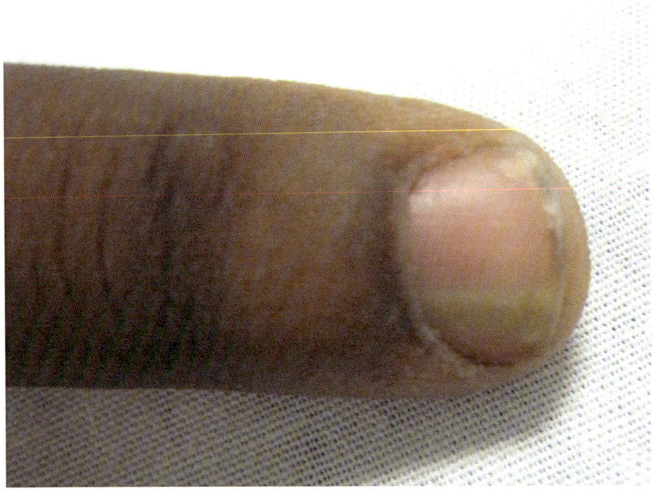

(b)

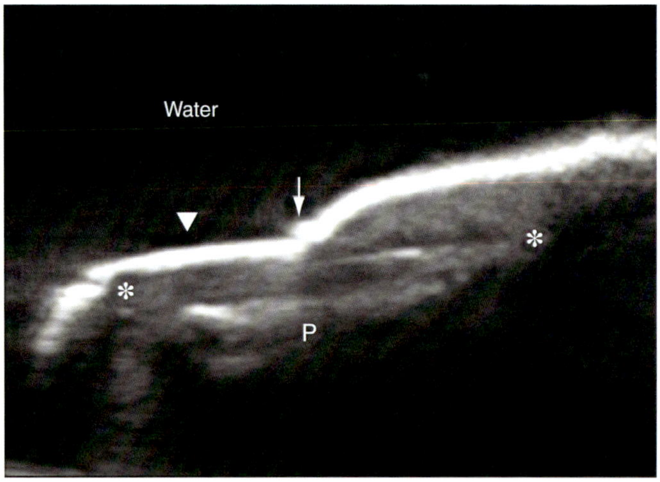

(c)

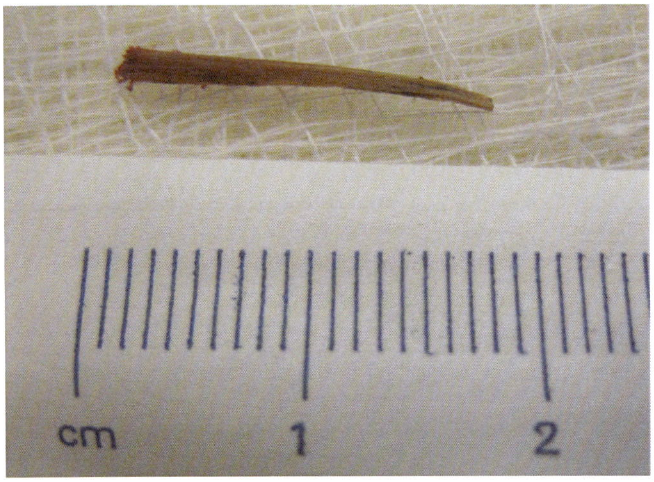

Figure 18.13 Splinter. (a) Patient's fingernail exhibiting discoloration. It is unclear whether there is a retained splinter. (b) Ultrasound image, utilizing a water bath, showing the splinter (**) under the nail (arrowhead), extending proximally past the eponychium (arrow). The splinter can be seen anterior to the phalanx (P). (c) The splinter retrieved from incision and drainage correlates with the size measured by ultrasound.

Selected references

Berger, T., Garrido, F., Green, J., *et al.* (2012) Bedside ultrasound performed by novices for the detection of abscess in ED patients with soft tissue infections. *Am J Emerg Med* **30**(8): 1569–73.

Blaivas, M., Adhikari, S. (2011) Unexpected findings on point-of-care superficial ultrasound imaging before incision and drainage. *J Ultrasound Med* **30**: 1425–30.

Friedman, D. I., Forti, R. J., Wall, S. P., *et al.* (2005) The utility of bedside ultrasound and patient perception in detecting soft tissue foreign bodies in children. *Pediatr Emerg Care* **21**(8): 487–92.

Marin, J., Alpern, E., Panebianco, N. L., *et al.* (2011) Assessment of a training curriculum for emergency ultrasound for pediatric soft tissue infections. *Acad Emerg Med* **18**(2): 174–82.

Orlinsky, M., Knittel, P., Feit, T., *et al.* (2000) The comparative accuracy of radiolucent foreign body detection using ultrasonography. *Am J Emerg Med* **18**(4): 401–3.

Ramirez-Schrempp, D., Dorfman, D. H., Baker, W. E., *et al.* (2009) Ultrasound soft-tissue applications in the pediatric emergency department: to drain or not to drain? *Pediatr Emerg Care* **25**(1): 44–8.

Sivitz, A. B., Lam, S. H., Ramirez-Schrempp, D., *et al.* (2009) Effect of bedside ultrasound on management of pediatric soft-tissue infection. *J Emerg Med* **39**(5): 637–43.

Squire, B. T., Fox, J. C., Anderson, C. (2005) ABSCESS: applied bedside sonography for convenient evaluation of superficial soft tissue infections. *Acad Emerg Med* **12**(7): 601–6.

Tayal, V. S., Hasan, N., Norton, H. J., *et al.* (2006) The effect of soft-tissue ultrasound on the management of cellulitis in the emergency department. *Acad Emerg* **13**(4): 384–8.

Teng, M., Doniger, S. J. (2012) Subungual wooden splinter visualized with bedside sonography. *Pediatr Emerg Care* **28**(4): 392–4.

Chapter

19 Orthopedics: extremity fractures, reductions, and arthrocentesis

Antonio Riera and Lei Chen

Objectives/indications

Children often present to the emergency department with orthopedic pathologies, such as bone fractures and joint effusions. Ultrasound can serve as a useful adjunct to the physical examination and radiography, in the assessment and management of pediatric orthopedic conditions. In order to identify a potential fracture or effusion, the current standard of practice is to obtain plain radiographs. If a reduction in the emergency department is necessary, either fluoroscopy or serial radiographs are utilized to confirm appropriate alignment of the reduced bone. All of these involve the exposure to ionizing radiation. However, ultrasound has the potential to decrease radiation exposure associated with the assessment and reduction of fractures.

Forearm fractures account for almost half of all pediatric fractures, with two-thirds of all forearm fractures located distally. The most common mechanism of injury is a fall on an outstretched hand, otherwise known as a "FOOSH." Children are also more at risk for forearm fractures than adults, since they have a relatively large amount of cartilage and collagen, which reduces the tensile strength of bone. This leads to certain fractures, such as greenstick fractures and torus fractures, that are not observed in adults. In addition, the presence of growth plates (physes) can be associated with fractures that are not readily visible on initial radiographic studies. These are referred to as Salter–Harris Type I fractures. It is likely that, for this reason, investigations have focused on using ultrasound to assess forearm fractures in children. Other reported sites for assessment by ultrasonography include ankle fractures, rib fractures, clavicle fractures, and even skull fractures. There are, however, limitations with ultrasound in reliably detecting compound injuries, fractures adjacent to joints, fractures involving the small bones of the hands and feet, non-displaced epiphyseal fractures (Salter–Harris I), or small injuries with a fracture line of less than 1 mm.

In addition to identifying fractures, ultrasound guidance may be helpful for fracture reductions. Ultrasound guidance offers several potential advantages over fluoroscopy or blind reduction. Most notably, there is no ionizing radiation involved. Portable ultrasound units are smaller and easier to set up, when compared to traditional, large fluoroscopy units. Finally, repeated studies can be performed relatively quickly without involving further radiation. The use of ultrasound is especially helpful in departments that do not have access to fluoroscopy, since real-time ultrasound guidance allows for the evaluation of the adequacy of reduction, obviating the need to obtain additional radiographs, which are often required with blind reductions. This is especially helpful in austere environments and developing countries, where radiographs may be limited or unavailable.

In addition, the emergency physician often encounters a child with a potential hip or knee effusion. Hip effusions may be seen in benign conditions, such as toxic synovitis, or pathologic conditions, such as with septic arthritis. When faced with a child with a suspected hip or knee effusion, it is crucial to expeditiously evaluate the child for septic arthritis, since, when left untreated, it rapidly progresses to the destruction of cartilage. The synovial fluid should be obtained for analysis and culture, which often requires irrigation in the operating room and intravenous antibiotics. Ultrasound guidance has the potential to identify such effusions, and allow for improved success and decreased complications associated with arthrocentesis.

In this chapter, we discuss the key components of point-of-care ultrasound for orthopedic injuries: the assessment and reduction of fractures, and the identification and aspiration of joint effusions.

FRACTURES: ASSESSMENT AND REDUCTION

Background

The literature has described point-of-care ultrasound as being an accurate modality to diagnose long-bone fractures. There have been several studies investigating forearm fractures. Chinnock *et al.* found similar overall success rates of ultrasound-guided distal forearm fracture reductions, when compared with traditional fracture reduction (83 vs. 80%). When compared with post-reduction radiographs, the emergency department physician-performed post-reduction ultrasound had a sensitivity of 94% and specificity of 56%. Interestingly, four patients in the traditional group required further sedation for repeat reduction, whereas there were none in the ultrasound group.

The use of point-of-care ultrasound for pediatric orthopedic emergencies is a relatively new modality, with most of the research in the emergency setting having been published within the last few years. The majority of pediatric studies have focused

Pediatric Emergency and Critical Care Ultrasound, ed. Stephanie J. Doniger. Published by Cambridge University Press.

on utilizing ultrasound to diagnose and to guide reductions for forearm fractures, since it is the most common fracture with which children present. Point-of-care ultrasound performed by trained emergency medicine physicians is both a reliable and a convenient method to diagnose and guide the reduction of forearm fractures in children. Chen *et al.* found that ultrasound revealed the correct type and location of a fracture in 96% of patients. When compared with radiographs, the sensitivity and specificity for ultrasound in the detection of forearm fractures was 97% and 100% respectively. For subjects that underwent ultrasound-guided fracture reduction, 92% had adequate alignment on post-reduction radiographs after the first attempt. Due to the severity and displacement of fractures, it was unclear whether the physical examination influenced the ultrasound results. Therefore, Chaar-Alvarez *et al.* evaluated non-angulated distal forearm fractures. When compared with traditional radiographs, ultrasound had an overall accuracy of 94%, and a sensitivity and specificity of 96% and 93% respectively. Ultrasound was actually less painful, when compared with obtaining traditional radiographs (mean Wong-Baker FACES® score 1.7 vs. 1.2, $P = 0.004$).

Further studies have shown that point-of-care ultrasound for extremity long-bone injuries may be comparable to radiography for fracture identification, in predicting the need for reduction, and in assessing adequacy of reduction. Ultrasound has been used to identify occult fractures not seen on radiographs. Performing ultrasound directly over regions of pain and swelling can be useful for diagnosing occult fractures of immature bones in pediatric-aged children. Sites of occult fractures included the elbow, knee, ischium, distal fibula, proximal femur, and humeral shaft. Ultrasonography clearly demonstrated cortical discontinuity in 92% of these cases. Indirect signs of fracture that were appreciated on ultrasound included step-off deformities, bone fragment avulsions, double-line appearance of cortical margins, and irregularities of bony surfaces. In addition, this technique has been introduced as a potential screening tool for long-bone fractures in pediatric trauma patients. A small study showed that the sensitivity was 89%, specificity 100%, with positive and negative predictive values of 100% and 97% respectively in detecting fractures. Further, ultrasound can aid in the assessment of need for fracture reduction. Barata *et al.* evaluated both upper- and lower-extremity fractures. Ultrasound detected long-bone fractures with a sensitivity of 95.3% and specificity of 85.5%. Ultrasound identified the need for reduction with a sensitivity of 100% and specificity of 97.3%. A recent study even suggests that point-of-care ultrasonography can be utilized for the evaluation of elbow fractures. Rabiner *et al.* showed a sensitivity of 98% and specificity of 70%, when ultrasound is compared with conventional radiographs. Overall, these studies suggest that ultrasound may play a larger role in decreasing the number of radiographs pediatric patients are exposed to in the future. It is also a helpful modality in situations where radiographs are of limited availability. Further studies need to be performed in order to assess the impact of this technology on actual clinical practice.

Technique

Transducer selection and orientation

When performing an assessment of long-bone fractures, a linear-array, high-frequency (5–10 MHz) transducer is typically preferred (Figure S3.3a). When the suspected injury is near a joint (such as the wrist), the conventional method for longitudinal image acquisition is to have the indicator oriented towards the direction of the closest joint.

Patient position and preparation

The patient should be in a position of comfort. Adequate analgesia should be given prior to performing ultrasonography. In order to further decrease pain, a liberal amount of ultrasound gel should be applied to the suspected fracture site, in order to minimize the degree of contact between the transducer and the injured extremity.

Ultrasound imaging

Longitudinal and transverse images should always be obtained (Figure 19.1). There are benefits to obtaining an additional "orthogonal" view during transverse image acquisition. First, this additional view allows for a more complete, multidimensional evaluation. Second, it can help guide and expedite the proper orientation for longitudinal image acquisition. Third, it may provide useful information such as the angle and direction of distal fragment displacement, providing a more complete assessment when determining the adequacy of fracture reduction.

Once the transducer is oriented in the correct position, the following findings suggest the presence of a long-bone fracture:

1. Disruption and irregularity of the hyperechoic bony cortex;
2. Step-off or "skipping" deformities;
3. Overlap or "bayoneting" of fracture fragments; and/or
4. The presence of avulsion fragments.

Ultrasound-guided procedure

Ultrasound may be performed during, and following the reduction of fractures. Dynamic imaging throughout the reduction provides a real-time visualization and reassessment of the reduction technique (Figure 19.2).

Training and education

Training and competency for emergency physicians in ultrasound-guided fracture identification and fracture reduction should be established. Until proper credentialing standards are in place, point-of-care ultrasound for these types of injuries should be verified with a confirmatory study by the radiology department. A collaborative approach with the institution's orthopedic surgery and radiology departments should be undertaken and will help ensure that high-quality images are obtained and interpreted by experienced providers in a timely fashion for the betterment of patient care.

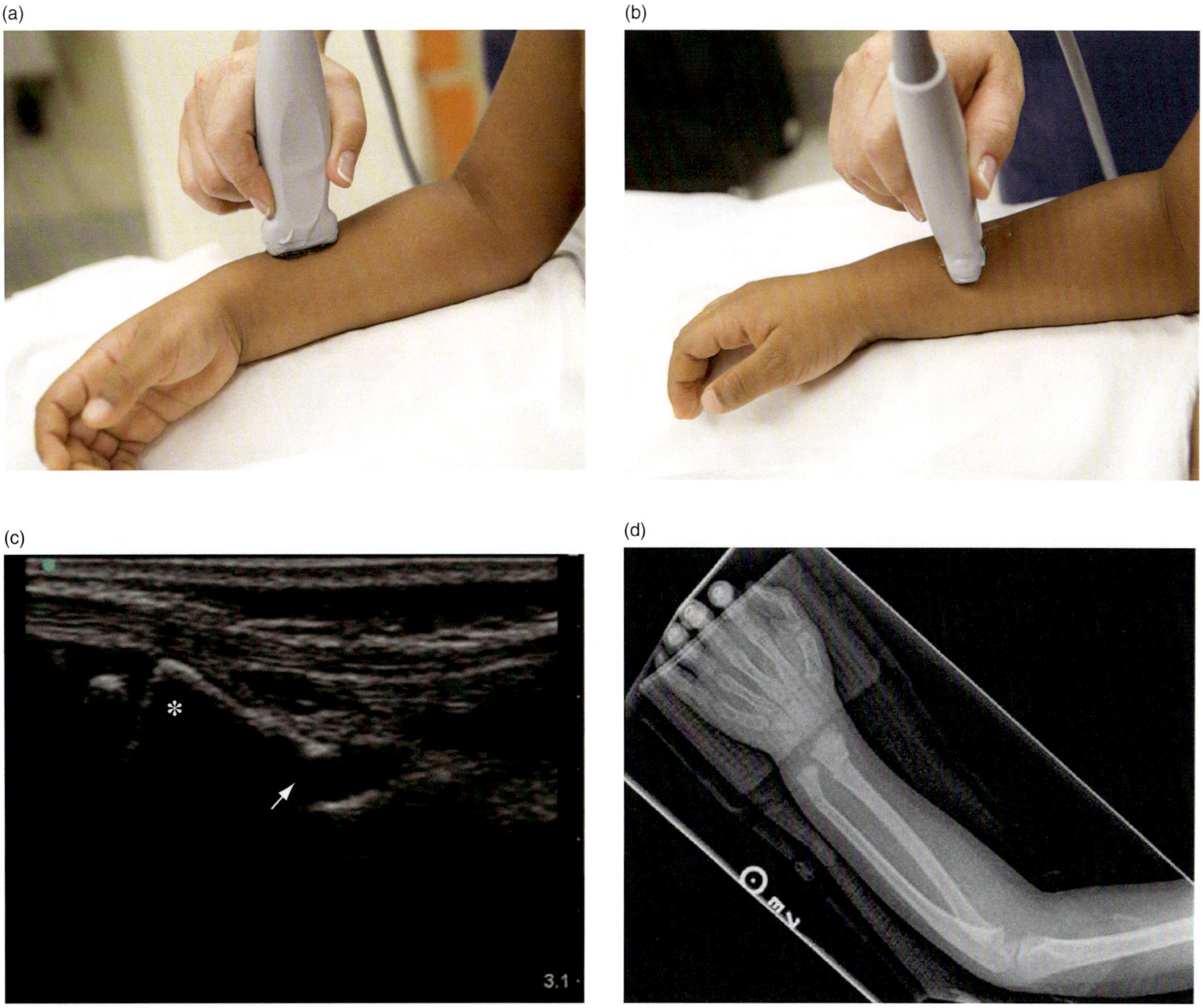

Figure 19.1 Distal forearm fracture. (a) Transducer orientation along the long-axis of the bone, with the indicator oriented distally towards the wrist. (b) Transducer orientation along the short-axis or transverse view of the bone. (c) Longitudinal ultrasound image showing a disruption in the bony cortex, consistent with a fracture site and displacement of the distal fragment. The metaphysis (*), with the echogenic epiphysis, is adjacent to the fracture site. (d) Forearm radiographs performed later confirmed the presence of both a distal radius and ulna fracture.

Specific scanning techniques

Forearm

Anatomy

The forearm comprises the radius and ulna running in parallel and held together by an interosseus membrane and a network of various flexor and extensor muscles (Figure 19.3).

Technique

A short-axis, or transverse view is obtained by placing the transducer perpendicular to the bone (Figure 19.4a). Longitudinal views in the volar, lateral, and dorsal planes may be required to best localize and characterize the fracture site.

Lower extremity

Anatomy

The lower extremity comprises the tibia and fibula running in parallel. Like the forearm, there is an intraosseous membrane (Figure 19.5).

Technique

At least two views of the lower-extremity long bones should be obtained. Position the transducer parallel to the long-axis of the bone and scan above and below the suspected fracture site. Then, orient the transducer perpendicular to the bone, in order to obtain the short-axis view. Again, scan above and below the suspected site of fracture. Disruption of the bony cortex may be visualized as a “step off” of the hyperechoic bone cortex (Figure 19.6).

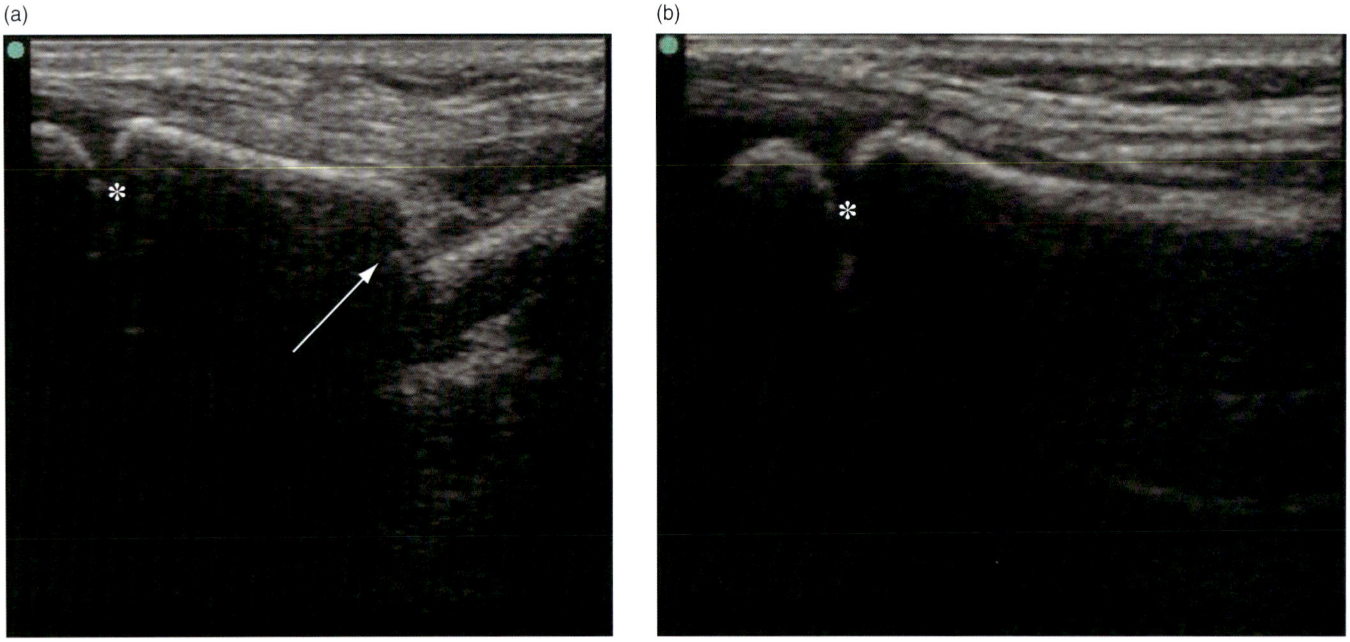

Figure 19.2 Distal radius fracture reduction. (a) Longitudinal ultrasound images of a distal radius fracture (arrow). (b) Longitudinal view of the radius, following a closed reduction. Note that the cortical discontinuity (arrow) in the pre-procedural ultrasound is not evident on the post-reduction image. The physis is visible on both images with the epiphysis (*).

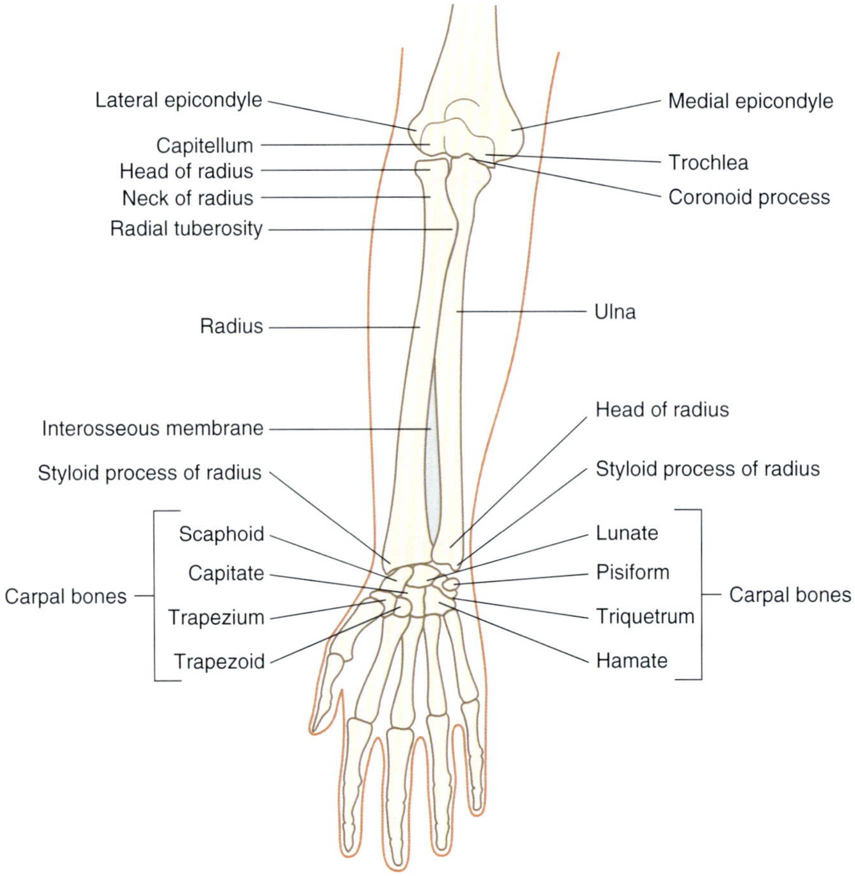

Figure 19.3 *Artwork created by Emily Evans © Cambridge University Press.*

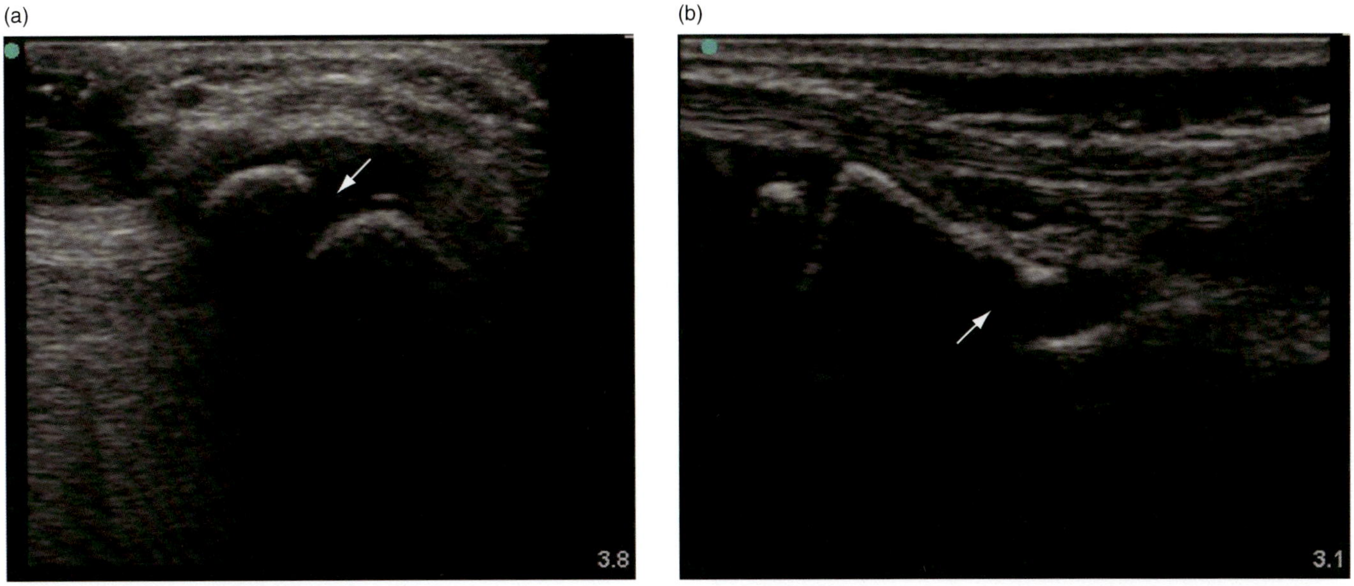

Figure 19.4 Forearm fracture. (a) Short-axis or transverse view of the radius. (b) Long-axis or longitudinal view of the radius. Note the disruption and displacement of the hyperechoic bony cortex (arrow) consistent with a fracture.

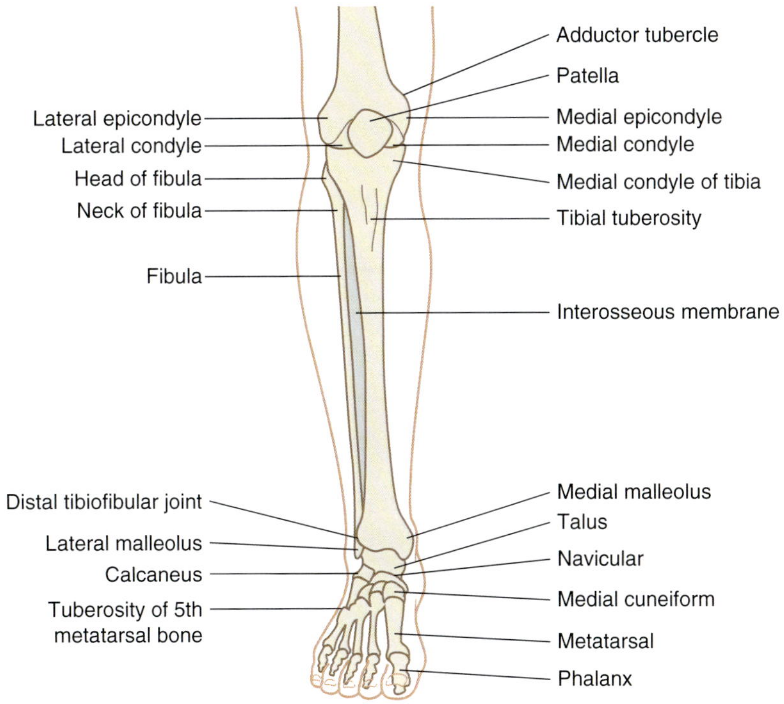

Figure 19.5 *Artwork created by Emily Evans © Cambridge University Press.*

Scanning tips

Pitfalls

- Careful consideration of the transducer indicator orientation should be taken into account during image interpretation.
- Growth plates or small bones may be confused for fractures.
- Not using sufficient analgesia or gel may lead to patient discomfort and the inability to obtain adequate ultrasound images.

Tips to improve scanning

✓ Use liberal amounts of ultrasound gel in order to minimize pain, or consider using a stand-off pad or water bath, when appropriate.

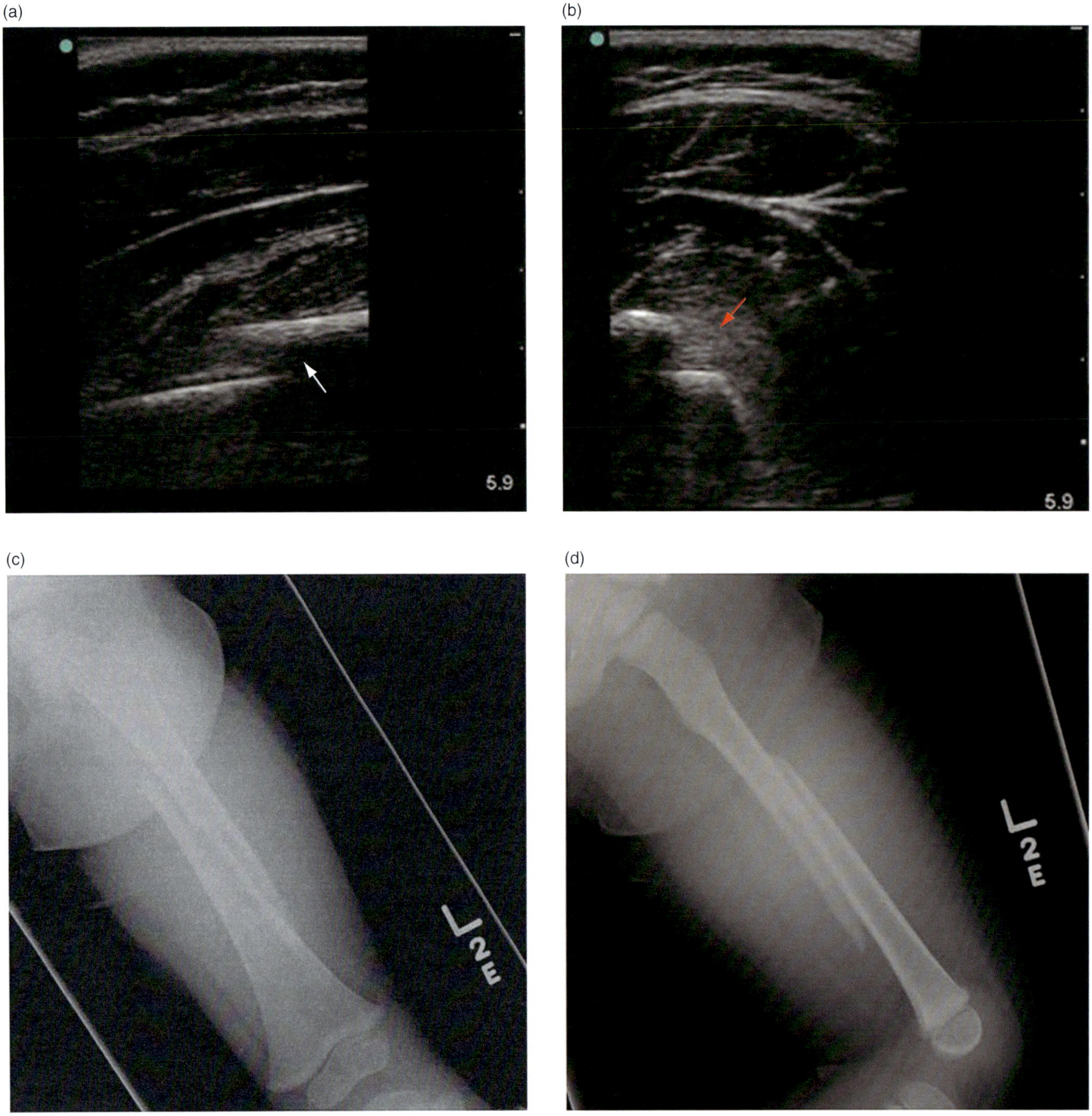

Figure 19.6 Femur fracture. (a) Longitudinal ultrasound view of the femur, with a notable deep discontinuity of the hyperechoic line (arrow), representing a fracture. (b) The fracture site (arrow) is again visible on the transverse view. (c,d) Corresponding AP and lateral radiographs of the mid-shaft, spiral femur fracture.

- ✓ Always obtain both longitudinal and transverse views in order to maximize sensitivity. An additional "orthogonal view" may be helpful.
- ✓ Knowledge of the distal forearm anatomy and growth plates should help guide interpretation of "gaps" between hyperechoic bony structures.
- ✓ It is often helpful to perform ultrasonography on the contralateral unaffected side for comparison, especially when findings are in question.

ARTHROCENTESIS

Background

In adult patients, ultrasound has been used to identify joint effusions, and to distinguish them from soft tissue abnormalities. Ultrasound has also been utilized to guide arthrocentesis. Wiler *et al.* compared the use of ultrasound-guided knee arthrocentesis to a landmark approach. No significant difference in arthrocentesis success rates were noted between the two groups, and no significant difference was found in the amount of fluid obtained. However, the ultrasound-guided group had lower overall pain scores, a shorter total procedure time, and greater confidence in procedural performance by novice providers.

In pediatric patients, ultrasound has been used to detect hip effusions. Tsung *et al.* presented a case series which suggested that point-of-care ultrasonography might expedite decision-making and the disposition of children with hip effusions in the emergency department. More recently, Viera *et al.* showed that, with focused training, PEM physicians are able to use point-of-care ultrasound to accurately identify hip effusions in pediatric patients. For the emergency physician provider, these findings suggest that point-of-care ultrasonography is more useful in identifying, rather than ruling out, pediatric hip effusions. When compared with radiographs, performing ultrasonography on *symptomatic* hips had a sensitivity and specificity of 85% and 93% respectively, and negative and PPVs of 88% and 92% respectively. For *all* hips, the sensitivity and specificity were 80% and 98% respectively, and negative and PPVs were 93% and 92% respectively.

Technique

Transducer selection and orientation

When performing a sonographic assessment for joint effusions, a linear-array, high-frequency (5–10 MHz) transducer is typically preferred (Figure S3.3a). In those patients with a greater amount of soft tissue (i.e. obesity, greater muscle mass, etc.), a lower-frequency (2–5 MHz), curvilinear transducer may be required.

Patient position and preparation

The patient should be lying in a position of comfort. In order to identify joint effusions, no sterile preparation is required. However, in order to perform ultrasound-guided arthrocentesis, the site and transducer should be prepared in a sterile fashion.

Ultrasound imaging

When performing ultrasonography to identify joint effusions, it is important to identify sonographic landmarks specific to that location. Bone will appear hyperechoic with posterior shadowing, while cartilage will appear hypoechoic. Further, it is also crucial to localize surrounding structures including nerves and blood vessels, especially when preparing to perform ultrasound-assisted or ultrasound-guided arthrocentesis. Finally, an effusion will appear as a hypoechoic or anechoic fluid collection. It is often useful to compare the patient's contralateral, unaffected side.

Ultrasound-guided procedure

Once an effusion has been identified, the optimal site for needle entry should be determined based on the largest amount of hypoechoic fluid visualized, and avoidance of surrounding neurovascular structures. First, the region should be prepared in typical sterile fashion. The transducer should also be prepared in a sterile fashion, with a sterile sleeve (Figure S3.7). Then, local anesthetic should be administered prior to the arthrocentesis. Local anesthetic should be administered to the epidermis and subcutaneous tissues, along the trajectory of planned needle insertion. Care should be taken to identify surrounding blood vessels in order to prevent injury during the procedure. Next, under direct visualization, a 20- or 22-gauge needle can be advanced through the long-axis of the ultrasound beam from a skin entry site at the inferior border of the transducer (Figure S3.11). The needle is advanced at an angle of about 45° from the skin towards the anterior synovial recess. Finally, the synovial space has been entered once the syringe starts to fill with fluid.

Specific scanning techniques

Hip

Anatomy

The hip joint is a synovial joint formed by the articulation between the femoral head and the cup-shaped acetabulum of the pelvis (Figure 19.7). The joint is enclosed within a strong, fibrous capsule. Extracapsular ligaments, such as the iliofemoral anteriorly and the ischiofemoral posteriorly, provide further protection and stability. Multiple muscle attachments surround the hip joint, which allow for various movements including flexion, extension, abduction, adduction, and internal and external rotation.

Technique

With the patient lying in the supine position, the linear transducer is typically oriented in an oblique sagittal plane parallel to the long-axis of the femoral neck. The patient's leg can be positioned in slight abduction and external rotation (Figure 19.8a). A slight internal rotation may relax the anterior portion of the joint capsule, allowing for fluid to collect in the anterior compartment of the joint capsule.

Prior to transducer placement, identify the greater trochanter as a surface anatomic landmark. The transducer is placed parallel to the long-axis of the femoral neck, which can be found just below the inguinal ligament and lateral to the femoral vessels. The surrounding landmarks of the femoral triangle should be identified.

The transducer is positioned with the indicator pointing superomedially, along an imaginary line extending from the greater trochanter towards the umbilicus (Figure 19.8a). Once the transducer is oriented in the correct position, sonographic landmarks of the hip joint are easily found. The femoral head can be identified as a curved, hyperechoic line. The femoral neck can be identified as a hyperechoic

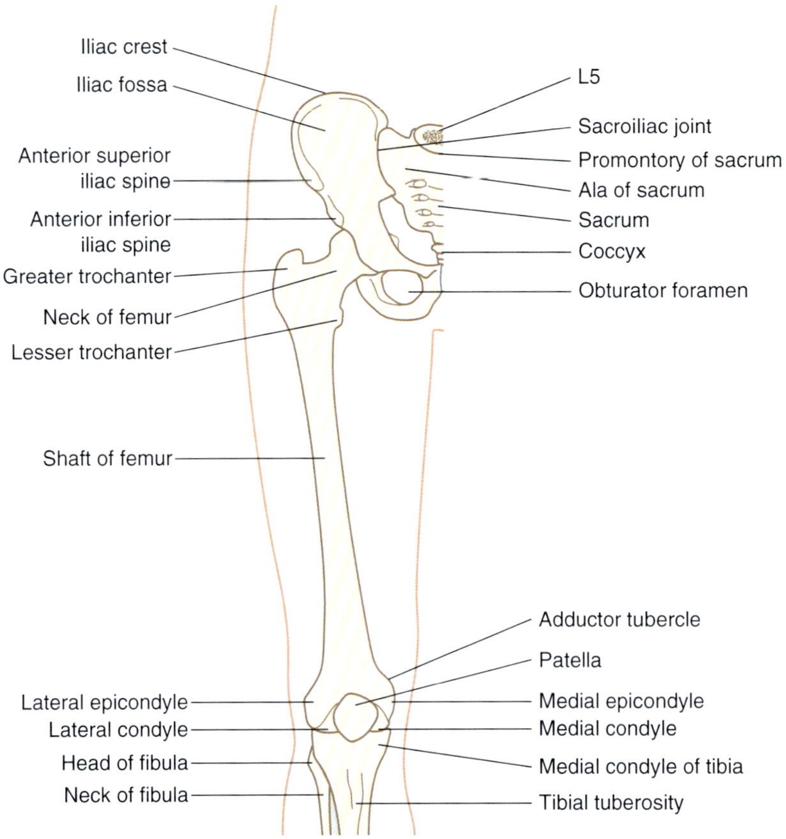

Figure 19.7 *Artwork created by Emily Evans © Cambridge University Press.*

line lateral to the femoral head and slanting downward. The articular cartilage between the femoral head and acetabulum is seen as a hypoechoic strip, above the femoral head (Figure 19.8b).

In the normal hip joint, the joint capsule appears as a hyperechoic band that runs above the femoral head and the proximal femoral neck (Figure 19.8b). In the presence of a hip effusion, the joint capsule is displaced and there is a hypoechoic or anechoic fluid collection in the anterior synovial recess just distal to the femoral head and anterior to the femoral neck (Figure 19.8c). Criteria for the diagnosis of a hip effusion include:

1. an anterior–posterior fluid collection of greater than **5 mm**, or
2. a fluid collection **difference of greater than 2 mm** when compared to the contralateral hip.

Ultrasound-guided procedure

During ultrasound-guided arthrocentesis, it is crucial to avoid the femoral vessels (Figure 19.9). This is typically achieved by placing the transducer in a transverse orientation, below the inguinal ligament with the indicator oriented towards the patient's left. After the medially located femoral vessels are identified, the transducer can once again be repositioned as described, with the indicator oriented superiomedially along the long-axis of the femoral neck.

Knee

Anatomy

The knee joint (Figure 19.10) is a complex joint formed by three articulations: the medial femoral condyle to medial meniscus, the lateral femoral condyle to lateral meniscus, and the patella to femur. The joint is supported by four collateral ligaments (anterior, posterior, medial, and lateral) and is stabilized by the quadriceps tendon, the pes anserinus, the semimembranosus muscle, the popliteal muscle and ligament, the iliotibial tract, and the biceps femoris muscle. This intricate collection of joint attachments allows for its wide range of movements, including flexion, extension, internal and external rotation, abduction, and adduction. The knee has the largest synovial cavity out of all the joints in the body, and extends from the suprapatellar bursa to the intra-articular space. The suprapatellar bursa lies deep to the quadriceps tendon and has a direct communication with the knee joint. This is clinically important, because any fluid collection of the suprapatellar bursa implies that a knee effusion is also present. This is in contrast to the prepatellar bursa, which has no direct communication with the knee joint.

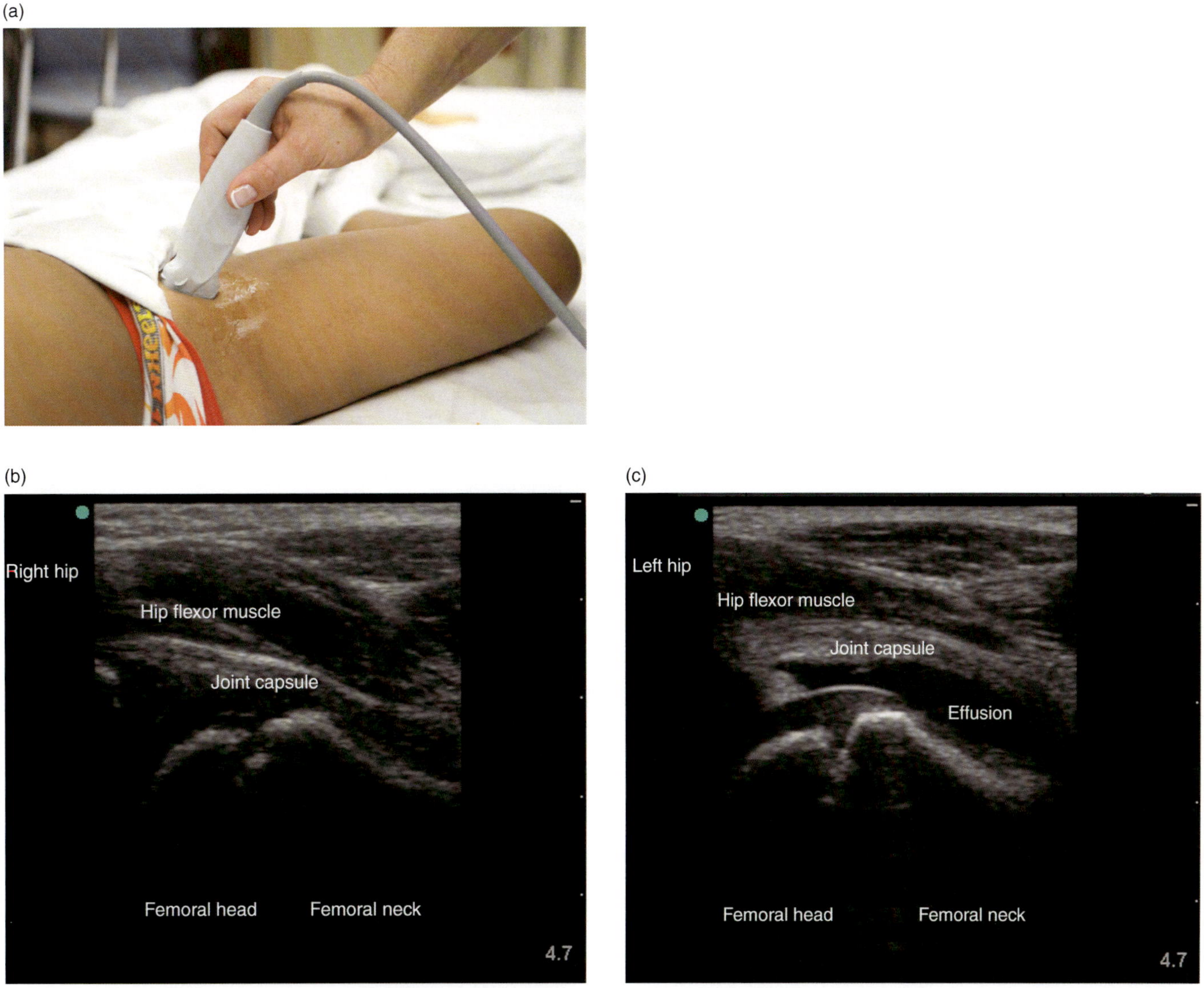

Figure 19.8 Hip imaging, longitudinal view. (a) Transducer positioning: longitudinal view along the long-axis of the femoral neck. The indicator is oriented towards the acetabulum. (b) Ultrasound of the hip along the long-axis of the femoral neck. A normal hip image from the patient's unaffected side is shown. The hyperechoic joint capsule is identified superficial to the femoral head. (c) In the affected side, the hip effusion (*) is visualized as an anechoic fluid collection displacing the joint capsule and tracking along the femoral neck. Note the similar image orientation represented by the left and right sides.

Technique

The anterior approach provides excellent visualization of the joint space, considering the lack of blood vessels and nerves that run in this region. With the patient lying in the supine position, a towel roll is placed under the knee to provide slight 30–45° flexion (Figure 19.11a). Prior to transducer placement, identify the patella as a surface anatomic landmark. The transducer is placed superior to the patella, longitudinally along the midline over the quadriceps. The indicator is oriented proximally, or towards the patient's head. Gentle pressure should be applied, as excessive downward force on the transducer could compress the suprapatellar bursa and mask a small effusion.

Once the transducer is oriented in the correct position, sonographic landmarks of the knee joint are easily found. In a normal knee joint, the quadriceps tendon and its attachment to the patella should be visualized (Figure 19.11b). The patella can be identified as a hyperechoic line, with a posterior acoustic shadow. The quadriceps tendon can be identified as a thick, hyperechoic stripe immediately adjacent to the patella. Below the quadriceps tendon, the suprapatellar bursa can be identified as a thin, hypoechoic line. An enlargement of this hypoechoic bursa **by more than 2 mm** is indicative of a knee effusion. In order to optimize image acquisition of a fluid collection, one can move the transducer to the medial or lateral side of the patella along the same longitudinal plane. In addition, gentle pressure over a suspected effusion often reveals compressibility, and is useful in the identification of an effusion (Figure 19.12).

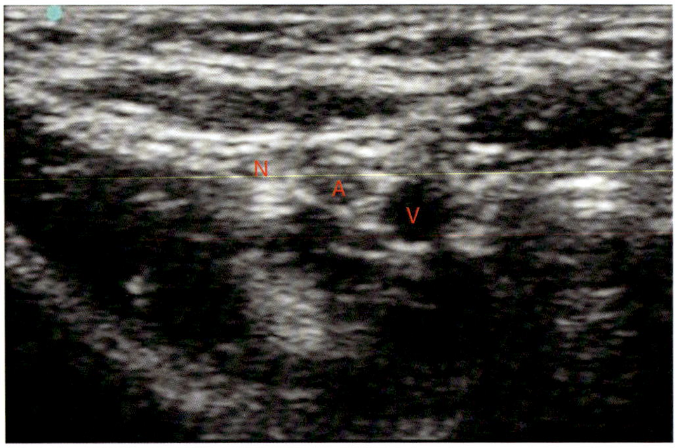

Figure 19.9 The femoral triangle. Transverse ultrasound image of the right femoral vein (V), artery (A), and nerve (N) (medial to lateral) in a three-year-old boy. These structures should be identified in order to avoid inadvertent injury during aspiration of a hip effusion.

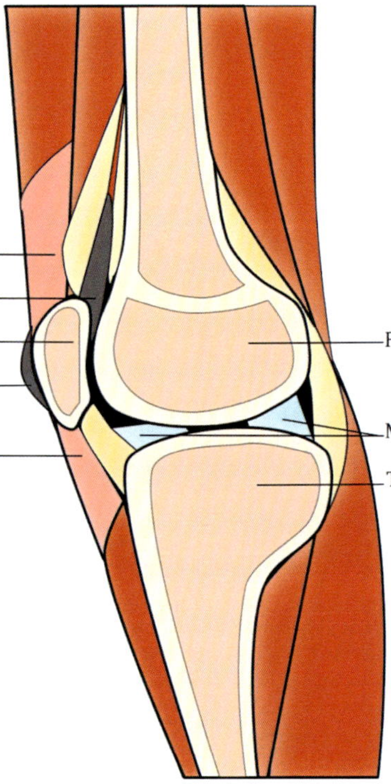

Figure 19.10 Anatomy of the knee.

(a)

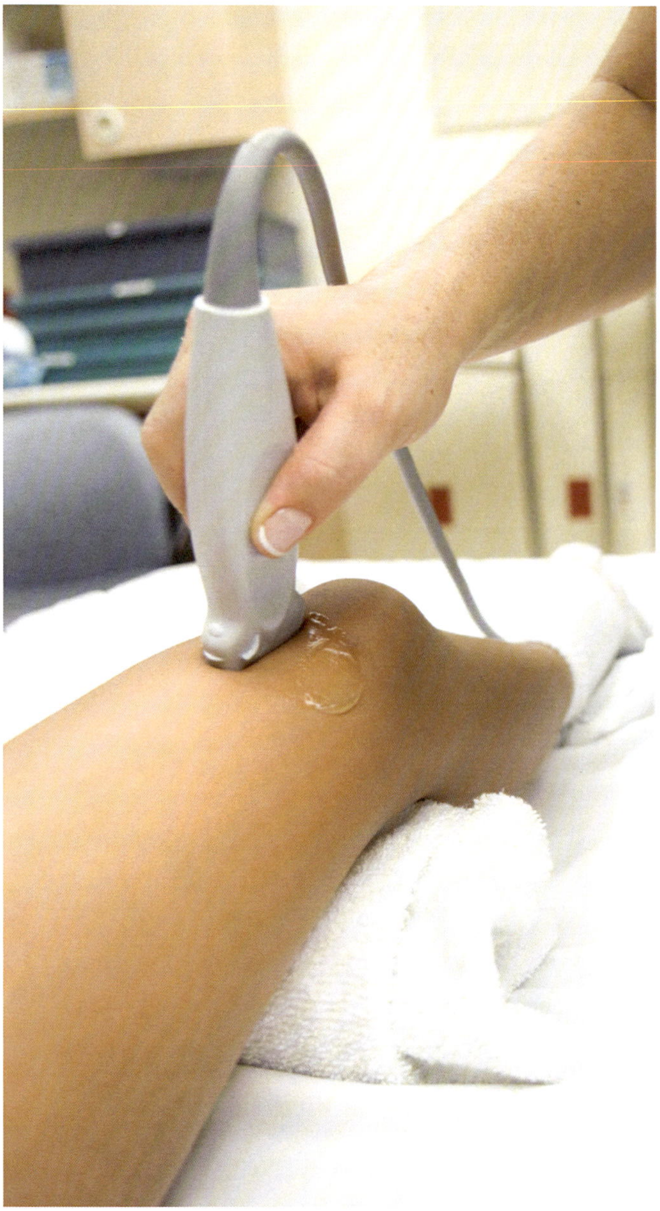

Figure 19.11 Knee imaging, suprapatellar views. (a) Transducer positioning: longitudinal suprapatellar view. Note the indicator is oriented towards the patient's head. (b) Ultrasound image of a normal right knee. The hyperechoic quadriceps tendon is seen extending inferiorly to the patella (arrowhead) attachment site. Note the acoustic shadowing posterior to the patella. (c) Ultrasound image of an abnormal left knee, in the same patient. The affected knee has a large, anechoic suprapatellar fluid collection (*) between the quadriceps tendon and the distal femur.

Ultrasound-guided procedure

Once a knee effusion has been identified, ultrasound can help locate the area of the largest fluid collection on either side of the patella. The supralateral approach is generally regarded as the safest and most effective technique. If a large effusion is present, a small towel roll can be placed under the knee to create about 15–20° of flexion. The midpoint of the lateral border of the patella should then be identified. For ultrasound assistance, the needle entry site may be marked with a pen just below the patellar border. For real-time ultrasound guidance, the needle should be visualized as it enters the synovial space. An 18-gauge needle attached to a 30 mL syringe is then inserted perpendicular to the long-axis of the leg, behind the midpoint of the patella. Care should be taken to direct the needle slightly posterior to the patella and slightly cephalad towards the intra-condylar notch. Inserting or directing the needle in a more caudal approach may lead to a greater risk of injury to the meniscus and surrounding cartilage. Pull back on the syringe plunger while advancing the syringe. As the synovial space is entered, the syringe will fill with fluid.

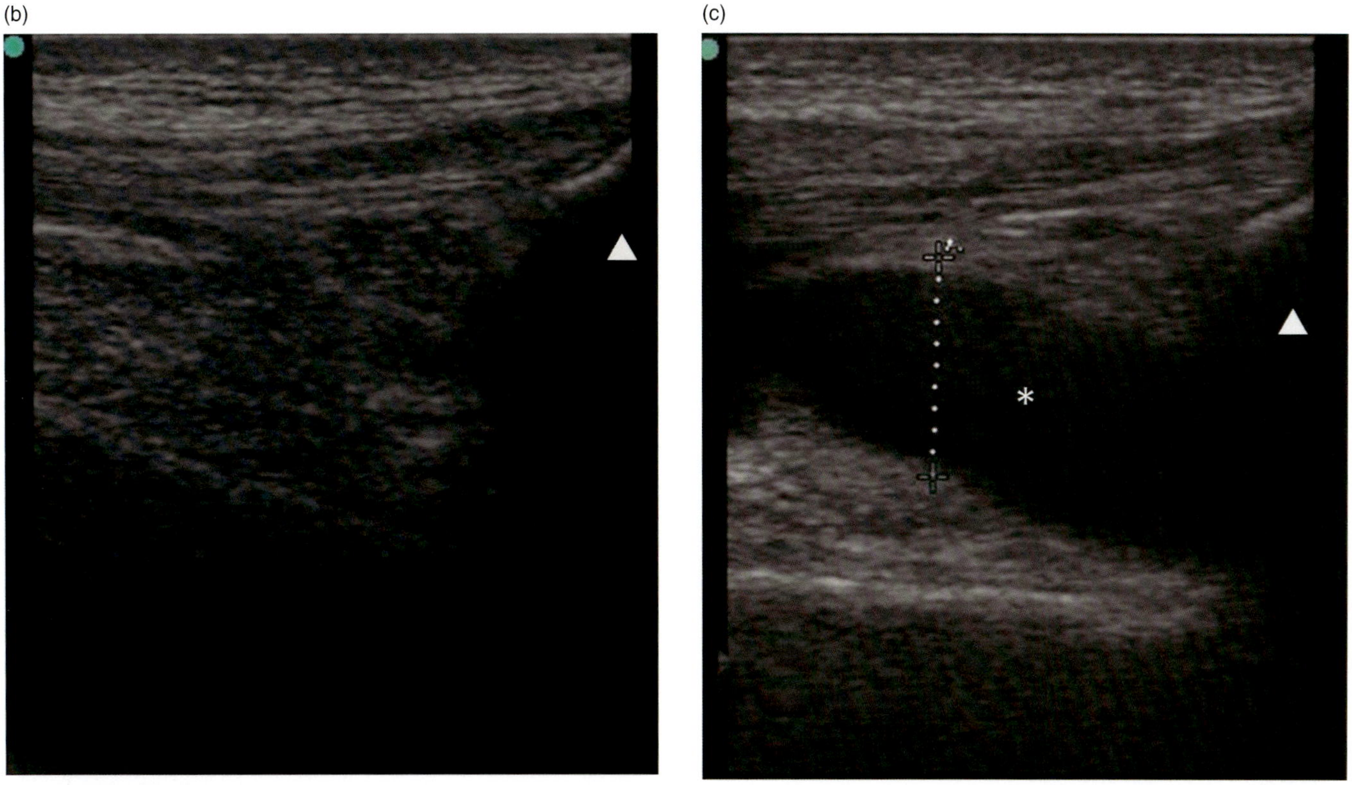

Figure 19.11 (cont.)

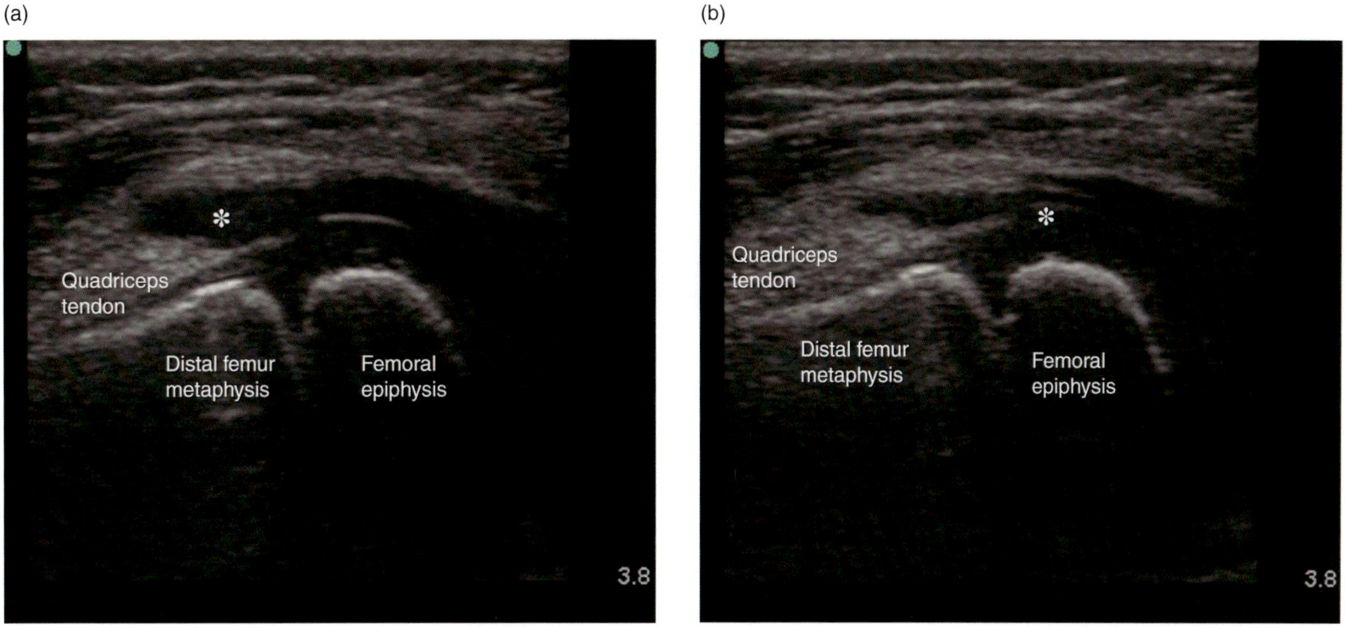

Figure 19.12 Suprapatellar effusion. (a) Suprapatellar view with anechoic fluid collection (*) consistent with an effusion. (b) Compression by the ultrasound transducer shows compressibility of this fluid collection (*).

Scanning tips

Pitfalls

- If one applies too much pressure on the transducer, small or superficial effusions may be compressed, leading to a false-negative interpretation.
- The hypoechoic articular cartilage over the femoral head may be mistaken as an effusion. In a true hip effusion, the hypoechoic collection will cross the femoral head and extend inferiorly along the course of the femoral neck.
- Arthrocentesis is contraindicated if cellulitis is present over the site of needle entry. Other relative contraindications

to performing arthrocentesis include known or suspected bacteremia, coagulopathic states, and the presence of prosthetic joints – in which case risks and benefits of the procedure should be discussed with an orthopedic surgeon.

- Smaller effusions may be more difficult to aspirate with the knee in a semi-flexed position. In such instances, performing the arthrocentesis with the knee in full extension may yield greater fluid acquisition success rates.
- The patella is ossified from a single center, which usually makes its radiographic appearance in the second or third year, but may be delayed until the sixth year of life. This limitation is important to note during suprapatellar image acquisition and interpretation in young children and infants.

Tips to improve scanning

✓ Remember to orient the transducer at an oblique angle in order to obtain an adequate longitudinal view of the femoral neck.

✓ Locating femoral vessels medially is an important landmark.

✓ Avoid exerting excessive pressure, which may mask the presence of a small effusion.

✓ Scan the knee while in 30–45° of flexion.

✓ In order to optimize image acquisition of a knee effusion, one can move the transducer to the medial or lateral side of the patella along the same longitudinal plane.

✓ When performing joint arthrocentesis, pull back on the plunger. As the synovial space is entered, the syringe will fill with fluid.

Cases

1. A six-year-old boy presents to the emergency department with right knee swelling and a limp. One week prior to presentation, he was playing outdoors and his mother noticed a "pimple" on the skin, just below the patella. His mother "popped the pimple" and expressed clear fluid. Three days later, the knee became red and swollen. The child has had tactile fevers at home which have been treated with acetaminophen. On the day of presentation, the knee had become extremely swollen; the child developed considerable pain, and began limping. On physical examination, the patient is afebrile. The right knee has good range of motion, but there is erythema, warmth, and swelling over the patella extending down to the site of the initial pustular lesion. There is concern for the presence of a joint effusion. Knee radiography reveals no fracture or evidence of osteomyelitis. An ultrasound examination reveals a 1 × 0.8 cm lesion corresponding with the pustule,

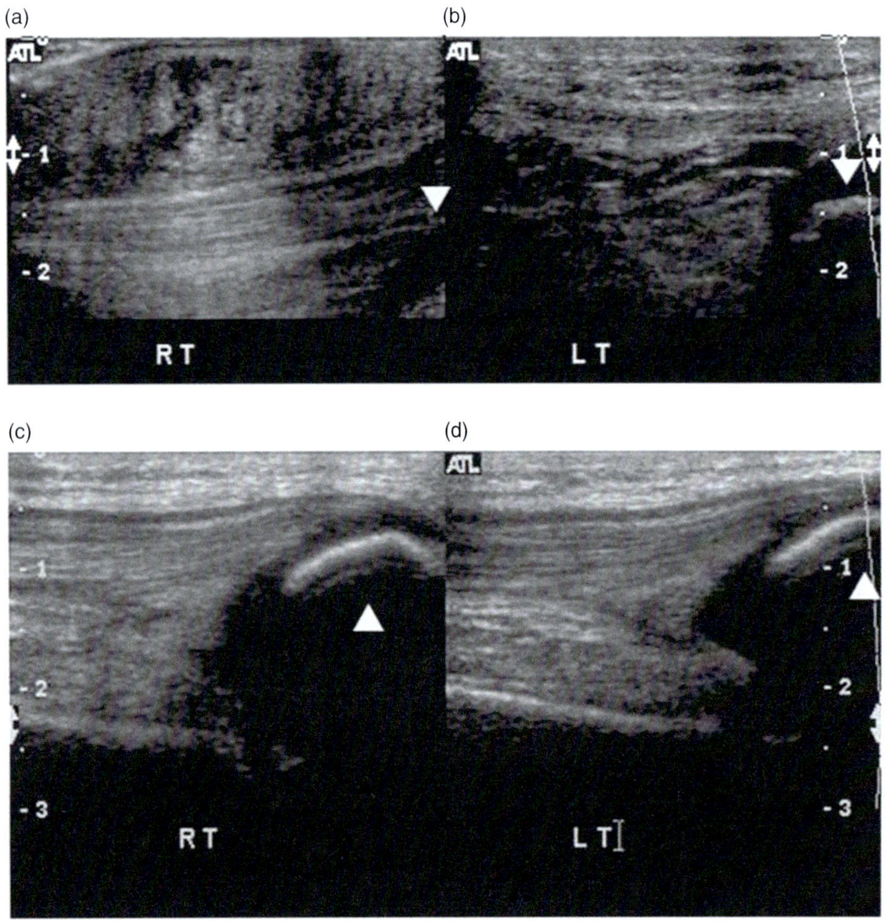

Figure 19.13 **Case 1: normal prepatellar ultrasound.** (a,b) Transverse view of bilateral anterior knees over the prepatellar space. (c,d) Longitudinal suprapatellar views of bilateral knees are negative for effusion. The patella (arrowhead) can be seen as hyperechoic with posterior shadowing.

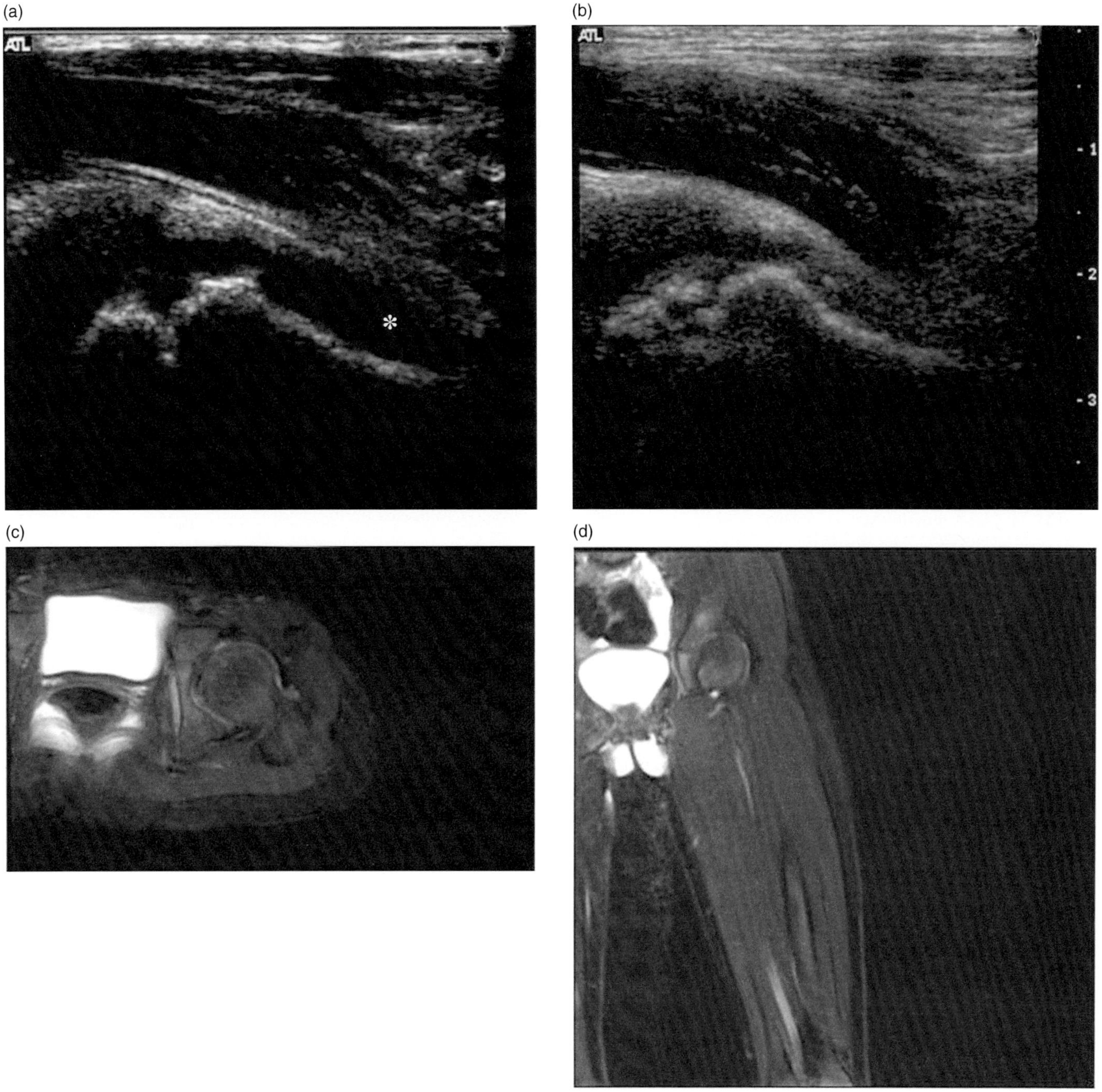

Figure 19.14 Case 2: left hip effusion. (a) Ultrasound of the left hip reveals a moderate-sized effusion coursing anterior to the femoral neck. (b) A comparison ultrasound is performed on the contralateral hip, demonstrating the absence of an effusion. (c,d) MRI of the left hip (T2-weighted images) showing edematous changes of the acetabulum, consistent with osteomyelitis.

without a significant abscess collection (Figure 19.13a,b), and the absence of a suprapatellar effusion (Figure 19.13c,d). A diagnosis of prepatellar bursitis/cellulitis is suspected. After orthopedic consultation, the decision is made to perform an incision and drainage over the superficial pustule and to defer arthrocentesis. A copious amount of purulent discharge is noted, and the cavity is packed with ¼ inch gauze. The culture subsequently grows MRSA, and the patient is successfully treated with a course of clindamycin.

This case highlights the utility of ultrasound in evaluating the presence of an effusion. Given the absence of an effusion in this patient, unnecessary procedure was avoided. The clinician and consultant were able to determine confidently that the infection did not extend into the joint.

2. A five-year-old girl presents to the emergency department with left hip pain and fever to 38.9 °C at home. The hip pain has become gradually worse over the course of the past 24 hours and has progressed to the point that she can no longer bear weight. On physical examination, the patient is well appearing with temperature of 38.4 °C and otherwise has normal vital signs for her age. Significant left

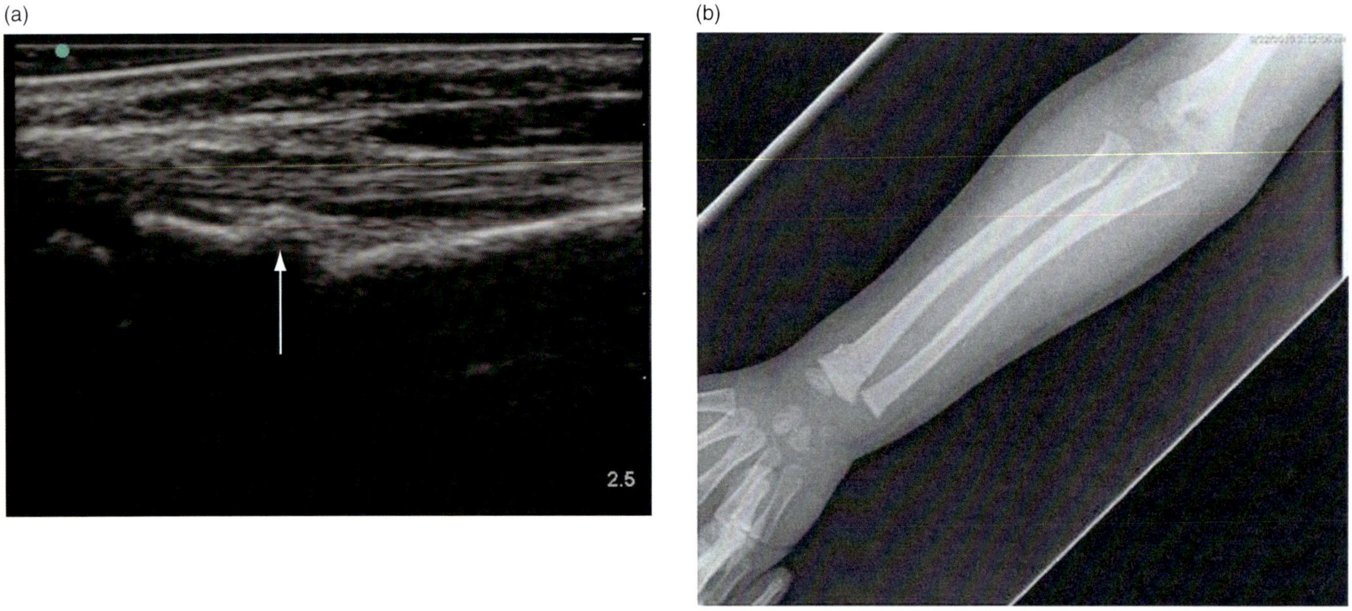

Figure 19.15 **Case 3: torus fracture**. (a) The longitudinal ultrasound image shows a buckling of the metaphysis (arrow). (b) Corresponding radiograph showing the fracture. Note the extension of the fracture line into the growth plate.

hip pain is elicited with internal and external rotation. There is no overlying erythema, warmth, or swelling, and the remainder of her extremity and joint examination is unremarkable. Hip radiography is normal. A point-of-care ultrasound examination is performed, which reveals a moderate left hip effusion with synovial thickening (Figure 19.14a). Aspiration is performed under ultrasound guidance with the following results: red blood cell count: 650 RBC/μL, white blood cell count: 23,100 WBC/μL (61% granulocytes), and a negative gram stain. After orthopedic consultation, the decision is made to defer operative management. She is given a dose of intravenous oxacillin, and is admitted. Almost immediately after being admitted, she regains full range of motion and weight bearing of her left hip. She is presumed to have either transient synovitis or an inflammatory arthritis and is then discharged home. However, after 48 hours, the child is seen by her pediatrician, who notes asymmetric hip range of motion. An MRI is obtained, which reveals marrow and subperiosteal edema of the left acetabulum consistent with osteomyelitis (Figure 19.14c,d). A peripherally inserted central catheter (PICC) line is placed and she receives a four-week course of intravenous oxacillin. She recovers uneventfully, with normal inflammatory markers at completion of her antibiotic course.

Point-of-care ultrasonography can identify the presence of a hip effusion. However, based on sonographic findings, one often cannot distinguish between a benign transient synovitis, and a more serious etiology such as septic hip or osteomyelitis.

3. An eight-year-old boy presents to the pediatric emergency department after falling on an outstretched arm while running (FOOSH). On physical examination, there is no obvious deformity, but there is significant tenderness to palpation overlying the distal radius and ulna, with decreased pronation and supination secondary to pain. A point-of-care ultrasound is performed which identifies a torus fracture (Figure 19.15a). This finding correlates with the radiograph which is obtained (Figure 19.15b). A volar splint is placed, and the patient is referred to orthopedics as an outpatient for follow-up.

   This case shows the use of point-of-care ultrasonography in one of the most common of pediatric fractures. It is important to scan in both longitudinal and transverse planes, and interrogate all regions that are painful.

Summary/key points

1. Linear, high-frequency transducers are utilized for the assessment of fractures, for ultrasound-guided fracture reductions, the identification of a joint effusion, and for guidance for arthrocentesis.
2. Bone is easily identified via ultrasound as a linear, hyperechoic structure. Any discontinuity or irregularity in the cortex is highly suggestive and usually consistent with a fracture or injury to the bony cortex.
3. Fractures may be identified by: disruption or irregularity of the hyperechoic bony cortex, step-off or "skipping" deformities, overlap or "bayoneting" of fracture fragments, and/or the presence of avulsion fragments.
4. Effusions are easily identified via ultrasound as a collection of hypoechoic or anechoic fluid.
5. A hip effusion is defined as an anterior–posterior fluid collection of greater than **5 mm**, or a fluid collection **difference of greater than 2 mm** when compared to the unaffected contralateral hip.

Selected references

Barata, I., Spencer, R., Suppiah, A., *et al.* (2012) Emergency ultrasound in the diagnosis of pediatric long-bone fractures. *Pediatr Emerg Care* **28**: 1154–7.

Chaar-Alvarez, F. M., Warkentine, F., Cross, K., *et al.* (2011) Bedside ultrasound diagnosis of nonangulated distal forearm fractures in the Pediatric Emergency Department. *Pediatr Emerg Care* **27**(11): 1027–32.

Chen, L., Kim, Y., Moore, C. L. (2007) Diagnosis and guided reduction of forearm fractures in children using bedside ultrasound. *Pediatr Emerg Care* **23**: 528–31.

Chinnock, B., Khaletskiy, A., Kuo, K., *et al.* (2011) Ultrasound-guided reduction of distal radius fractures. *J Emerg Med* **40**(3): 308–12.

Patel, D. D., Blumberg, S. M., Crain, E. F. (2009) The utility of bedside ultrasonography in identifying fractures and guiding fracture reduction in children. *Pediatr Emerg Care* **25**: 221–5.

Rabiner, J. E., Khine, H., Avner, J. R., *et al.* (2013) Accuracy of point-of-care ultrasonography for diagnosis of elbow fractures in children. *Ann Emerg Med* **61**(1): 9–17.

Sinha, T. P., Bhoi, S., Kumar, S., *et al.* (2011) Diagnostic accuracy of bedside emergency ultrasound screening for fractures in pediatric trauma patients. *J Emerg Trauma Shock* **4**(4): 443–5.

Tsung, J. W., Blaivas, M. (2008) Emergency department diagnosis of pediatric hip effusion and guided arthrocentesis using point-of-care ultrasound. *J Emerg Med* **35**: 393–9.

Vieira, R. L., Levy, J. A. (2010) Bedside ultrasonography to identify hip effusions in pediatric patients. *Ann Emerg Med* **55**: 284–9.

Wiler, J. L., Constantino, T. G., Filippone, L., *et al.* (2010) Comparison of ultrasound-guided and standard landmark techniques for knee arthrocentesis. *J Emerg Med* **39**(1): 76–82.

Chapter

20 Peripheral nerve blocks

Jason W. Fischer

Objectives/indications

Regional anesthesia provides effective and safe analgesia for otherwise challenging pain control scenarios. However, regional anesthesia has failed to gain popularity or clinical prominence in pediatric patients for several reasons. Traditional techniques of nerve localization, which include the use of surface landmarks, nerve stimulation, and paresthesia induction, are often inaccurate and unpleasant for patients. In addition, anatomic assumptions based on surface landmarks may lead to unreliable nerve blockade, unpredictable onset times, longer procedure duration, and the risk of serious adverse events.

The use of ultrasound guidance in regional anesthesia provides the opportunity to greatly improve pain control management for pediatric patients. Current ultrasound technology allows the physician to visualize peripheral nerves and their surrounding anatomy in real time. Growing enthusiasm for point-of-care ultrasound and the emergence of this technology has led to a renaissance in peripheral nerve blockade (PNB), and an evolution in the treatment of emergent pediatric pain. The forearm nerve block, femoral nerve block, and popliteal sciatic nerve block in particular, are easily adopted and can create an immediate impact in patient care. The goal of the ultrasound-guided nerve blocks is to provide safe and effective pain control for pediatric patients.

Background

The clinical benefits of regional anesthesia have long been recognized in the medical literature. The majority of studies of point-of-care ultrasound for peripheral nerve blocks in the emergency department have been in adult patients. Peripheral nerve blockade has demonstrated fewer serious side effects, shorter emergency department lengths of stay, less monitoring, enhanced cost-effectiveness, and greater patient satisfaction when compared to alternative methods of pain control. These methods include local anesthesia, parenteral opioids, procedural sedation, or general anesthesia.

Studies have shown that emergency physicians can reliably identify target nerves, and distinguish them from adjacent structures. Ultrasound guidance has many advantages over conventional blind or landmark techniques of regional anesthesia. The real-time ultrasound visualization of the target nerve allows the physician to confirm that the anesthetic agent is being delivered to the appropriate location, at an adequate volume. The circumferential spread of agent around the nerve is assured. This greatly increases both success rates and the reliability of onset times and block duration. The reliability gained eliminates the possibility that a second or third block attempt will be required to achieve successful anesthesia. This saves considerable procedure time, when compared to the traditional blind techniques, which often require multiple attempts, followed by periods of observation and testing, to achieve a successful block.

Most importantly, ultrasound guidance leads to improved patient safety with decreased complication rates. Ultrasound guidance impacts complication rates and patient safety in two ways. First, the visualization of anesthetic agent location and spread reduces the volume of anesthetic agent needed for a successful block. This is often a significant reduction of the anesthetic volume classically used in blind techniques. The precise delivery of less anesthetic decreases the risk of local anesthetic neurotoxicity or pressure-induced neural ischemia from intraneural injection. The real-time visualization of the needle tip and the target nerve decreases neuronal injury caused by mechanical nerve trauma or nerve ischemia. Moreover, direct visualization allows for the identification of structures surrounding the target nerve. This reduces the risk of accidental vascular puncture with subsequent hematoma formation. Moreover, this visualization decreases intravascular injection of anesthetic agents, which can lead to serious adverse effects such as seizure, hypotension, or cardiac arrest.

This technology has only begun to emerge as a viable pain management alternative to conventional pain management control measures such as procedural sedation. Further study is needed to characterize the impact and limitations of this technique in the pediatric emergency department setting. However, ultrasound-guided peripheral nerve blocks have shown great promise and have the potential to revolutionize pain management in injured children.

Technique

Transducer selection and orientation

A high-frequency (10–15 MHz) linear transducer is ideal for all pediatric PNBs (Figure S3.3a). This allows for higher resolution and better visualization of the superficial target nerve(s) and

Pediatric Emergency and Critical Care Ultrasound, ed. Stephanie J. Doniger. Published by Cambridge University Press.

surrounding structures. Other transducers may be utilized, but image quality may be reduced or inadequate for the procedure. For instance, a low-frequency, curvilinear transducer may be required for the imaging of the sciatic nerve within the popliteal fossa in obese patients. However, care must be taken when using low-frequency transducers with needle insertion and injection given that the image is curved.

The transducer should be adequately cleaned prior to and following its use. A sleeve or transparent covering of the user's choosing may be applied to the transducer (Figures S3.5–7).

Patient position and preparation

For each PNB, the patient is placed in a position of comfort that allows the physician access to the target nerve. Infants, toddlers, and young children may require an extremity board or a papoose in order to limit movement of the affected limb. The ultrasound monitor and the injection site are then aligned in the operator's direct line of vision to eliminate any unnecessary head movement during the procedure, and to allow for ease of needle redirection when necessary (Figure S3.4a). The operator should be in an ergonomic position of comfort to perform the procedure. Finally, the patient's skin should be cleaned and prepared similar to that of other ultrasound-guided procedures.

Patient and caregiver satisfaction and comfort can be increased through the use of adjunctive agents prior to any PNB. For instance, topical anesthetic creams, ointments, and sprays, can be applied to the skin to decrease discomfort with needle puncture. In addition, the intranasal delivery of anxiolytics such as midazolam (0.4 mg/kg, maximum 10 mg), or analgesics such as fentanyl (1.5 μg/kg), can effectively decrease patient anxiety or pain prior to the nerve block. Their rapid onset of action, and the absence of requiring vascular access, make these agents ideal adjuncts. Finally, caregivers should be invited to remain present and offer support during the procedure, as they are able and without disruption. Specialized resources such as child life specialists should be utilized whenever available.

Ultrasound imaging

Procedural success is partially dependent upon obtaining adequate image quality in nerve localization and the identification of surrounding anatomy. This is often best accomplished by selecting the manufacturer software preset for nerve blocks. Further manipulation of depth, gain, and focal zones may be necessary.

Peripheral nerves appear in the long-axis, or longitudinal, plane as hyperechoic or bright, tubular structures. They may be difficult to distinguish from layers of soft tissue, muscle, and ligaments. In the short-axis, or transverse plane, the peripheral nerve appears round or elliptical with hypoechoic fascicles in a hyperechoic homogeneous background. This is often described as "honeycomb" in appearance (Figure 20.1). It is important to distinguish nerves from surrounding vascular structures. This may be easily accomplished with grayscale compression or the color Doppler function.

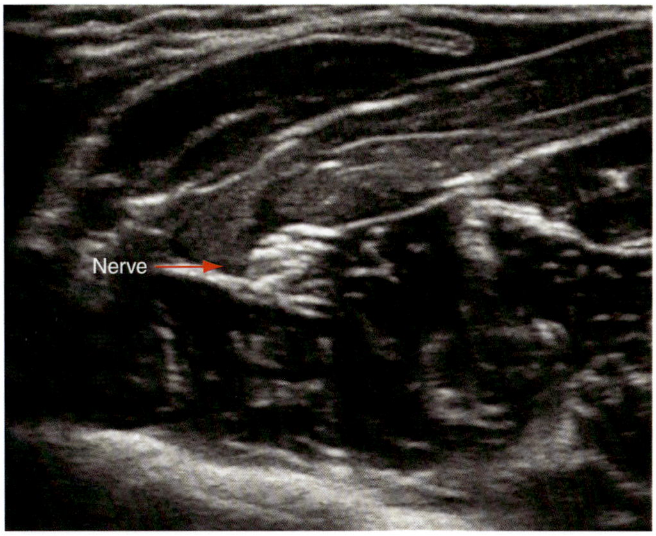

Figure 20.1 **A peripheral nerve in short-axis or transverse view**: hypoechoic fascicles in a hyperechoic background, often described as "honeycomb" in appearance.

Ultrasound-guided procedure

The selection of an anesthetic agent should be tailored to the specific goals of the PNB. In general, lidocaine provides faster onset times, while bupivacaine and ropivacaine provide longer duration of action. This distinction becomes important when longer durations of anesthesia are preferred, such as with complex lacerations. Situations in which shorter durations of anesthesia are preferred include fractures with a risk of compartment syndrome. There is no evidence to date that any particular anesthetic agent is superior to another in terms of efficacy, or that any significant benefit is gained by mixing different agents together.

First, one must determine the appropriate anesthetic agent and calculate the maximum amount to be used. Ultrasound guidance has allowed providers to deliver lower volumes of anesthetic agent than were classically used with the landmark techniques without sacrificing nerve block quality. For this reason, current dosing recommendations are based upon the maximum safe dose of the agent, and do not reflect the optimal dose for an effective block (Table 20.1). It is important to note that the volume of distribution of anesthetic agents is greater in children than in adults, allowing them to tolerate higher doses on a mg/kg basis without peak plasma levels reaching toxic thresholds. The exception is an infant less than six months of age. In this age group, the volume of distribution is reduced due to lower protein-binding capacity and depressed hepatic metabolism. It is for these reasons that the dose of amide agents should be reduced by 50% in this age group, to safely reduce peak plasma levels and to avoid systemic toxicity.

Next, the appropriate needles should be chosen. A small-bore needle such as a 27- or 30-gauge needle is generally used for a pediatric PNB. The needle length is dependent upon the depth of the optimal injection site, and should be measured during sonographic nerve identification. A small needle size decreases patient pain during skin puncture and limits the injection rate, both of which are major sources of patient discomfort. However, a smaller needle size can affect the ease of needle visualization by ultrasound. A smaller needle can be challenging to maintain in plane, requiring both very subtle hand movements and a high degree of hand–eye coordination. One may also use injection syringes or similar syringe attachments, which may aid in needle control.

Then, the operator should determine the path for the needle that best avoids surrounding structures. The needle is then inserted using the long-axis, or in-plane, approach (Figure 20.2a) in order to maximize the visualization of the needle and its tip. The needle will appear longitudinally on the screen in this orientation, as it travels under the transducer (Figure 20.2b). Real-time ultrasound visualization of the needle tip is essential during the entire procedure, in order to eliminate the possibility of accidental puncture of surrounding vascular structures. The needle tip location can be confirmed by injecting small amounts of anesthetic agent as the needle is advanced. This is called the "step down" approach, in which hypoechoic spread should occur at the needle tip. Failure to visualize this phenomenon indicates that the needle tip is out of plane and must be found and redirected, prior to further needle advancement or injection at the target nerve.

Occasionally, a short-axis, or out-of-plane, approach is necessary when performing a PNB on small infants (Figure 20.3). The needle may be too short to reach the target nerve from the edge of the transducer using the in-plane approach, depending upon the size of the transducer, the needle, and the patient. Care should be taken using the short-axis, or out-of-plane, approach in this circumstance, as it is much more challenging to correctly identify the needle tip, which appears as a hyperechoic or bright dot. The "step down" approach is often helpful in identifying the needle tip in the short-axis.

Finally, it is critical at the time of injection to precisely deliver the anesthetic agent circumferentially around the entire target nerve for optimal efficacy. Ideally, the target nerve will float or bathe in the hypoechoic anesthesia, making the nerve's hyperechoic structure more prominent and distinct (Figure 20.4). The syringe plunger should always be drawn back prior to any injection, to avoid intravascular injection.

Table 20.1 Recommended dosing of anesthetic agents.

Anesthetic agent	Recommended dose (mL/kg)	Onset[a]	Duration[b] (h)
Lidocaine 2%	0.25–0.5	Fast	0.75–2
Bupivacaine 0.25%	0.25–0.5	Intermediate	1.5–8
Ropivacaine 0.2%	0.25–0.5	Intermediate	1.5–8

[a] Onset times are described qualitatively relative to other common anesthetic agents.
[b] Wide variation in duration depending on age of patient, location, technique, and whether combined with an adjuvant.

Training and education

The ability to successfully execute a PNB using ultrasound guidance requires that the provider be trained both to identify the target nerve, and to deliver the anesthetic agent accurately and safely. It is strongly advised that appropriate training should be sought for both aspects of the procedure on phantom models, prior to performing in the clinical setting. Special attention should be given to the physical act of needle insertion and injection while in plane with the ultrasound transducer, using a single hand (the single-operator method). The quantity and quality of training to ensure overall procedural competence and proficiency remains unclear.

Specific scanning techniques

Forearm nerve block

Anatomy

It is important to become familiar with the anatomy of the forearm (Figure 20.5). Vascular structures run throughout the forearm, and are located close to the radial and ulnar nerves within their neurovascular bundles. These arteries and veins must be identified, in order to avoid unnecessary puncture and associated complications.

(a)

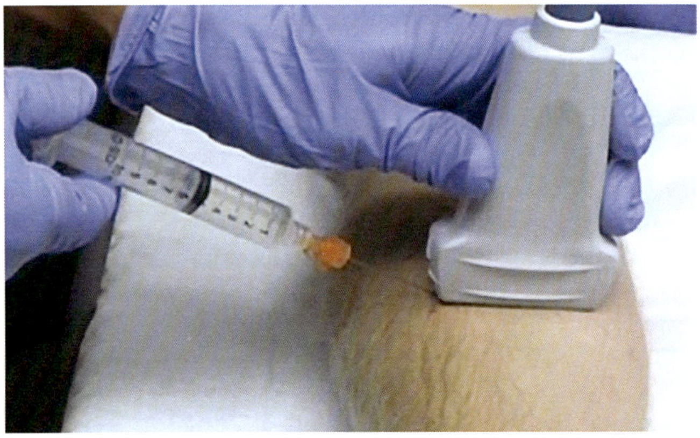

(b)

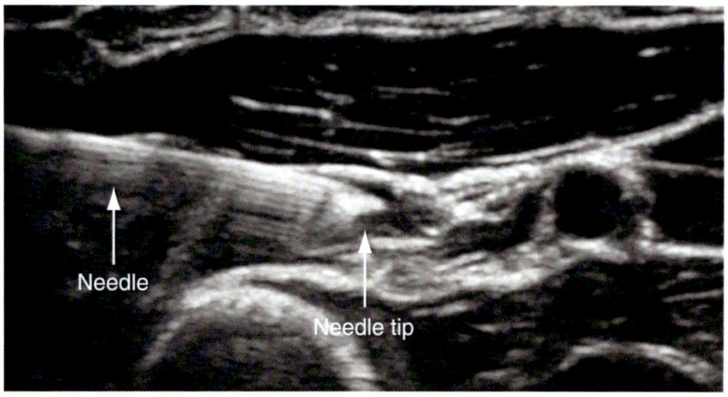

Figure 20.2 The in-plane or long-axis approach to peripheral nerve blocks. (a) The preferred needle orientation is shown in plane with the transducer. (b) The needle appears longitudinally on the screen. *Courtesy of William Soares, MD.*

(a)

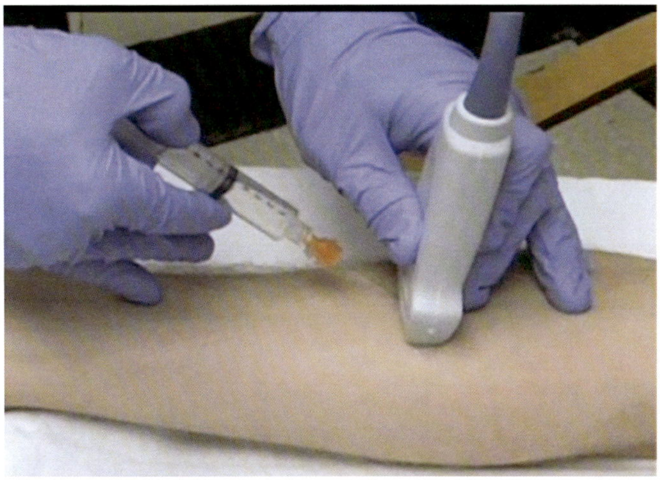

(b)

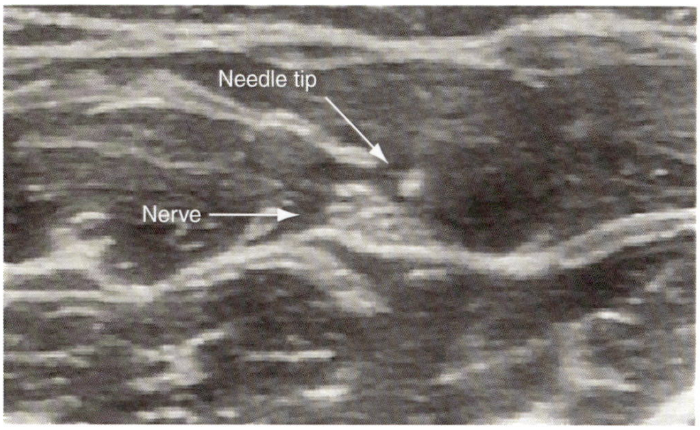

Figure 20.3 The out-of-plane or short-axis needle orientation. (a) Needle orientation is shown out-of-plane with the transducer. (b) The needle appears as a hyperechoic or bright dot on ultrasound.

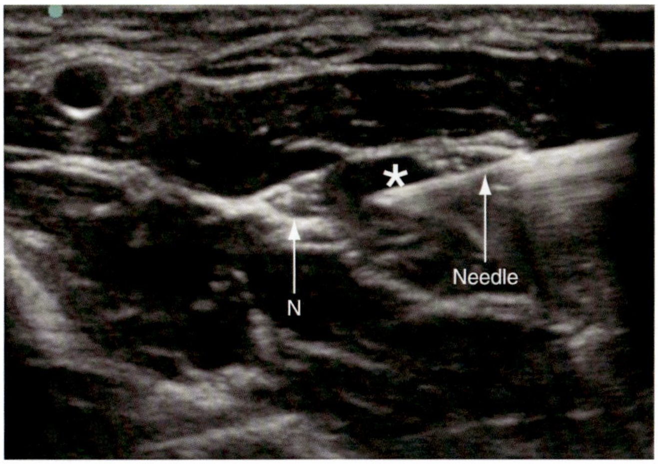

Figure 20.4 Injection of anesthetic agent circumferentially around a target nerve. Anesthetic agent is shown being delivered at the median nerve (N). The anesthetic agent appears hypoechoic or dark (*) on the ultrasound screen. Ideally, anesthetic agent will surround the target nerve at completion of the procedure. *Courtesy of William Soares, MD.*

The innervation of the hand must be conceptualized in three dimensions. Three nerves innervate the hand: the median nerve, the ulnar nerve, and the radial nerve. The selection of these nerves for blockade is dependent upon the location within the hand that the provider intends to anesthetize (Figure 20.6). For example, a deep palmar laceration may require a radial nerve blockade and a median nerve blockade, in order to guarantee the complete anesthesia of all deep structures. The routine blockade of all three nerves ensures a successful outcome, regardless of anatomical variation of the nerves and their innervation within the hand.

Technique

In order to sonographically identify the three target nerves in the forearm, a systemic approach is utilized. The transducer is placed at the distal forearm and moved proximally to the mid-forearm (Figure 20.7). Once the nerve is identified, the transducer should be firmly anchored. Even subtle movement of the transducer may result in the loss of needle visualization and prolonged time to complete the procedure.

The radial nerve is identified on ultrasonography using a two-step procedure. First, the transducer is placed over the radial artery at the wrist, so that the artery can be seen in a transverse orientation, or cross-section. Then, the transducer is moved proximally to the mid-forearm, keeping the radial artery in the middle of the screen. The radial nerve is located adjacent to the radial side of the radial artery (Figure 20.8). Targeting the radial nerve in the mid-forearm is often adequate for a successful block. If the radial nerve is blocked too distally, a branch of the radial nerve may be missed, leading to incomplete anesthesia.

The ulnar nerve is identified using the same two-step procedure in identifying the radial nerve. However, the transducer is initially placed at the distal ulnar artery. The ulnar nerve is visualized adjacent to the ulnar side of the ulnar artery (Figure 20.9).

The median nerve does not have an associated median artery, except in rare anatomical variants. For this reason, the transducer is centered over the volar wrist, between the ulnar and radial arteries, and then moved proximally. The median nerve is visualized in the mid-forearm among the flexor digitorum muscle bundles (Figure 20.10).

In order to enhance the visualization of the forearm nerves, it may be necessary to immobilize the forearm in infants and toddlers. Immobilizing the fingers of their affected hand may eliminate movement of the flexor muscles and tendons within the forearm, which can radically alter the position of all three target nerves. In addition, target nerves may be difficult to identify in the distal forearm, due to their close proximity to flexor tendons, which have a similar ultrasonographic appearance. Visualizing the target nerve more proximally usually resolves this issue.

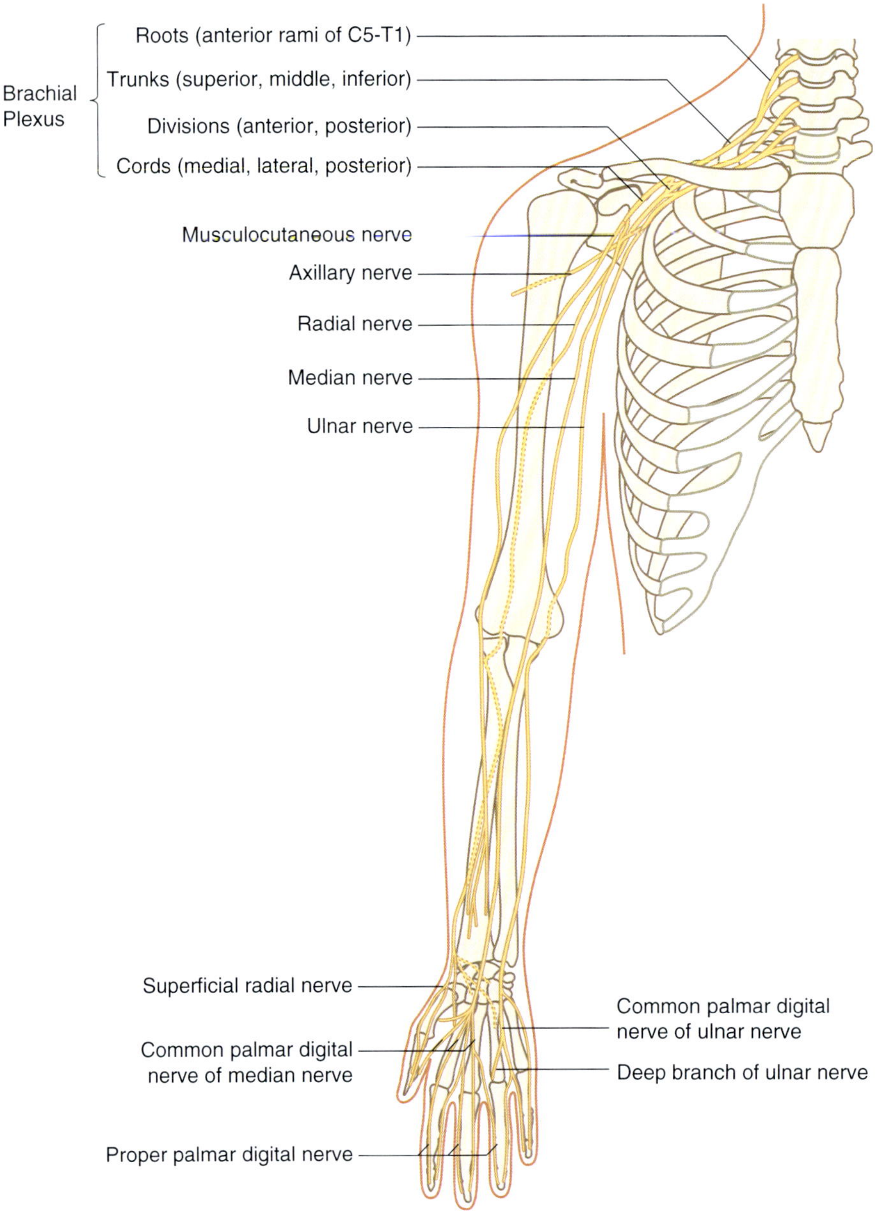

Figure 20.5 Anatomy of the forearm. It is important to be familiar with the radial nerve, the ulnar nerve, and the median nerve, and their associated neurovascular bundles. *Artwork created by Emily Evans © Cambridge University Press.*

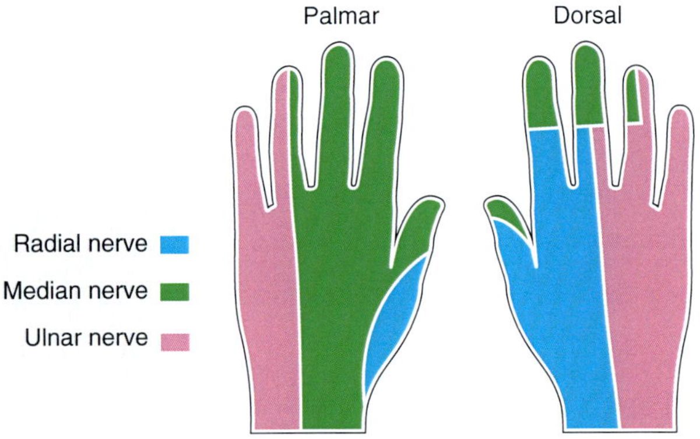

Figure 20.6 The nerve innervation of the hand. Shown is the median, radial, and ulnar nerve distribution of the hand. *Artwork created by Emily Evans © Cambridge University Press.*

Femoral nerve block

Anatomy

The femoral nerve block is selected for anesthesia of the thigh and hip. The femoral nerve innervates the skin and soft tissue of the anterior thigh (Figure 20.11a) and the majority of the femur osteotome (Figure 20.11b). The region of anesthesia can be increased for the proximal hip and thigh by blocking the lateral femoral cutaneous and obturator nerves in addition to the femoral nerve. The femoral neurovascular bundle contains the femoral nerve, the femoral artery, and the femoral vein and is found in the femoral triangle (Figure 20.12a). These prominent femoral vessels travel on a parallel course, adjacent to the femoral nerve. The fascia lata is the most superficial fascial layer, and is superficial to the neurovascular structures. The fascia iliaca lies deep to the fascia lata surrounding the

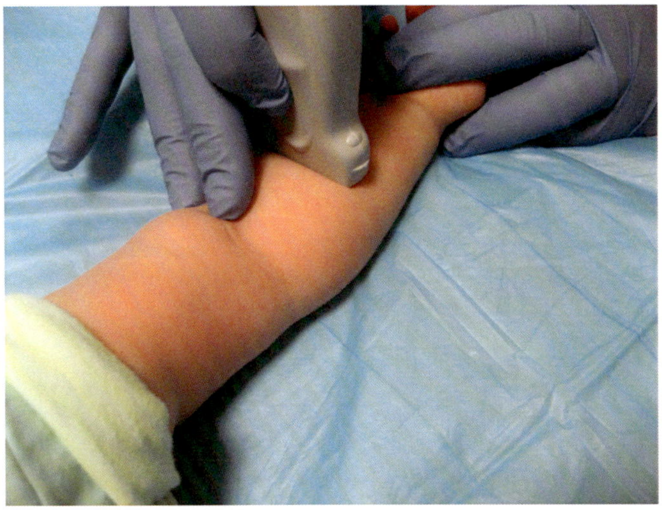

Figure 20.7 Transducer placement, the median nerve. Transducer placement is shown on the forearm for the identification of the median nerve.

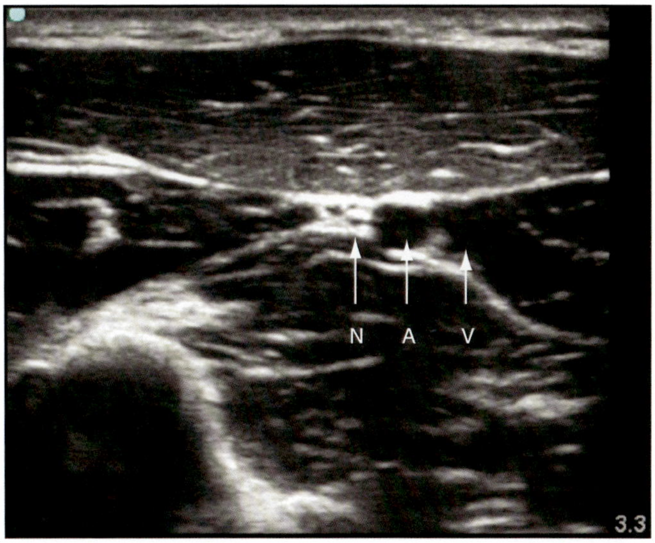

Figure 20.8 The radial nerve (N) is located on the radial side of the radial artery (A) and radial vein (V).

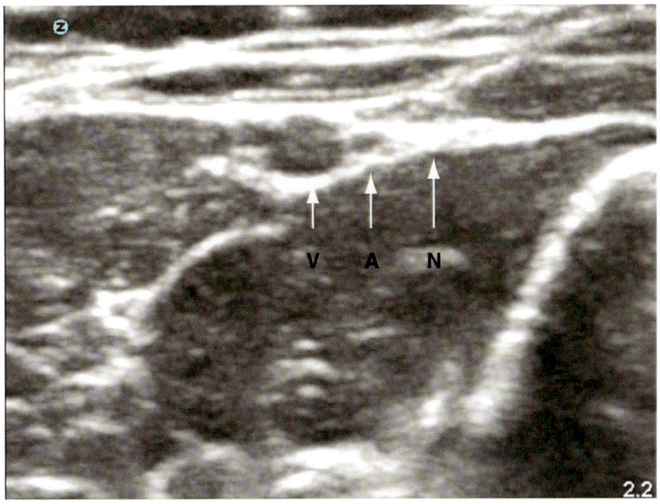

Figure 20.9 The ulnar nerve (N) is located on the ulnar side of the ulnar artery (A) and ulnar vein (V).

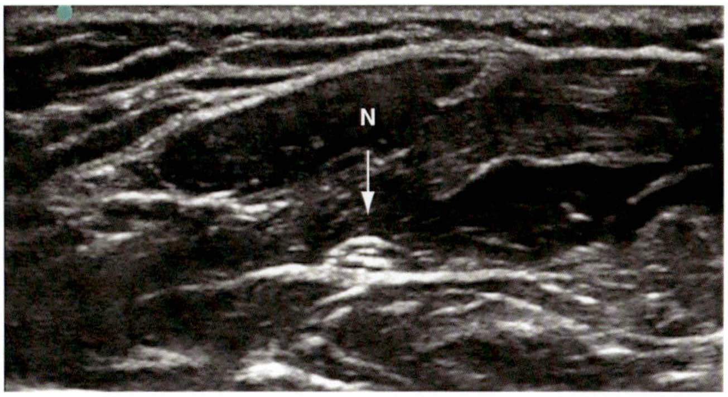

Figure 20.10 The median nerve (N) is visualized in the mid-forearm among the flexor digitorum muscle bundles.

neurovascular bundle, and may separate the femoral nerve from the adjacent vascular structures (Figure 20.12b).

Technique

The transducer is positioned parallel to the inguinal crease and perpendicular to the nerve axis (Figure 20.13). Lateral rotation of the hip on the affected side facilitates both nerve identification and injection, by creating more space for the physician to operate. On ultrasonography, the femoral nerve is most easily identified by first visualizing the neurovascular bundle at the level of the inguinal crease. The femoral nerve appears triangular in shape and may be of variable size. It is positioned lateral to the large, anechoic, round and pulsatile femoral artery and below the linear, hyperechoic fascia lata and fascia iliaca (Figure 20.14).

An optimal injection site is selected at the most proximal aspect of the femoral nerve, in which the nerve is separated from the adjacent vessels. In order to attain circumferential spread around the femoral nerve, needle redirection is often required. Half of the anesthetic agent dose may be injected on each side of the femoral nerve to achieve this goal. In addition, operators can increase the region of anesthesia to include the entire proximal hip and the entire anterior thigh, by targeting the lateral femoral cutaneous and obturator nerves. This may be performed with either a block of each individual nerve, a "three-in-one" block, or a fascia iliaca block. A failed femoral block is most commonly the result of anesthetic agent being delivered on the opposite side of the fascia lata or fascia iliaca from the target femoral nerve. The fascial planes must be identified and penetrated by the needle to ensure success.

Popliteal sciatic nerve block

Anatomy

The sciatic nerve bifurcates at the level of the popliteal fossa, into the common peroneal and tibial nerves (Figure 20.15). These nerves innervate the lower extremity below the knee, with the exception of a small segment of the medial aspect of the leg innervated by the saphenous nerve (Figure 20.16). Vascular structures run throughout the popliteal fossa; the

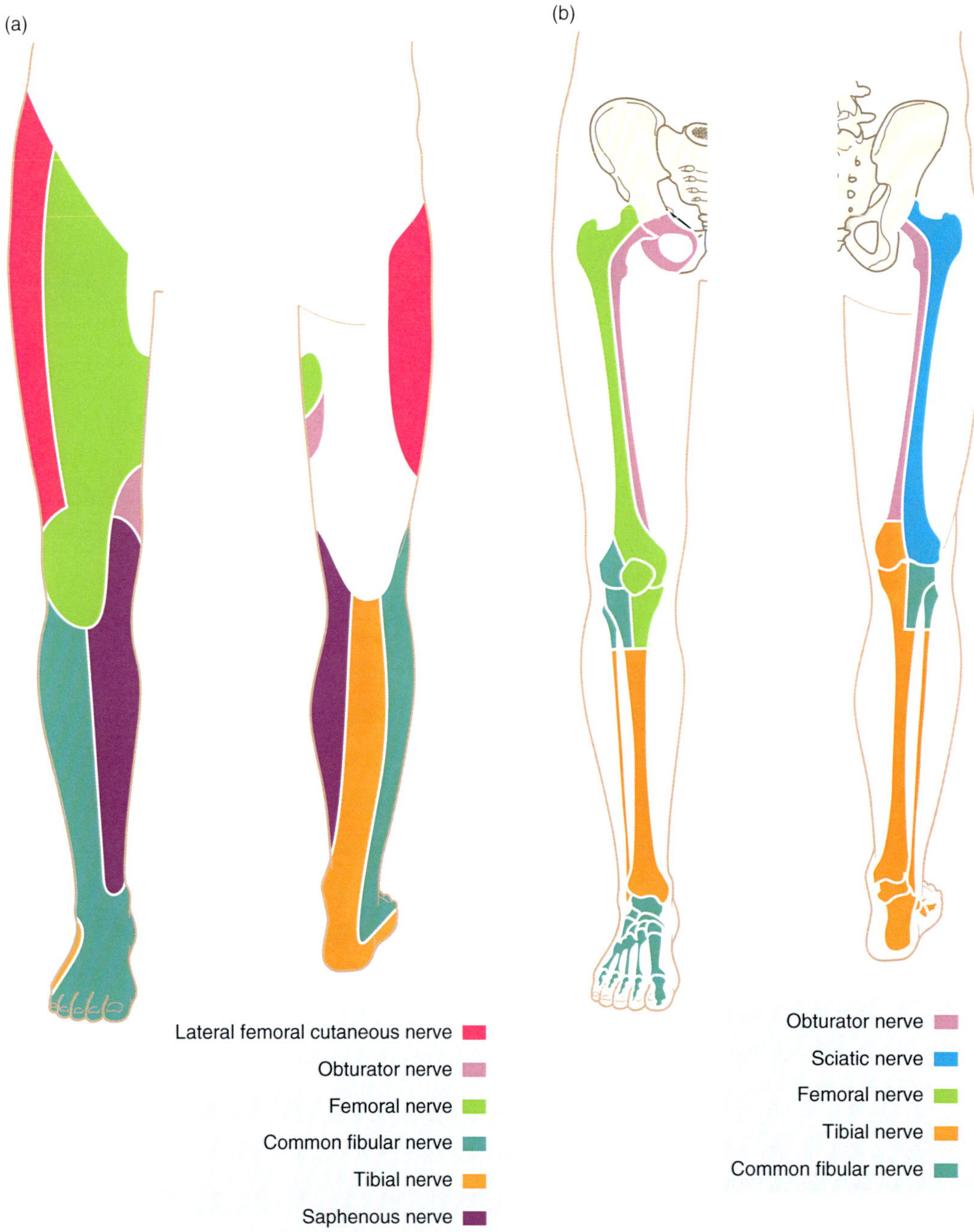

Figure 20.11 The nerve innervation of the lower-extremity skin (a) and bone (b). *Artwork created by Emily Evans © Cambridge University Press.*

popliteal artery and vein are located adjacent to the sciatic nerve. These arteries and veins must be identified and avoided.

Technique

The ideal patient positioning for a popliteal sciatic nerve block is in a lateral or prone position. A supine position can be used, but requires the affected limb to be manipulated into an elevated position, which proves to be challenging for needle insertion. The transducer is positioned transversely at the base of the popliteal fossa (Figure 20.17). On ultrasound, the prominent popliteal blood vessels are identified first and provide a reference landmark. The sciatic nerve appears superior to the popliteal artery and vein, at the level of the popliteal fossa (Figure 20.18). The sciatic nerve should be traced both proximally and distally, to identify the bifurcation, which often occurs before the level of the popliteal crease. This tracing is important and ensures that the branches of the sciatic nerve have not been mistaken for the target sciatic nerve.

The sciatic nerve can be difficult to visualize if the transducer is not held perpendicular to the target nerve. Improper patient positioning, and an inability to extend the knee due to pain, may limit transducer positioning. If the sciatic nerve is not easily visualized after locating the popliteal vessels, the physician should slowly scan caudally until the nerve appears. In addition, tendons can be easily mistaken for the sciatic nerve within the popliteal fossa. Rotating the transducer and

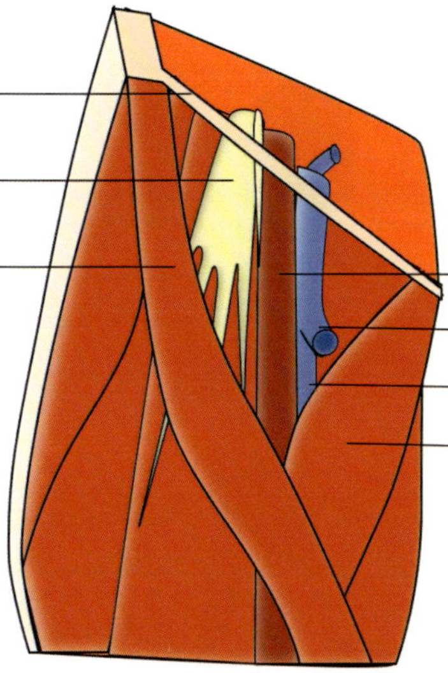

Figure 20.12 **Anatomy of the femoral triangle.** (a) The femoral nerve (N) is located adjacent to the femoral artery (A) and femoral vein (V). *Illustration by Laura Berg, MD.* (b) The course of the femoral nerve with its associated branches and surrounding nerves.

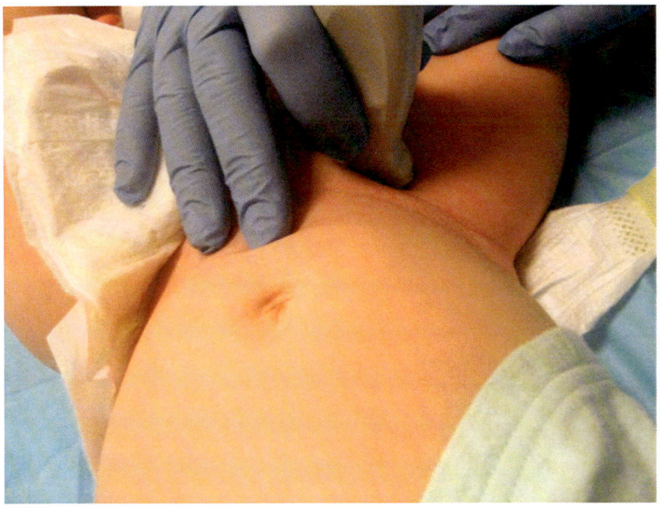

Figure 20.13 **Transducer placement, the femoral nerve.** Transducer placement is shown on the inguinal crease for the identification of the femoral nerve.

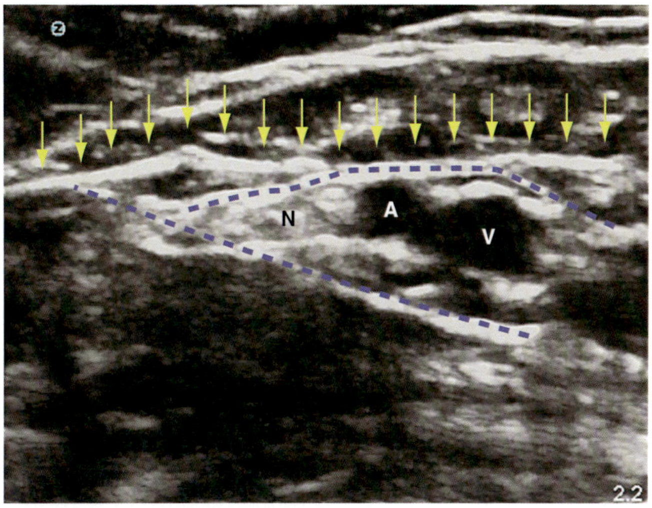

Figure 20.14 **The femoral nerve** (N). The femoral nerve (N) is located adjacent to the femoral artery (A) and femoral vein (V). The fascia lata (yellow arrows) is the most superficial fascial layer, with the fascia iliaca (broken line) lying deep and surrounding the bundle.

tracing the nerve in the longitudinal plane can help avoid confusion.

Finally, the puncture site is often at the tip of the triangle formed by the popliteal crease at the base and the biceps femoris and semimembranosus muscles. Depending on which site is identified as the more optimal site for the procedure, the anesthetic agent can be effectively injected at the site of the sciatic nerve bifurcation, or after the bifurcation. The circumferential spread of anesthetic agent around each branch will create a "double doughnut" sign, with each nerve appearing more distinct.

Scanning tips

Pitfalls

- It is important to distinguish peripheral nerves from surrounding vascular structures and tendons. Color Doppler ultrasound may be able to further identify blood vessels. Visualizing the target nerve more proximally may resolve the issue.
- Always trace the nerves proximally and distally to identify the bifurcation of the nerves. This ensures that the branches of the nerve have not been mistaken for the target nerve.
- The femoral neurovascular bundle contains two large vessels, the femoral artery and vein, which must be carefully avoided given the potential harm caused by intravascular injection of anesthetic agents.
- A failed femoral block is most commonly the result of anesthetic agent being delivered on the opposite side of the fascia lata or fascia iliaca from the target femoral nerve. The fascial planes must be identified and penetrated by the needle to ensure success.

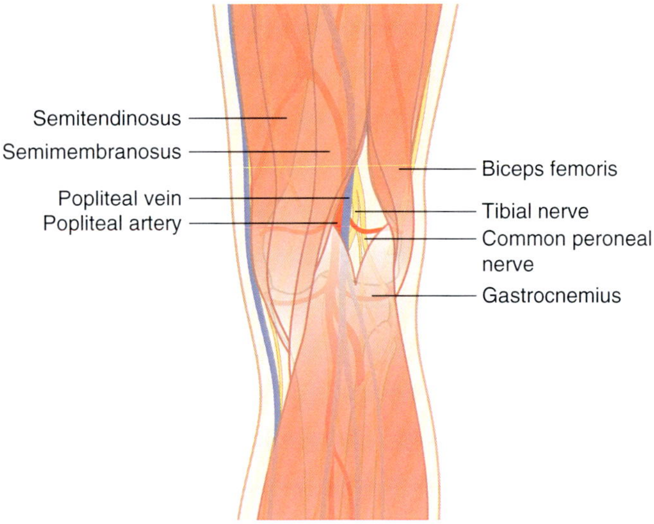

Figure 20.15 Anatomy of the popliteal fossa. *Artwork created by Emily Evans © Cambridge University Press.*

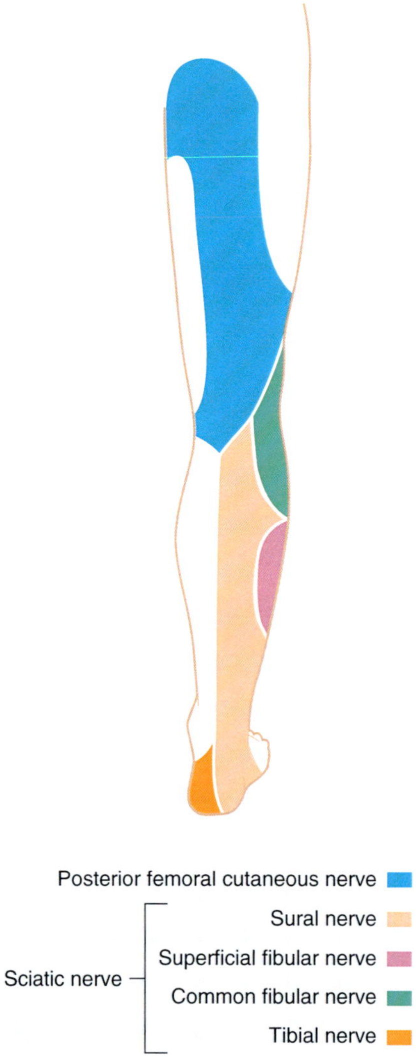

Figure 20.16 Innervation of the popliteal nerve. *Artwork created by Emily Evans © Cambridge University Press.*

Tips to improve scanning

✓ When choosing which nerve to block, it is important to be familiar with the innervations of each particular nerve.

✓ Needle tip location can be confirmed by injecting small amounts of anesthetic agent as the needle is advanced. This is called the "step down" approach.

✓ It is critical at the time of injection to precisely deliver the anesthetic agent circumferentially around the entire target nerve for optimal efficacy. Ideally, the target nerve floats or bathes in hypoechoic anesthetic agent, making its hyperechoic structure more prominent and distinct.

✓ Infants and toddlers often require the fingers of their affected hand to be immobilized, in order to eliminate movement of the flexor muscles and tendons within the forearm, which can radically alter the position of all three target nerves. Once the nerve is identified, the transducer should be firmly anchored.

✓ Circumferential spread around the femoral nerve often requires redirection of the needle. Delivery of half of the anesthetic agent dose on each side of the femoral nerve can help achieve this goal. To increase anesthesia, lateral femoral cutaneous and obturator nerves may be targeted with an individual nerve block, a "three-in-one" block, or a fascia iliaca block.

Cases

1. A nine-month-old, otherwise healthy male presents to the emergency department with severe left hand pain for the past 30 minutes. The boy had submerged his hand into his mother's hot coffee while sitting on her lap at home. He has been inconsolable since being burned, despite receiving ibuprofen and the application of a cool washcloth. On physical examination, the child is in acute distress. He has partial thickness burns to a majority of the dorsal and ventral surfaces of the left hand with circumferential involvement of the fingers. There are several areas of blistered skin. Neurologic and vascular examinations of the hand are normal.

   Intranasal fentanyl (1.5 μg/kg) is given immediately upon arrival, and topical anesthetic applied to his ventral left forearm under a transparent dressing. An ultrasound-guided nerve block of the left median, ulnar, and radial forearm nerves is performed. Exactly 1 mL of 2% lidocaine is injected in plane at each site, using a 30-gauge needle, and observed to surround each target nerve using real-time ultrasound visualization (Figure 20.19). No complications occur during the procedure. Complete pain relief is achieved within 8 minutes of the injection, and no additional analgesia is required for 90 minutes.

   This case highlights the utility of peripheral nerve blockade in the management of burns. Analgesia is often difficult to obtain with narcotic agents. In this situation, the administration of intranasyl fentanyl offered immediate analgesia, while facilitating the nerve block procedure. In

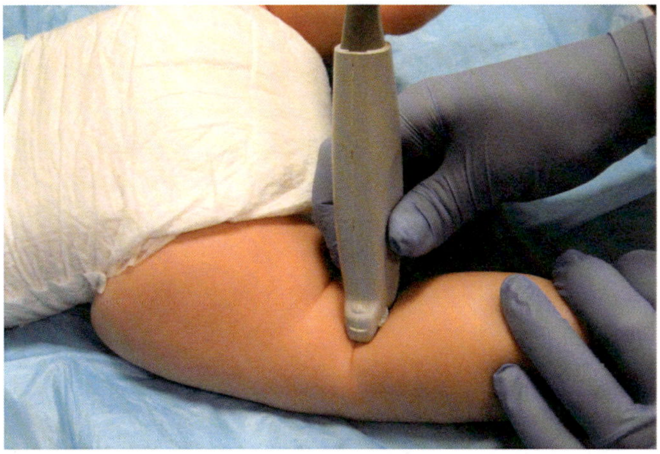

Figure 20.17 Transducer placement, sciatic nerve. Transducer placement is shown on the popliteal fossa for identification of the sciatic nerve.

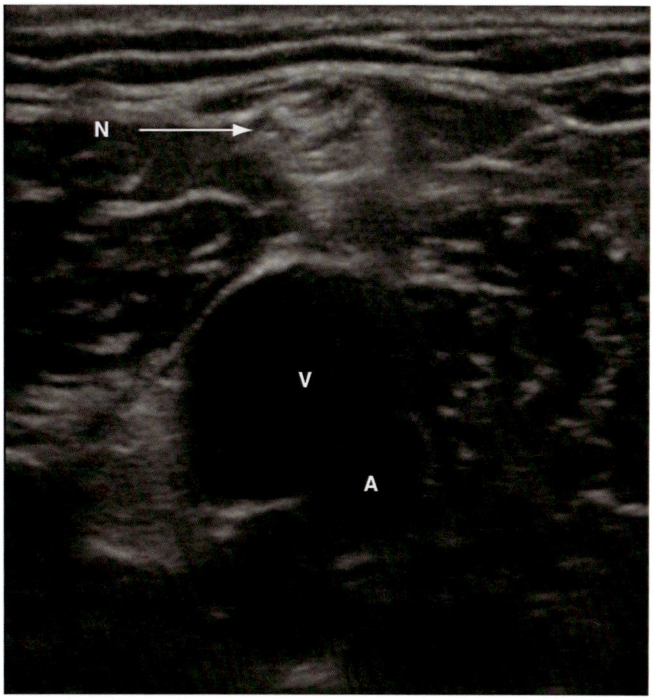

Figure 20.18 The sciatic nerve (N) appears on the ultrasound screen to be located superior to the popliteal artery (A) and popliteal vein (V). *Courtesy of Dr. Arun Nagdev, MD.*

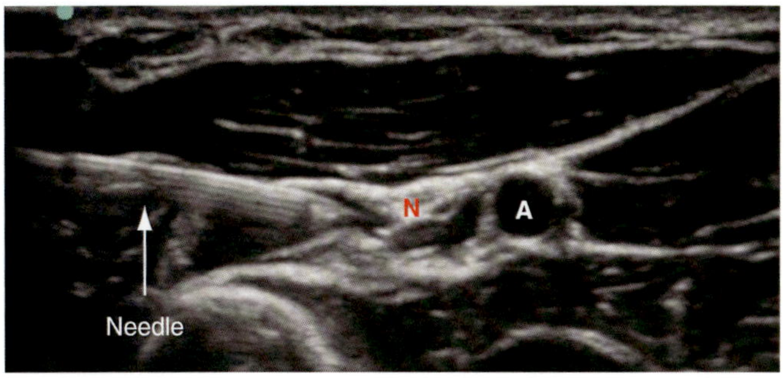

Figure 20.19 Case 1, radial nerve block. The radial nerve (N) and artery (A) are seen, along with the needle in its long axis.

this situation, lidocaine was chosen as the anesthetic agent to achieve early pain control, without masking a potential late-onset compartment syndrome.

2. A seven-month-old female presents to the emergency department with a complaint of right thigh pain. The patient's mother states that the girl has been in severe distress since she returned home three hours ago, and that the right thigh appeares swollen. The patient had been in the care of the mother's boyfriend who said he witnessed the child roll off the couch. On physical examination the patient is in acute distress, and there is marked swelling of the right thigh. She has considerable tenderness with palpation of the right thigh and significant pain with both active and passive range of motion at the right hip. Neurologic and vascular examinations of the right leg are normal.

   Intranasal fentanyl (1.5 μg/kg) is given immediately upon arrival, and topical anesthetic applied to her right inguinal area under a transparent dressing. A radiograph shows a proximal femur fracture (Figure 20.20). The orthopedics service was consulted. The medical social worker is also contacted for suspicion of non-accidental trauma. An ultrasound-guided nerve block of the right femoral nerve is then performed. The target nerve and the surrounding structures including the femoral artery, femoral vein, fascia lata, and fascia iliaca are identified (Figure 20.14). Exactly 3 mL of bupivacaine 0.25% is injected in plane, using a 27-gauge needle, and observed to surround the target nerve under real-time ultrasound guidance. There are no complications. Complete pain relief is achieved within 10 minutes of the injection. The patient is admitted and placed in a Pavlik harness. No additional analgesia is required for 180 minutes following the procedure.

   This case shows how a femoral nerve block can provide effective analgesia in an injury that is often difficult to attain adequate analgesia. Intranasal fentanyl is a useful adjunct to be administered prior to performing the nerve block.

3. A six-year-old female presents to the emergency department after stepping on a broken glass and cutting her foot at home. The patient is unable to walk on the right foot due to pain. The broken glass is intact, without any missing pieces, and she denies a foreign-body sensation. On physical examination the patient is in mild distress. She has a 5 cm complex laceration to her right sole without tendon or bony involvement. Bleeding from the wound is minimal, and there is no apparent foreign body. She is unable to bear any weight. Neurologic and vascular examination of the right foot are normal.

   Intranasal fentanyl (1.5 μg/kg) is given immediately upon arrival, and topical anesthetic applied to her right popliteal fossa under a transparent dressing. A radiograph of the right foot shows no radioopaque foreign body or bony injury. An ultrasound-guided nerve block of the right sciatic nerve is then performed. The target nerve, its bifurcation, and the surrounding structures including the popliteal artery and popliteal vein are identified. Exactly 5 mL of bupivacaine 0.25% is injected in plane, using a 27-gauge needle, and observed to surround the target nerve using real-time ultrasound visualization (Figure 20.21). There are no complications. Complete pain

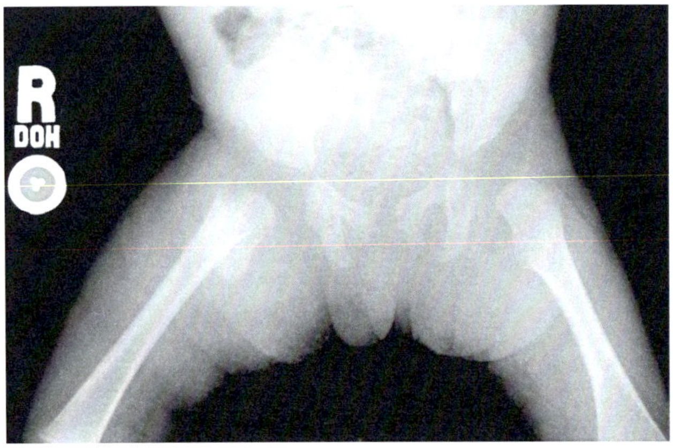

Figure 20.20 **Case 2**: An acute fracture of the right femur in a seven-month-old girl caused by non-accidental trauma is shown.

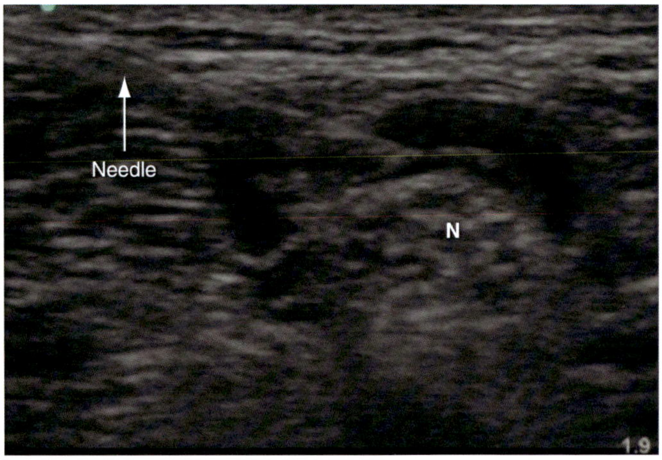

Figure 20.21 **Case 3, popliteal sciatic nerve block.** A popliteal sciatic nerve block is performed in the in-plane approach. In the ultrasound image, the needle is visualized in its long-axis, with its target nerve (N).

relief is achieved within 10 minutes of the injection. The laceration is then irrigated, explored, and repaired without discomfort. No additional analgesia is required for 180 minutes following the procedure.

This is a case where a sciatic nerve block is extremely helpful in attaining pain relief. After adequate anesthesia is attained, the laceration is able to be adequately irrigated, explored, and repaired. As this is a complex laceration, the choice of Bupivacaine is ideal, due to its long duration of action.

Summary/key points

1. Ultrasound-guided regional anesthesia, or peripheral nerve blocks, provide a safe and effective method of emergent pediatric pain control for traditionally challenging injuries, pathologies, and procedures.
2. Proper patient positioning and the use of adjunct analgesia can improve both success rates and patient satisfaction.
3. A high-resolution, linear transducer provides the highest quality image of peripheral nerves and their surrounding anatomy. Occasionally, in obese patients, a low-frequency transducer may need to be used. Care must be taken with injection, since the transducer and image are curved.
4. Prior to the injection of an anesthetic agent, target nerves and surrounding structures (i.e. arteries, veins, and tendons) should be located and identified.
5. The needle tip must be visualized throughout the entire procedure to ensure accurate anesthetic agent delivery, and to prevent unnecessary complications. A long-axis, or in-plane, orientation is preferred.

Selected references

Bhoi, S., Sinha, T. P., Rodha, M., *et al.* (2012) Feasibility and safety of ultrasound-guided nerve block for management of limb injuries by emergency care physicians. *J Emerg Trauma Shock* **5** (1): 28–32.

Christos, S. C., Chiampas, G., Offman, R., Rifenburg, R. (2010) Ultrasound-guided three-in-one nerve block for femur fractures. *West J Emerg Med* **11**(4): 310–13.

Ganesh, A., Gurnaney, H. (2009) Ultrasound guidance for pediatric peripheral nerve blockade. *Anesthesiol Clin* **27**: 197–212.

Ivani, G., Mossetti, V. (2009) Pediatric regional anesthesia. *Minerva Anesthesiol* **75**(10): 577–83.

Liebmann, O., Price, D., Mills, C., *et al.* (2006) Feasibility of forearm ultrasonography-guided nerve blocks of the radial, ulnar, and median nerves for hand procedures in the emergency department. *Ann Emerg Med* **48**: 558–62.

Mariano, E., Ilfeld, B., Cheng, G., *et al.* (2008) Feasibility of ultrasound-guided peripheral nerve block catheters for pain control on pediatric medical missions in developing countries. *Paediatr Anaesth* **18**: 598.

Neal, J. M., Brull, R., Chan, V. W. S., *et al.* (2010) The ASRA evidence-based medicine assessment of ultrasound-guided regional anesthesia and pain medicine. *Reg Anesth Pain Med* **35**(2 Suppl): S1–9.

Neal, J. M., Gerancher, J. C., Hebl, J. R., *et al.* (2009) Upper extremity regional anesthesia: essentials of our current understanding, 2008. *Reg Anesth Pain Med* **34**: 134–70.

Sites, B., Brull, R. (2006) Ultrasound guidance in peripheral regional anesthesia: philosophy, evidence-based medicine, and techniques. *Curr Opin Anaesthesiol* **19**: 630.

Tsui, B., Suresh, S. (2010) Ultrasound imaging for regional anesthesia in infants, children, and adolescents: a review of current literature and its application in the practice of extremity and trunk blocks. *Anesthesiology* **112**: 473–92.

Chapter 21

Pericardiocentesis, thoracentesis, and paracentesis

Rebecca L. Vieira

Objectives/indications

The presence of a pericardial effusion, pleural effusion, or ascites may warrant emergent drainage via pericardiocentesis, thoracentesis, or paracentesis, respectively. Though these are rare conditions in children, point-of-care ultrasound may assist in decreasing the complications associated with these procedures. The indications for pericardiocentesis, thoracentesis, and paracentesis are well summarized by the Society of Cardiovascular and Interventional Radiology Standards of Practice Committee as "the presence of an abnormal fluid collection with suspicion that the fluid is infected, the need for fluid characterization, or suspicion that the collection is producing clinically relevant symptoms." Pericardiocentesis, thoracentesis, and paracentesis in children are especially complicated by their relatively small size and lack of cooperation compared to adults. Moreover, children often require procedural sedation in order to perform these procedures. The risks and benefits of procedural sedation should be considered carefully for each patient.

Clinically significant pericardial effusions are rare in children and can result from trauma, neoplasm, collagen vascular disease, or infection. A significant proportion of pericardial effusions in children are idiopathic. An abnormal fluid collection may develop in the pericardial sac either acutely or chronically. When fluid accumulation is acute, small pericardial effusions can result in tamponade. When fluid accumulation is chronic, the pericardium can actually accommodate large effusions without cardiovascular compromise. Tamponade occurs when pressure from the pericardial fluid impairs ventricular filling during diastole, which can compromise normal circulatory function and lead to the rapid deterioration of the patient. The classic clinical triad of hypotension, elevated systemic venous pressure, and muffled heart sounds is unreliable and lacks specificity. While relatively uncommon, when tamponade with cardiovascular compromise is present, an emergent aspiration of fluid from the pericardial sac, or pericardiocentesis, is indicated. Pericardiocenteses have been performed since the 1840s, but traditional "blind" approaches are associated with significant complications. Whether performed on an emergent or semi-elective basis in a controlled setting, ultrasound is recommended to identify pericardial effusions, and to guide pericardiocentesis.

In contrast, pleural effusions are not uncommon in pediatric patients. The most common causes of pleural effusions in otherwise healthy children are pulmonary infections such as parapneumonic effusions. Other causes of pleural effusions include congestive heart failure, malignancy, and renal disease. Point-of-care ultrasound is a valuable tool in the diagnosis and characterization of these effusions. If an abnormal fluid collection is identified in the pleural space (by ultrasound or by other imaging modalities), ultrasound may be used to assist in performing thoracentesis. The two main indications for thoracentesis are (1) to obtain pleural fluid for diagnostic purposes and (2) to drain pleural fluid that is compromising normal respiratory function. When thoracentesis is performed for diagnostic purposes, it is generally performed on a semi-elective basis in a controlled setting, such as the operating room. However, thoracentesis may need to be performed more emergently, when it is required to alleviate respiratory compromise.

Finally, ascites is a rare condition in pediatrics. Causes of ascites in children include hepatocellular disease, congestive heart failure, cardiac abnormalities, infection, pancreatic disease, and low albumin states. While reasonably safe in adults, paracentesis is a relatively uncommon procedure performed in pediatric patients. However, paracentesis may be indicated to aid in the diagnostic evaluation of patients who present with ascites, and especially when bacterial peritonitis is suspected. Paracentesis may also be performed to alleviate symptoms caused by ascites, such as pain or respiratory distress.

Although pediatric-specific literature is scarce, using point-of-care ultrasound to assist in pericardiocentesis, thoracentesis, and paracentesis may increase the safety and likelihood for procedural success. The principles of ultrasound assistance for these procedures are similar for pediatric patients and adults. However, adjustments may need to be made for children because of their relatively small size. For each procedure, ultrasound may be used to mark the optimal incision site (ultrasound assistance) or to actively guide needle insertion (ultrasound guidance). When using real-time ultrasound guidance, novice users should strongly consider using a dual-operator approach, with one person operating the ultrasound device and the other performing the procedure.

Pediatric Emergency and Critical Care Ultrasound, ed. Stephanie J. Doniger. Published by Cambridge University Press.

PERICARDIOCENTESIS

Background

Conventionally, pericardiocentesis that is performed by the non-cardiologist is performed using the landmark technique, with a subxiphoid approach. Complications of this technique are common and include myocardial injury, coronary artery laceration, pneumothorax, dysrhythmias, injury to the diaphragm and subdiaphragmatic organs, and even death. Most of the literature supporting ultrasound assistance and ultrasound guidance for pericardiocentesis derives from the interventional cardiology literature, where pericardiocentesis is performed in a controlled environment, on a semi-elective basis. In this setting, echocardiographically guided pericardiocentesis has been used to identify the optimal site for needle placement, and has been shown to increase success rates and reduce complications of the procedure. Tsang *et al.* studied 1127 ultrasound-guided pericardiocenteses and demonstrated an overall success rate of 97%, with a complication rate of 4.7% (major 1.2%; minor 3.5%). In addition, echocardiographically guided pericardiocentesis has also been found to be safe in pediatric patients. As a result, echocardiographic guidance has become standard for pericardiocentesis in cardiology.

While the principles of echocardiographically guided pericardiocentesis can be extrapolated to the pediatric intensive care and emergency department settings, more research is needed to support the routine use of point-of-care ultrasound to assist in pericardiocentesis in these settings. Based on the established literature thus far, the American Society of Echocardiography Consensus Statement specifically recommends that, when emergent pericardiocentesis is indicated in the emergency department, an ultrasound first be performed in order to determine the best needle trajectory, followed by ultrasound-guided pericardiocentesis. In hemodynamically unstable patients with pericardial effusions, a comprehensive echocardiogram need not be performed.

Anatomy

The anatomy of the heart is discussed in Chapter 5 (Figure 5.1). The heart is surrounded by the inner visceral and outer parietal pericardium. Normally, a trace amount of physiologic fluid provides lubrication between these two layers, in the pericardial sac. A pericardial effusion develops between these two layers.

Technique

Transducer selection and orientation

A low-frequency, phased-array transducer should be used to obtain the standard cardiac views (see Chapter 5). The parasternal long-axis or apical views are preferred when performing ultrasound-guided pericardiocentesis, since they provide a more direct anatomic approach. In the parasternal long-axis view, the indicator is oriented towards the patient's left hip (Figure 21.1a). Alternatively, in the subxiphoid view, the transducer is flattened, below the xiphoid process, with the indicator oriented towards the patient's right side (Figure 21.2a).

(a)

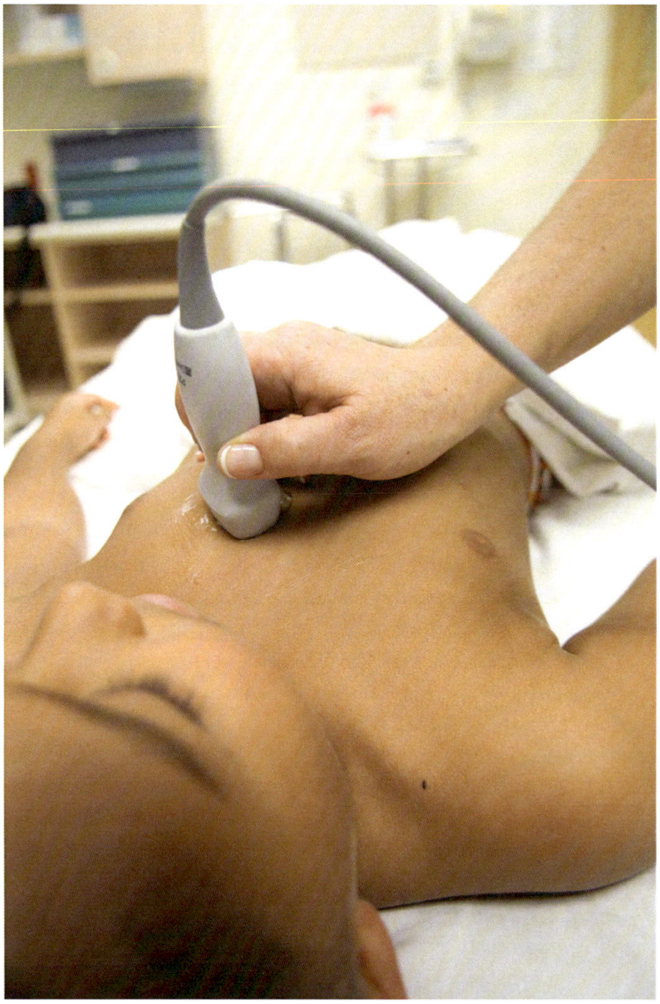

(b)

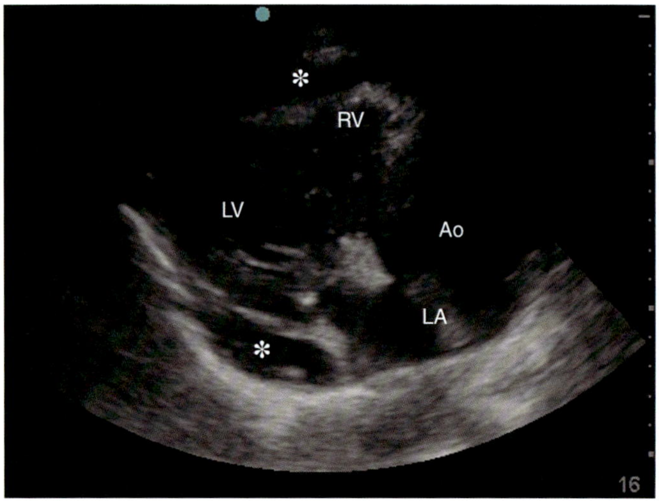

Figure 21.1 The evaluation of a pericardial effusion, parasternal long-axis view. (a) Transducer placement. (b) Ultrasound image of a pericardial effusion (*). Note the effusion appears as an anechoic stripe between the two layers of the pericardium. This effusion is loculated and does not extend circumferentially around the heart. Other structures seen are the left ventricle (LV), right ventricle (RV), left atrium (LA), and aorta (Ao).

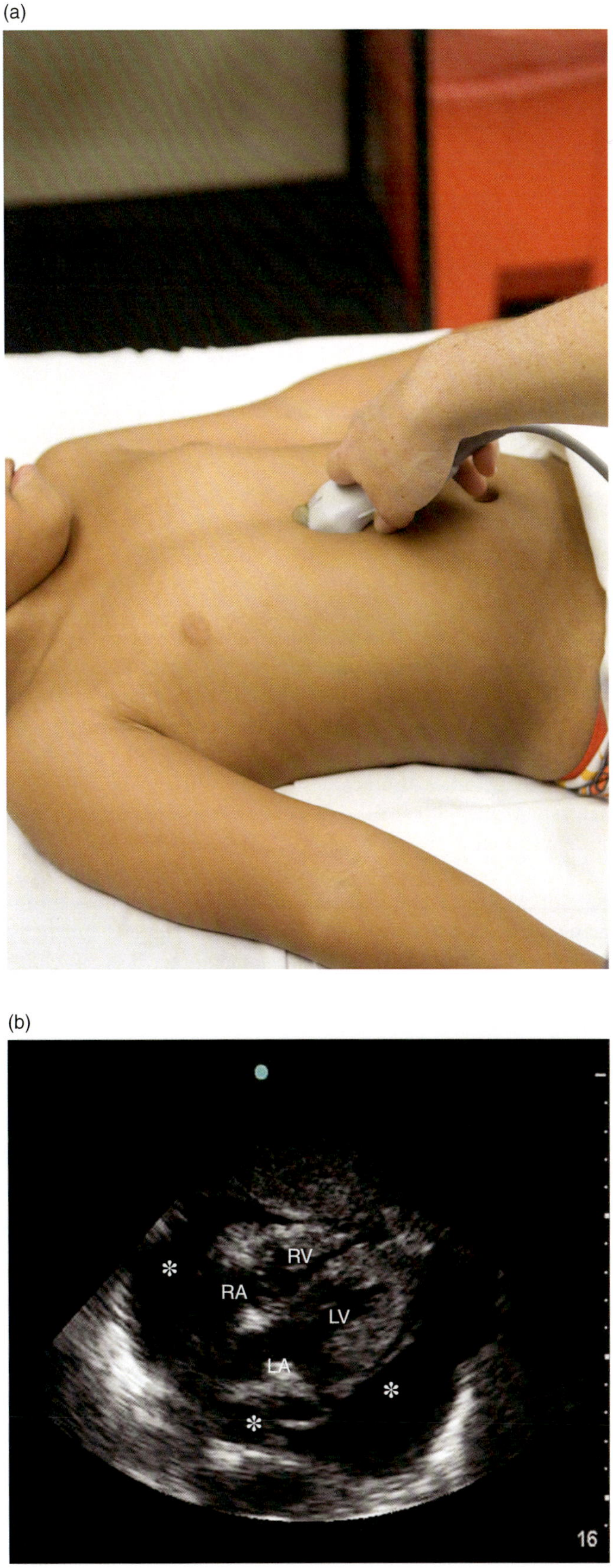

Figure 21.2 **The evaluation for a pericardial effusion, subxiphoid view.** (a) Transducer placement. (b) Ultrasound image of a pericardial effusion (*). Other structures visualized are the right atrium (RA), right ventricle (RV), left atrium (LA), and left ventricle (LV). *Ultrasound image courtesy of Jason Levy, MD RDMS.*

Patient position and preparation

If clinically feasible, the patient should be positioned in an upright, seated, or a left-lateral decubitus position. When performing pericardiocentesis, sterile preparation of the patient and transducer should be carried out whenever possible.

Ultrasound imaging

Both the parasternal long-axis (Figure 21.1b) and the subxiphoid (Figure 21.2b) views can confirm the presence of a pericardial effusion, can delineate the extent of the effusion, and can identify the relationship of the fluid to the chest wall. Pericardial fluid will appear as an anechoic or hypoechoic stripe between the two layers of the pericardium. When tamponade is clinically suspected, the sonographic findings of right ventricular diastolic collapse, a circumferential pericardial effusion, and hyperdynamic heart support the diagnosis. Because physical examination findings for tamponade are unreliable, point-of-care ultrasound can be used to rapidly confirm the presence of a pericardial effusion and assess its hemodynamic effects prior to performing pericardiocentesis.

Ultrasound-guided procedure

When using ultrasound, the optimal needle placement for pericardiocentesis is the location where the effusion is closest to the transducer and the fluid collection is the greatest. For the static technique, the angle of interrogation of the transducer and depth from the skin to the pericardial fluid should be noted and used to determine the angle and the depth of needle insertion. This site can be marked on the patient's skin prior to the procedure.

Alternatively, if the patient's clinical status permits, ultrasound guidance may be utilized, in which real-time imaging visualizes the needle insertion and advancement (Figure 21.3). This offers the advantage of the direct visualization of the needle and the ability to redirect the needle's approach in real time, and decreases the uncertainty about the accuracy of the needle's position within the pericardial space. With ultrasound guidance, the parasternal long-axis approach is preferred, since it involves a more direct anatomic approach. This is in contrast to the blind methods, which traditionally utilize a subxiphoid approach, and involve a needle trajectory directly through the liver. The injection of agitated saline may help localize the needle during the ultrasound-guided procedure.

Training and education

When training practitioners to perform ultrasound-assisted and ultrasound-guided pericardiocentesis, it is important to first become proficient in performing cardiac ultrasound and obtaining the different views of the heart (see Chapter 5). Commercially available simulators and phantom models may be utilized to demonstrate pericardial effusions, with the ability to practice the procedure. Recently, Zerth *et al.* described a low-cost, easily constructed task trainer to simulate ultrasound-guided pericardiocentesis (Figure 21.4).

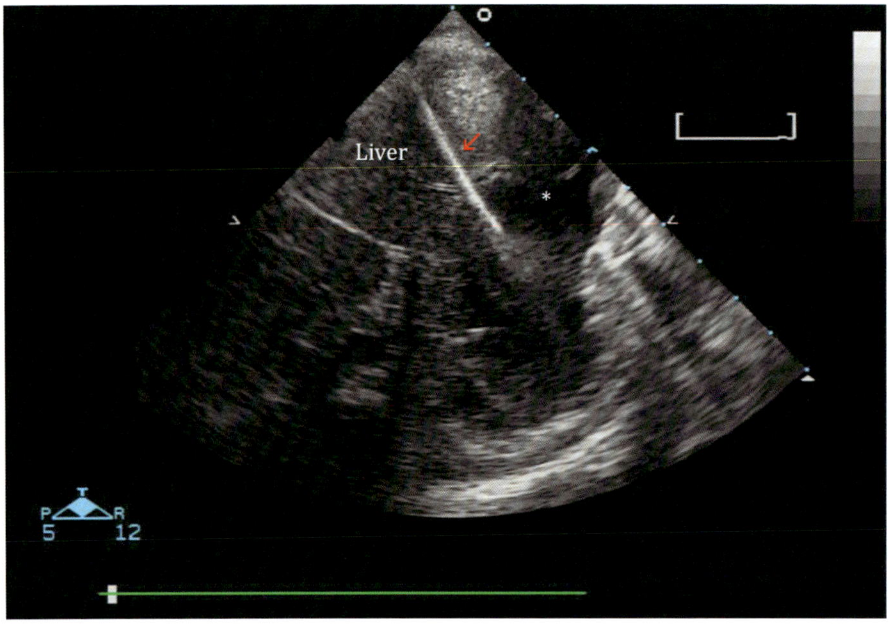

Figure 21.3 Pericardiocentesis. Real-time ultrasound guidance shows the needle (arrow) entering the pericardial space to drain a pericardial effusion (*). *Image courtesy of Mahmoud Elbarbarry, MD MSc PhD.*

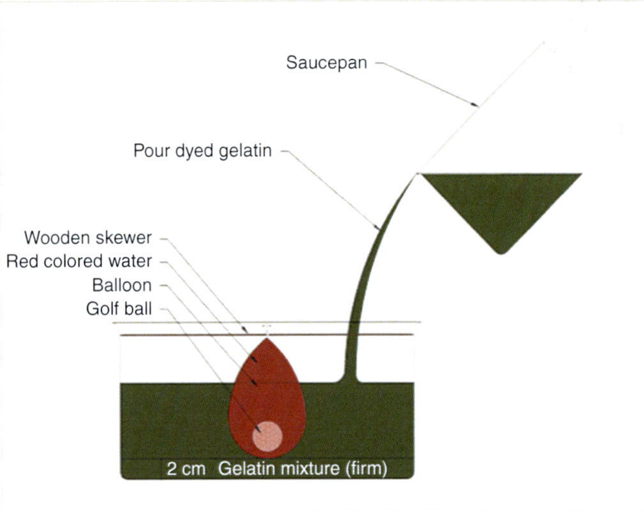

Figure 21.4 Homemade model for pericardiocentesis. Low-cost materials include a gelatin mixture, colored water, golf ball, balloon, and wooden skewer. *Source (copyright): Zerth, H., Harwood, R., Tommasso, L., Girzadas, D. V. Jr. (2011) An inexpensive, easily constructed, reusable task trainer simulating ultrasound-guided pericardiocentesis. J Emerg Med 43(6): 1066–9.*

THORACENTESIS

Background

Historically, thoracentesis has been performed using a landmark technique in conjunction with physical examination and X-ray findings. Complications of thoracentesis include pneumothorax, hemothorax, lung laceration, hepatic laceration, and splenic laceration. Failures, or "dry taps," are not uncommon.

Several studies have shown an advantage to ultrasound-assisted thoracentesis in adult patients. The use of ultrasound to mark the needle insertion site immediately prior to performing thoracentesis has been shown to reduce the rate of pneumothorax and to increase the accuracy of the insertion site. The risk of an iatrogenic pneumothorax after ultrasound-guided thoracentesis is 0 to 2.5%, in contrast to blind approaches, where the risk ranges from 4 to 30%. Ultrasound has also been used to assist successful thoracentesis following failed attempts by traditional techniques. It is especially useful in patients in whom a thoracentesis is expected to be difficult, such as patients with small or loculated effusions, and mechanically ventilated patients.

While ultrasound has been used to identify pleural effusions in children, there are no known pediatric-specific studies comparing ultrasound-assisted to traditional thoracentesis. Further, it is extremely rare to require emergent thoracentesis in children; the procedure is most often performed in the controlled operating room setting.

Anatomy

As discussed in Chapter 6, the lung is surrounded by two layers of pleura: the inner visceral pleura and the more superficial parietal pleura. A trace amount of physiologic fluid provides lubrication between these two layers during normal respiration. Abnormal fluid can collect in the potential space between the parietal and visceral pleura as a result of infection, inflammation, congestive heart failure, or anatomic abnormalities. Pleural fluid initially collects in the potential space known as the costodiaphragmatic recess. In an upright or prone patient, pleural fluid will first accumulate in the most dependent parts of the pleural space, posteriorly and inferiorly.

Technique

Transducer selection and orientation

The selection of the appropriate transducer depends on the patient's size and the operator's preference. In adults, evaluation of the pleural space is often performed with a curvilinear, low-frequency (2–5 MHz) transducer. However, in children, the

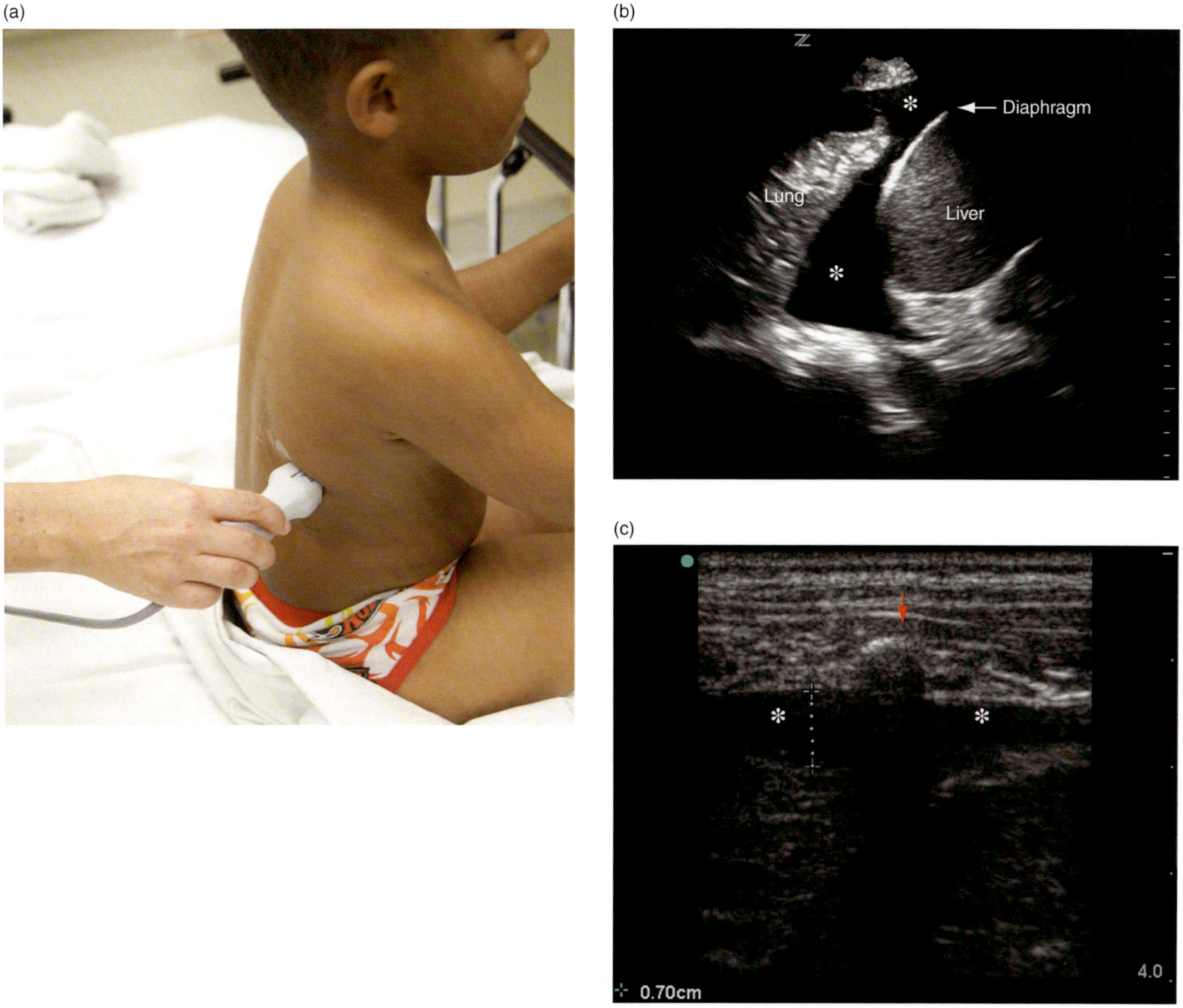

Figure 21.5 The evaluation of pleural effusions; preparation for thoracentesis. (a) Transducer placement. (b) Ultrasound image of a pleural effusion (*) with the phased-array transducer. Surrounding structures include the liver, lung, and diaphragm. (c) Ultrasound image of a pleural effusion (*) with the linear transducer. A rib and its posterior shadow (red arrow) can be seen and aid in the identification of the pleural line. A pleural effusion (*) appears as a hypoechoic or an anechoic collection between the two pleural layers. *Ultrasound images courtesy of James Hwang, MD RDMS.*

smaller footprint of the phased-array transducer may provide better views through the relatively small intercostal spaces. Alternatively, a high-frequency, linear transducer may be utilized when less penetration is needed. The transducer is positioned with the indicator towards the patient's right or the patient's head.

Patient position and preparation

To evaluate the presence of a pleural effusion, the patient should be seated upright whenever possible (Figure 21.5a). In order to improve image acquisition and patient comfort, the patient can lean slightly forward over a bedside table or chair for support, with his/her arms positioned forward or over the head. In patients who cannot be seated upright, such as mechanically ventilated patients, ultrasound may be performed with the patient prone or in the lateral decubitus position (affected side up) with the ipsilateral arm brought across the chest.

When performing a thoracentesis, the most common location is the mid/lateral back, with the patient in a seated position. Alternatively, with a supine patient, the head of the bed should be elevated to 30–45°, and the needle entry should be at the mid-axillary line. When preparing a patient for a thoracentesis, the patient's skin should be prepared in a sterile fashion. The transducer should also be covered with a sterile sheath (Figure S3.5).

Ultrasound imaging

Approaching the patient from behind, the sonographer should interrogate the area laterally from the anterior axillary line to the paravertebral space, and axially from the diaphragm to the superior margin of the effusion. The liver, spleen, and kidneys serve as helpful landmarks inferiorly (Figure 21.5b).

The evaluation of the thorax is complicated by the highly reflective ribs and reverberation artifacts from air within the lung. Normally, the two layers of the pleura are visualized as thin, hyperechoic, linear structures deep to the soft tissue and muscles of the chest wall. A pleural effusion appears as a hypoechoic or anechoic fluid collection between the two layers of the pleura (Figure 21.5b,c). However, it is important to note that thickened pleura can also appear anechoic. One of the early signs of the presence of a pleural effusion is the loss of the mirror-image artifact at the right and left upper quadrants. To definitively identify the presence of a pleural effusion, one must witness dynamic changes in the shape of the fluid collection, and motion within the echogenic space during respirations.

Ultrasound-guided procedure

It is important to identify surrounding structures such as the liver, spleen, and diaphragm in order to avoid puncturing them during thoracentesis. It is also important to avoid the intercostal vein, artery, and nerve. Once these structures are identified, measure the depth from the skin to the parietal pleura. It is recommended that a visceral to parietal distance be at least **10 mm** in order to minimize risks associated with ultrasound-guided thoracentesis. An absolute contraindication to performing an ultrasound-guided thoracentesis includes the incursion of lung or diaphragm during the respiratory cycle into the sonographic window.

Once a pleural effusion is identified, either skin marking prior to thoracentesis or direct visualization of the needle may be performed. Most studies demonstrating the advantage of the use of ultrasound versus traditional approaches actually use pre-procedure marking rather than dynamic visualization. For the static technique, ultrasound is first performed in order to evaluate the effusion and the ideal location for needle-entry is marked with a surgical pen. Then, the transducer may be tilted in different directions in order to plan the best needle trajectory. The angle of interrogation of the transducer and depth from the skin to the pleural fluid should be noted and used to determine the angle and depth of needle insertion. Thoracentesis should be performed immediately following site marking without repositioning the patient; changes in patient positioning or the respiratory cycle may change the positioning of the pleural effusion relative to the skin markings.

Alternatively, a dynamic technique may be used. Following the identification and marking of the optimal incision site, the patient and transducer should be positioned to actively visualize and guide needle insertion and advancement. This offers the advantage of visualization of important structures, such as the diaphragm, lung, and liver or spleen, during the procedure, and the ability to view and adjust the needle's trajectory in real time.

Training and education

It is important to understand ultrasound of the lung and the identification of pleural effusions, prior to performing ultrasound-assisted or ultrasound-guided thoracentesis. It has been recommended to utilize simulation scenarios – both with ultrasound phantoms and cadaveric models. A recent study suggested that procedural competency with thoracentesis would include didactic training, simulation, ultrasound guidance, competency testing, and performance feedback.

PARACENTESIS

Background

The use of ultrasound to identify, characterize, and quantify ascites is well recognized. Ascites accumulates in gravity-dependent regions, as is the case with hemoperitoneum in trauma (see Chapter 4). Historically, paracentesis has been performed using a landmark or "blind" technique, with the left lower quadrant as the most commonly cited location for incision. Complications of paracentesis include abdominal wall hematoma, hollow viscous perforation, and perforation of major vascular structures. Failure to obtain fluid using the landmark technique is common, especially when the diagnosis of ascites is suspected based on physical examination findings alone.

In adults, it has been suggested that ultrasound can aid in identifying the optimal needle entry site for paracentesis. When an insignificant amount of ascites is identified on ultrasound, unnecessary attempts at paracentesis are avoided. Further, ultrasound can identify intraperitoneal structures, thereby making the procedure safer. Point-of-care ultrasound has been successfully used to guide paracentesis when traditional "blind" techniques have failed. Nazeer *et al.* studied ultrasound-guided versus the landmark technique for paracentesis in the emergency department. Ultrasound guidance demonstrated a 95% success rate, compared to the 65% success rate without the use of ultrasound. Of the failed attempts in the landmark group, ultrasound successfully guided drainage in all but two patients. These patients did not have fluid present on ultrasound.

To our knowledge, there is no pediatric-specific literature related to ultrasound assistance for paracentesis. This may be due in part to the fact that paracentesis is an uncommonly performed procedure in children in the emergency department or critical care settings.

Anatomy

As discussed in Chapter 4, free fluid in the abdomen collects in the most dependent regions (Figures 4.1, 4.2). In the supine patient, these regions include Morison's pouch, the splenorenal recess, the right and left paracolic gutters, the rectovesical pouch in males, and the pouch of Douglas in females. Previous surgeries, adhesions, and infection can result in variations in the location of fluid collections and loculated fluid collections.

Technique

Transducer selection and orientation

A low-frequency (2–5 MHz), curvilinear or phased-array transducer should be used. The peritoneal cavity should be evaluated for free fluid using an approach similar to the FAST examination (Figure 21.6a–c). In addition to the right upper quadrant, left upper quadrant, and suprapubic views, the right and left lower quadrants should be evaluated.

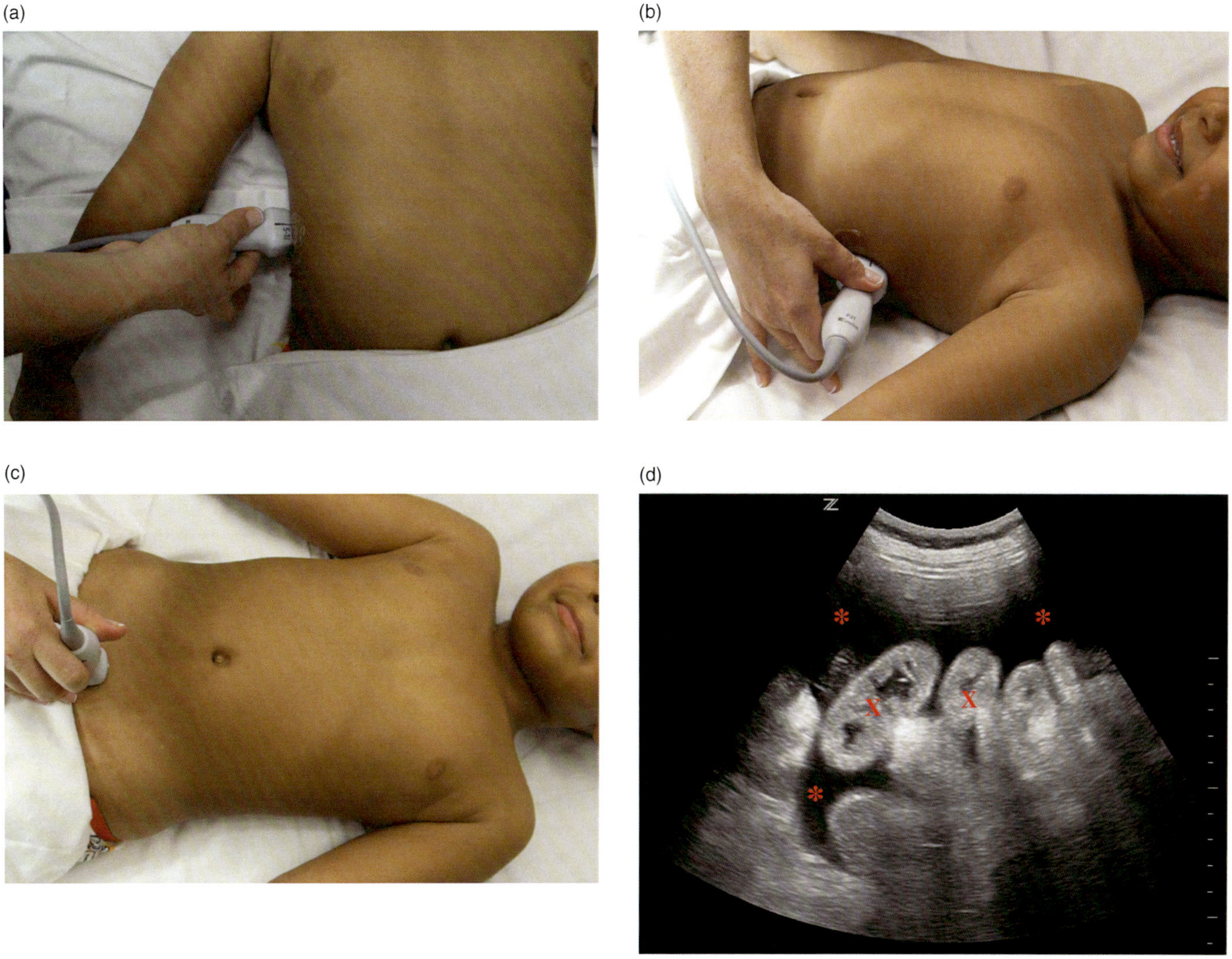

Figure 21.6 The evaluation of ascites; preparation for paracentesis. (a) Transducer placement, right upper quadrant view. (b) Transducer placement, left upper quadrant view. (c) Transducer placement, suprapubic view. (d) Ultrasound image of ascites (*) with clearly identifiable bowel loops (X). *Ultrasound image courtesy of James Hwang, MD RDMS.*

Patient position and preparation

The patient should be positioned either supine or seated, based on physician preference. When performing paracentesis, the patient's skin should be prepared in a sterile fashion. The transducer should be covered with a sterile probe cover (Figure S3.5).

Ultrasound imaging

Ascites fluid appears as anechoic or hypoechoic fluid, depending on the type of fluid (Figure 21.6d). Occasional echogenic strands may be visualized. It is important to identify bowel and vascular structures when determining the ideal location to perform paracentesis.

Ultrasound-guided procedure

Once ascites is identified (using point-of-care ultrasound or other imaging modalities), ultrasound can be used to assist in performing the paracentesis. If the diagnosis of ascites is suspected based on physical examination findings alone, it should be confirmed using point-of-care ultrasound. The safety and success of paracentesis depends on the identification of an acoustic window that does not contain any important intra-abdominal structures in the expected trajectory of the needle. The window should be observed to be free of floating viscera for a period of time, as the position of bowel within free fluid can change significantly. The inferior epigastric artery, which normally travels along the lateral third of the rectus muscle, should be avoided.

For the static technique (ultrasound assistance), the ideal site is marked with a surgical pen. The best site is the largest and deepest pocket of fluid, far away from floating bowel loops and vascular structures. The angle of interrogation of the transducer, and the depth from the skin to the ascites fluid, should be noted and used to direct the angle and depth of needle insertion. Paracentesis should be performed immediately following site marking without repositioning the patient.

Alternatively, a dynamic technique (ultrasound guidance) may be used. Following site identification, skin marking, and sterile preparation, the transducer can be positioned to actively guide needle insertion and advancement. This offers the advantage of visualization of important structures, such as floating viscera, during the procedure, and the ability to view and adjust the needle's approach in real time.

Training and education

There is a paucity of literature specifically discussing training and education with regards to the performance of paracentesis and ultrasound-guided paracentesis. However, adequate training in the identification of intraperitoneal fluid such as in the FAST examination is important. There may be a future role of simulation in the training of practitioners to perform paracentesis with the use of utlrasonography.

Scanning tips

Pitfalls

- Changing the patient's position between the marking of the acoustic window and performing the procedure when using the static technique may lead to movement of fluid, and the inadvertent puncture of surrounding structures.
- Failure to observe changes in the position of important structures relative to the acoustic window during the respiratory cycle.
- Mistaking other fluid-filled structures, such as bowel and bladder, for intraperitoneal fluid.
- Failure to immobilize or sedate the patient adequately during the procedure.

Tips to improve scanning

✓ Consider using a higher-frequency transducer for smaller children when less depth is needed.

✓ A phased-array transducer may provide better windows than a curvilinear transducer in smaller children. It also has a smaller footprint, which may easily image between the small intercostal spaces.

✓ Always identify the most favorable location for an incision site and surrounding structures.

✓ When encountering difficulty in identifying an acoustic window, interrogate the area of interest using the low-frequency transducer. Once the window is found, consider switching to the linear transducer for real-time guidance.

✓ Note the distance between the skin and the superficial aspect of the fluid collection to assess the necessary needle depth. Try to mimic the transducer's angle when inserting and advancing the needle.

Cases

1. A two-year-old male is brought in by paramedics to the emergency department in full cardiac arrest, with cardiac compressions in progress. Limited history is available of the patient, but he recently had repair of an unknown congenital heart lesion. Upon arrival, the patient is intubated, and vascular access is obtained. It is difficult to ascertain whether the patient has palpable pulses. A focused point-of-care ultrasound of the heart is performed, which exhibits a large circumferential pericardial effusion on subxiphoid view (Figure 21.7a). There is diastolic collapse of the right ventricle and poor contractility of the heart. Given the patient's clinical presentation and sonographic evidence of cardiac tamponade, the decision is made to perform an emergent pericardiocentesis. The parasternal long-axis view is obtained (Figure 21.7b), with the largest region of fluid identified. A needle is inserted with real-time ultrasound guidance, and pericardial fluid is aspirated. The patient is then stabilized, and brought to the PICU. Ultimately, the cardiothoracic surgeon places a pericardial drain in the operating room, in order to prevent the acute recurrence of this effusion.

   Point-of-care ultrasound is ideal for determining whether cardiac activity is present, and whether a pericardial effusion

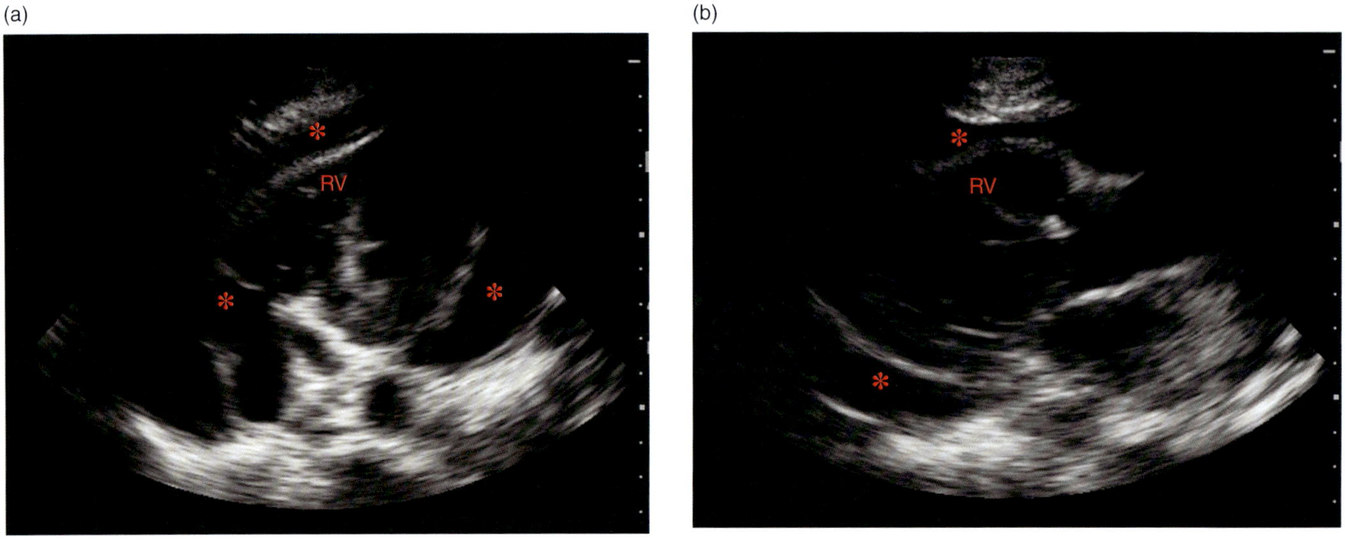

Figure 21.7 **Case 1**: cardiac ultrasound performed at the (a) subxiphoid region and the (b) parasternal long-axis view, which demonstrates a large circumferential pericardial effusion (*). There is notable diastolic right ventricular (RV) collapse and sonographic evidence of tamponade, which is most evident in video clips.

is present. In this situation, a focused cardiac ultrasound rapidly revealed the presence of a circumferential pericardial effusion with signs of tamponade. Physical examination findings of tamponade are often unreliable. Further, point-of-care ultrasound can be used to improve the safety and success of performing an emergent pericardiocentesis.

2. A 15-year-old African American male with sickle cell trait presents to the emergency department with acute anterior chest pain, which is worse with deep inspiration. He has had tactile fevers at home, and developed shortness of breath just prior to his arrival. On presentation, his vital signs are: T 39.2 °C, HR 156 bpm, RR 22/min, BP 110/60. A point-of-care ultrasound of his heart is performed, which demonstrates a hyperdynamic heart, but there is no pericardial effusion, and normal contractility. An assessment of his IVC is performed in order to determine whether dehydration is a cause of his tachycardia. The IVC shows significant respiratory variation, with near-complete collapse with inspiration. Aggressive intravenous fluid administration is initiated. Finally, a limited lung ultrasound is performed in order to assess for the presence of a pleural effusion. There is a significant pleural effusion on the left (Figure 21.8), with a small effusion on the right. An upright portable radiograph confirms this finding. The patient rapidly deteriorates, becomes hypotensive, and is admitted to the PICU. Ultrasound is performed in order to determine the ideal placement for chest tube drainage of the right hemithorax. A chest tube is successfully placed without complications. Subsequent fluid cultures and clinical course reveal a septic patient with necrotizing staphylococcal pneumonia.

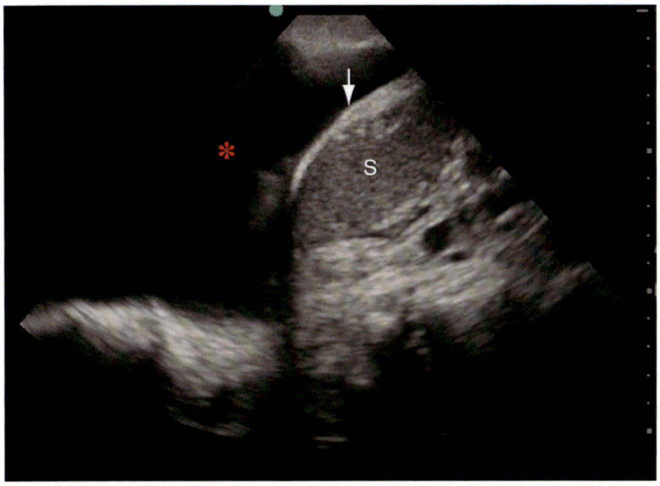

Figure 21.8 **Case 2: Pleural effusion**. Ultrasound performed at the left upper quadrant, demonstrating a large left pleural effusion (*). Note the loss of the mirror image artifact of the spleen (S), and the anechoic fluid collection superior, or cephalad, to the diaphragm (arrow).

This case demonstrates the utlity of point-of-care ultrasound in evaluating the patient with dyspnea and tachycardia. While the differential diagnosis is broad for these presenting complaints, ultrasound can rapidly narrow the differential diagnosis and guide clinical management. In this scenario, the patient is tachycardic and short of breath. The point-of-care ultrasound is able to identify that this is largely due to his fever and dehydration, rather than cardiac compromise. More telling is the lung ultrasonography that is performed, which reveals pleural effusions. This is found at the bedside, long before portable radiographs are able to be performed and interpreted.

3. A four-year-old girl with nephrotic syndrome presents to the emergency department with acute abdominal distension, severe abdominal pain, and fevers. On physical examination, she is febrile to 41.2 °C, tachycardic, diaphoretic, and in acute respiratory distress. You perform a point-of-care ultrasound, which reveals a significant amount of intraperitoneal fluid in all fields. Given the concern for acute respiratory distress and potential decompensation, it is decided to perform an ultrasound-assisted paracentesis. The largest pocket of fluid is identified in the suprapubic region. The bladder (Figure 21.9a) and surrounding bowel (Figure 21.9b) are identified, in order

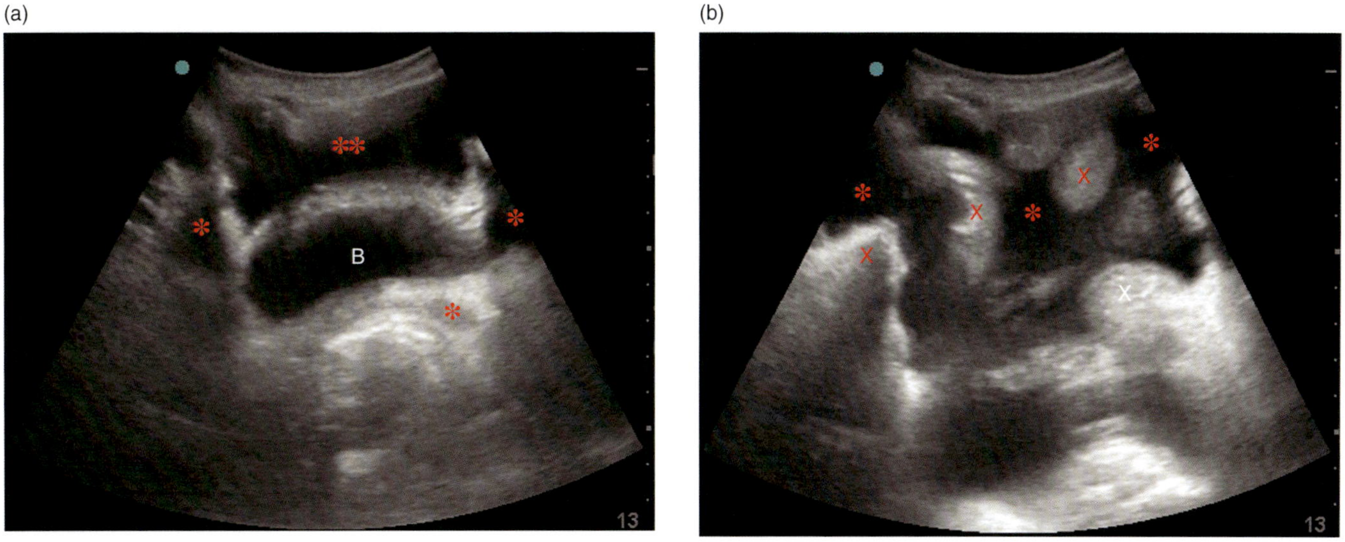

Figure 21.9 **Case 3: ascites**. (a) ultrasound performed at the suprapubic region with several regions of free fluid or ascites (*), with the largest fluid collection (**) anterior and superficial to the bladder (B). (b) Ultrasound of surrounding bowel (x) identified, in order to avoid puncture.

to avoid puncturing them. The depth from the skin to the most superficial portion of the fluid collection is identified, and the skin is marked. The needle trajectory is at the same angle as the ultrasound transducer. The needle is visualized as entering the fluid pocket under real-time ultrasound guidance, and 250 mL of purulent fluid is removed and sent for culture. There is minimal bleeding at the needle puncture site, with no complications. The patient has improvement in her respiratory status, and is started on intravenous antibiotics. Laboratory studies reveal acute bacterial peritonitis as the etiology of the ascites fluid and her clinical presentation.

This case demonstrates the utility of point-of-care ultrasound in identifying the presence of intraperitoneal fluid. Once this fluid is identified, ultrasound-guided drainage can be performed emergently in order to alleviate the patient's respiratory distress. Ultrasound guidance improves the safety profile of the procedure and prevents the inadvertent puncture of surrounding intraperitoneal structures.

Summary/key points

1. Pericardiocentesis, thoracentesis, and paracentesis are uncommonly performed procedures in pediatric patients. However, the use of ultrasound can help decrease the complications associated with performing these procedures.
2. It is always important to identify the ideal site for needle entry and aspiration of fluid. This site avoids inadvertently puncturing surrounding structures.
3. When performing these procedures, a static approach (ultrasound assistance) may be utilized, in which the incision site and needle trajectory are identified, and the skin is marked prior to performing the procedure. A dynamic approach (ultrasound guidance) visualizes the needle as it enters the fluid space and allows for real-time needle localization and needle redirection.
4. Once the site for aspiration is identified, avoid repositioning of the patient in order to avoid the movement of important structures into the path of the needle.
5. Further studies need to be performed regarding the role of ultrasound for pericardiocentesis, thoracentesis, and paracentesis in pediatric patients.

Selected references

Bard, C., Lafortune, M., Breton, G. (1986) Ascites: ultrasound guidance or blind paracentesis? *Can Med Assoc J* **135**(3): 209–10.

Duncan, D. R., Morgenthaler, T. I., Rhy, J. H., *et al.* (2009) Reducing iatrogenic risk in thoracentesis: establishing best practice via experiential training in a zero-risk environment. *Chest* **135**(5): 1315–20.

Jones, P. W., Moyers, J. P., Rogers, J. T., *et al.* (2003) Ultrasound-guided thoracentesis: is it a safer method? *Chest* **123**(2): 418–23.

Labovitz, A. J., Noble, V. E., Bierig, M., *et al.* (2010) Focused cardiac ultrasound in the emergent setting: a consensus statement of the Society of Echocardiography and American College of Emergency Physicians. *J Am Soc Echocardiogr* **23**(12): 1225–30.

Lichtenstein, D., Hulot, J. S., Rabiller, A., *et al.* (1999) Feasibility and safety of ultrasound-aided thoracentesis in mechanically ventilated patients. *Intensive Care Med* **25**(9): 955–8.

Nazeer, S. R., Dewbre, H., Miller, A. H. (2005) Ultrasound-assisted paracentesis performed by emergency physicians vs. the traditional technique: a prospective, randomized study. *Am J Emerg Med* **3**(3): 363–7.

Patel, P. A., Ernst, F. R., Gunnarsson, C. L. (2012) Ultrasonography guidance reduces complications and costs associated with thoracentesis procedures. *J Clin Ultrasound* **40**(3): 135–41.

Tsang, T. S., El-Najdawi, E. K., Seward, J. B., *et al.* (1998) Percutaneous echocardiographically guided pericardiocentesis in pediatric patients: evaluation of safety and efficacy. *J Am Soc Echocardiogr* **11**(11): 1072–7.

Tsang, T. S., Enriquez-Sarano, M., Freeman, W. K., *et al.* (2002) Consecutive 1127 therapeutic echocardiographically guided pericardiocentesis: clinical profile, practice patterns, and outcomes spanning 21 years. *Mayo Clin Proc* **77**(5): 429–36.

Zerth, H., Harwood, R., Tommasso, L., Girzadas, D. V. Jr. (2011) An inexpensive, easily constructed, reusable task trainer simulating ultrasound-guided pericardiocentesis. *J Emerg Med* **43**(6): 1066–9.

Chapter

22 Cutting-edge procedures: the airway

Randall T. Rhyne, Jamie A. Jenkins, and Beatrice Hoffmann

Objectives/indications

The applications of ultrasound for procedural assistance and guidance are rapidly evolving. One of the basic principles of pediatric emergency and critical care medicine is to establish and maintain the airway during resuscitation. When intubation is indicated, point-of-care ultrasound provides a rapid, direct, and real-time method for confirming proper endotracheal tube (ETT) placement within the trachea. In situations where direct visualization of the ETT passing through the vocal cords is not possible, ultrasound may provide advantages over traditional secondary means of confirming ETT placement.

In situations of chest trauma, thoracostomy tubes, or chest tubes, are often indicated as an adjunct to airway management. Traditional methods of confirming proper placement include radiographs and CT scan. More recently, it has been suggested that ultrasound may be a useful means by which the correct placement of intrathoracic thoracostomy tubes may be confirmed.

The objectives of this chapter are to describe how point-of-care ultrasound may be utilized to evaluate proper endotracheal tube placement within the larynx and trachea, and proper thoracostomy tube positioning within the thoracic cavity. While these are novel applications, the suggested techniques for performing these applications are reviewed. Further research needs to be performed in order to validate these applications.

ENDOTRACHEAL TUBE PLACEMENT

Background

Endotracheal tube (ETT) placement is often indicated in order to establish and stabilize an airway during resuscitations. Traditional methods by which a clinician may confirm proper ETT placement include auscultation, capnography, and chest radiography.

Recently, ultrasound was also introduced to serve as an adjunct to traditional methods of ETT confirmation. Since ultrasound of the airway is an emerging indication for point-of-care sonography, there are relatively few studies on using ultrasound for ETT confirmation. Thus far, when compared to the traditional methods of auscultation and capnography, airway ultrasound is more sensitive in detecting esophageal intubation. In addition, ultrasound is more rapid when compared to conventional chest radiography. Prior literature focuses on the indirect signs of proper endotracheal tube placement, which include the evaluation of bilateral lung expansion following intubation (see Chapter 6).

Several small studies evaluating ultrasound's ability to determine correct ETT placement have been performed in the controlled environments of intensive care units and operating rooms. In both pediatric and adult patients, sonography has been shown to be both 100% sensitive and specific in confirming the intratracheal position of the ETT. Research in the uncontrolled environment of the adult emergency department has shown that bedside sonography may be highly accurate in determining endotracheal versus esophageal intubation. Further studies need to be performed in pediatric patients in the emergency department.

Anatomy

Key structures of the larynx and hypopharynx are important to be familiar with. Most important is the relationship between the trachea, esophagus, and external anatomic landmarks (Figure 22.1).

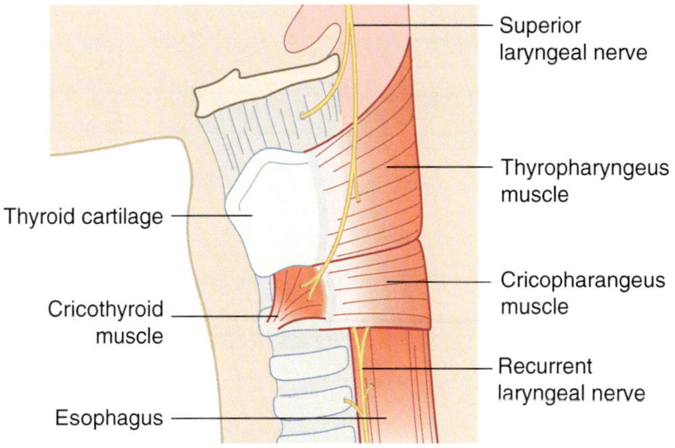

Figure 22.1 Anatomy of the larynx. External landmarks. It is important to recognize the location of the trachea in relation to the esophagus. *Artwork created by Emily Evans © Cambridge University Press.*

Pediatric Emergency and Critical Care Ultrasound, ed. Stephanie J. Doniger. Published by Cambridge University Press.

(a)

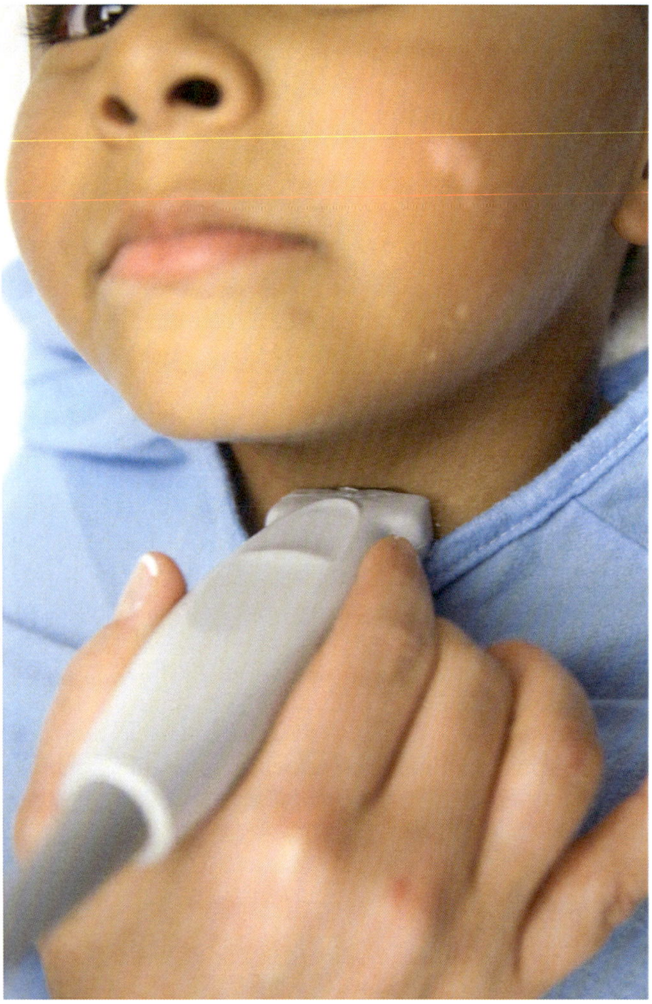

Technique

Transducer selection and orientation

The superficial location of the upper airway structures makes ultrasound visualization with a high-frequency (5–10 MHz), linear transducer ideal. The indicator should be oriented towards the patient's right side.

Patient position and preparation

Proper patient positioning is the key to a successful intubation and should be at the discretion of the individual performing the intubation. Frequently, the sonographer is positioned at the right-hand side of the patient, holding the transducer over the anterior neck of the patient (Figure 22.2a).

Ultrasound imaging

The vocal cords can be located by placing the transducer midline on the anterior neck at the level of the mid-thyroid or just below the thyroid (Figure 22.2a), and scanning cephalad to the level of the thyroid cartilage. The vocal cords appear as hyperechoic, linear structures in the shape of an inverted "V," and can be observed to open or close with respiration and phonation. In the transverse view, the trachea appears as a midline, hypoechoic structure with a brightly echogenic line immediately behind it representing air in the tracheal lumen. The tracheal rings can best be appreciated in the long-axis view. The esophagus appears as a collapsed, oval, multilayered structure immediately to the left of the trachea and posterior to the left thyroid lobe (Figure 22.2b,c). It is important to note that the position of the esophagus relative to the trachea may differ depending on the level at which it is being visualized.

Ultrasound-guided procedure

Ultrasound may be performed simultaneously during intubation, or following intubation. It may be preferred to perform

(b)

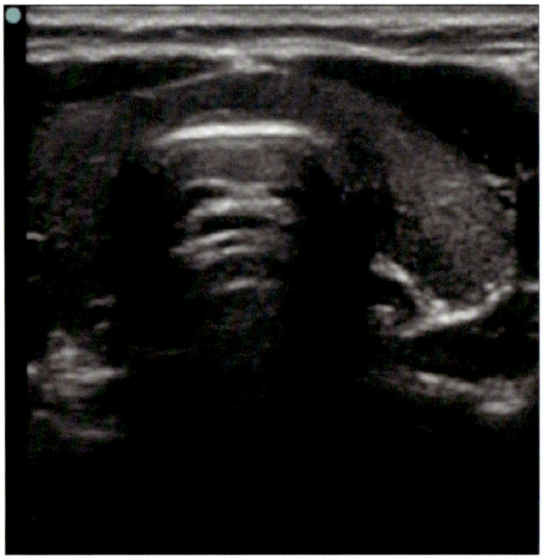

(c)

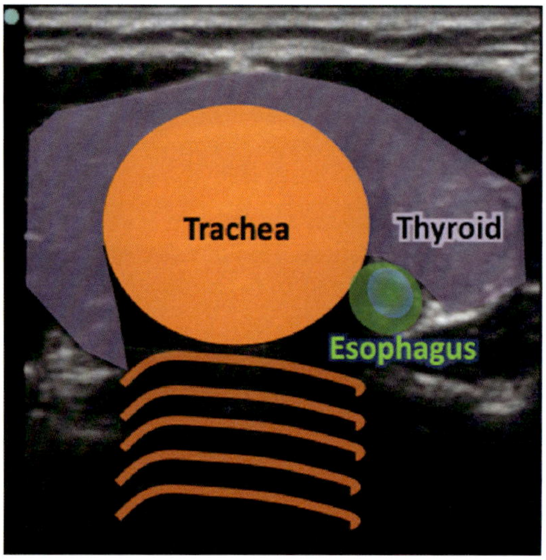

Figure 22.2 Sonography of the airway. (a) Transducer position for localizing the lower cervical trachea and esophagus. The transducer is positioned at the height of C6 or the isthmus of the thyroid gland. If the transducer is moved more cephalad, the sonographer can also attempt to provide cricoid pressure with the transducer. (b) Ultrasound image of the lower neck anatomy. (c) Illustration depicting important structures: the trachea, esophagus, and thyroid. *Reprinted with permission, Beatrice Hoffmann, MD PhD.*

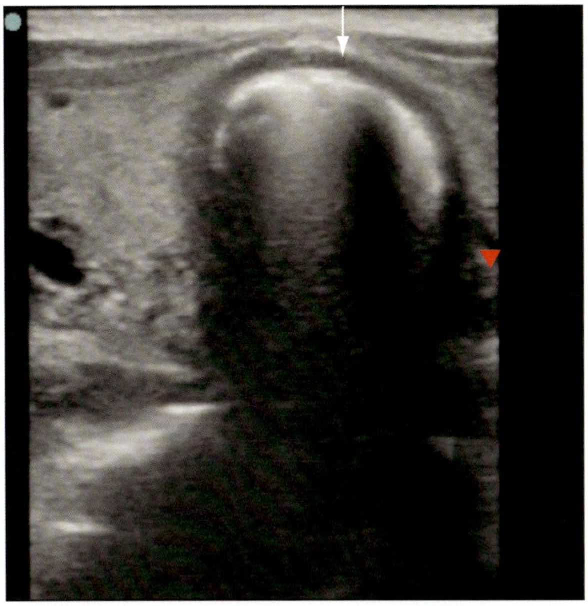

Figure 22.3 Tracheal intubation. Ultrasound image showing the trachea (arrow) and an empty esophagus (arrowhead) without visualization of the actual ETT. *Reprinted with permission, Beatrice Hoffmann, MD PhD.*

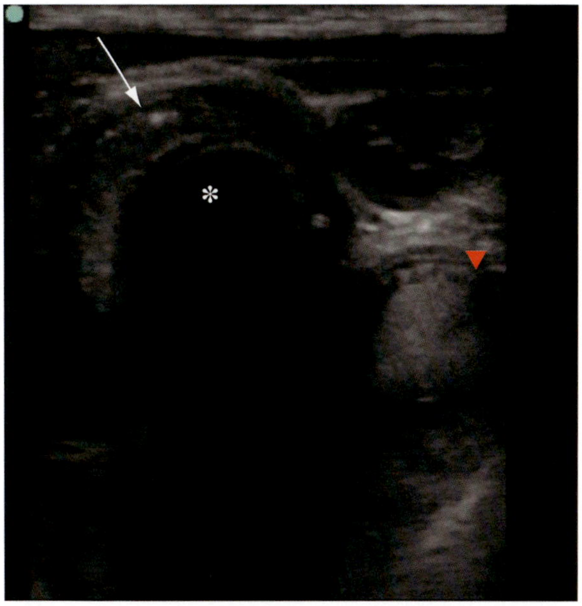

Figure 22.4 Tracheal intubation with a fluid-filled airway after drowning. Fluid-filled trachea (arrow), fluid-filled esophagus (arrowhead). The dark lumen of the ETT (*) can also be visualized. *Reprinted with permission, Beatrice Hoffmann, MD PhD.*

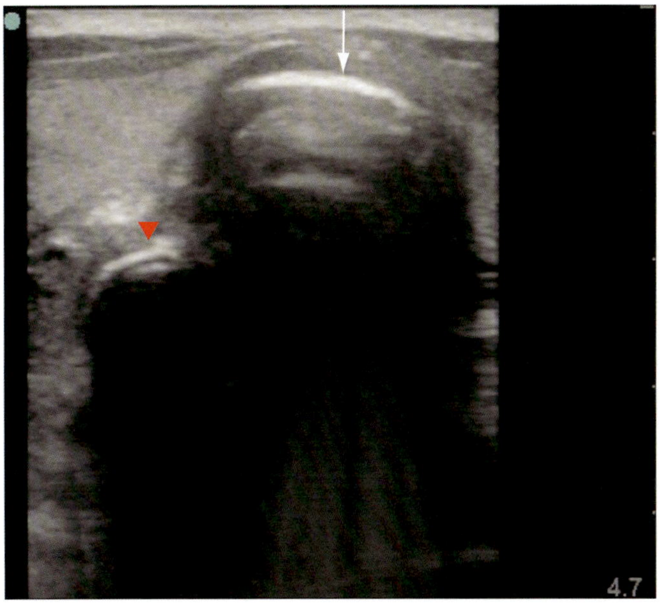

Figure 22.5 Esophageal intubation: "double trachea" sign. The stented open esophagus (arrowhead) appears similar to a second trachea (arrow). *Reprinted with permission, Beatrice Hoffmann, MD PhD.*

real-time visualization during intubation, since the ETT is rarely visualized within the trachea following intubation. This is due to the fact that the air between the wall of the trachea and the ETT causes an acoustic impedance mismatch (Figure 22.3). Exceptions include near-drowning patients and those with significant airway secretions, where this air is replaced by fluid (Figure 22.4). In order to improve the direct visualization of the ETT, one may fill the ETT cuff with normal saline. Other secondary signs of successful intubation include normal bilateral lung sliding on lung ultrasound (see Chapter 6).

In order to perform simultaneous, real-time visualization, some investigators suggest observing the region of the larynx simultaneously for a brief "widening" or distortion of the glottis as the ETT is passed. Others have shown successful sonographic detection of tracheal and esophageal intubations with positioning of the transducer close to the middle or inferior aspect of the thyroid in midline. In this location, the trachea and often the esophagus can both be identified and monitored during intubation. The sonographer can observe a brief and transient "flush" at the anterior aspect of the trachea, as the ETT is passed into the trachea, while the esophagus remains empty.

In contrast, improper ETT placement, or esophageal intubation, must be considered if distortion of the glottis and upper trachea is not noted during intubation. On ultrasound, an esophageal intubation can be recognized by the visualization of the "double trachea" sign. The esophagus that is stented open by an errant ETT which appears as curved echogenic lines with posterior acoustic shadowing located lateral to the trachea, giving the appearance of a second trachea (Figure 22.5).

CHEST TUBE PLACEMENT

Background

The incidence of chest trauma is estimated at 12 persons per million of the population per day. The majority can be adequately managed medically with thoracostomy tubes, or chest tubes. Mechanical ventilation is sometimes necessary. Chest tubes may be placed to drain a hemothorax or pneumothorax, which may be compromising a patient's adequate ventilation. Chest tubes have been shown to be malpositioned in up to 20% of cases, with increasing numbers seen

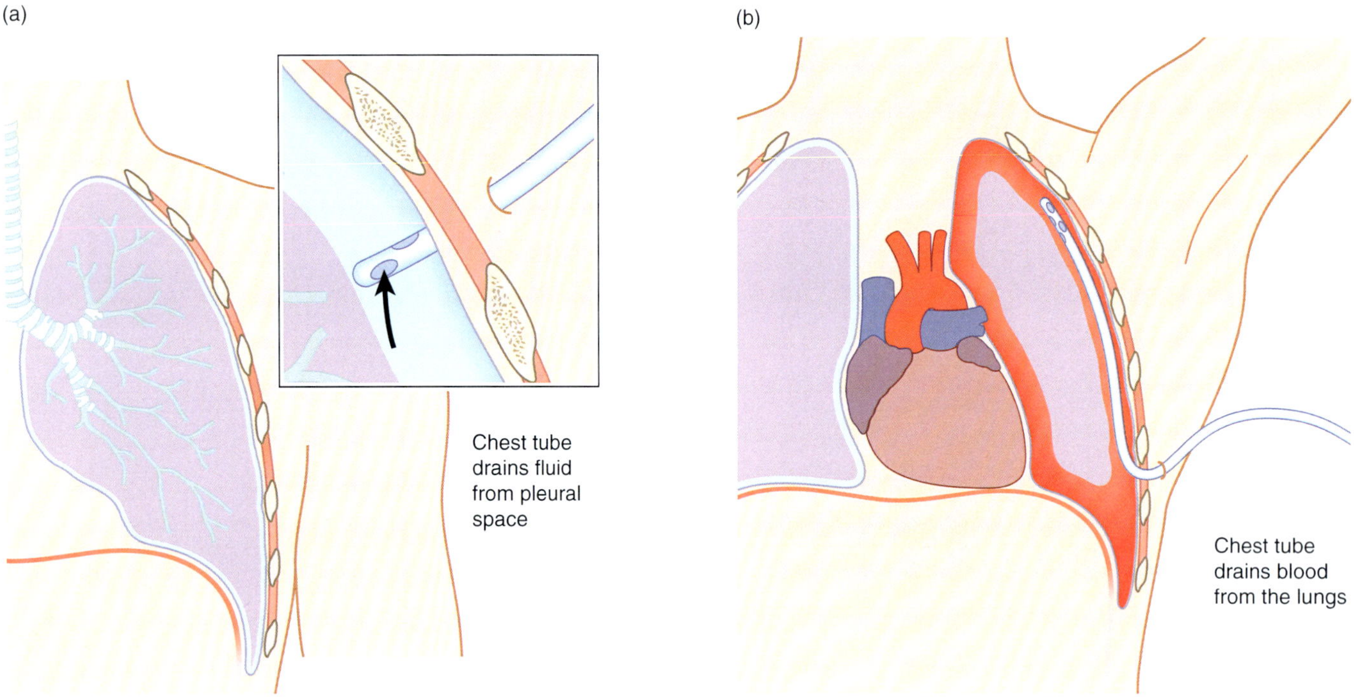

Figure 22.6 Anatomic representation of thoracostomy tube placement. (a) A thoracostomy, or chest tube is placed in order to drain fluid or air from the pleural space. (b) A thoracostomy tube that is placed for a hemothorax should be more posteriorly directed. *Artwork created by Emily Evans © Cambridge University Press.*

at teaching hospitals and in emergent settings. In order to identify proper chest tube placement, the American College of Surgeons recommends chest radiographs as the initial imaging modality of choice. This is controversial since chest computed tomography (CT) scans may be better in determining chest tube malpositioning and have been determined to be the gold standard. However, both techniques expose the patient to ionizing radiation and require further time, resources, and expense. If repositioning of chest tubes is required, the patient is exposed to additional pain, more invasive procedures, and increased risk of infection. Further associated complications include empyemas, tension pneumothorax, lung contusions, and vascular injury.

Recent studies have determined that ultrasound has the ability to determine the chest tube position at its entrance into the pleural space. Jenkins *et al.* conducted a small study, which showed the ability to identify an intrathoracic chest tube on ultrasound. While no malpositioned tubes were investigated, it can be inferred that, if the chest tube can be visualized, it likely is within subcutaneous tissues of the chest wall. If it disappears from view beyond the pleural line, it can be inferred that it is within the pleural space. Further investigation needs to be performed with larger studies, malpositioned tubes, and pediatric patients.

Anatomy

A chest tube is placed in the thoracic cavity to drain air or fluid from the pleural space. Important landmarks are the ribs, intercostal vessels and nerves, and the pleura (Figure 22.6a,b).

Technique

Transducer selection and orientation

Linear transducers have a greater spatial resolution and are, therefore, better able to distinguish between objects within the subcutaneous space. In order to visualize the chest tube entering the pleural space for proper placement, it is important to vizualize the chest tube in relation to the subcutaneous structures. While the low-frequency transducers may also be utilized, the linear transducer more accurately illustrates the chest tube as it courses through the subcutaneous tissue into the pleural space.

The views necessary for determining proper chest tube placement are that of the chest tube at its insertion into the pleural space in both transverse and longitduinal views. Initially, the linear transducer should be placed adjacent to the chest tube insertion site, perpendicular to the tube, evaluating it in the transverse orientation (Figure 22.7a). Then, the transducer should be oriented parallel to the chest tube, or in the longitudinal orientation (Figure 22.8a).

Patient position and preparation

The ideal patient positioning is supine or semi-recumbent position. Whenever possible, the transducer should be prepared in a sterile fashion (Figure S3.7).

Ultrasound imaging

In the transverse view, the chest tube appears as an anechoic, circular with posterior shadowing in two-dimensional

(a) (b)

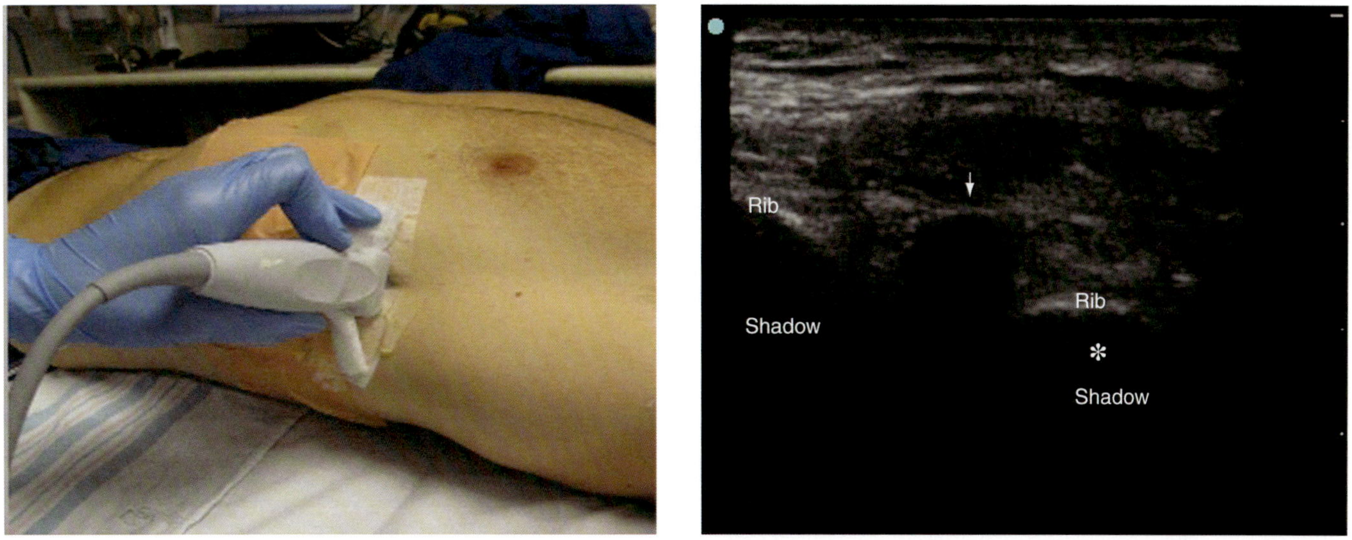

Figure 22.7 Thoracostomy tube imaging, transverse view. (a) The thoracostomy tube is first identified in the transverse view by placing the transducer perpendicular to the tube insertion site. (b) Transverse view of the thoracostomy tube (arrow) using the linear transducer. The tube appears as a thinly curved echo with posterior shadowing. A rib can be seen adjacent to the thoracostomy tube, with a hyperechoic curved echo with posterior shadowing. In this image, an anechoic pleural effusion (*) can be seen posterior, or deep, to the ribs and thoracostomy tube.

(a) (b)

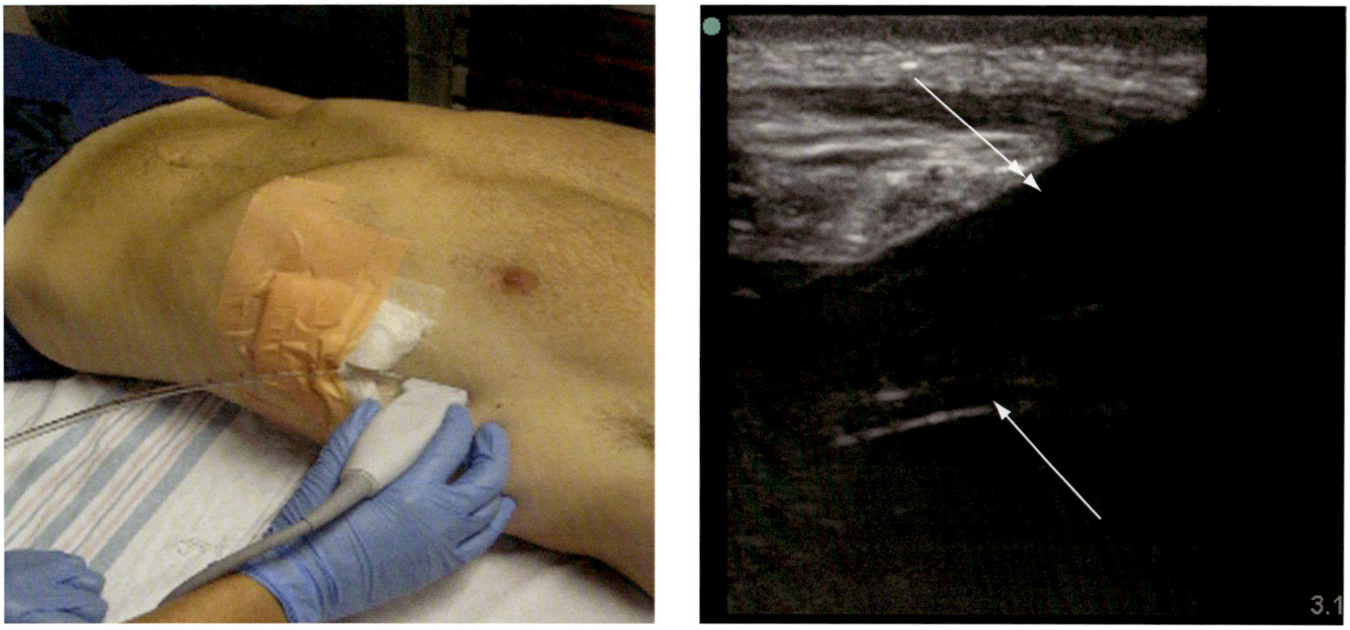

Figure 22.8 Thoracostomy tube imaging, longitudinal view. (a) The thoracostomy tube is identified in the longitudinal view by placing the transducer parallel to the tube insertion site. (b) Longitudinal view of the thoracostomy tube using the linear transducer. The tube appears as a linear anechoic structure that courses through the subcutaneous tissues and into the pleural space (double white arrow). The visceral pleura is also seen (arrow).

gray scale (Figure 22.7b). Once the chest tube is identified, the transducer should then be advanced along the pathway of the chest tube, visualizing the chest tube course through the subcutaneous tissue, passing the hyperechoic pleural line and entering the pleural space. Then, in order to obtain the longitudinal view, the transducer is placed parallel to the chest tube, and advanced to visualize the chest tube entering into the pleural space (Figure 22.8b). Lastly, for additional confirmation, M-mode should be used to elicit the characteristic "black out" sign (Figure 22.9a). This is in contrast to the pattern shown in Figure 22.9b, which is typical of a pneumothorax, the "stratosphere" sign.

Ultrasound-guided procedure

Thus far, only static evaluation of chest tube placement has been investigated. No studies have addressed the use of real-time ultrasound visualization during chest tube placement.

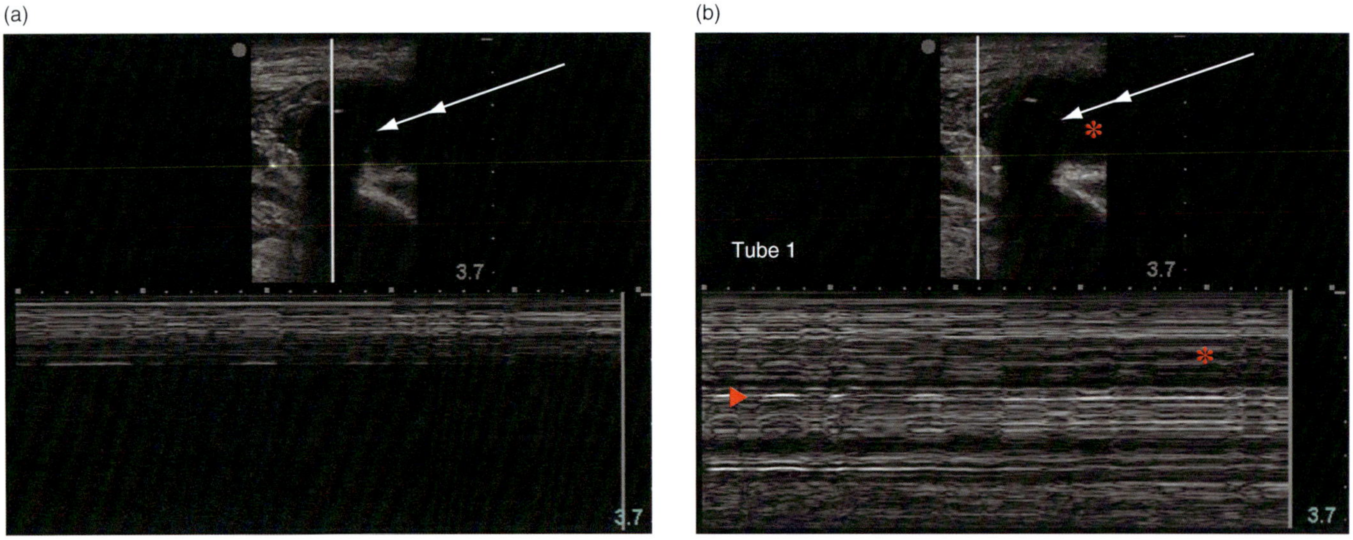

Figure 22.9 **M-mode** images with the linear transducer. (a) The thoracostomy tube appears in transverse view as an anechoic, circular structure with posterior shadowing (double white arrow). When the M-mode cursor is placed on top of the tube there is a distinct absence of waveform. This characteristic pattern is referred to as the "black out" sign. (b) With the M-mode cursor positioned to the lateral aspect of the tube, a "stratosphere" sign is present, indicating pneumothorax. The visceral pleura is also seen (arrowhead). A pleural effusion (*) can be seen just above the visceral pleura (*).

Scanning tips

Pitfalls

- It is important to recognize situations where the clinical utility of airway ultrasound may be limited. Edema, neck masses, or subcutaneous emphysema can make upper airway ultrasound difficult due to the distortion of normal anatomy.
- Real-time sonographic ETT confirmation can be difficult in patients with short necks, or who are unable to fully extend their necks. Proper transducer placement may interfere with direct laryngoscopy.
- Acoustic impedance mismatch prevents the ETT from being directly visualized on ultrasound. Proper endotracheal placement is the absence of the tube in the esophagus.
- In some cases, the esophagus may reside directly posterior to the trachea, which may make esophageal intubation difficult to detect.
- There have been limited studies that show that ultrasound can detect intrathoracic chest tube placement. A malpositioned tube is not actually visualized, but inferred by its disappearance beyond the pleural line.

Tips to improve scanning

✓ Real-time, simultaneous scanning during endotracheal intubation enhances visualization of proper endotracheal tube placement. A widening or distortion of the epiglottis may be visualized.

✓ In order to enhance visualization of the ETT, one may fill the ETT cuff with saline.

✓ To improve scanning of a chest tube it is important to start scanning at its insertion site and follow it through the subcutaneous tissues to its entrance into the pleural space.

✓ Visualize the chest tube in transverse and longitudinal views. M-mode of the chest tube creates a typical "black out" sign.

Case

1. An 11-year-old male is brought in by EMS after being found floating face down in a neighbor's swimming pool. Upon EMS arrival, the patient is apneic and pulseless at the scene and receives bystander CPR. Paramedics intubates the patient and continues CPR during transport to the emergency department; however, they report poor O_2 saturation, and a massive amount of fluid is suctioned from the ETT tube. The paramedics communicate uncertainly of the correct tube placement on arrival in the emergency department. In the emergency department, the patient is still in cardiac arrest and pediatric advanced life support (PALS) is initiated. During the primary survey, the emergency physician is unable to visualize the ETT by direct laryngoscopy due to the presence of massive fluid and secretions in the oropharynx and larynx, and both auscultation for breath sounds and colorimetric CO_2 detection are equivocal. A second emergency physician performs simulataneous airway ultrasound of the patient, which shows the ETT within the tracheal lumen and an empty esophagus (Figure 22.4). After confirming intratracheal placement of the ETT using ultrasound, the primary survey is continued. After additional rounds of PALS the patient has return of spontaneous circulation and is admitted to the ICU.

This case highlights the utility of point-of-care ultrasonography incorporated into resuscitation. This cutting-edge technique serves an additional confirmatory method for endotracheal tube placement.

Summary/key points

1. Limited studies have shown that ultrasound offers a rapid and accurate method of providing real-time confirmation of proper endotracheal tube placement. Other means of ETT confirmation should be used in conjunction with ultrasound.
2. A high frequency 5–10 MHz, linear transducer transducer is ideal for airway ultrasound due to the superficial nature of the airway structures. This transducer is used both for confirmation of endotracheal tube placement and for visualizing chest tubes.
3. The ETT itself is frequently not visualized within the trachea, but detection of an ETT within the esophagus or an empty esophagus post-intubation seems to have a very high predictive value for esophageal or tracheal intubation, respectively.
4. Point-of-care ultrasound may be able to determine proper chest tube positioning as well as distinguish the chest tube from surrounding subcutaneous tissue. Ultrasound imaging of a chest tube creates a unique M-mode appearance termed the "black out" sign.
5. Identify the chest tube in both transverse and longitudinal planes. Advance the transducer along the length of the chest tube and watch it course through subcutaneous tissue, pass through the pleural line, and enter the intrathoracic region.

Selected references

Chou, H., Tseng, W., Wang, C., *et al.* (2011) Tracheal rapid ultrasound exam (T.R.U.E.) for confirming endotracheal tube placement during emergency intubation. *Resuscitation* **82**(10): 1279–84.

Hoffmann, B., Gullett, J. P. (2010) Emergency ultrasound for the detection of esophageal intubation. *Acad Emerg Med* **17**(4): 464–5.

Jenkins, J. A., Gharahbaghian, L., Doniger, S. J., *et al.* (2012) Sonographic Identification of Tube Thoracostomy Study (SITTS): confirmation of intrathoracic placement. *West J Emerg Med* **13**(4): 305–11.

Kool, D. R., Blickman, J. G. (2007) Advanced Trauma Life Support. ABCDE from a radiological point of view. *Emerg Radiol* **14**(3): 135–41.

Marciniak, B., Fayoux, P., Hebrard, A., *et al.* (2009) Airway management in children: ultrasonography assessment of tracheal intubation in real time? *Anesth Analg* **108**(2): 461–5.

Muslu, B., Sert, H., Kaya, A., *et al.* (2011) Use of sonography for rapid identification of esophageal and tracheal intubations in adult patients. *J Ultrasound Med* **30**(5): 671–6.

Raphael, D. T., Conard, F. U. (1987) Ultrasound confirmation of endotracheal tube placement. *J Clin Ultrasound* **15**(7): 459–62.

Rowan, K. R., Kirkpatrick, A. W., Lui, D., *et al.* (2002) Traumatic pneumothorax detection with thoracic US: correlation with chest radiography and CT – initial experience. *Radiology* **225**: 210–14.

Tsung, J. W., Fenster, D., Kessler, D. O., Novik, J. (2012) Dynamic anatomic relationship of the esophagus and trachea on sonography: implications for endotracheal tube confirmation in children. *J Ultrasound Med* **31**(9): 1365–70.

Werner, S. L., Smith, C. E., Goldstein, J. R., *et al.* (2007) Pilot study to evaluate the accuracy of ultrasonography in confirming endotracheal tube placement. *Ann Emerg Med* **49**(1): 75–80.

S4 Introduction

Stephanie J. Doniger

Worldwide, point-of-care ultrasonography has become integrated in the practice of critical care physicians, both in the neonatal intensive care unit (NICU) and the pediatric intensive care unit (PICU). In the NICU in particular, a recent survey showed that there is variation with regards to the level of use of point-of-care ultrasonography among neonatologists worldwide. Some NICUs have very limited capabilities of performing ultrasonography, while others are fully integrated. The most common uses in the NICU include functional echocardiography (fECHO), also referred to as targeted neonatal echocardiography (TnECHO). Other common uses include cranial ultrasonography and the identification of umbilical line positioning. Regardless of the levels of incorporation of point-of-care ultrasound into their practice, neonatologists worldwide have introduced this technology with close ongoing collaboration with subspecialists, such as the pediatric cardiologists. There is also variable use of point-of-care ultrasound in the PICU. The majority of the applications utilized focus on cardiac function and central line placement

When dealing with a critically ill patient, an integrated approach is useful in incorporating point-of-care ultrasonography into the clinical assessment. In these patients, the rapid identification and treatment of causes of hemodynamic instability or cardiac arrest is crucial. Through the use of cardiac ultrasound, lung ultrasound, and the IVC evaluation, one can distinguish between the different types of shock (i.e. cardiogenic vs. hypovolemic). It can further distinguish between different causes of acute dyspnea. In those patients presenting in cardiac arrest, ultrasonography can be instrumental in identifying reversible causes of pulseless electrical activity (PEA). As a result of the utility of integrated ultrasonography in critically ill patients, it has been suggested that point-of-care ultrasonography be incorporated into the resuscitation sequence as: Airway (A), Breathing (B), Circulation (C), Defibrillation (D), and exposure (E) (Figure S4.1). This concept was also included in the updated Advanced Pediatric Life Support (APLS) guidelines.

There is a great deal of similarity between the various indications for the use of ultrasonography in critical care and in the emergency department. Nevertheless, the circumstances faced in the ICUs may have some peculiarities, which include:

1. Patients stay longer in the ICU, and this may warrant repetitive scans.
2. The scan can be more monitoring in scope, rather than diagnostic.
3. Scans are utilized for early goal-directed therapy.
4. Ultrasonography-guided procedures in the ICU may differ from the types of procedure performed in the emergency department.
5. Elective scans (rather than emergent) are considered.

This section highlights the uses of point-of-care ultrasonography in the neonatal and pediatric critical care units. Initially, we discuss pathology specific to neonatal populations, then describe the use of ultrasonography in those critically ill neonates and children requiring hemodynamic and ventilatory support.

Selected references

Arntfield, R.T., Millington, S.J. (2012) Point of care cardiac ultrasound applications in the emergency department and intensive care unit – a review. *Curr Cardiol Rev* **8**(2): 98–108.

Copetti, R., Copetti, P., Reissig, A. (2012) Clinical integrated ultrasound of the thorax including causes of shock in nontraumatic critically ill patients. A practical approach. *Ultrasound Med Biol* **38**(3): 349–59.

Doniger, S. J., Chen, L. (2012) Ultrasonography for novices. In Fuchs, S., Yamamoto, L., eds. *APLS: The Pediatric Emergency Medicine Resource.* [Online] 5th edn. Burlington, MA: Jones & Bartlett Learning.

Evans, N., Gournay, V., Cabanas, F., *et al.* (2011) Point-of-care ultrasound in the neonatal intensive care unit: international perspectives. *Semin Fetal Neonatal Med* **16**: 61–8.

Lambert, R.L., Boker, J.R., Maffei, F.A. (2011) National survey of bedside ultrasound use in pediatric critical care. *Pediatr Crit Care Med* **12**(6): 655–9.

Manno, E., Navana, M., Faccio, L., *et al.* (2012) Deep impact of ultrasound in the intensive care unit: the "ICU sound" protocl. *Anesthesiology* **117**(4): 801–9.

Neri, L., Storti, E., Lichtenstein, D. (2007) Toward an ultrasound curriculum for critical care medicine. *Crit Care Med* **35**(5): S290–304.

Prekker, M.E., Scott, N.L., Har, D., *et al.* (2013) Point-of-care ultrasound to estimate central venous pressure: a comparison of three techniques. *Crit Care Med* **41**(3): 833–41.

Srinivasan, S., Cornell, T. T. (2011) Bedside ultrasound in pediatric critical care: a review. *Pediatr Crit Care Med* **12**(6): 667–74.

Via, G., Storti, E., Gulati, G., *et al.* (2012) Lung ultrasound in the ICU: from diagnostic instrument to respiratory monitoring tool. *Minerva Anestesiol* **78**(11): 1282–96.

Pediatric Emergency and Critical Care Ultrasound, ed. Stephanie J. Doniger. Published by Cambridge University Press.

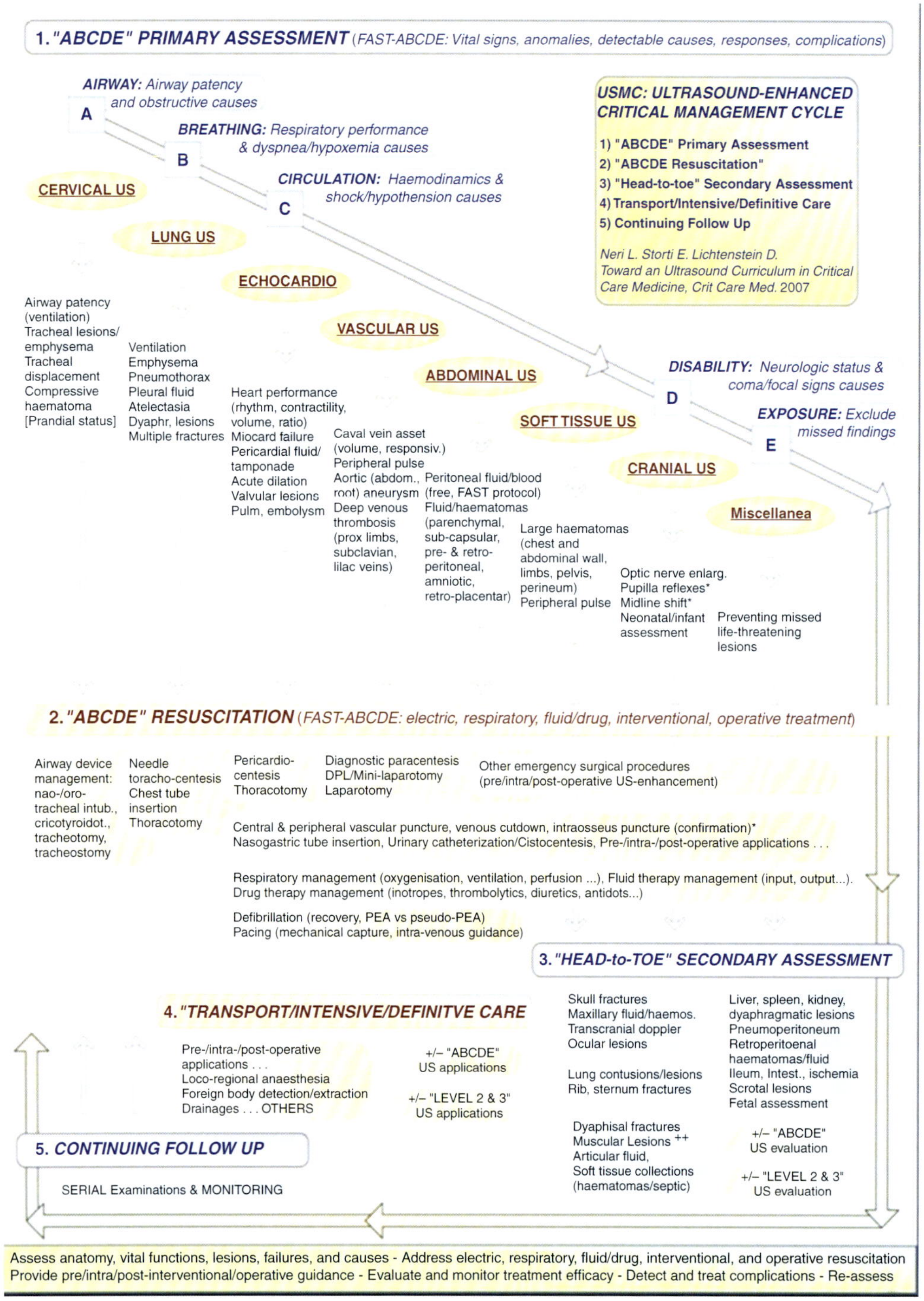

Figure S4.1 ABCD curriculum. Incorporating ultrasonography into the ABCD assessment. *Source (copyright): Neri, L., Storti, E., Lichtenstein, D. (2007) Toward an ultrasound curriculum for critical care medicine. Crit Care Med* ***35****(5): S290–304.*

Chapter

23

Neonates and infants

Alaa A. Eldemerdash, Mahmoud Elbarbary, and Stephanie J. Doniger

Objectives/indications

Both premature infants and full-term infants may present with pathology distinct to the neonatal period. The majority of these entities occur in the critically ill neonate, in the neonatal intensive care unit (NICU).

This chapter is a brief overview of the application of point-of-care ultrasonography in this unique population. The majority of research originates from the radiology and surgical literature. However, worldwide, neonatologists are increasingly incorporating this technology into their practice at the bedside, in order to rapidly diagnose life-threatening conditions in the smallest and most fragile of patients.

ABDOMINAL EMERGENCIES: NECROTIZING ENTEROCOLITIS

Background

Necrotizing enterocolitis (NEC) is an acquired condition of diffuse necrotic injury to the mucosal and submucosal layers of the bowel. It is the most common gastrointestinal emergency of all infants admitted to a NICU, and is the most serious gastrointestinal disorder that occurs during the neonatal period. Necrotizing enterocolitis affects mostly the extremely low-birth-weight (ELBW) infants, but can occur in full-term infants as well. The mortality rate for NEC is estimated to be 10–30%, or 11.5 to 12.3 per 100,000 infant deaths, greatly exceeding that of other gastrointestinal surgical disorders. Approximately 20% of babies with NEC will require surgical intervention, either for advanced disease or due to delay in diagnosis. Their mortality rate increases to 50%. Those that survive often have long-term problems including short-gut syndrome, growth impairment, and adverse neurodevelopmental outcomes.

The challenge with NEC is that most infants present with nonspecific symptoms, such as feeding intolerance and abdominal distension. For infants presenting with these complaints, feeds are often held and radiographs are obtained. Radiographic findings are important in the staging of NEC and determine the need for surgical intervention. The pathognomonic finding on plain radiographs is pneumatosis intestinalis. However, this finding is often absent or difficult to identify. Bohnhorst *et al.* showed that the sensitivity and specificity of pneumatosis intestinalis on abdominal radiographs was 75% and 91% respectively. When ultrasound and radiographs are combined, the sensitivity increases to 89%. Ultrasound imaging can identify portal venous gas, which is pathognomic for NEC. With new grading criteria for NEC, ultrasonography has a high specificity for the suspicion of NEC: approaching 100%. In addition, with the application of specific radiologic criteria, the diagnostic sensitivity reaches 90%.

Technique

Point-of-care questions

1. Is air present in the portal system?

Transducer selection and orientation

Ultrasound imaging should be performed with the linear transducer (5–10 MHz, most commonly 7.5 MHz), with a small footprint. The higher frequency provides better resolution, while sacrificing penetration.

A suggested protocol is to scan the liver and portal vein in both the longitudinal and transverse views. Dördelmann *et al.* suggested a scan time of approximately 3 minutes, with a mean of 4.5 minutes (Figure 23.1a).

Ultrasound imaging

Those babies suspected of having NEC may have an ultrasound evaluation, which can detect air bubbles moving through the wall of the intestine, otherwise known as pneumatosis intestinalis (Figure 23.1b). The ultrasound finding of air in the portal system can also be indicative of NEC. Sonographic findings of portal venous gas involve the trapping of air in the small branches of the portal vein inside the liver. This appears as dense granular echogenicities within the liver parenchyma. Portal venous gas may also be visualized as continuously streaming echogenic dots in the bloodstream. Doppler may also be helpful in detecting hyperemia or decreased blood flow in the wall of the intestine (Figure 23.2). These ultrasound findings, along with other clinical signs, can assist in making the diagnosis of NEC prior to bowel perforation and development of peritonitis.

Pediatric Emergency and Critical Care Ultrasound, ed. Stephanie J. Doniger. Published by Cambridge University Press.

(a)

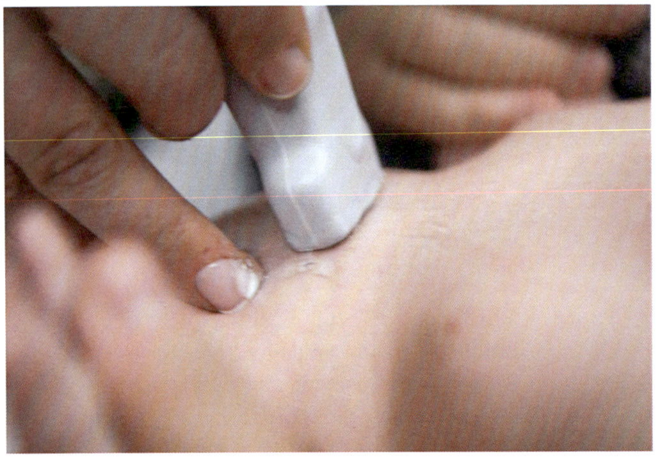

(b)

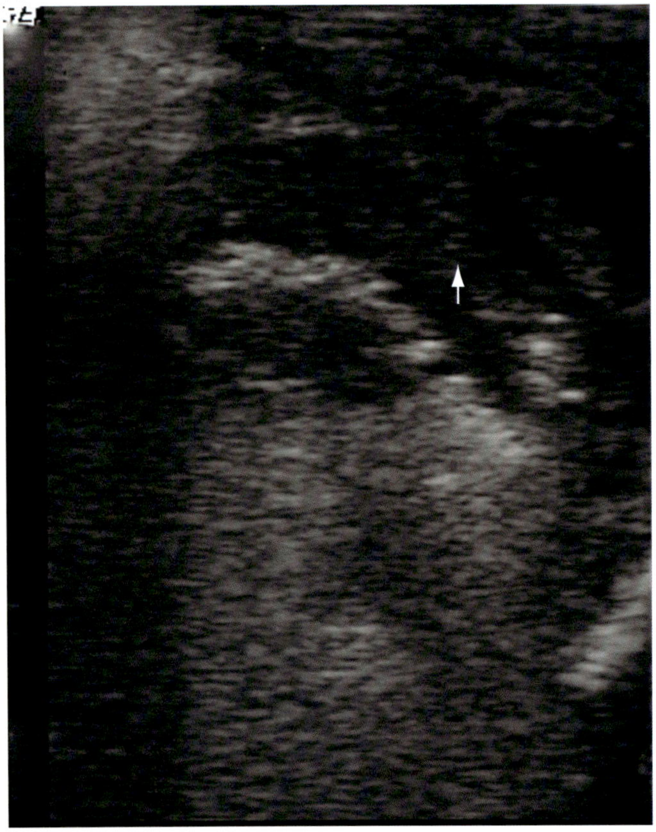

(c)

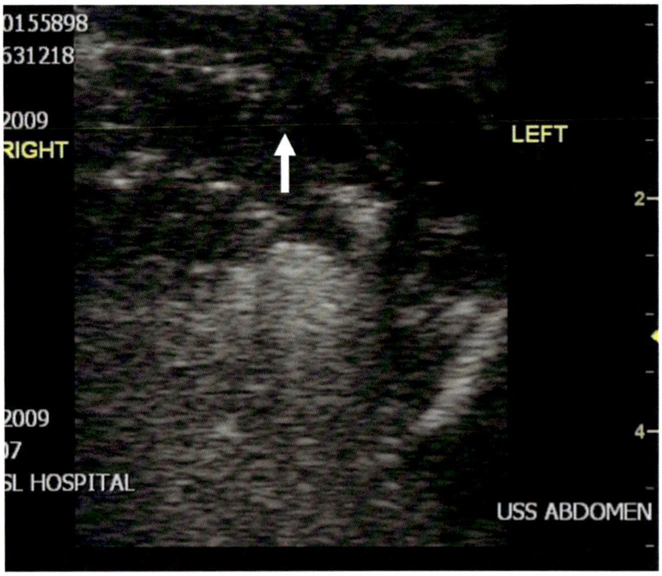

Figure 23.1 The evaluation for NEC. (a) Transducer placement. (b) Ultrasound image shows white dots with shadows (white arrow), indicative of air bubbles in the wall of the intestine. (c) Portal venous gas can also be visualized by ultrasound. Air bubbles appear hyperechoic (arrows). *Ultrasound image courtesy of Michael Jones, MD RDMS FACEP.*

ABDOMINAL EMERGENCIES: BOWEL OBSTRUCTION, MALROTATION WITH VOLVULUS

Background

Neonatal bowel obstruction is a serious condition that can be complicated by intestinal perforation. Early radiologic studies in cases of neonatal bowel obstruction are needed to rule out intestinal malrotation with midgut volvulus. Intestinal malrotation is a congenital anomaly that involves an abnormal position of the small bowel: the small bowel is predominantly on the right side of the abdomen, the cecum is displaced, and the ligament of Treitz is displaced inferiorly and to the right. With malrotation, volvulus may occur, when there is a twisting of the bowel, that obstructs the mesenteric blood vessels, thereby causing intestinal ischemia. As many as 40% of infants with malrotation with volvulus present within the first week of life. It is often difficult to differentiate malrotation from other causes of intestinal obstruction such as intestinal atresia. Volvulus is fatal, if not surgically corrected within hours.

An Upper GI Series is the gold standard for evaluating for malrotation, and can determine the length of the mesenteric base. Ultrasonography can be helpful in diagnosing malrotation and volvulus. With malrotation, there is an abnormal position of the duodenojejunal junction, to the right of midline. Studies have suggested that an inversion of the superior mesenteric vein

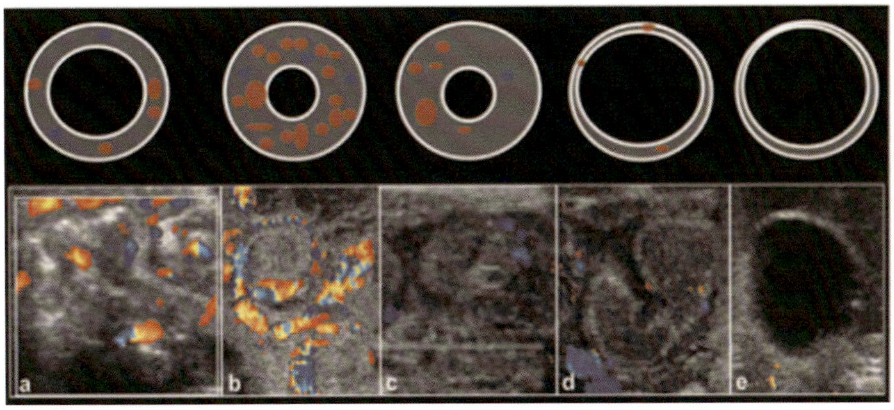

Figure 23.2 Doppler for necrotizing enterocolitis (NEC). The sequential changes in bowel wall thickness and perfusion in NEC, seen with transverse bowel sections (top) and color Doppler sonograms (bottom). (a) There is normal flow to normal bowel. The diagram shows normal bowel wall thickness and perfusion. (b) The changes of NEC are shown with bowel wall thickening and hyperemia. (c) The bowel wall thickening persists, but the perfusion has diminished. (d) As the process progresses, the mucosa starts to slough, and the bowel wall becomes much thinner; some perfusion persists. (e) Sloughing continues, the bowel wall becomes asymmetrically thinned, and blood flow ceases. *Source (copyright): Epelman, M., Daneman, A., Navarro, O. M.,* et al. *(2007) Necrotizing enterocolitis: review of state-of- the-art imaging findings with pathologic correlation. RadioGraphics 27: 285–305.*

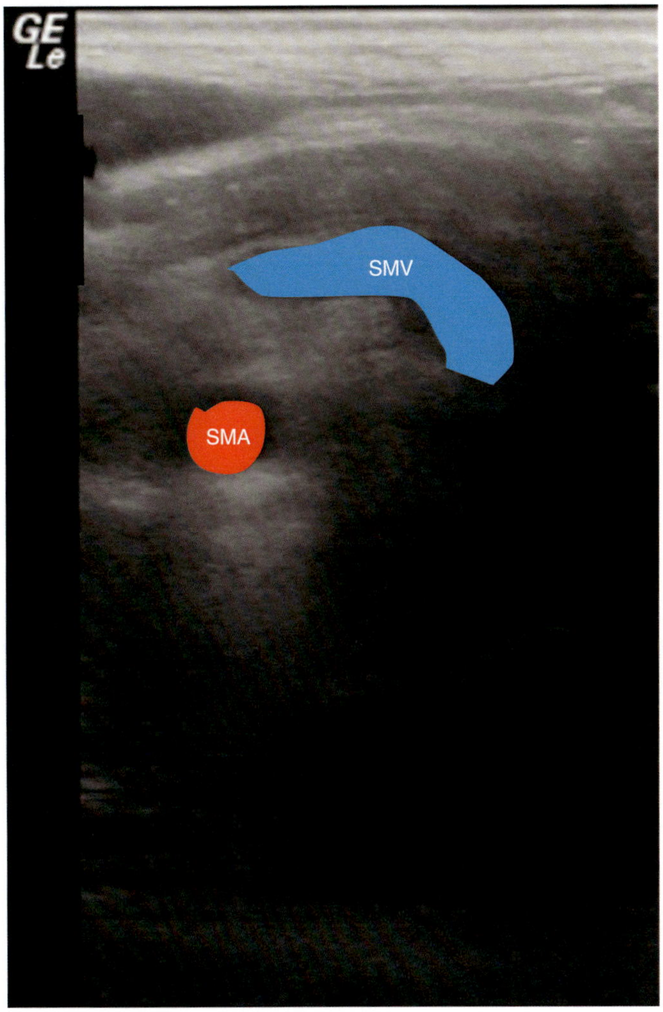

Figure 23.3 Malrotation with volvulus. Ultrasound image showing the "whirlpool" sign which involves the bowel and mesentery wrapping in a clockwise fashion around the superior mesenteric artery (SMA). Malrotation can also include the inversion of the SMA and SMV.

(SMV) and superior mesenteric artery (SMA) on ultrasound is diagnostic in nearly 100% of patients. In situations where the SMV lies anterior to the SMA, the incidence of malrotation decreases to 25–28%. Orzech *et al.* showed that, when compared with the gold standard of an Upper GI Series, ultrasonography had a false-positive rate of 15% and a false-negative rate of 2%. In those patients who had a negative ultrasound but positive Upper GI Series, there were no patients who had malrotation with midgut volvulus. Therefore, ultrasonography can serve as a good screening tool. Those patients with an abnormal ultrasound should have an upper GI study or go to the operating room, depending on their clinical presentation and consultation by a pediatric surgeon.

Technique

Point-of-care questions

1. Are dilated loops of bowel present?
2. Is the SMV to the left of the SMA?

Transducer selection and orientation

The evaluation for bowel obstruction, and malrotation with volvulus, differs a bit from other evaluations of the bowel. For the most part, ultrasound of the bowel is performed with a linear, high-frequency transducer (see Chapter 10). In contrast, the evaluation for bowel obstruction and for malrotation involves the lower-frequency transducers. For children, a low-frequency (2–5 MHz) curved-array transducer should be utilized; while a higher-frequency (4–8 MHz) micro-convex transducer should be utilized for newborns (Figure 23.3a). A methodic evaluation of the bowel should be utilized. The "mowing the lawn" approach has been suggested (Figure 23.3b).

Ultrasound imaging

A distal small-bowel or large-bowel obstruction will show multiple, dilated loops of fluid-filled bowel throughout the abdomen (Figure 23.3c). Ultrasound can further distinguish between causes of bowel obstruction, including meconium ileus and ileal atresia. In meconium ileus, the bowel loops are filled with echogenic inspissated material. In contrast, in ileal atresia, bowel loops are filled with hypoechoic or anechoic fluid. With intestinal atresia ultrasonography will demonstrate a dilated, fluid-filled intestinal loop adjacent to a very narrow loop of unused intestine.

Sonographic features of malrotation include the superior mesenteric vein positioned to the left of the superior mesenteric artery. The "whirlpool" sign can be visualized on ultrasound (Figure 23.4),

(a)

(b)

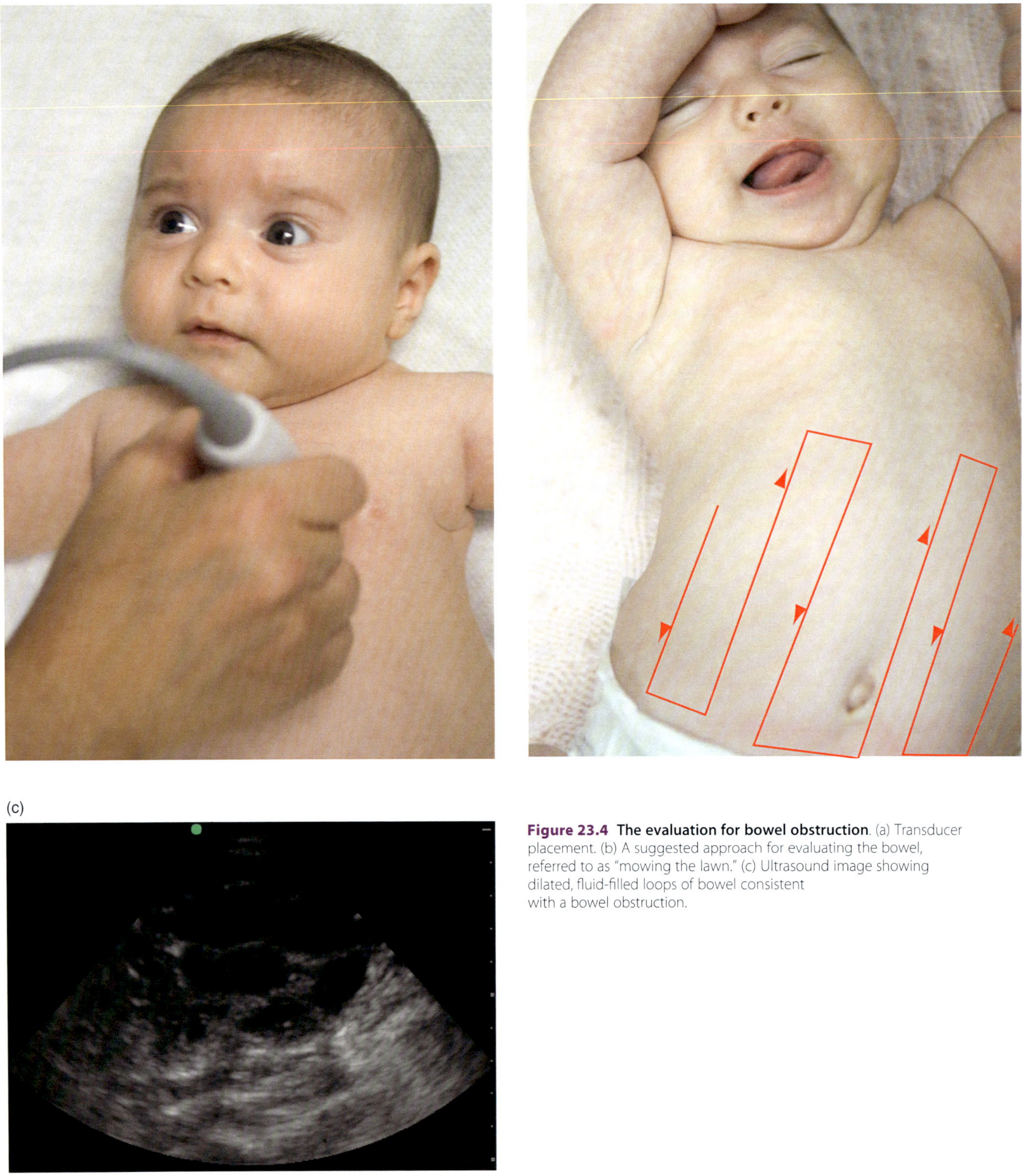

(c)

Figure 23.4 The evaluation for bowel obstruction. (a) Transducer placement. (b) A suggested approach for evaluating the bowel, referred to as "mowing the lawn." (c) Ultrasound image showing dilated, fluid-filled loops of bowel consistent with a bowel obstruction.

which is pathognomonic for malrotation. It involves the bowel and mesentery wrapping in a clockwise fashion around the SMA. The "whirlpool" sign has a sensitivity of only 45.5% and negative predictive power of 71.4%, but specificity of 99% and PPV of 97.1%. Other sonographic features of malrotation with volvulus include duodenal dilatation with a tapering configuration, fixed midline bowel, and dilatation of the distal SMV.

Scanning tips

Pitfalls

- Bowel gas can obstruct the view of the SMA and SMV, and decrease the sensitivity of the sonographic demonstration of bowel.

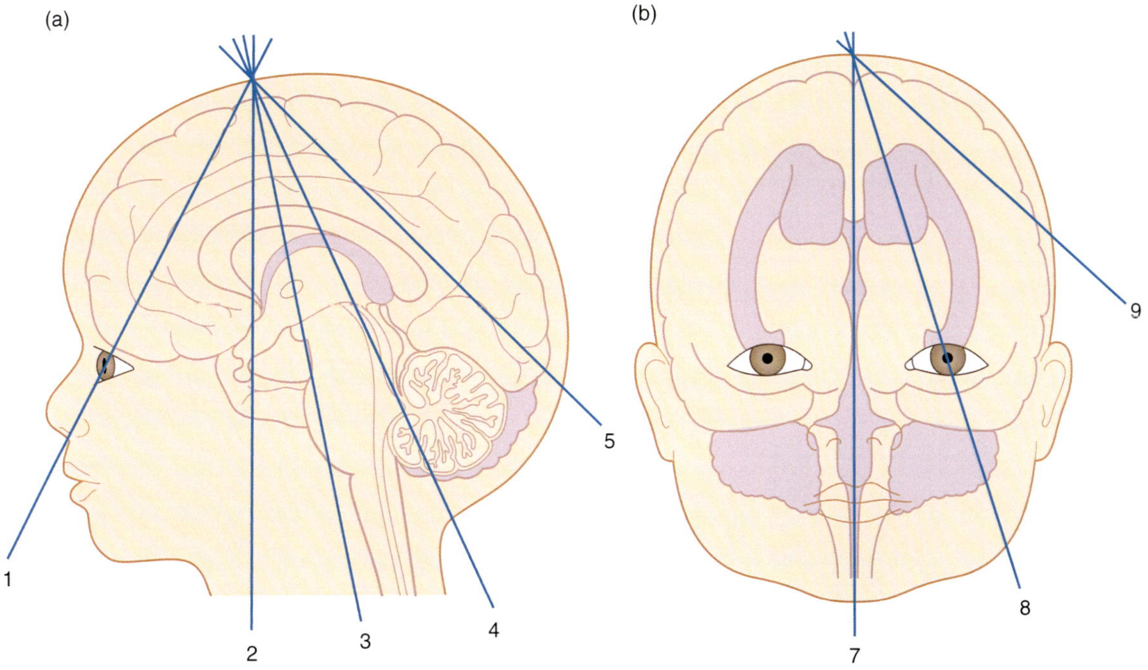

Figure 23.5 Scanning planes for cranial ultrasound examination. (a) The six coronal planes of scanning. (b) The sagittal and parasagittal planes of scanning. *Artwork created by Emily Evans © Cambridge University Press.*

- If the transducer is not maintained perfectly midline, there may be an oblique, inaccurate evaluation of the vessels.

Tips to improve scanning

✓ Apply gentle pressure to displace bowel gas and to better visualize vessels.

✓ Utilize the lower-frequency transducer to evaluate for bowel obstruction and malrotation.

✓ Ensure that the transducer is kept perfectly midline when evaluating the vessels.

✓ In order to improve visualization of bowel, 50 mL of distilled water may be instilled by nasograstric tube.

✓ Look for portal venous gas in order to diagnose NEC.

✓ Bowel obstruction will exhibit dilated, fluid-filled loops of bowel.

✓ Look for the inversion of the SMA/SMV and the "whirlpool sign," which are suggestive of malrotation.

CRANIAL ULTRASOUND: IVH, HYDROCEPHALUS

Background

Preterm infants, particularly ELBW, are at high risk for many complications of prematurity. A sudden clinical deterioration can happen in the first few days of life, due to various causes. Severe intraventricular hemorrhage (IVH) is an important complication that can occur in ELBW infants. Its incidence is inversely related to gestational age, and occurs in 20–25% of low-birth-weight infants, and 1% of term infants. Intraventricular hemorrhage is due to impaired autoregulatory ability, which can result in rapid alterations in cerebral blood flow and large changes in cerebral blood pressure. These sudden changes can result in hemorrhage inside the lateral ventricles and hemorrhagic infarctions in the brain parenchyma adjacent to the lateral ventricles. The most severe form of IVH is a Grade IV intraventricular hemorrhage, which can manifest as a sudden clinical deterioration with metabolic acidosis, hypotension, apnea, and bradycardia. Other problems of prematurity include sepsis, pneumothorax, and patent ductus arteriosus. While these may all present with a similar clinical picture, it is important to differentiate between them, in order to best guide definitive treatment in an expeditious manner.

Following an intraventricular hemorrhage, one-third of neonates may develop post-hemorrhagic hydrocephalus. Hydrocephalus involves the dilatation of ventricles and eventually progresses to increased intracranial pressure, thereby causing damage to brain tissue and delayed neurodevelopment. Approximately 35% of neonates with post-hemorrhagic ventricular dilatation will need some sort of intervention, such as serial lumbar punctures or the placement of a ventriculoperitoneal shunt. Hydrocephalus may also be present in conditions such as congenital hydrocephalus and infections such as toxoplasmosis.

Ultrasound screenings are the benchmark for the detection of intraventricular hemorrhage and hydrocephalus in neonates. Ultrasonography can also identify pre-existing structural abnormalities or evidence of longstanding damage. It can further identify focal regions of hemorrhage and infarction. Ultrasound imaging results may assist in targeting other examinations such as MRI. Even once treatment has been initiated for hydrocephalus, serial cranial ultrasound measurements may be performed. Ultrasound has the potential to have a prognostic

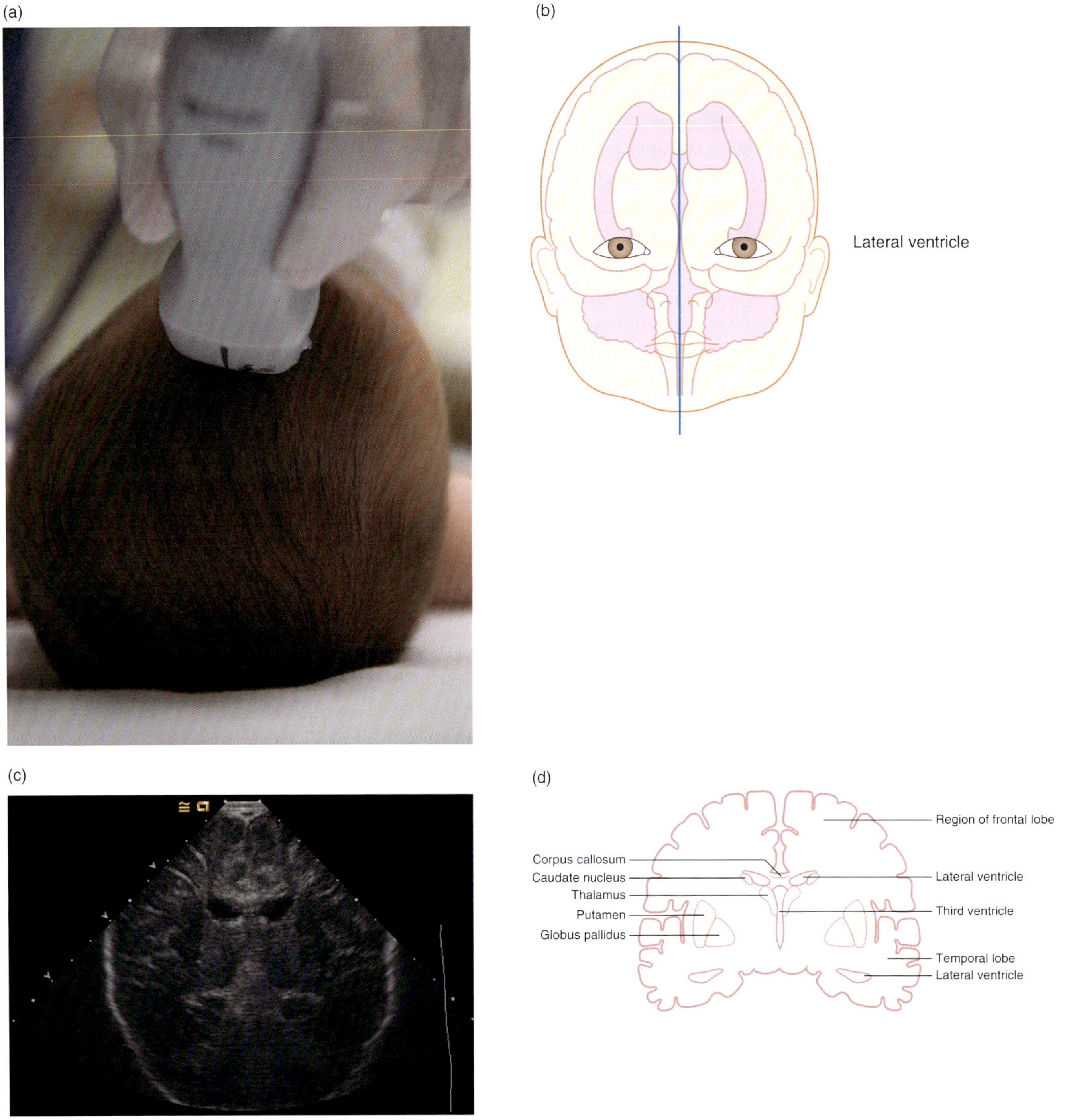

Figure 23.6 Cranial ultrasonography, coronal view. (a) Transducer placement over the anterior fontanelle, with the indicator oriented towards the patient's right side. (b) Anatomy of the neonatal brain, coronal view. (c) Ultrasound image of a normal coronal view of the neonatal brain. (d) Illustration depicting structures seen in the ultrasound image. *Artwork created by Emily Evans © Cambridge University Press.*

value with regards to neurodevelopmental outcomes in these high-risk neonates.

Anatomy

When performing ultrasonography of the neonatal brain, it is important to be familiar with the basic structures and ventricles in the coronal (Figure 23.6d) and sagittal orientations (Figure 23.7d).

Technique

Point-of-care questions

1. Are dilated ventricles present?
2. Is a visible intraventricular hemorrhage present?
3. Is a scalp hematoma present?

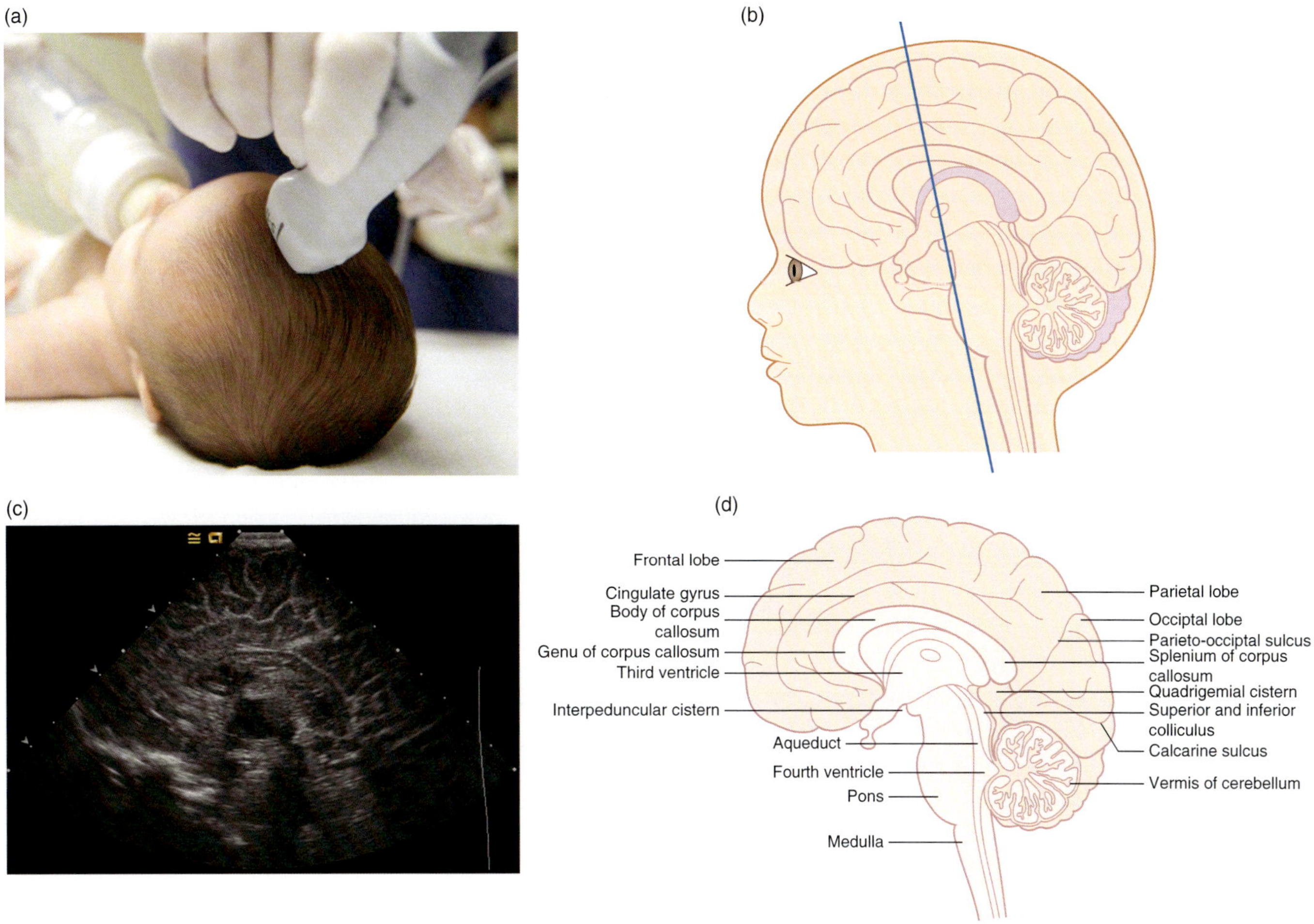

Figure 23.7 Cranial imaging, sagittal view. (a) Transducer placement over the anterior fontanelle, with the indicator oriented towards the patient's front (anterior). (b) Anatomy of the neonatal brain, sagittal view. (c) Ultrasound image of a normal sagittal view of the neonatal brain. (d) Illustration depicting structures seen in the ultrasound image. *Artwork created by Emily Evans © Cambridge University Press.*

Transducer selection and orientation

Using a transducer that fits at the infant's open anterior fontanel can easily yield the diagnosis. A phased-array transducer is often ideal for this type of imaging. In order to assess for the presence of a scalp hematoma, a linear, high-frequency transducer is utilized.

For a comprehensive cranial ultrasound examination, the brain should be evaluated at six coronal levels, in addition to the sagittal and parasagittal planes (Figure 23.5). Start by placing the transducer on the anterior fontanelle, with the indicator oriented towards the patient's right side (Figure 23.6a). The resulting coronal ultrasound image will mimic the orientation as seen on tomography. Then, in order to obtain the sagittal view, rotate the indicator towards the patient's anterior, front side (Figure 23.7a). Set the depth so that the base of the skull is visualized on the bottom of the ultrasound image. The depth is usually approximately 7 cm. Different levels can be obtained by angling the transducer. Then, rotate the transducer 90° in order to obtain the sagittal and parasagittal views.

Ultrasound imaging

A normal coronal (Figure 23.6c) and sagittal view (Figure 23.7c) of the neonatal brain shows small ventricles. In general, blood appears hyperechoic. A germinal matrix intraventricular hemorrhage appears as an echoreflective area in the caudothalamic groove (Figure 23.8). However, the interobserver agreement for this evaluation is relatively poor. Ultrasound is limited in reliability in detecting lesions of less than 0.5 cm. However, the sensitivity and specificity for detecting lesions of greater than 0.5 cm are 100% and 91% respectively. Ultrasound is the modality of choice for detecting ventriculomegaly. It is easily reproduced with minimal inter- and intra-observer variability. Additional findings may include calcifications, as seen in infections such as toxoplasmosis. Hyperechoic, calcified lesions may be identified at the basal ganglia, cortex, and periventricular white matter.

Scalp hematomas will appear hypoechoic or anechoic. They are easily visible anterior to the skull, which appears as a hyperechoic line (Figure 23.9). Compression with the transducer can determine whether the fluid collection is compressible. This

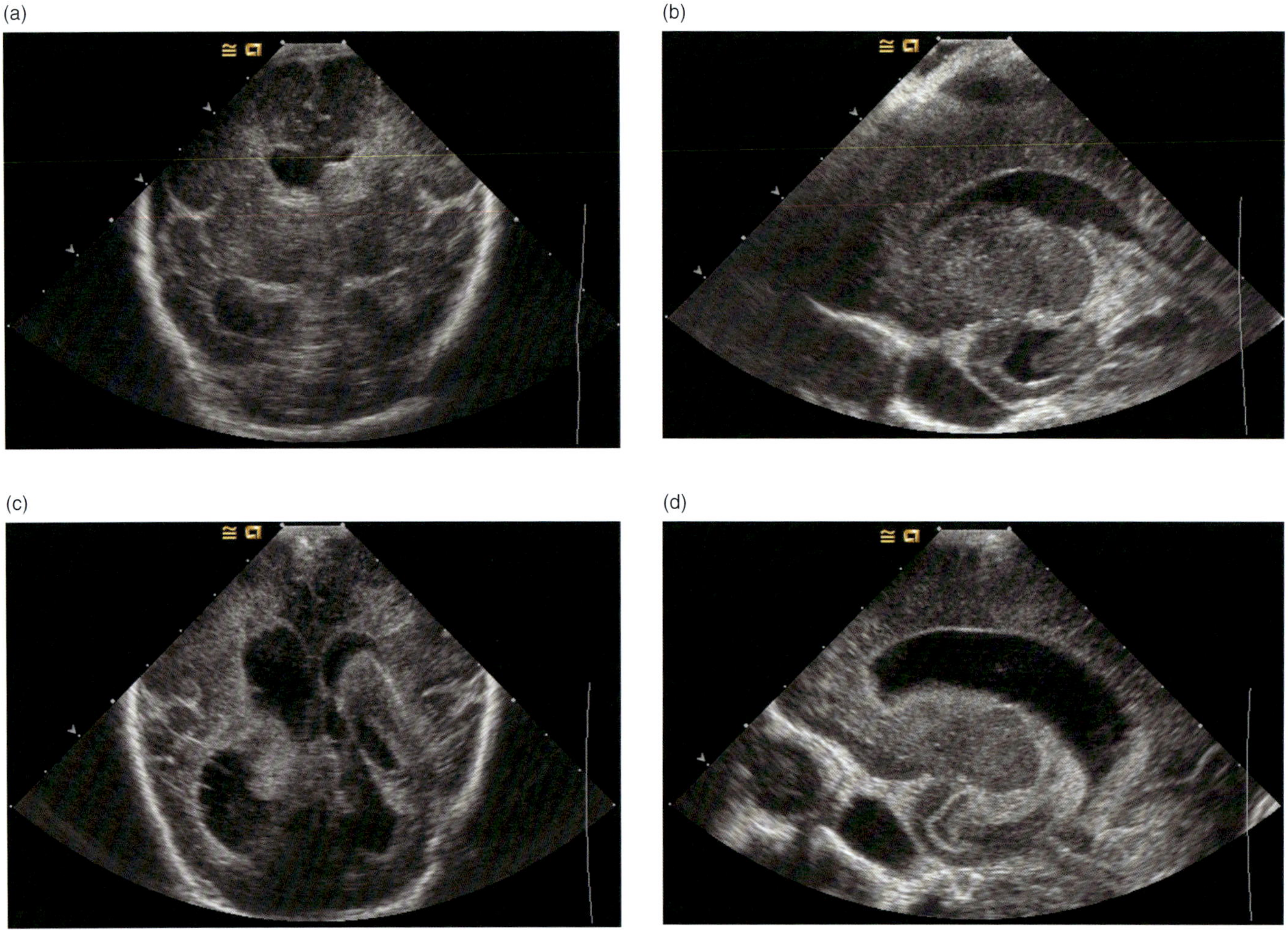

Figure 23.8 Intraventricular hemorrhage (IVH). (a) Coronal view of bilateral germinal matrix and intraventricular hemorrhage, left greater than right. (b) Sagittal view of intraventricular hemorrhage. (c) Coronal view of evolution of germinal matrix and intraventricular hemorrhage, with ventricular dilatation one week later. (d) Coronal view of evolving intraventricular hemorrhage with ventricular dilatation.

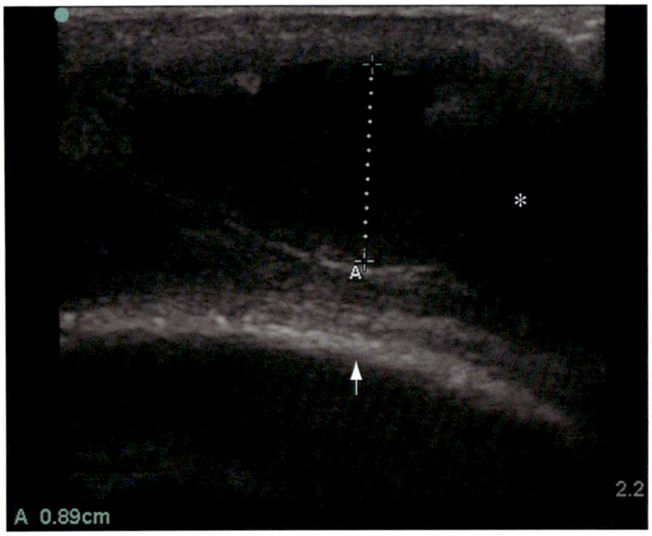

Figure 23.9 Scalp hematoma. The anechoic fluid collection (*.....) is visualized anterior to the hyperechoic skull (arrow).

technique may also be utilized in order to assess for the presence of skull fractures, which will appear as hypoechoic discontinuities in the bony cortex. It is important to note that fractures can often be mistaken for normal suture lines. When in doubt, perform ultrasonography of the contralateral side for comparison.

Measurements

With hydrocephalus, clinical signs such as a tense fontanelle or the "sunsetting" phenomenon are often unreliable. The sonographic measurements of the ventricular size (Table 23.1) are much more reliable. The ventricular index (VI) is the most commonly performed and reliable of measurements. Other measurements include the thalamo-occipital distance (TOD) and the anterior horn width (AHW). Additional, more-detailed measurements such as area and volume measurements have been performed. There may be some variation between genders of 0.1–0.6 mm, which is clinically insignificant. There may also be asymmetry of the lateral ventricles, of which the clinical significance is unclear, but is probably a normal physiologic variant. The ventricular index is obtained in the coronal view, at the level of the third ventricle. The index is the distance between the falx and the lateral wall of the anterior horn (Figure 23.10).

Table 23.1 Measurements of ventricular size. The three most commonly used measurements include the ventricular index (VI), anterior horn width (AHW), and thalamo-occipital distance (TOD).

Measurement	Abnormal (<33 weeks gestational age)
Ventricular index (VI)	4 mm above 97th percentile (see curve in Figure 23.11)
Anterior horn width (AHW)	>4 mm
Thalamo-occipital distance (TOD)	>26 mm

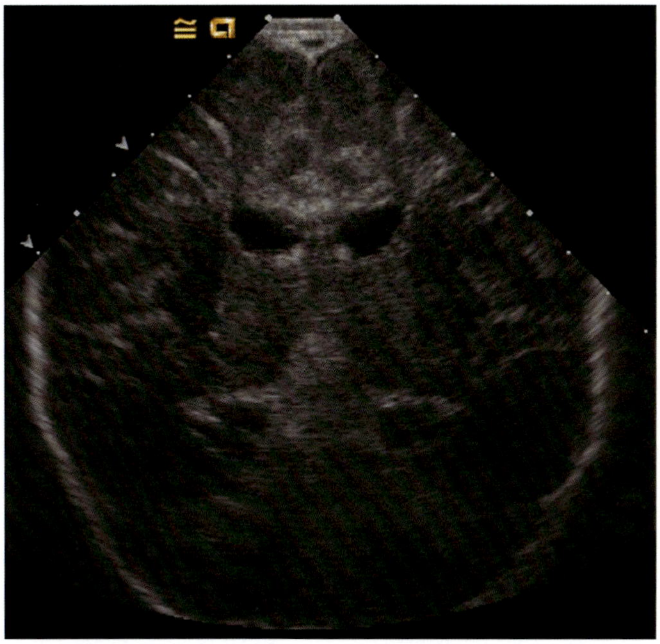

Figure 23.10 **The ventricular index (VI) measurement.**

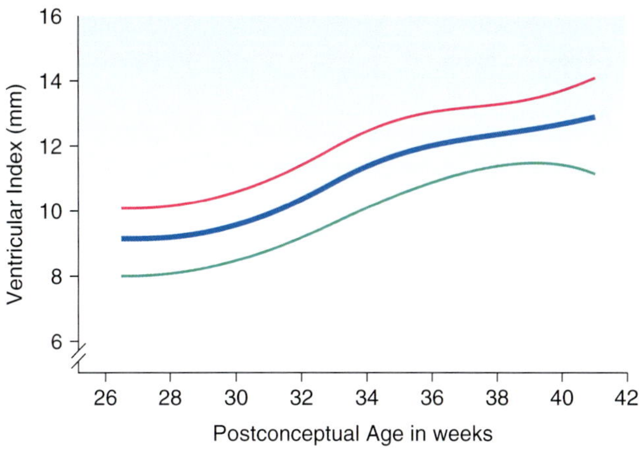

Figure 23.11 **Centile chart of the Levene ventricular index (VI).** *Reproduced with permission from Levene, M. I. (1981) Measurement of the growth of the lateral ventricles in preterm infants with real-time ultrasound. Arch Dis Child 56(12): 900–4.*

Scanning tips

Pitfalls

- Improper depth settings: the depth should be set so that the base of the skull is visualized at the bottom of the image.
- Small fontanelles may prohibit scanning of the brain.
- Incorrect settings of TGC can lose detail of the brain.
- Ultrasound is limited in detecting lesions of less than 0.5 cm.

Tips to improve scanning

✓ Use a phased-array transducer at the anterior fontanelle.

✓ Obtain both coronal and sagittal images, and tilt the transducer in order to visualize the brain at different levels.

✓ Avoid too much gain in order to decrease artifact.

✓ For concern of hemorrhage or ventricular dilatation, obtain consultation with radiologists; consider neurosurgical consultation. Further imaging studies may need to be obtained.

CARDIORESPIRATORY: TRANSIENT TACHYPNEA OF THE NEWBORN (TTN), RESPIRATORY DISTRESS SYNDROME (RDS)

Background

Transient tachypnea of the newborn (TTN), also referred to as type II respiratory distress syndrome (RDS) or "wet lungs", can usually be diagnosed in the first few hours after birth. Transient tachypnea of the newborn involves the delayed clearance of fluid from the alveoli and interstitium. Thirty to fifty percent of all neonates with respiratory distress will have a clinical course consistent with TTN. It has a low morbidity but can also be severe. TTN is a mild form of RDS, and it is important to differentiate it from other cardiopulmonary disorders early in its course. TTN can occur in premature infants because their lungs are not yet fully developed; it can also occur in full-term babies. It is not possible to detect, prenatally, whether a child will have it. However, those newborns at higher risk for developing TTN include those who are delivered by cesarean section or born to mothers with diabetes or asthma, and those who are small for gestational age.

This is in contrast to respiratory distress syndrome, also referred to as hyaline membrane disease, which is a severe form of neonatal respiratory distress. Respiratory distress syndrome occurs almost exclusively in premature infants, and is largely due to the insufficiency of pulmonary surfactant.

Chest radiographs are the gold standard for the diagnoses of both TTN and RDS. Typical findings of TTN on radiographs include fluid in the fissures and prominent perihilar streaking. Other findings may include patchy infiltrates and reticulonodular opacities. These abnormalities usually resolve by 72 hours of life. For RDS, typical radiographic findings include "ground glass" appearance, and air bronchograms. These findings, however, are not seen exclusively in RDS.

Recently, Copetti *et al.* applied point-of-care ultrasound to evaluate neonates with respiratory distress and found that the "double lung point" was only present in those infants with TTN. Copetti *et al.* also used ultrasound to characterize findings seen

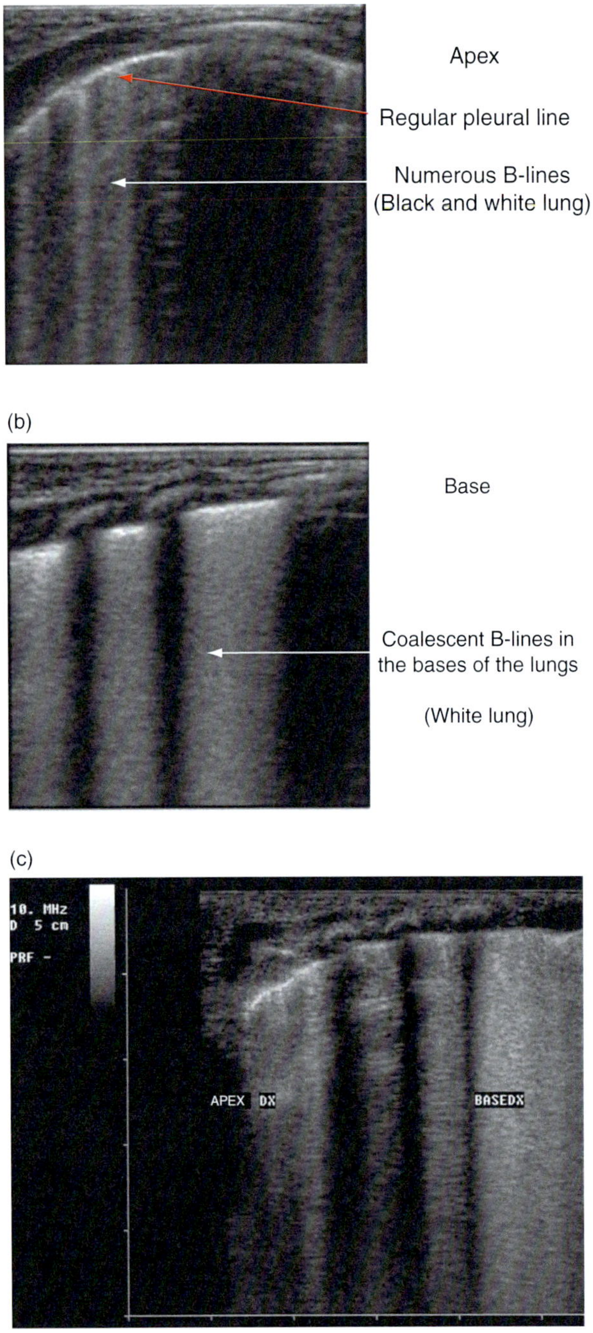

Figure 23.12 Transient tachypnea of the newborn (TTN). The "double lung point." (a) The normal pleural line (red arrow) can be visualized. At the apex, numerous B-lines are visible (white arrow). (b) At the base, coalescent B-lines (arrow) are present. (c) Ultrasound image showing both the apex and base.Note the transducer is oriented with the indicator towards the neonate's head.

in RDS. When compared with healthy newborns, infants with RDS had several sonographic signs that yielded a sensitivity and specificity of 100%. Given the high sensitivity and specificity of the presence of these signs, lung ultrasound might be a helpful screening method for RDS. This technique may also serve as guiding the early administration of surfactant to preterm infants found to have RDS. While ultrasonography is useful, it cannot entirely replace chest radiographs. This is due to the fact that certain acute complications of RDS, including pneumomediastinum, interstitial emphysema, and pneumopericardium, cannot be seen with ultrasound.

Technique

Point-of-care questions

1. Is a double lung point present?
2. Is an echogenic "white lung" present? Are more than 7 B-lines present, 3mm apart?
3. Is a thickened pleural line present?
4. Are "spared areas" present in a non-homogenous lung?

Transducer selection and orientation

A high-frequency, (5–10 MHz), linear transducer is utilized to assess for the presence of TTN. Longitudinal and transverse views should be obtained of the anterior, posterior, and lateral chest walls (see Chapter 6).

Ultrasound imaging

Copetti and Cattarossi described a unique sonographic sign, referred to as the "double lung point" (Figure 23.12). In infants with TTN, lung sonography shows a difference in lung echogenicities between the upper and lower lung areas. There are very compact, comet-tail artifacts in the inferior fields, while comet-tail artifacts are rare in the superior fields. This finding was called the "double lung point" and was not observed in healthy infants, or infants with respiratory distress syndrome, atelectasis, pneumothorax, pneumonia, or pulmonary hemorrhage. The sensitivity and specificity of the "double lung point" were both 100% for the diagnosis of TTN. It is worth knowing that, in normal babies delivered by cesarean section, one can find multiple B-lines bilaterally that disappear in a few days.

For infants with RDS, several findings were consistently shown. These include:

1. "White lung," created by multiple (>7) compact B-lines less than 3 mm apart. This depicts alveolar-interstitial edema (Figure 23.13);
2. Pleural line abnormalities: small subpleural consolidations (Figure 23.13), thickening (greater than 0.5 mm), irregularity and coarse appearance; and
3. The absence of "spared areas," or areas with a normal pattern.

CARDIORESPIRATORY: PATENT DUCTUS ARTERIOSUS (PDA)

Background

A patent ductus arteriosus (PDA) is the delayed closure of the ductus arteriosus. Its frequency is high in premature infants, ranging from 54% in infants of less than 34 weeks gestational age to 65% in infants of less than 26 weeks gestational age. The treatment of a PDA often requires pharmacologic or surgical closure. A PDA is associated with increased risk of necrotizing

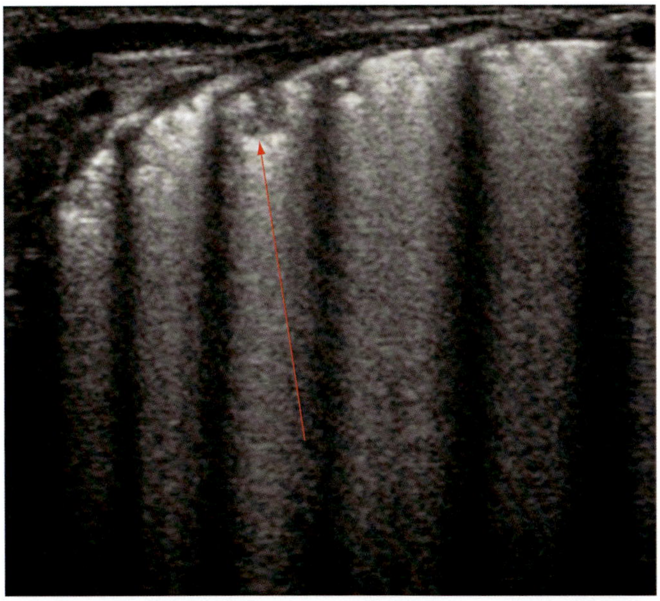

Figure 23.13 Respiratory distress syndrome (RDS). Findings include attenuation, irregularity, and a coarse/thickened pleural line. In addition, multiple, small, subpleural consolidations can be present (arrow). The ultrasound image shows the lung parenchyma which is referred to as "white lung" in RDS.

enterocolitis, intraventricular hemorrhage, bronchopulmonary dysplasia, and bronchopulmonary hemorrhage. In addition, the presentation of neonatal shock can be due to the closure of the ductus arteriosus in some ductal-dependent cardiac lesions such as severe aortic coarctation, pulmonary atresia, and transposition of great arteries. Physical examination findings are often include: a cardiac murmur on auscultation, bounding pulses, and a wide pulse pressure. However, physical examination findings are unreliable and inadequate in diagnosing a PDA. The gold standard for the diagnosis of a PDA is formal echocardiography interpreted by pediatric cardiologists.

Point-of-care ultrasound can help in establishing the diagnosis of a PDA as well as in monitoring the effect of pharmacologic therapy in either keeping the PDA open with prostaglandin or closing it with indomethacin. The identification of the presence of a PDA is especially important in those infants with intracardiac, ductal-dependent lesions. When the PDA begins to close, the patient may abruptly decompensate. The infusion of prostaglandin may be life-saving in these neonates. Additionally, a neonate can suffer from heart failure and become ventilator dependent in the absence of intracardiac lesions, simply due to the presence of a large PDA with left-to-right shunt.

A pilot study examined point-of-care ultrasound performed by neonatologists compared with pediatric cardiologists, to detect PDAs. After limited instruction, neonatologists were able to detect PDAs with moderate accuracy. When moderate to large PDAs were present, their accuracy increased. A recent study showed that serial echocardiography performed by neonatologists allowed for a significantly earlier identification and treatment of PDAs. In those babies in whom a PDA was identified, there was a decreased number of those who subsequently developed severe IVH and less overall ventilator days. For those patients in whom a PDA was not present, hospital days were shorter. While further research needs to be performed, this offers a promising adjunct to the neonatologist's assessment and management in the NICU.

Anatomy

A PDA involves an abnormal connection between the aorta and pulmonary artery (Figure 23.14b).

Technique

Point-of-care question

1. Is a PDA present?

Transducer selection and orientation

A high-frequency (4–8 MHz), micro-convex, or neonatal transducer is often utilized (Figure 23.15). All views of the focused cardiac ultrasound should be obtained (see Chapter 5), including the parasternal long-axis, parasternal short-axis, apical four-chamber, and subcostal views. The additional view of the suprasternal approach is of great value. For the suprasternal view, the transducer is placed at the suprasternal notch, oriented towards the patient's right hip, or 7 o'clock (see Figure 23.14a). It is often necessary to tilt the transducer downward, towards the patient's feet. This orientation is to maintain imaging consistency with the other views described in Chapter 5. Note that the technique the cardiologists use is to have the indicator oriented towards the patient's left shoulder, or 2 o'clock.

Ultrasound imaging

The assessment for the presence of a PDA includes: the left atrial size, and the left ventricular size and function. The use of Doppler and continuous pulsed-wave Doppler can be especially helpful in denoting the magnitude of shunting across the PDA and detecting the direction of blood flow to help evaluate for pulmonary hypertension (right-to-left) (Figure 23.14d). Color Doppler can estimate the ductus size. This is measured at the narrowest point of the jet, known as the vena contracta. In addition, the velocity and character of the ductus Doppler signal and the amount of retrograde abdominal flow can be evaluated.

Scanning tips

Pitfalls

- Physical examination findings are often unreliable in diagnosing a PDA.
- Smaller PDAs are often difficult to identify on ultrasonography.

Tips to improve scanning

✓ The suprasternal view is helpful in evaluating for the presence of a PDA.

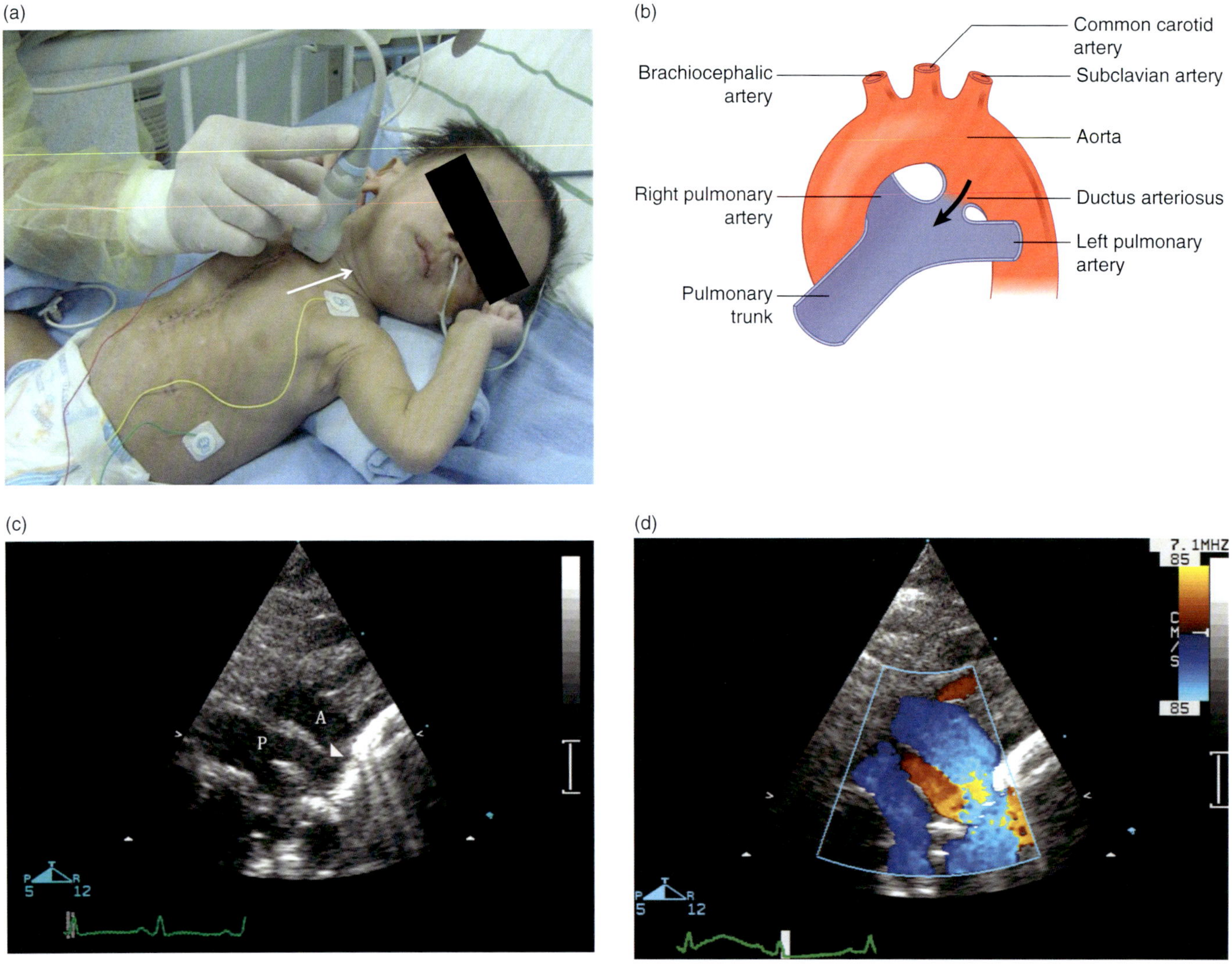

Figure 23.14 The evaluation for a PDA, suprasternal view. (a) Transducer placement. (b) Illustration depicting a PDA. *Artwork created by Emily Evans © Cambridge University Press.* (c) Ultrasound image showing the PDA (arrowhead), the connection between the aorta (A) and pulmonary artery (P). (d) The use of color Doppler to assess the PDA.

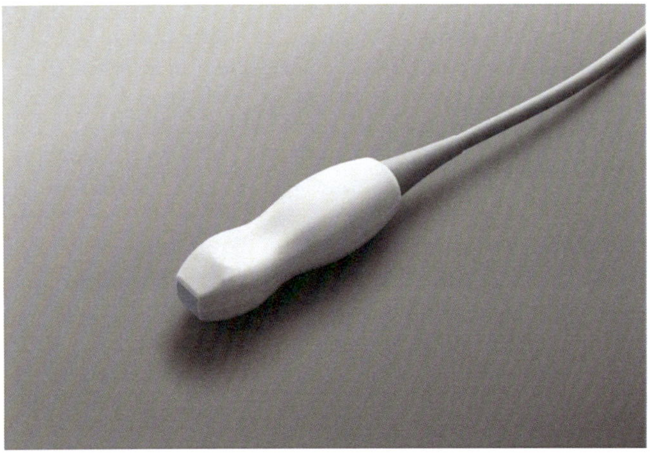

Figure 23.15 Micro-convex or neonatal transducer. This transducer has a high frequency and small footprint, ideal for imaging neonates and small infants. *Image courtesy of Sonosite, Inc*

- ✓ The use of Doppler and continuous pulsed-wave Doppler can be helpful in evaluating the magnitude of the shunt and the direction of blood flow through the PDA.
- ✓ Perform repeated evaluations, in order to detect smaller PDAs.
- ✓ Consult a pediatric cardiologist and obtain formal echocardiography when intracardiac lesions are suspected.

PROCEDURAL GUIDANCE: UMBILICAL LINES

Background

In addition to procedures routinely performed in the emergency room, additional procedures performed in the ICU can be facilitated by ultrasound. Lumbar puncture (see Chapter 17), paracentesis, pericardiocentesis (see Chapter 21), and line insertions are of special interest. Abcess drainage, gallbladder drainage, suprapubic drainage, and trans-hepatic lines are often

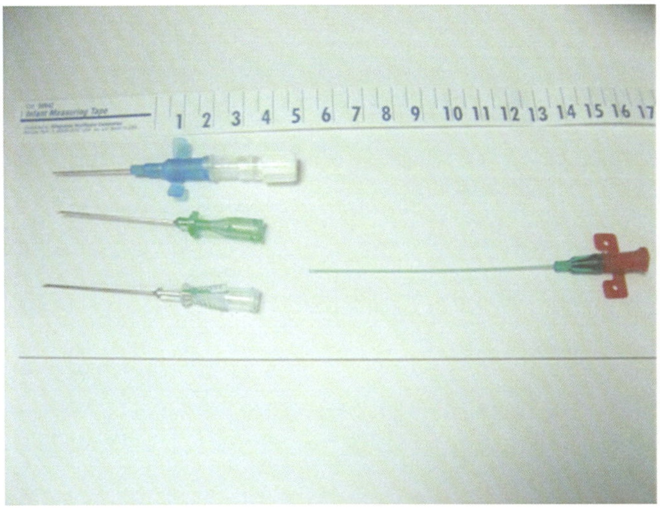

Figure 23.16 **Cannulas** used for neonatal line placement.

guided by ultrasound and performed by an interventional radiologist in the critical care setting.

Of particular interest in the neonatal population is the use of ultrasonography for PICC line and umbilical line placement. As discussed in Chapter 15, ultrasound assistance and ultrasound guidance can be utilized to improve success and decrease the complications associated with central line placement. The same principles may be applied to umbilical line placements in neonates. For PICC line placement in neonates, it is important to use a separate 22G–24G canula and baby wire instead of the central line introducer kit (Figure 23.16).

Traditionally, umbilical lines are placed and the distance advanced is estimated based on a shoulder–umbilicus length graph or a regression equation based on birth weight. Catheters are traditionally placed and advanced blindly. Following umbilical line placement, portable radiographs are performed in order to determine the location of the catheter tip. Often multiple radiographs need to be performed when the initial positioning is not ideal. Alternatively, point-of-care ultrasound was recently introduced in order to determine the location of the catheter tip. A prospective, randomized trial compared traditional blinded attempts with ultrasound guidance for umbilical arterial and venous lines. Radiographs were obtained to confirm positioning. Ultrasound saved 64 minutes, and reduced the number of radiographs performed. In umbilical venous lines there was a decrease in the number of line manipulations; while in the arterial lines there was no difference.

Technique

Transducer selection and orientation

A high-frequency (5–10 MHz), linear transducer, preferably with a small footprint, is utilized. The optimal targeted location of umbilical line placement is at the mid-chest to identify the IVC–right atrium junction for the umbilical venous catheter, and the T7–9 segment of the descending thoracic aorta for the umbilical arterial catheter.

For arterial catheters, ultrasonography is performed in the mid-chest, in the sagittal plane (with the indicator towards the patient's head) in order to locate the catheter tip. For venous catheters, ultrasonography is performed in the sagittal plane as well, but on the anterior side of the right abdomen (Figure 23.17a). The liver is utilized as an acoustic window to visualize the catheter. If the tip is improperly positioned, it can be manipulated under real-time ultrasound guidance, until suitable positioning is attained. One should consider obtaining a radiograph to confirm placement.

Patient position and preparation

The patient should be prepared in a sterile fashion, with sterile drapes. In additon, the transducer should be pepared in a sterile fashion, with a sterile sheath and sterile gel (Figures S3.5,6).

Ultrasound imaging

The use of point-of-care ultrasound has been reported for umbilical line placement. Initially, the line is placed via traditional techniques. The short-axis technique provides a view of surrounding structures and allows operation even in a small field. The long-axis allows better needle visualization and depth throughout the cannulation (Figure 23.17b). A combined short-axis and long-axis approach is sometimes used (see Chapter S3).

After securing the catheter, ultrasonography is performed in order to locate the catheter tip. The injection of a small amount of sterile saline through the catheter tip may improve visualization on ultrasonography, since this creates turbulence with the injection. For umbilical arterial lines, identify the T7–9 segment of the descending aorta. For umbilical venous lines, identify the IVC–right atrial junction (Figure 23.17b).

Scanning tips

Pitfalls

- The umbilical catheter tip may be difficult to localize.
- Malpositioned catheters are common; identify the catheter tip and redirect under real-time guidance.

Tips to improve scanning

✓ Identify the IVC–right atrium junction for the umbilical venous catheter, and the T7–9 segment of the descending thoracic aorta for the umbilical arterial catheter.

✓ Sometimes a combination of a short-axis and long-axis approach may be helpful.

✓ The injection of saline through the umbilical catheter may improve visualization of the catheter tip, by creating turbulence.

(a)

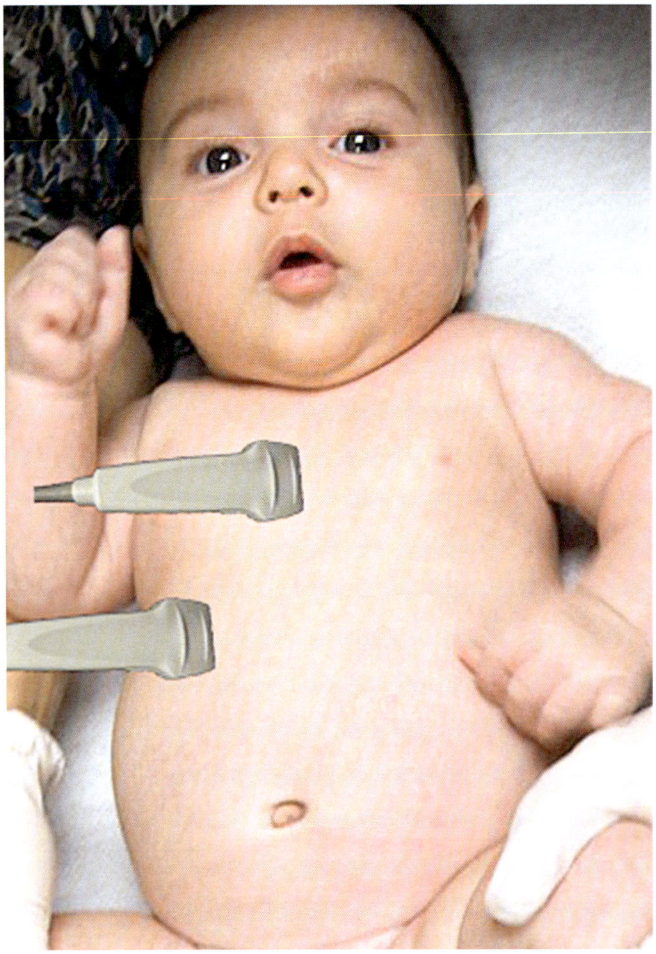

(b)

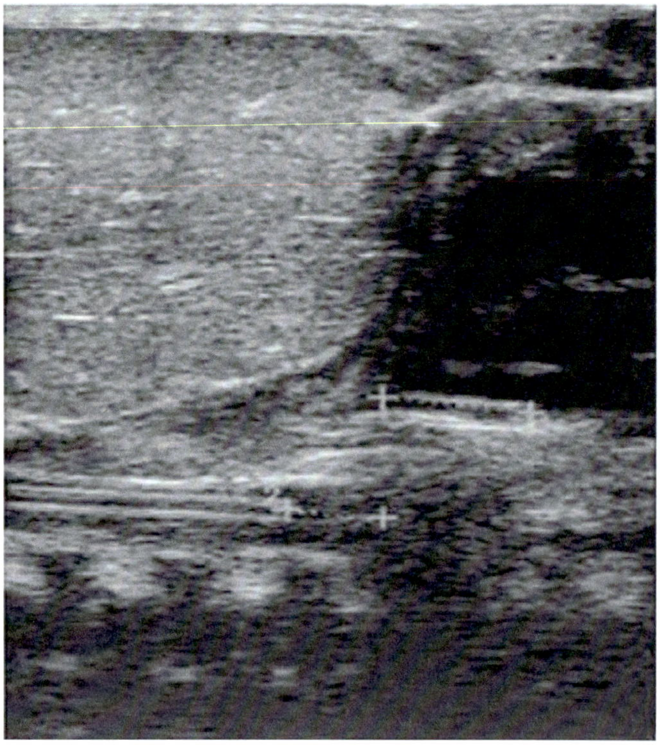

(c)

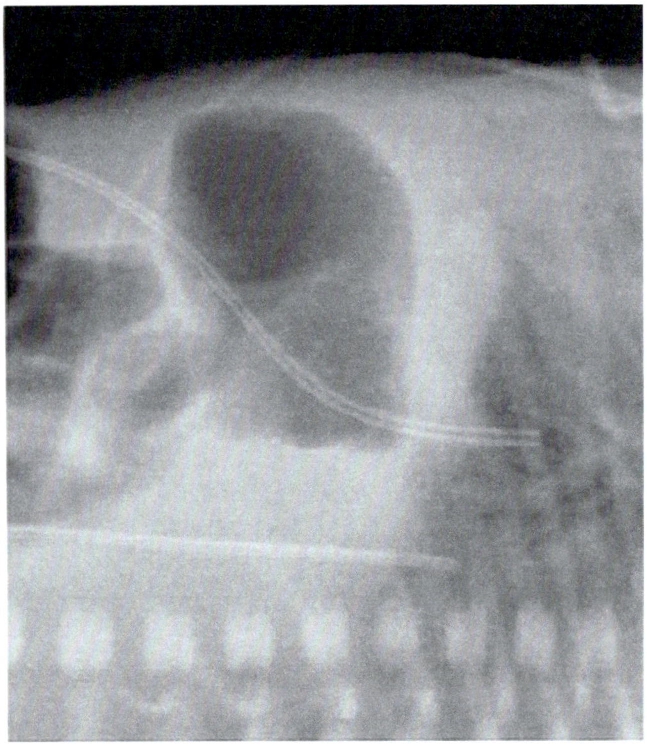

Figure 23.17 Umbilical line placement. (a) Transducer placement at the mid-chest for an umbilical venous catheter, and at the right upper quadrant for the umbilical artery. (b) Ultrasound image, longitudinal view, showing the umbilical venous line at the T7–9 segment of the descending thoracic aorta, and the arterial line at the IVC–right atrial junction. (c) Corresponding radiograph showing line placement. The catheter tip for a venous line should be at the T7–9 segment of the descending aorta; while the catheter tip for an arterial line should be at the IVC–right atrial junction. *Source for (b) and (c) (copyright): Fleming, S. E., Kim, J. H. (2011) Ultrasound-guided umbilical line catheterization. J Perinatol 34: 344–9.*

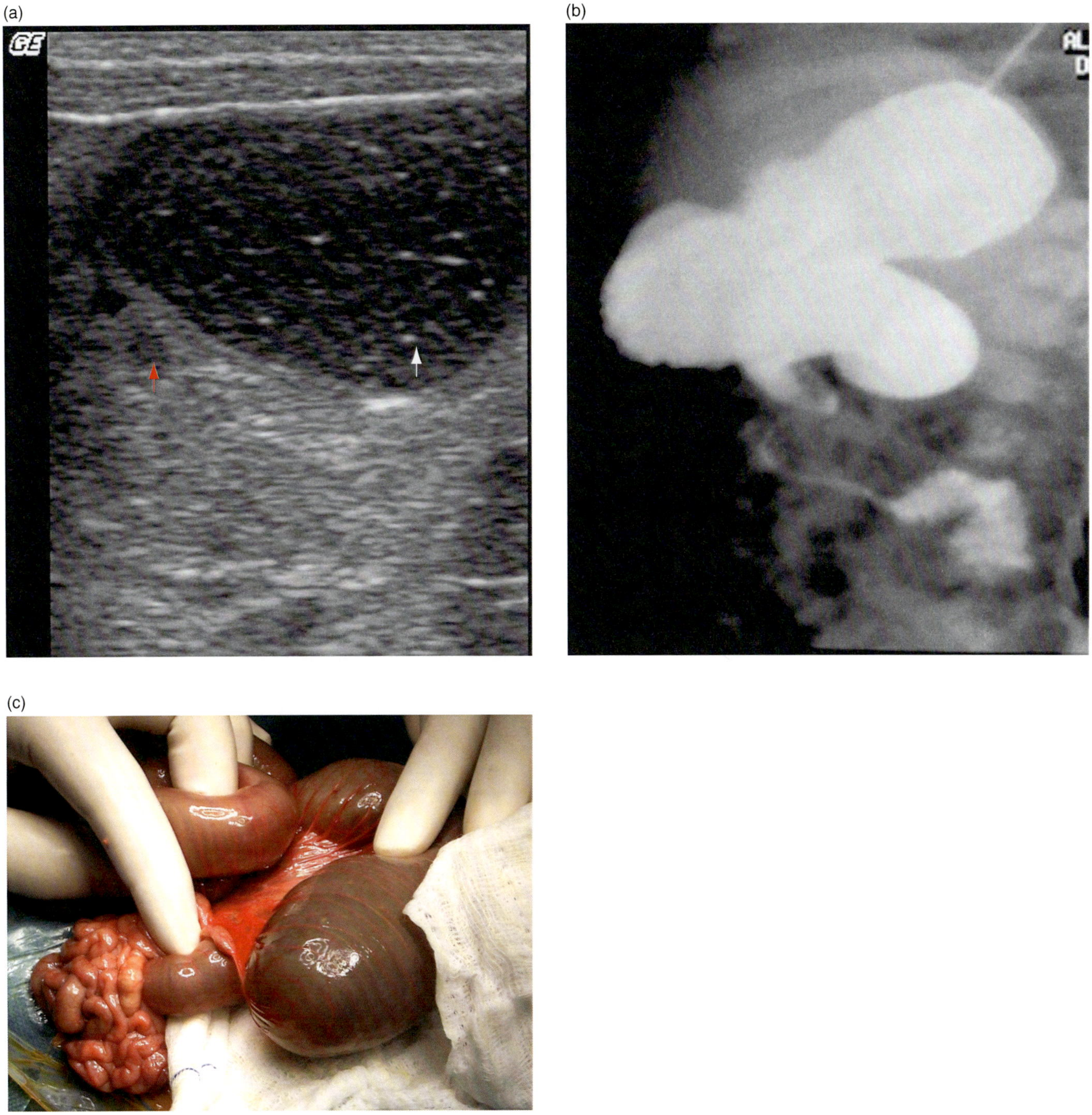

Figure 23.18 **Case 1: bowel obstruction**. (a) Ultrasound of the abdomen showing dilated intestinal loop (white arrow) and adjacent narrow loop (red arrow). (b) Upper GI contrast study showing a dilated proximal bowel and a narrow segment. (c) Intraoperative photo.

Cases

1. A seven-day-old baby in the NICU was born prematurely at 26 weeks gestation, and was of low birth weight. He suddenly develops abdominal distension and vomiting. As a result, his feeds are held. Point-of-care ultrasonography is performed in order to assess for possible causes of the vomiting, including NEC, bowel obstruction, and malrotation with volvulus. The point-of-care ultrasound (Figure 23.18a) reveals dilated, fluid-filled loops of bowel, indicative of a bowel obstruction. An Upper GI Series is then performed (Figure 23.18b) confirmed these findings. As a result, the patient is brought to the operating room, where the obstruction is found (Figure 23.18c).

Ultrasonography can be extremely useful in evaluating the cause of vomiting in a neonate. Necrotizing enterocolitis will demonstrate portal venous gas, while malrotation with volvulus can cause an inversion of the

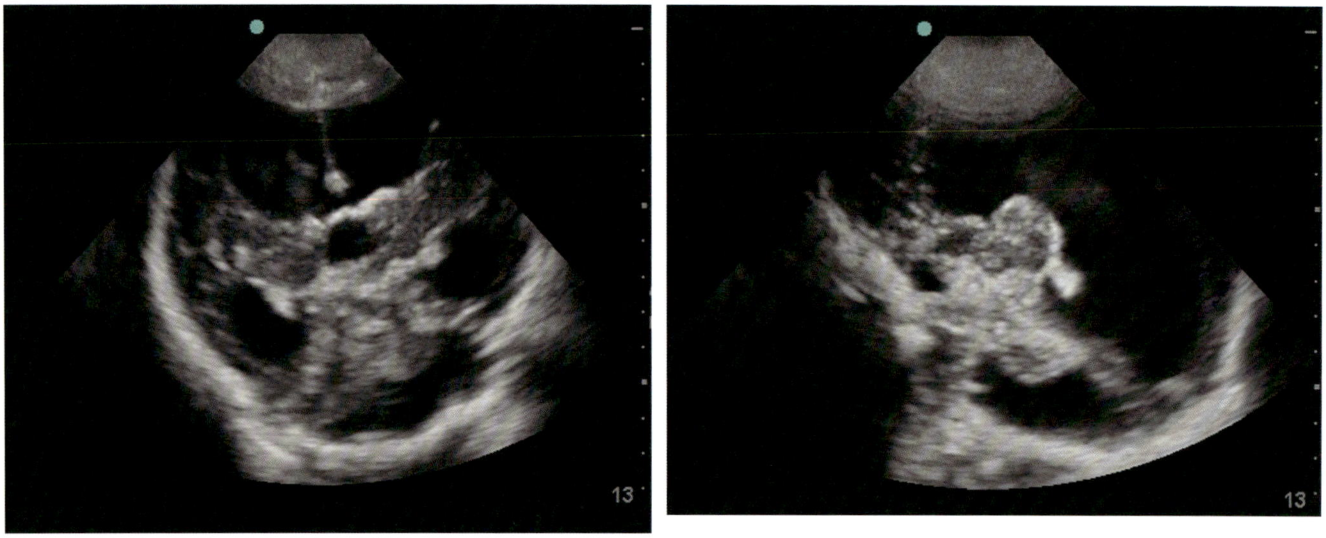

Figure 23.19 **Case 2: hydrocephalus**. (a) Coronal view of the brain. (b) Sagittal view of the brain, showing markedly dilated ventricles, which are anechoic.

SMA/SMV and the "whirlpool" sign. In this case, sonographic findings suggestive of a bowel obstruction prompted the neonatologists to obtain an upper GI with contrast study and consultation from their pediatric surgeon.

2. A two-week-old boy, who was born at 37 weeks gestation, was admitted to the NICU, for weight gain, was discharged from the NICU, and has been well. He now presents to the emergency department, with progressively worsening irritability, and worsening of his reflux. His mother notices that he seems to be "only looking down." He has been afebrile. On examination, his vital signs are normal. He has a full fontanelle, with an apparent downward gaze. A point-of-care cranial ultrasound is performed, which shows markedly dilated ventricles (Figure 23.19). Neurosurgery is immediately consulted, and he is admitted to the NICU while awaiting the placement of a ventriculoperitoneal shunt.

   Point-of-care ultrasonography can be helpful in evaluating those premature infants at risk for developing IVH and post-hemorrhagic hydrocephalus. Ultrasound can be helpful later, if there is clinical concern for the development of hydrocephalus. This baby clinically has "sun-setting," which is suggestive of hydrocephalus. The immediate result of dilated ventricles on ultrasonography helped to mobilize the neurosurgical team and the operating room, long before a CT scan would be available.

Summary/key points

1. Necrotizing enterocolitis is the most common gastrointestinal emergency of all infants admitted to a neonatal intensive care unit. Portal venous air can be identified on ultrasonography, with the linear high-frequency transducer.
2. An important cause of bowel obstruction is malrotation with volvulus. In contrast to other bowel studies, a lower-frequency transducer is utilized. Findings are the "whirlpool" sign and inversion of the SMA/SMV.
3. Preterm infants are especially susceptible to developing IVH and subsequent hydrocephalus. Point-of-care ultrasonography can be utilized to evaluate for the presence of hemorrhage and dilatation of the ventricles. The ventricular index (VI) is the most accurate measurement for hydrocephalus.
4. A higher-frequency micro-convex or neonatal transducer may be utilized with the help of color and continuous pulsed-wave Doppler to identify a PDA.
5. Ultrasonography can be utilized for procedural guidance in the NICU. It can be especially helpful for localizing the catheter tip during the placement of umbilical lines.

Selected references

Bohnhorst, B., Kuebler, J. F., Rau, G., *et al.* (2011) Portal venous gas detected by ultrasound differentiates surgical NEC from other acquired neonatal intestinal diseases. *Eur J Pediatr Surg* **21**(1): 12–17.

Brouwer, M. J., de Vries, L. S., Pistorius, L., *et al.* (2010) Ultrasound measurements of the lateral ventricles in neonates: why, how, and when? A systematic review. *Acta Paediatr* **99**(9): 1298–1306.

Chao, H. C., Kong, M. S., Chen, J. Y., *et al.* (2000) Sonographic features related to volvulus in neonatal intestinal malrotation. *J Ultrasound Med* **19**(6): 371–6.

Copetti, R., Cattarossi, L. (2007) The 'double lung point': an ultrasound sign diagnostic of transient tachypnea of the newborn. *Neonatology* **91**(3): 203–9.

Copetti, R., Cattarossi, L., Macagno, F., *et al.* (2008) Lung ultrasound in respiratory distress syndrome: a useful tool for early diagnosis. *Neonatology* **94**(1): 52–9.

Dördelmann, M., Rau, F., Bartels, D., *et al.* (2009) Evaluation of portal venous gas detected by ultrasound examination for diagnosis of necrotising enterocolitis. *Arch Dis Child Fetal Neonatal Ed* **93**(3): F183–7.

Fleming, S. E., Kim, J. H. (2011) Ultrasound-guided umbilical line catheterization. *J Perinatol* **34**: 344–9.

Lee, H. C., Silverman, N., Hintz, S. R. (2007) Diagnosis of a patent ductus arteriosus by a neonatologist with a compact, portable ultrasound machine. *J Perinatol* **27**: 291–6.

Mahaeshwari, P., Abograra, A., Shamam, O. (2009) Sonographic evaluation of gastrointestinal obstruction in infants: a pictoral essay. *J Pediatr Surg* **44**(10): 2037–42.

Rennie, J. M., Hagmann, C. F., Robertson, N. J. (2008) *Neonatal Cerebral Investigation*. New York: Cambridge University Press.

Chapter 24

The critically ill: respiratory and hemodynamic support

Mahmoud Elbarbary

An integral part of critical care is the management of patients who need hemodynamic and respiratory support. In pediatric patients in particular, the monitoring of these patients in order to provide appropriate, targeted therapy can be challenging. It often requires invasive monitoring, since physical examination findings and clinical signs are often equivocal and provide insufficient information.

Point-of-care ultrasonography can be helpful in rapidly determining the causes of respiratory failure and hemodynamic compromise. Lung ultrasound (Chapter 6) and cardiac ultrasound (Chapter 5) play an important role in the evaluation of the critically ill neonates and children. Once patients are placed on ventilators and pressor therapy, ultrasonography can further provide ongoing monitoring in order to determine the adequacy of support, so as to target therapies.

RESPIRATORY SUPPORT

Background

In addition to determining whether a patient has a pneumothorax or pleural effusion (Chapter 6), lung ultrasonography can be helpful in identifying causes of acute respiratory failure. Lichtenstein introduced the BLUE protocol, which is an integrated approach that involves a three-minute interrogation of the lung. The goal of the BLUE protocol is to identify the cause of respiratory distress and impending respiratory failure, in order to provide appropriate relief to dyspneic patients. This involves a step-by-step approach, involving three signs with a binary answer, creating patterns consistent with pulmonary edema, interstitial syndromes, pulmonary emboli, pneumothoraces, pleural effusions, asthma/chronic obstructive diseases, and pneumonia/consolidations.

Ultimately, those patients who do not respond to therapies need to have respiratory support. This may be achieved by administering positive pressure through continuous positive airway pressure (CPAP) or by endotracheal intubation. Intubation is especially helpful in providing support for respiratory failure, but also for those with hemodynamic compromise. Positive pressure ventilation, in general, helps the impaired left ventricle (LV) due to the reduction of the transmural pressure across the LV free wall, thereby reducing the LV afterload. This is based on the formula:

$$\textbf{Transmural P} = \textbf{Systemic P} - \textbf{Intrathoracic P}$$

Where P is pressure.

In contrast, the positive pressure ventilation will constitute, in general, a burden on the impaired right ventricle (RV) because of the reduction of the preload and increase of RV afterload.

Ultrasound can aid in optimizing positive pressure ventilation, in order to achieve the maximum benefit and avoid the side effects of it on the ventricles. Combined lung (Chapter 6) and heart (Chapter 5) ultrasonography can be used to optimize the settings of positive end expiratory pressure (PEEP), and minimize the deleterious effects on the RV. The titration of optimum PEEP can help the RV by opening the collapsed alveoli and improving the functional residual capacity, thereby reducing the pulmonary vascular resistance. A repetitive assessment by heart and lung ultrasound during positive pressure ventilation weaning will help in titrating both ventilator and circulatory support, in order to achieve success in this process by optimizing the heart–lung interaction.

Finally, in those patients who require prolonged ventilator support, point-of-care ultrasonography can identify particular conditions that may lead to difficulty in weaning patients from support. Diaphragmatic and vocal cord paralysis in particular, can lead to extubation failure.

Technique

Point-of-care questions

1. Are characteristic signs of respiratory failure present?
2. Is diaphragmatic paralysis present?
3. Is vocal cord paralysis present?
4. What is the preload?

Transducer selection and orientation

Lung ultrasonography may be performed utilizing either a low-frequency or a high-frequency transducer (Chapter 6). Cardiac ultrasonography is performed with a low-frequency transducer (Chapter 5). Small-footprint transducers, such as the micro-convex or phased-array transducers are ideal in performing these examinations in neonates and small children respectively (Figure 23.15).

The assessment of the vocal cords and diaphragm should be performed in a spontaneously breathing patient, in a supine position. For the ultrasound examination of the vocal cords,

Pediatric Emergency and Critical Care Ultrasound, ed. Stephanie J. Doniger. Published by Cambridge University Press.

a high-frequency (5–10 MHz) linear transducer is recommended. The patient should have minimal neck extension, in order to allow enough space for the transducer to be placed and gently manipulated. The transducer is placed in the axial (transverse) plane on the thyroid cartilage, which can be used as an acoustic landmark. For the evaluation of the diaphragm, a lower-frequency (2–5 MHz) curvilinear transducer is recommended, and evaluated in three windows: subcostal, and right and left subhepatic regions.

Ultrasound imaging

The cardiac preload can be approximated by calculating the end diastolic area (EDA). Measurements may be performed in the parasternal short-axis or the parasternal long-axis views. Using the caliper, trace along the endocardium to measure the area of the left ventricle at the end of diastole (Figure 24.1a). The calculation of preload is derived from the law of Laplace. A higher EDA implies a higher preload (Figure 24.1b). A left ventricle EDA index (LV EDA / BSA) of less than 5.5 cm^2/m^2, where BSA is body surface area, indicates significant hypovolemia.

$$\mathbf{EDA} = \frac{(\mathbf{LV\ EDV} \times \mathbf{LV\ EDR})}{\mathbf{2}h}$$

where h is ventricle thickness, EDV is the end diastolic volume, and EDR is the end diastolic radius.

Trans-mitral flow estimation of LV end diastolic pressure (EDP) can be utilized during the weaning process from mechanical ventilation.

When encountering difficulties weaning or extubating a child from ventilatory support, it is often useful to evaluate the vocal cords and diaphragm for dysfunction. During spontaneous respirations, the clinician should be able to see the movement of the diaphragm, so as to differentiate between paradoxically moving, non-moving, or a weakly moving hemidiaphragm. Evaluation by M-mode can also be helpful in determining whether diaphragmatic dysfunction is present (Figure 24.2). Vocal cord paralysis can also be evaluated (Figure 24.3).

Scanning tips

Pitfalls

- The EDA is only an approximation of the cardiac preload.
- Positive pressure ventilation will constitute, in general, a burden on the impaired right ventricle (RV) because of the reduction of the preload and increase in RV afterload.

Tips to improve scanning

✓ Combined lung and heart ultrasound may be utilized to obtain the optimum level of positive end expiratory pressure (PEEP).

✓ The cardiac preload can be approximated by calculating the end diastolic area (EDA).

✓ EDA measurements may be performed in the parasternal short-axis or the parasternal long-axis views.

✓ A higher EDA implies a higher cardiac preload.

✓ When encountering difficulty weaning or extubating a child from ventilator support, the evaluation of the diaphragm and vocal cords for dysfunction is helpful.

HEMODYNAMIC MANAGEMENT

Background

In order to assess for cardiovascular function, the heart rate, and invasive blood pressure monitoring, are often utilized. Clinical signs such as the capillary refill time and skin turgor are often unreliable. Indirect measurements such as urine output and serum lactate are also utilized, but are nonspecific. Functional echocardiography can be a valuable tool for assessing a rapidly changing hemodynamic status. It can characterize acute physiology, identify the exact nature of cardiovascular compromise, and guide therapeutic decisions. Functional echocardiography has become prevalent in neonatology, in particular, and can be utilized in order to assess cardiovascular physiology and function, and how they change over time. This involves the longitudinal assessment of myocardial function, systemic and pulmonary blood flow, intracardiac and extracardiac shunts, organ blood flow, and tissue perfusion. In neonates with a PDA, response to treatment may also be monitored (see Chapter 23). In addition, in those neonates and children with a high oxygen requirement, ultrasonography may be utilized to exclude the presence of structural heart disease, and monitor response to therapy. However, as with other applications of point-of-care ultrasonography, this is not meant to replace formal echocardiography performed by pediatric cardiologists. This bedside evaluation is meant to be an extension of the physical examination, and to be a functional evaluation over time.

The basic components of the hemodynamic assessment include cardiac function and fluid status. Goal-directed ultrasound may also be incorporated into the evaluation of undifferentiated hypotension in ICU patients. Lichtenstein introduced the FALLS protocol (Figure 24.4), which involves cardiac and lung ultrasonography in order to distinguish between the different types of shock: obstructive shock (tamponade, pulmonary embolism), cardiogenic shock, hypovolemic shock, and septic shock. As a result of findings found on ultrasonography, fluid therapy can be targeted, with the constant monitoring of lung artifacts. Moreover, point-of-care ultrasonography can facilitate the assessment, diagnosis, and optimization of interventions and follow the adequacy of interventions of these two components. Chapter 5 discusses the overall cardiac contractility. More in-depth measurements of the left ventricle and global systolic function include fraction shortening and ejection fraction, either by global visual assessment or by actual measurement. Additional parameters that are helpful in ICU settings include the Doppler assessment of trans-mitral flow that reflects the LV EDP and hence the left atrial pressure. This can be very useful in the assessment of different etiologic causes of pulmonary edema, and in titrating fluid and inotropes.

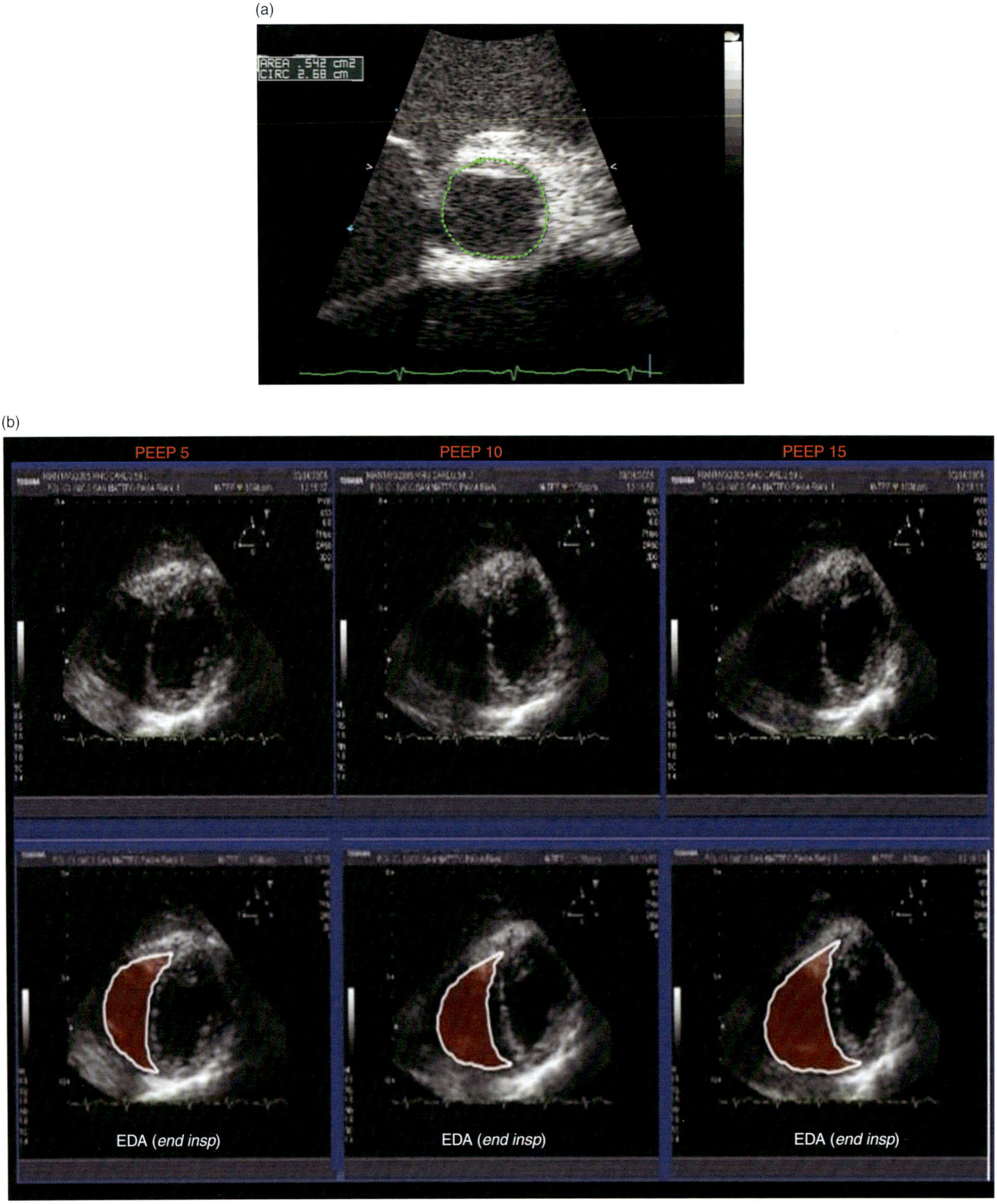

Figure 24.1 Left ventricular end diastolic area (EDA) as an estimation of preload. (a) Parasternal short-axis view. Using the caliper trace along the endocardium to measure the area of the LV at end diastole. (b) The effect of PEEP on EDA. Effects of PEEP of 5, 10, and 15 cm H_2O on the right ventricle.

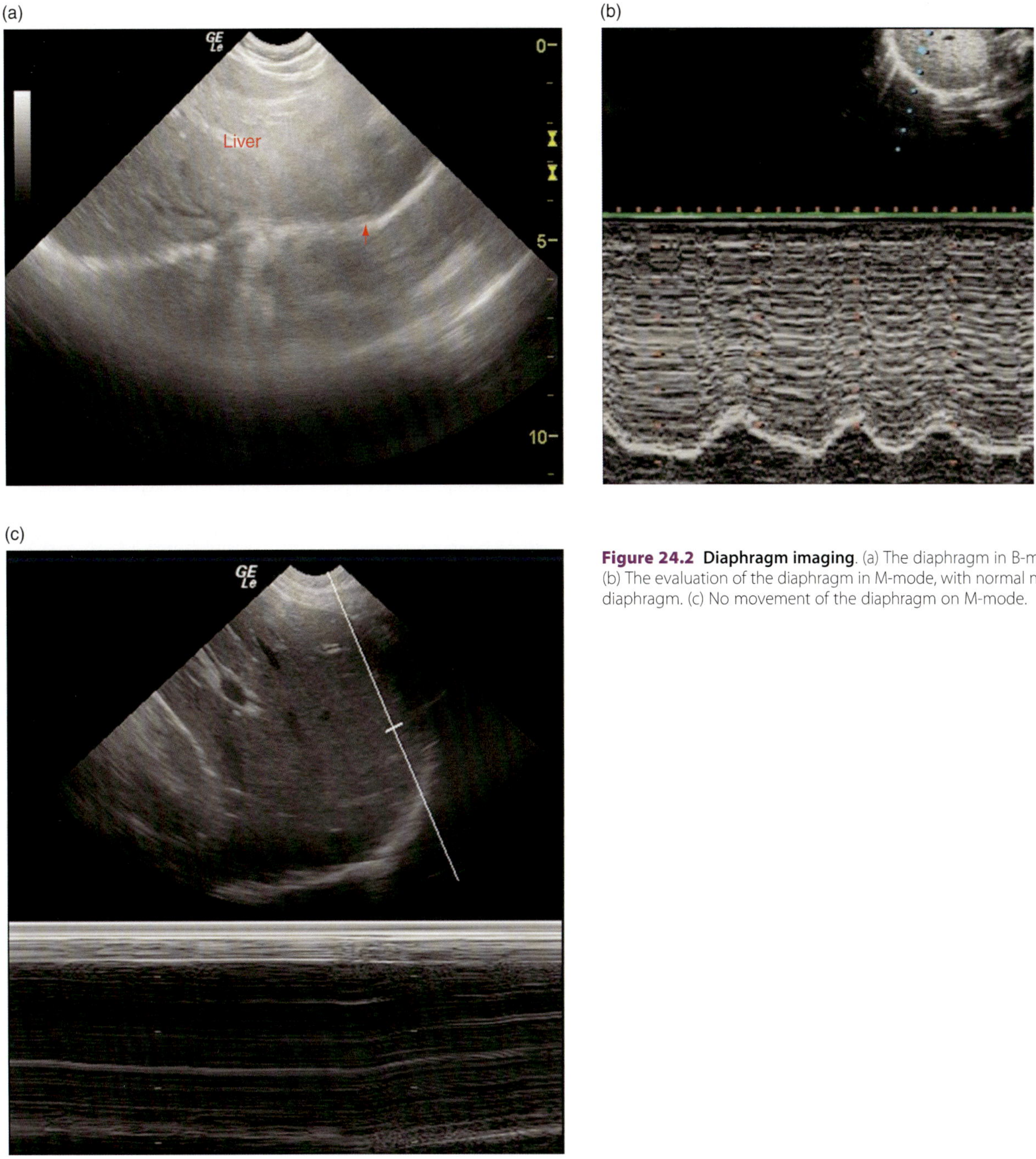

Figure 24.2 Diaphragm imaging. (a) The diaphragm in B-mode (arrow). (b) The evaluation of the diaphragm in M-mode, with normal movement of the diaphragm. (c) No movement of the diaphragm on M-mode.

Technique

Point-of-care questions

1. Is pre-existing cardiac disease present?
2. IVC evaluation: is the patient hypovolemic?
3. Is the RV hypokinetic/hyperkinetic?
4. Is the LV hypokinetic/hyperkinetic?
5. Measurements: cardiac output, ejection fraction, shortening fraction.

Transducer selection and orientation

The assessment of the hemodynamic status in critically ill neonates and children includes the cardiac examination (Chapter 5) and the IVC evaluation (Chapter 7). A low-frequency, phased-array or micro-convex transducer with a small footprint should be utilized. In order to assess for cardiac function, all views of the cardiac assessment should be obtained: the subxiphoid, parasternal long-axis, parasternal short-axis, and apical four-chamber (Figures 5.5–5.8), or five-chamber

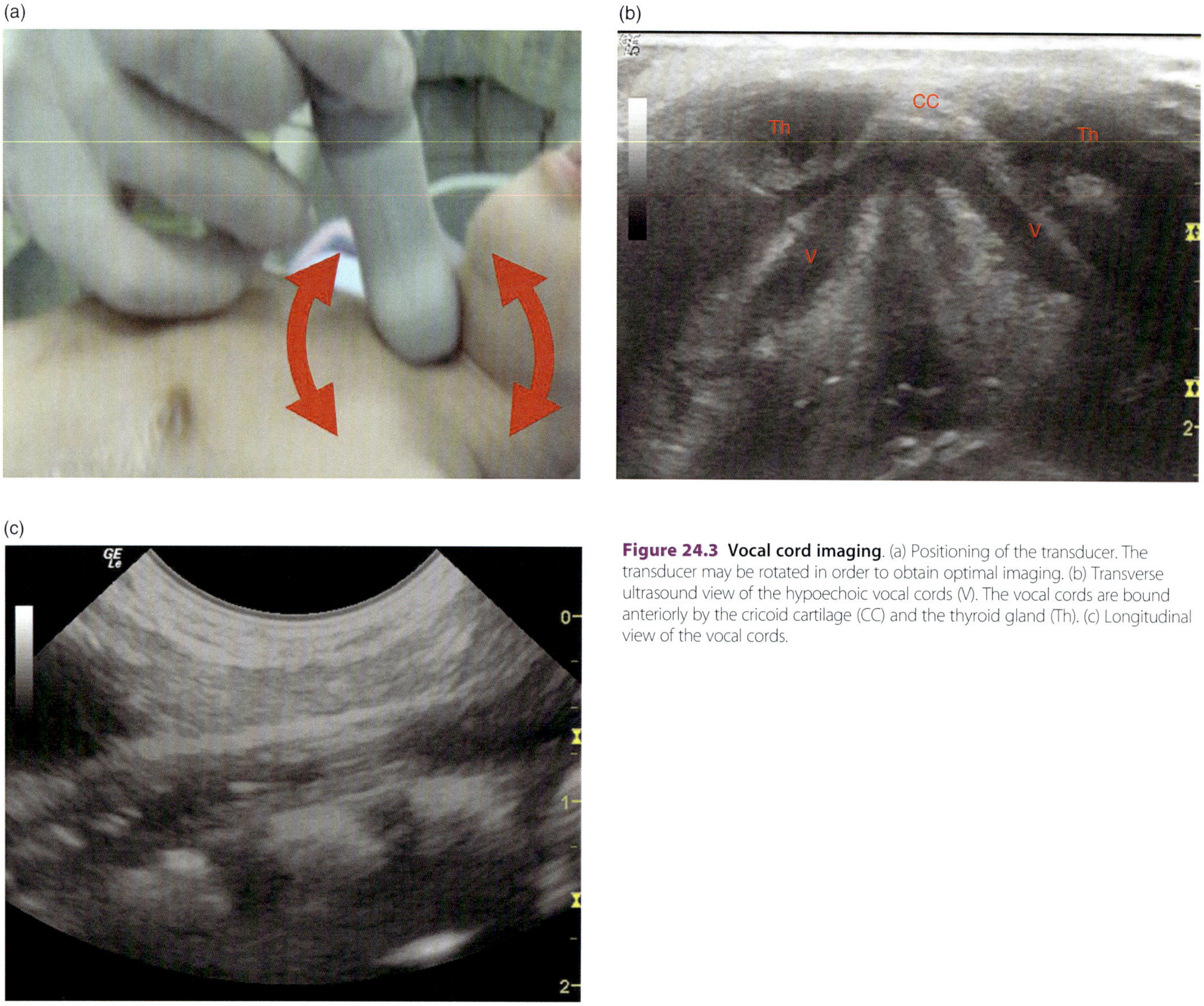

Figure 24.3 Vocal cord imaging. (a) Positioning of the transducer. The transducer may be rotated in order to obtain optimal imaging. (b) Transverse ultrasound view of the hypoechoic vocal cords (V). The vocal cords are bound anteriorly by the cricoid cartilage (CC) and the thyroid gland (Th). (c) Longitudinal view of the vocal cords.

views. In neonates, an additional suprasternal view should be obtained in order to assess for the presence of a PDA (Figure 23.14). For the evaluation of the IVC, the transducer should be oriented towards the patient's right and the patient's head in order to visualize the IVC in the transverse and longitudinal orientations (Figures 7.2, 7.3).

Ultrasound imaging

The hemodynamic assessment involves the global ventricular function (Chapter 5), and overall volume status (Chapter 7), as previously described. The combination of these two evaluations is essential in distinguishing between the different types of shock, and in monitoring the adequacy of therapy. This may be performed through four steps:

1. **Grossly ruling out pre-existing cardiac disease.** This is achieved by assessing for and ruling out the presence of gross dilatation/hypertrophy of the LV and RV, and identifying a valvular abnormality.
2. **Assessment of the IVC** for fluid status. In hypovolemia, inspiratory collapse is greater than 50% in spontaneous ventilation, and is greater than 20% in passive mechanical ventilation. Hypovolemia can be absolute (hemorrhage, dehydration, third spacing) or relative (sepsis, anaphylaxis, drugs). The responsiveness of the IVC to fluid therapy can guide titration of the amount of fluid to be administered. A dilated and fixed IVC may suggest pulmonary hypertension or tamponade.
3. **Assessment of the right ventricle (RV).** The right ventricle may be small and hyperkinetic or dilated and hypokinetic. The presence of a fixed, distended IVC with a small, hyperkinetic RV suggests tamponade. In contrast, a dilated and hypokinetic RV suggests pulmonary hypertension. There are additional confirmatory signs of both tamponade and pulmonary hypertension. For tamponade, these include right atrial diastolic collapse, a swinging heart, and a circumferential pericardial effusion. For pulmonary hypertension, the Doppler assessment of flow across the

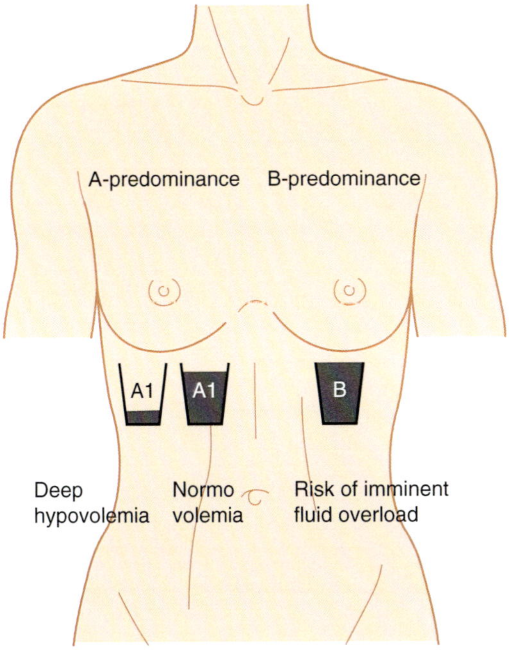

Figure 24.4 The FALLS protocol. *Artwork created by Emily Evans.* Based on: *Lichtenstein, D.(2012) Fluid administration limited by lung sonography: the place of lung ultrasound in assessment of acute circulatory failure (the FALLS protocol).* Expert Rev Resp Med ***6****(2): 155–62.*

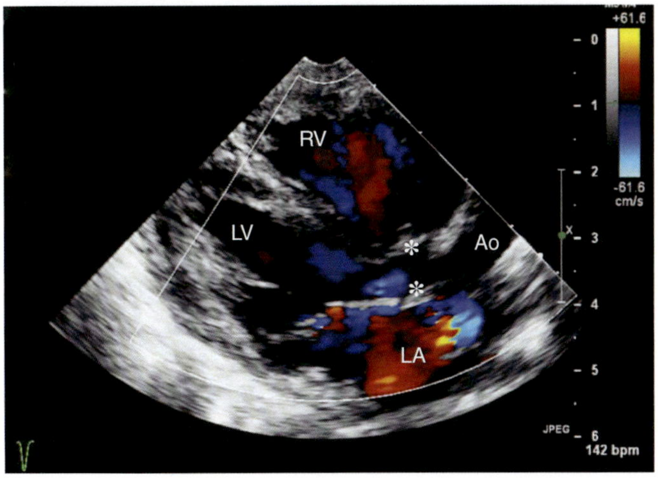

Figure 24.6 Parasternal long-axis view of the heart, with Doppler important structures visualized include the left ventricle (LV), right ventricle (RV), aorta (AO), left atrium (LA), and aortic root (**).

tricuspid valve can accurately estimate the pulmonary artery systolic pressure, in the absence of pulmonary valvular lesions. A septal shift towards the LV also confirms a high RV systolic pressure.

4. **Assessment of left ventricular (LV) function.** A hyperkinetic LV will be against the necessity to use ionotropes; while a hypokinetic LV would prompt the use of ionotropes. The combination of LV function with the fluid status will help in establishing the diagnosis, determining the need to start ionotropes, and monitoring management during infusions and follow-up of the patient.

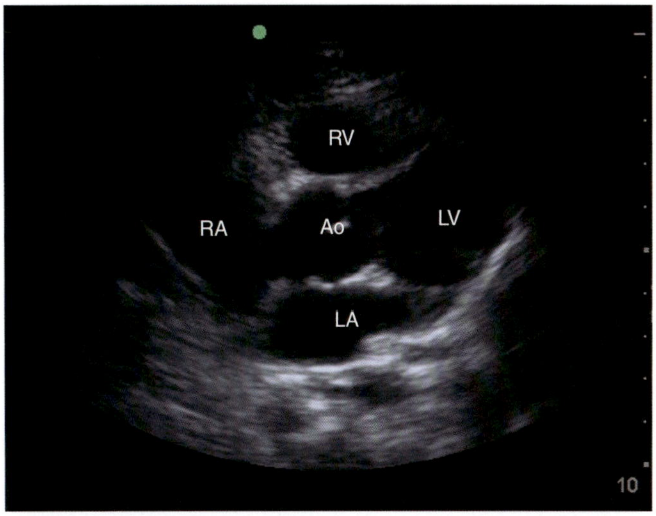

Figure 24.5 Apical five-chamber view of the heart. Right ventricle (RV), left ventricle (LV), right atrium (RA), left atrium (LA), and aorta (Ao).

Ultrasound imaging: measurements: LVO, RVO

Left and right ventricular outputs

A measurement of cardiac output can be performed. This involves a Doppler assessment of the left ventricular output (LVO) and right ventricular output (RVO). The LVO is the mean velocity of blood flow across the ascending aorta. This measurement is performed using the apical five-chamber view, using pulsed-wave Doppler. In Chapter 5, the apical four-chamber view is discussed. The apical five-chamber view is obtained by angling the transducer upwards, in order to have the aorta in the center of the four chambers (Figure 24.5). The diameter of the aortic root can be measured in the parasternal long-axis view (Figure 24.6).

Any cardiac value or outlet can be used to calculate cardiac output, but the left ventricular outflow tract (LVOT) is most commonly used, since the LVOT is similar to a cylinder. It is simple to calculate the volume of a cylinder using standard geometry (Figure 24.7a), using the aortic diameter (Figure 24.7b) and the velocity time integral (VTI), which is the measure of distance traveled by blood during a given beat. In order to measure the VTI, use continuous pulsed-wave Doppler, in the apical five-chamber view. First, obtain a waveform over three to four respiratory cycles, and freeze the image. Then, identify the largest and smallest waveforms over a single respiratory cycle. Next, go to calculations (aortic continuity equation) and trace the edge of the waveform with the trackball. Finally, the machine will calculate the VTIs for the two waveforms (Figure 24.7c). The velocity time integral variation is the difference between the maximum and minimum velocities.

Once the cross-sectional area (CSA) and VTI are calculated, they are multiplied by the heart rate (HR), and divided by the patient's weight (Figure 24.7b) in order to calculate the final cardiac output (CO).

$$CO = SV \times HR.$$

where SV is stroke volume.

(a)

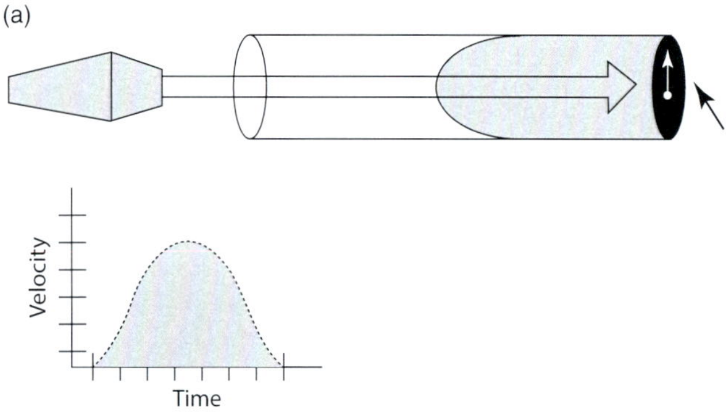

(b)

$$\text{Cylinder volume (Stroke volume)} = \text{Cross-sectional area (CSA)} \times \text{Height}$$

CSA: $\pi r^2 = \pi(D/2)^2$ (D = Aorta diameter)

Height: Velocity time integral (VTI) measured at the LVOT

$$\underset{(\text{mL/kg/min})}{\text{LVO}} = \frac{(\text{CSA} \times \text{VTI} \times \text{HR})}{\text{Weight}}$$

(c) (d)

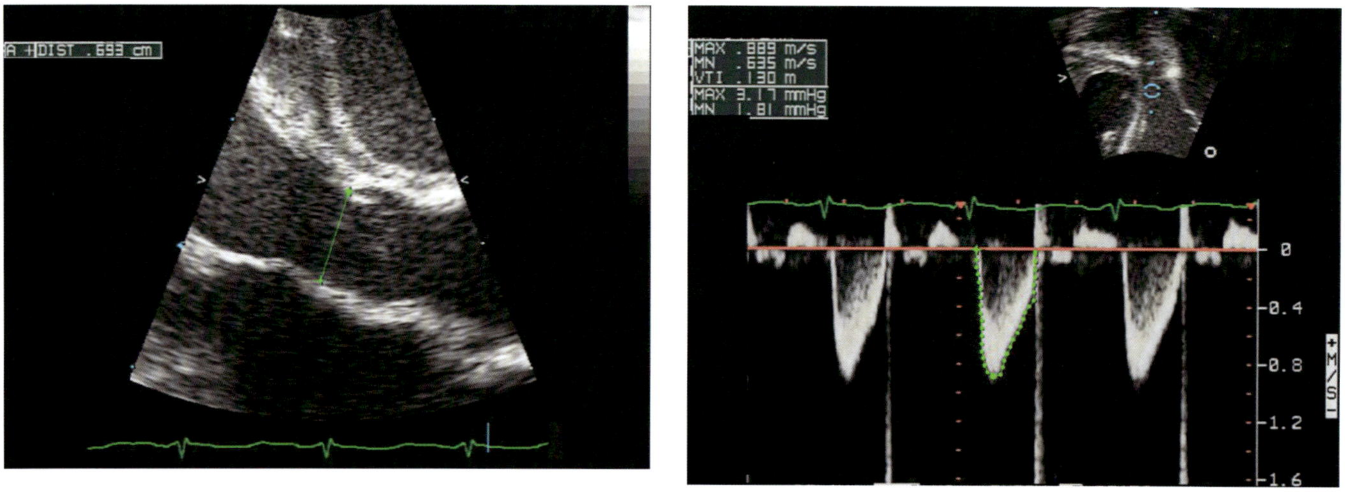

Figure 24.7 Cardiac output measurement at the LVOT. (a) Cylinder. (b) The calculation of a cylinder volume (stroke volume). (c) Measurement of the diameter of the aortic root. (d) Velocity time integral (VTI) measurement, using pulsed-wave Doppler.

The right ventricular output (RVO) reflects blood return from the systemic circulation. This is determined by using an oblique parasternal long-axis view to measure the pulmonary artery diameter. Other measurements may include the superior vena cava flow. This is a measure of systemic blood flow, which reflects venous return exclusively from the brain and upper body, and is not influenced by shunts. In order to perform this measurement, a subcostal approach or a high suprasternal view is utilized in order to measure the superior vena cava diameter. This measurement may provide insights into cerebral blood flow and cerebral injury.

Ejection and shortening fractions

The sonographic assessment of global systolic ventricular function includes the left ventricular ejection fraction (EF) and the left ventricular shortening fraction (SF). These measurements are performed in the short-axis view at the mid-papillary level. Both M-mode (Figure 24.8) and B-mode (Figure 24.9) are useful in performing these assessments.

The LV ejection fraction (EF) is the most commonly measured parameter of ventricular function, and evaluates cardiac performance in terms of contractility. The calculation of the ejection fraction deals with volumes, and is based on the approximation of the volume of the left ventricle cavity at the end of systole and at the end of diastole. When the left ventricle empties to more than half of its volume, this is a normal ejection fraction. A normal ejection fraction is 56–78%. Mild impairment is with an EF of 45–55%, moderate impairment 30–44%, and severe impairment $< 30\%$ (Figure 24.9).

$$\text{EF\%} = \frac{(\text{LV EDV} - \text{LV ESV})}{\text{LV EDV}} \times 100.$$

where EDV is end diastolic volume, and ESV is end systolic volume.

An additional measurement of cardiac performance includes the shortening fraction (SF), which is a measurement of the extent of LV shortening. Normal values of the shortening fraction range from 28 to 44%. Normal neonatal values range from 28 to 40%. It is important to note that the SF is an unreliable measurement in the first few days of life. It can be calculated by the formula:

$$\text{SF\%} = \frac{(\text{LV EDD} - \text{LV ESD})}{\text{LV EDD}} \times 100.$$

where EDD is the end diastolic dimension and ESD is the end systolic dimension.

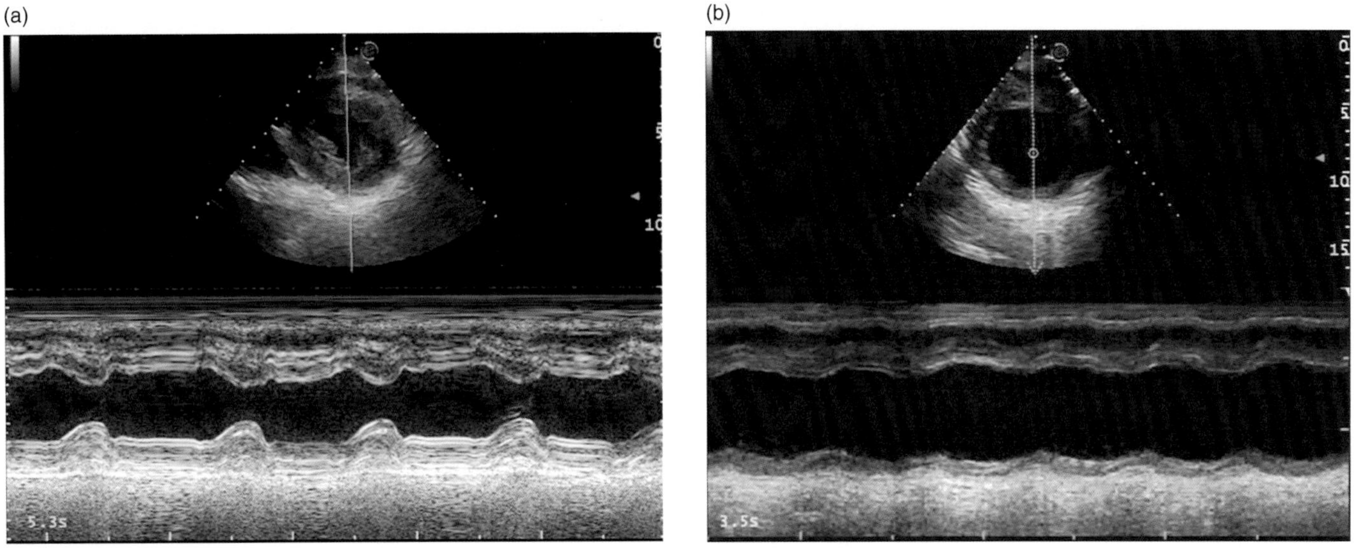

Figure 24.8 M-mode: left ventricular function (shortening fraction). (a) Good function of the LV. (b) Poor function of the LV.

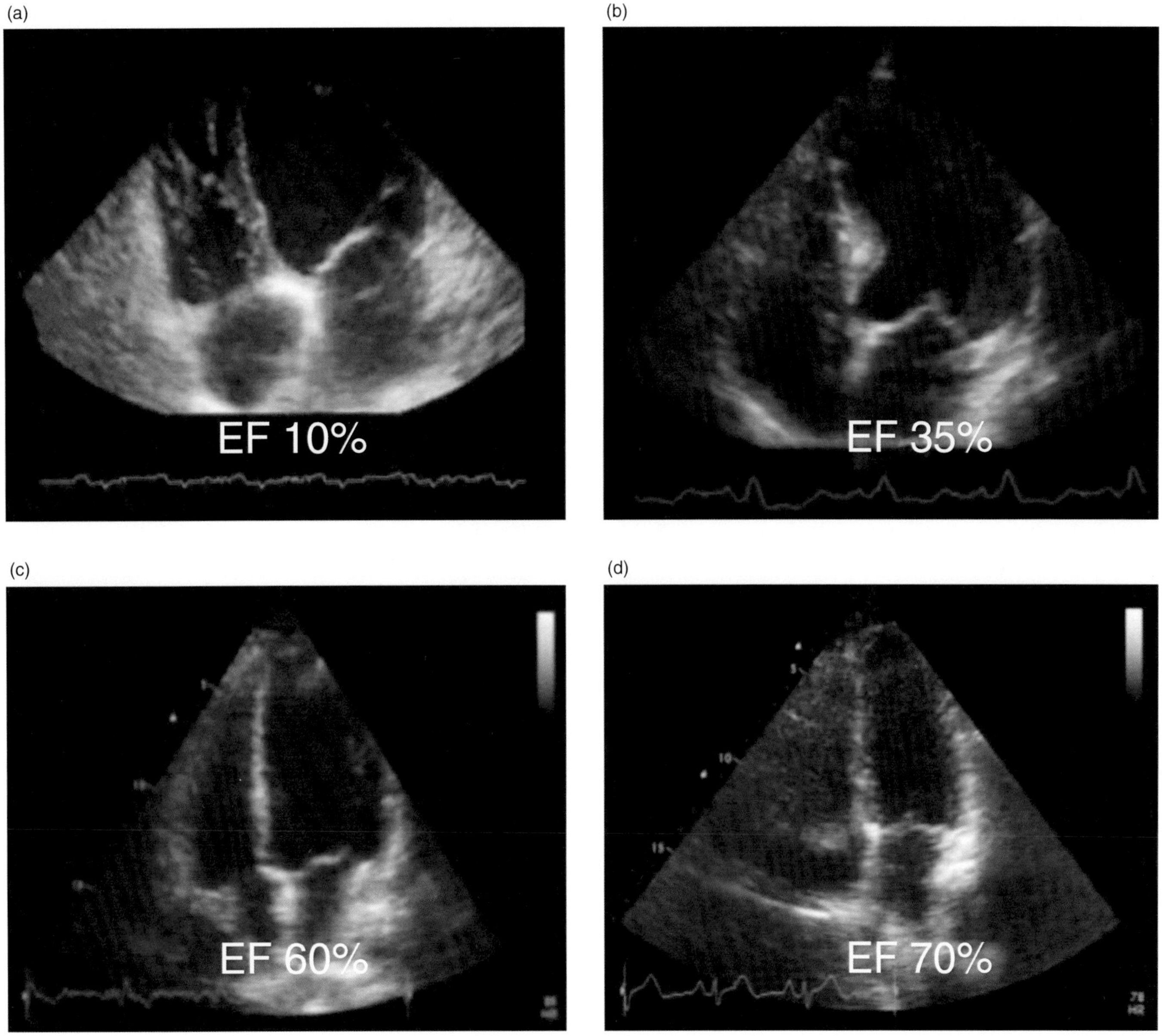

Figure 24.9 B-mode: left ventricular function (ejection fraction). (a) Ejection fraction 10%. (b) Ejection fraction 35%. (c) Ejection fraction 60%. (d) Ejection fraction 70%.

Scanning tips

Pitfalls

- The measurements of preload, ejection fraction, and shortening fraction involve complicated formulas and calculations.
- Point-of-care ultrasonography is not meant to replace formal echocardiography or consultation with a pediatric cardiologist.
- Shortening fraction calculations are unreliable in neonates, in the first few days of life.
- Echocardiography should not be used in the diagnosis or "ruling-out" of congenital heart disease. All neonates and children suspected of having congenital heart disease should have an initial formal echocardiogram performed by a pediatric cardiologist.

Tips to improve scanning

Functional echocardiography can be a valuable tool for assessing a rapidly changing hemodynamic status.

✓ The goal of the extended echocardiography assessment is a functional evaluation over time.

✓ The hemodynamic assessment includes: grossly ruling out pre-existing cardiac pathology, and the assessments of the IVC, right ventricle, and left ventricle.

✓ Measurements of EF and SF are performed in the short-axis, at the level of the papillary muscle. M-mode is helpful in performing measurements.

✓ The LV ejection fraction is the most commonly measured parameter of ventricular function, and evaluates cardiac performance in terms of contractility.

✓ A normal ejection fraction is 56–78%.

✓ Normal values of the shortening fraction range from 28 to 44%. Normal neonatal values range from 28 to 40%.

Cases

1. A 14-year-old boy presents with progressively worsening respiratory distress. Over the past three days, he has developed substernal chest pain and dyspnea. He has no prior past medical history. On examination, his vital signs are: T 40 °C, HR 138 bpm, RR 42/min, and BP 142/80 mmHg. He is diaphoretic, unable to lie backwards due to difficulty breathing, and is unable to speak in full sentences. Auscultation is limited, due to poor respiratory effort, but he has decreased breath sounds throughout all lung fields. On cardiac examination, his precordium is hyperdynamic, but there are no murmurs, gallops, or rubs auscultated. He has good peripheral perfusion. The remainder of his examination is unremarkable. A point-of-care ultrasound examination of the lung is performed, which shows a large left pleural effusion with consolidation (Figure 24.10a), and a small right pleural effusion. On cardiac ultrasonography, he has good contractility without a pericardial effusion. The evaluation of his IVC shows normal collapsibility. A portable chest radiograph is performed, at the request of the PICU (Figure 24.10b). It shows a large left pleural effusion. He is brought to the PICU and placed on antibiotics for a large pneumonia with empyema. He rapidly decompensates, and is shortly thereafter intubated. Ultimately, a video-assisted thoracoscopic surgery (VATS) procedure is performed, and culture reveals MRSA.

   Point-of-care ultrasonography can be useful in identifying the causes of acute dyspnea. Specific patterns

(a) (b)

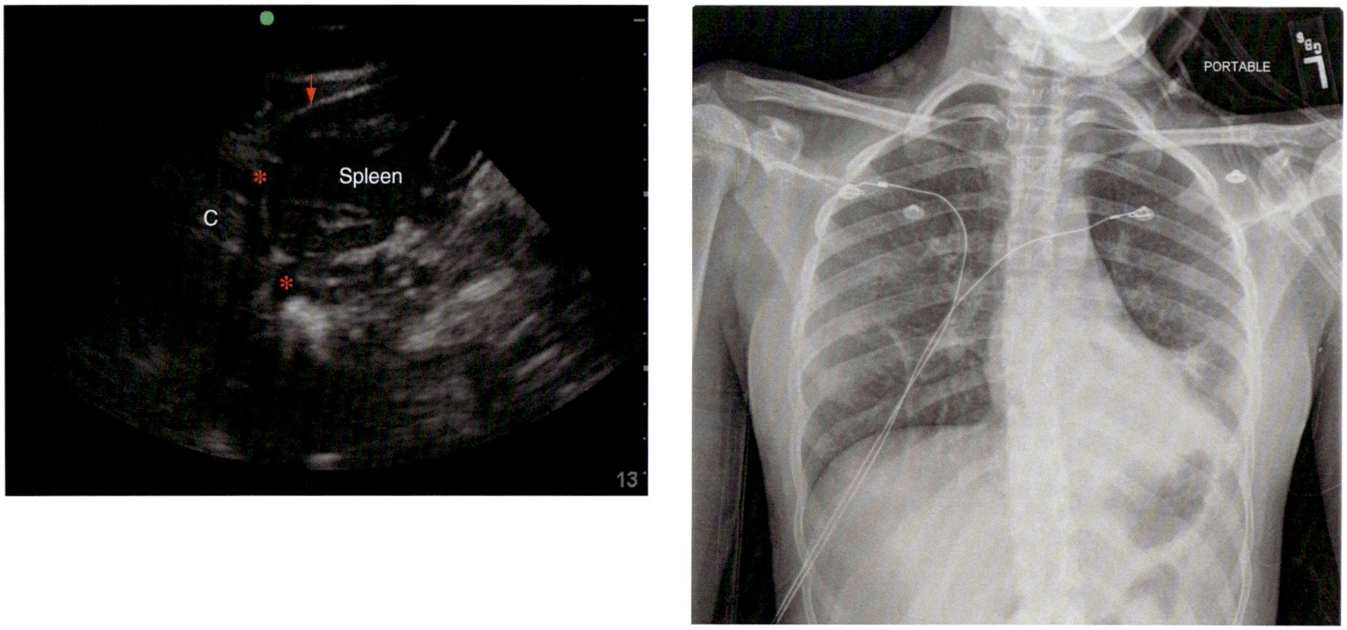

Figure 24.10 Case 1: pneumonia, empyema. (a) Ultrasound performed at the left upper quadrant, showing a pleural effusion (*) above the diaphragm (arrow), with consolidation (C). (b) Corresponding portable chest radiograph showing the left-sided pleural effusion.

can be visualized on ultrasonography that are consistent with pulmonary edema, interstitial syndromes, pulmonary emboli, pneumothoraces, pleural effusions, asthma/chronic obstructive diseases, and pneumonia/consolidations. Once patients are intubated, continued assessment may be performed in order to optimize positive pressure ventilation, and provide the appropriate amount of PEEP, without causing dysfunction to the right ventricle.

2. An eight-year-old girl presents with fever and altered mental status. She has had intermittent tactile fevers and vomiting. Her past medical history is significant for repaired congenital heart disease. However, her parents don't recall the specific lesion and all of her medical care was received out of the country. On presentation, her triage vital signs are: T 39°C, HR 162 bpm, RR 43/min, BP 82/60 mmHg. On examination, she is obtunded but withdraws from painful stimuli. She has poor peripheral perfusion. On auscultation, her lungs are clear. Her cardiac examination is notable for a II/VI systolic ejection murmur auscultated throughout the precordium. Point-of-care ultrasonograpy is performed in order to identify the type of shock this child is exhibiting. Lung ultrasonography is performed, and is normal without a pneumothorax, a pleural effusion, or a consolidation. On cardiac ultrasonography, the anatomy appears grossly normal. There is no pericardial effusion. On 2D views, the heart appears hyperdynamic with good contractility. The ejection fraction is further calculated as 57%, which is normal. Finally, an assessment of the IVC is performed, which shows greater than 50% collapsibility, consistent with dehydration.

   In patients presenting in shock, it is often difficult to identify the type of shock by history and physical examination alone. While a history of congenital heart disease might suggest cardiogenic shock, that is actually not the case in this child. Ultrasonography results reveal a hypovolemic shock, since the IVC shows greater than 50% collapsibility, with normal cardiac function. As a result of findings on ultrasonography, fluid therapy can be targeted. During therapy, repeated monitoring of lung artifacts can be performed. If the lungs show increased B-lines, then fluid resuscitation can be stopped. A stepwise, integrated approach is paramount in evaluating these patients, in order to identify the cause and provide appropriate, targeted therapy.

Summary/key points

1. Lung ultrasonography may be utilized to assess the cause of respiratory failure, and optimize positive pressure ventilation. It can also identify causes of difficulty in extubating a child, including diaphragmatic and vocal cord dysfunction.
2. The sonographic evaluation for hemodynamic assessment in critically ill neonates and children is meant to be an extension of the physical examination, and aid in targeted therapy and management. It is not meant to replace comprehensive echocardiography performed by pediatric cardiologists.
3. The overall hemodynamic assessment can be performed in four steps: ruling out pre-existing cardiac disease, assessment of the IVC, assessment of the LV, and assessment of the RV.
4. Cardiac output is best assessed by the evaluation of the left ventricular output (LVO). The LVO expressed in mL/kg/min is calculated by: (CSA × VTI × HR) divided by the patient's weight.
5. The ejection fraction is calculated by: [(LV EDV – LV ESV) / LV EDV] × 100. A normal ejection fraction is >55%, mild impairment 45–55%, moderate impairment 30–44%, and severe impairment <30%.

Selected references

Carr, B. G., Dean, A. J., Everett, W. W., *et al.* (2007) Intensivist bedside ultrasound (INBU) for volume assessment in the intensive care unit: a pilot study. *J Trauma* **63**(3): 495–502.

El-Khuffash, A. F., McNamara, P. J. (2010) Neonatologist-performed functional echocardiography in the neonatal intensive care unit. *Semin Fetal Neonatal Med* **16**: 50–60.

Kluckow, M., Seri, I., Evans, N. (2008) Echocardiography and the neonatologist. *Pediatr Cardiol* **29**: 1043–7.

Lichtenstein, D. (2009) Lung ultrasound in acute respiratory failure an introduction to the BLUE-protocol. *Minerva Anesthesiol* **75**(5): 313–17.

Lichtenstein, D. (2012) Fluid administration limited by lung sonography: the place of lung ultrasound in assessment of acute circulatory failure (the FALLS protocol). *Expert Rev Resp Med* **6**(2): 155–62.

Mark, D. G., Hayden, G. E., Ky, B., *et al.* (2009) Hand-carried echocardiography for assessment of left ventricular filling and ejection fraction in the surgical intensive care unit. *J Crit Care* **24**: 470. e1–7.

Sehgal, A., McNamara, P. J. (2008) Does point-of-care functional echocardiography enhance cardiovascular care in the NICU? *J Perinatol* **28**: 729–35.

Shaath, G. A., Jijeh, A., Alkurdi, A., *et al.* (2012) Ultrasonography assessment of vocal cords mobility in children after cardiac surgery. *J Saudi Heart Assoc* **24**(3): 187–90.

Spurney, C. F., Sable, C. A., Berger, J. T., *et al.* (2005) Use of a hand-carried ultrasound device by critical care physicians for the diagnosis of pericardial effusions, decreased cardiac function, and left ventricular enlargement in pediatric patients. *J Am Soc Echocardiogr* **18**(4): 313–19.

Vignon, P., Dugard, A., Abraham, J., *et al.* (2007) Focused training for goal-oriented hand-held echocardiography performed by noncardiologist residents in the intensive care unit. *Intensive Care Med* **33**: 1795–9.

Index